2012
YEAR BOOK OF
SPORTS MEDICINE®

The 2012 Year Book Series

Year Book of Anesthesiology and Pain Management™: Drs Chestnut, Abram, Black, Gravlee, Lien, Mathru, and Roizen

Year Book of Cardiology®: Drs Gersh, Cheitlin, Elliott, Gold, Graham, and Thourani

Year Book of Critical Care Medicine®: Drs Dries, Zanotti-Cavazzoni, Latenser, Martinez, Rincon, and Zwank

Year Book of Dermatology and Dermatologic Surgery™: Dr Del Rosso

Year Book of Diagnostic Radiology®: Drs Elster, Abbara, Oestreich, Offiah, Rosado de Christenson, Stephens, and Strickland

Year Book of Emergency Medicine®: Drs Hamilton, Bruno, Handly, Minczak, Mullin, Quintana, and Ramoska

Year Book of Endocrinology®: Drs Schott, Apovian, Clarke, Eugster, Ludlam, Meikle, Oetgen, Ovalle, Schteingart, and Toth

Year Book of Hand and Upper Limb Surgery®: Drs Yao, Adams, Isaacs, Lee, and Rizzo

Year Book of Medicine®: Drs Barker, Garrick, Gersh, Khardori, LeRoith, Panush, Talley, and Thigpen

Year Book of Neonatal and Perinatal Medicine®: Drs Fanaroff, Benitz, Donn, Neu, Papile, Polin, and Van Marter

Year Book of Neurology and Neurosurgery®: Drs Klimo, Minagar, Gandhi, House, Kevill, Liu, Mazia, Panagariya, Ragel, Riesenburger, Robottom, Schwendimann, Shafazand, Uhm, and Yang

Year Book of Obstetrics, Gynecology, and Women's Health®: Drs Dungan and Shulman

Year Book of Oncology®: Drs Arceci, Bauer, Chiorean, Gordon, Lawton, Murphy, Thigpen, and Tsao

Year Book of Ophthalmology®: Drs Rapuano, Cohen, Flanders, Hammersmith, Milman, Myers, Nagra, Nelson, Penne, Pyfer, Sergott, Shields, Talekar, and Vander

Year Book of Orthopedics®: Drs Morrey, Huddleston, Rose, Swiontkowski, and Trigg

Year Book of Otolaryngology-Head and Neck Surgery®: Drs Sindwani, Balough, Franco, Gapany, and Mitchell

Year Book of Pathology and Laboratory Medicine®: Drs Raab and Bissell

Year Book of Pediatrics®: Dr Stockman

Year Book of Plastic and Aesthetic Surgery™: Drs Miller, Gosman, Gurtner, Gutowski, Ruberg, Salisbury, and Smith

Year Book of Psychiatry and Applied Mental Health®: Drs Talbott, Ballenger, Buckley, Frances, Krupnick, and Mack

Year Book of Pulmonary Disease®: Drs Barker, Jones, Maurer, Spradley, Tanoue, and Willsie

Year Book of Sports Medicine®: Drs Shephard, Cantu, Feldman, Galea, Jankowski, Janssen, Lebrun, and Nieman

Year Book of Surgery®: Drs Copeland, Behrns, Daly, Eberlein, Fahey, Huber, Klodell, Mozingo, and Pruett

Year Book of Urology®: Drs Andriole and Coplen

Year Book of Vascular Surgery®: Drs Moneta, Gillespie, Starnes, and Watkins

2012
The Year Book of
SPORTS MEDICINE®

Editor-in-Chief
Roy J. Shephard, MD (Lond), PhD, DPE, LLD

Professor Emeritus of Applied Physiology, Faculty of Physical Education and Health, University of Toronto, Toronto, Ontario, Canada

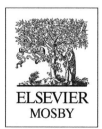

ELSEVIER
MOSBY

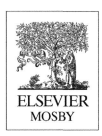

ELSEVIER
MOSBY

Vice President, Continuity Publishing: Kimberly Murphy
Editor: Jessica McCool
Production Supervisor, Electronic Year Books: Donna M. Skelton
Electronic Article Manager: Mike Sheets
Illustrations and Permissions Coordinator: Dawn Vohsen

2012 EDITION
Copyright 2012, Mosby, Inc. All rights reserved.

No part of this publication may be reproduced, stored in a retrieval system, or transmitted, in any form or by any means, electronic, mechanical, photocopying, recording, or otherwise, without prior written permission from the publisher.

Permission to photocopy or reproduce solely for internal or personal use is permitted for libraries or other users registered with the Copyright Clearance Center, provided that the base fee of $35.00 per chapter is paid directly to the Copyright Clearance Center, 21 Congress Street, Salem, MA 01970. This consent does not extend to other kinds of copying, such as copying for general distribution, for advertising or promotional purposes, for creating new collected works, or for resale.

Composition by TNQ Books and Journals Pvt Ltd, India

Editorial Office:
Elsevier, Inc.
Suite 1800
1600 John F. Kennedy Boulevard
Philadelphia, PA 19103-2899

International Standard Serial Number: 0162-0908
International Standard Book Number: 978-0-323-08894-7

Associate Editors

Robert C. Cantu, MA, MD, FACS, FAANS, FACSM
*Clinical Professor of Neurosurgery, Boston University School of Medicine;
Co-Director, Neurological Sports Injury Center at Brigham and Women's
Hospital; Neurosurgery Consultant, Boston College Eagles and Boston Cannons
Lacrosse Teams; Co-Director, Center for the Study of Traumatic Encephalopathy
(CSTE), Boston University Medical Center, Boston, Massachusetts; Co-Founder
and Chairman, Medical Advisory Board Sports Legacy Institute (SLI), Waltham,
Massachusetts; Chairman, Department of Surgery, Chief, Neurosurgery
Service, and Director, Service Sports Medicine, Emerson Hospital, Concord,
Massachusetts; Adjunct Professor, Exercise and Sport Science, University of
North Carolina; Medical Director, National Center for Catastrophic Sports
Injury, Research, Chapel Hill, North Carolina; Senior Advisor, National Football
League (NFL) Head, Neck and Spine Committee, New York, New York*

Debbie Ehrmann Feldman, PT, PhD
*Professor, Faculty of Medicine, School of Rehabilitation, Université de
Montréal; and Physiotherapist, Montreal Children's Hospital, McGill University
Health Centre, Montreal, Quebec, Canada*

Victoria Galea, PhD
*Associate Professor, School of Rehabilitation Science, Department of
Kinesiology and The Education Program in Anatomy, McMaster University,
Hamilton, Ontario, Canada*

Catherine M. Jankowski, PhD
*Assistant Research Professor, Division of Geriatric Medicine, University of
Colorado Denver, Aurora, Colorado*

Ian Janssen, PhD
*Associate Professor, School of Kinesiology and Health Studies, and Department
of Community Health and Epidemiology, Queen's University, Kingston,
Ontario, Canada*

Connie Lebrun, MDCM, MPE, CCFP, Dip Sport Med, FACSM
*Associate Professor, Faculty of Medicine and Dentistry, Department of Family
Medicine, Consultant Sports Medicine Physician, Glen Sather Sports Medicine
Clinic, University of Alberta, Edmonton, Alberta, Canada*

David C. Nieman, DrPH
*Professor, Appalachian State University, Boone, North Carolina; Director,
The Human Performance Laboratory, North Carolina Research Campus,
Kannapolis, North Carolina*

Table of Contents

Journals Represented

Journals represented in this YEAR BOOK are listed below.

Academic Emergency Medicine
Acta Paediatrica
Allergy
American Heart Journal
American Journal of Cardiology
American Journal of Clinical Nutrition
American Journal of Emergency Medicine
American Journal of Epidemiology
American Journal of Human Biology
American Journal of Preventive Medicine
American Journal of Public Health
American Journal of Sports Medicine
Annals of Internal Medicine
Annals of the Rheumatic Diseases
Annals of Thoracic Surgery
Applied Physiology, Nutrition and Metabolism
Archives of Internal Medicine
Archives of Pediatrics & Adolescent Medicine
Archives of Physical Medicine and Rehabilitation
Arthritis Care & Research (Hoboken)
Arthroscopy
Brain
Brain Research
Breast Cancer Research and Treatment
British Journal of Anaesthesia
British Journal of Cancer
British Journal of Sports Medicine
British Journal of Surgery
British Medical Journal
Burns
Canadian Medical Association Journal
Cancer Research
Chest
Circulation
Clinical Biomechanics
Clinical Endocrinology (Oxford)
Clinical Journal of Sport Medicine
Clinical Pediatrics
Clinical Pediatrics (Philadelphia)
Deutsche Zeitschrift fuer Sportmedizin
Developmental Medicine and Child Neurology
Diabetes Care
European Heart Journal
European Journal of Applied Physiology
European Respiratory Journal

European Urology
Heart
Hypertension
International Journal of Cardiology
International Journal of Obesity
International Journal of Sports Medicine
Journal of Applied Physiology
Journal of Athletic Training
Journal of Autism and Developmental Disorders
Journal of Bone and Joint Surgery (American)
Journal of Bone Mineral Research
Journal of Child Psychology and Psychiatry
Journal of Clinical Endocrinology & Metabolism
Journal of Clinical Psychopharmacology
Journal of Emergency Medicine
Journal of Neurological Sciences
Journal of Neurology, Neurosurgery, and Psychiatry
Journal of Orthopaedic and Sports Physical Therapy
Journal of Pain
Journal of Pediatric Surgery
Journal of Pediatrics
Journal of the American College of Cardiology
Journal of the American Geriatrics Society
Journal of the American Medical Association
Journal of Trauma
Journal of Urology
Lancet
Maturitas
Medicine and Science in Sports and Exercise
Neurology
Neuron
Neuroradiology
Neurosurgery
New England Journal of Medicine
Obesity Reviews
Obstetrics & Gynecology
Pain
Pediatric Exercise Science
Pediatric Research
Pediatrics
Preventive Medicine
Proceedings of the National Academy of Sciences of the United States of America
Psychologie Medicale
Research In Developmental Disabilities
Resolution in Autism Spectrum Disorders
Scandinavian Journal of Medicine & Science In Sports
Sleep
Spine
Spine Journal
Sports Medicine

Stroke
World Neurosurgery

STANDARD ABBREVIATIONS

The following terms are abbreviated in this edition: acquired immunodeficiency syndrome (AIDS), cardiopulmonary resuscitation (CPR), central nervous system (CNS), cerebrospinal fluid (CSF), computed tomography (CT), deoxyribonucleic acid (DNA), electrocardiography (ECG), health maintenance organization (HMO), human immunodeficiency virus (HIV), intensive care unit (ICU), intramuscular (IM), intravenous (IV), magnetic resonance (MR) imaging (MRI), ribonucleic acid (RNA), and ultrasound (US).

NOTE

The YEAR BOOK OF SPORTS MEDICINE is a literature survey service providing abstracts of articles published in the professional literature. Every effort is made to assure the accuracy of the information presented in these pages. Neither the editors nor the publisher of the YEAR BOOK OF SPORTS MEDICINE can be responsible for errors in the original materials. The editors' comments are their own opinions. Mention of specific products within this publication does not constitute endorsement.

To facilitate the use of the YEAR BOOK OF SPORTS MEDICINE as a reference tool, all illustrations and tables included in this publication are now identified as they appear in the original article. This change is meant to help the reader recognize that any illustration or table appearing in the YEAR BOOK OF SPORTS MEDICINE may be only one of many in the original article. For this reason, figure and table numbers will often appear to be out of sequence within the YEAR BOOK OF SPORTS MEDICINE.

Will Active Commuting Solve the Problems of the City-Dweller in 2012?

Roy J. Shephard, M.D., Ph.D., D.P.E

Faculty of Physical Education & Health, University of Toronto, Toronto, Ontario

Introduction

There has been extensive research on "active commuting" (travel to and from school or work on foot or on bicycle) during the past two years,[1-10] and a growing number of authors believe the encouragement of active transportation would solve several of the problems that face city-dwellers in 2012: low levels of personal fitness and associated "lifestyle diseases," a growing prevalence of obesity,[11,12] congested streets and associated accumulations of greenhouses gases.[13,14]

Certainly, much of the world's population is no longer undertaking sufficient physical activity to optimize health, maintain function into old age and optimize the quality of life (see, for example, a recent accelerometry study from Statistics Canada[15]). Nevertheless, we lack a clear consensus on the most effective method of tackling this problem. For individuals who have already developed appropriate motor skills and enjoy competition, the answer may be to encourage participation in a traditional team or individual sport. But in most countries, this is not very practical for the population as a whole.[16] Such an approach would make enormous demands for land (e.g. for the construction of soccer pitches), and huge capital investments in other sports facilities such as gymnasia, skating rinks and tennis courts. Health Canada has thus shifted its public health emphasis from involvement in sport to advocating "active living," the incorporation of adequate amounts of physical activity into normal daily life (see, for example, the Web site of the Canadian Coalition for Active Living, www. activeliving.ca). In the U.S., similar policies are advocated, for instance the Leadership for Healthy Communities program of the Robert Wood Johnson Foundation (www.activelivingleadership.org), and the Healthy People 2010 recommendation that walking be used as a means of personal transportation.[17]

From the viewpoint of public health, active commuting has several advantages relative to other possible forms of physical activity. Active commuters do not require any preliminary medical clearance, and they have no need to purchase expensive equipment or clothing. With a little forethought, the walk or cycle trip to work can be combined with other pleasant activities that enhance mental health,[18,19] such as conversation with a colleague, admiring urban architecture or studying the wonders of nature. The distance covered each week, the associated time commitment, and thus the intensity of effort are known with much greater precision than for most types of exercise. A formal exercise prescription is easily neglected when a person becomes busy, but it is difficult to "forget" the journey to work or school. A decreased use of cars could make a useful contribution to meeting urban targets for the reduction of "greenhouse" gases (www.davidsuzuki.org/Climate_Change/Kyoto/). In the face of ever-rising costs of gasoline, personal savings would be a further welcome dividend, and city-wide economic benefits might be anticipated, such as a reduced need for expenditures on freeways, bus systems and subways. Precise fiscal calculations remain somewhat suspect. Nevertheless, one Canadian analyst estimated that the 7.8% of Canadian workers who currently engage in active commuting save the national economy some $2 billion per year,[20] and a recent study from New York suggested that the use of public transit and associated walking would save each participant some $5500 per year in obesity-related medical costs alone.[21]

This article examines active commuting from the perspective of its effectiveness in maintaining and enhancing patient health. It evaluates such transportation in the context of the currently recommended minimum volume and intensity of physical activity. It compares the relative merits of walking and cycling, and examines secular trends in both modes of transportation. It then considers the role that physicians can play in augmenting active commuting, reviews empirical data on associated changes in population health, and finally suggests some areas requiring further research.

The Currently Recommended Minimum Volume and Intensity of Physical Activity

Issues concerning the minimum volume and intensity of physical activity needed for population health were considered in the lead article of the 2004 YEAR BOOK OF SPORTS MEDICINE,[22] and in a recent issue of the journal "Applied Physiology, Nutrition and Metabolism."[23] Expert groups in the U.S. have concluded that the minimum recommendation for adults is to take 30 minutes of moderately vigorous physical activity on most days of the week.[24] For a number of years, groups in Canada and elsewhere argued that this recommendation was insufficient. Adults needed to exercise for a minimum of 60 or even 90 minutes per day, particularly if the current epidemic of obesity was to be contained,[25-28] and the minimum requirement was thought to be even greater in children.[29] However, for reasons discussed below, the U.S. view has now been endorsed.

Most recommendations for the daily dose of physical activity were intended mainly to reduce an individual's risk of premature all-cause and cardiovascular mortality. Estimates are based heavily on questionnaires completed by male Harvard alumni at the behest of the late Ralph Paffenbarger and his associates. Multiple analyses of this data set have found favorable outcomes among individuals reporting what has been interpreted as a gross energy exercise expenditure of between 2 and 8 MJ per week; the most frequently cited recommendation is to engage in physical activity demanding a total of at least 4 MJ per week.[19-30] However, there are some important limitations to these estimates. Firstly, the proposed minimum energy expenditure is a gross rather than a net weekly figure, so that the active component of the total is greater for short periods of vigorous activity than for longer periods of moderate activity. Secondly, most people over-report their activity when using a questionnaire,[31] a problem recently highlighted by comparisons between questionnaire and accelerometer data for the Canadian population.[15] The original observations of Paffenbarger and associates were cross-sectional in type. Subsequent reports have also looked at changes in reported volumes of physical activity over periods of 10 years or longer, but it remains uncertain whether the positive health outcomes seen in those apparently becoming more active reflects altered behavior, or whether the dual assessments allow a clearer identification of active individuals. The conclusions drawn from Paffenbarger's original questionnaire data were reinforced by treadmill endurance times collected on another highly selected population, individuals attending the Cooper Fitness Clinic in Dallas, TX. Again, a high and/or an improved treadmill score was associated with improved health outcomes.[32,33] Treadmill endurance time was interpreted as an index of the individual's cardiorespiratory fitness, although clearly scores also depend on body mass and thus obesity.

The minimum volume and intensity of activity needed for good health thus continue to be a source of vigorous debate. In the past year, both Health Canada/Canadian Society of Exercise Physiology[34] and the World Health Organization[35] have drastically reduced their minimum recommendation for adults, from 60 or more minutes per day to a total of only 150 minutes per week. Reasons given for this change include a possible over-estimation of physical activity in the original questionnaire studies, and a recognition that since few of the current population are within reach of the previous standards, insistence on such activity levels might be counter-productive.[15] Nevertheless, Health Canada acknowledges that relative to the current recommendation, "greater health benefits appear to occur with higher volumes and/or intensities of activity."[34]

A minimum intensity of activity seems as important as a minimum volume, particularly if the goal is to maintain or enhance a patient's cardiovascular health. However, there have been varied interpretations of the words "moderately vigorous activity," as found in many of the consensus recommendations. The Centers for Disease Control and the American College of Sports Medicine have suggested that moderate activity encompasses a broad range of energy expenditures, from 3-6 METs (metabolic equivalents).[36] In recommending appropriate intensities, expert groups have not always taken sufficient account of such variables as the age, sex, and initial physical condition of the exerciser.[37,38] Certainly, if a program aims to enhance cardiorespiratory health, the intensity must reach the training zone, at least 50 percent of the individual's maximal oxygen intake, or an oxygen consumption of at least 20-25 ml/[kg.min] (6-7 METs) in a young adult, decreasing to 12-15 ml/[kg.min] (3-4 METs) as an individual reaches the age of retirement.[19] How likely is active commuting to meet these demands?

Physical demands of walking

A commuter normally walks at a speed of about 5 km/hour, except in hot weather, or when traveling on inner city routes with busy intersections. The *gross* energy expenditure when walking at this pace on a smooth and level path is about 18 kJ/min.[39] Thus, a total energy expenditure of 4 MJ/week would be reached by walking 1.9 km (22 minutes in each direction) on 5 days per week; the total, 220 minutes of moderately vigorous activity per week, seems a likely commuting pattern for many city workers, and it offers the middle-aged commuter a not unreasonable recommendation in terms of either distance or time commitments.[40] Indeed, if the local bus service is infrequent, it may be quicker to walk this distance than to wait for public transportation. The likely intensity of effort is more problematic from the viewpoint of improving cardiovascular health, at least in younger patients. Even without halts at traffic lights, the *gross* oxygen cost on a level city street (around 12.5 ml/[kg.min]) would amount to only 30-35% of maximal oxygen intake in a moderately fit young man. In contrast, the same walking speed would bring a 65-year-old commuter to the lower end of the aerobic training zone, about 50% of his or her maximal aerobic power.

This does not necessarily imply that walking to work must be rejected as an ineffective recommendation for a young patient. Several simple tactics can enhance cardiovascular benefits. If the pace is increased to 6.4 km/hour, the *gross* oxygen cost rises to about 16.2 ml/[kg.min], with some saving of commuting time, and little change in the total energy expended in covering what is necessarily a fixed distance. The intensity of effort can be further increased by the choice of a hilly route; if the previous pace of walking is maintained, a 5% (1 in 20) incline boosts the rate of energy expenditure by about 50%.[39,41] Roughness of terrain is another important variable, and after a heavy snowfall there can be a 2-3 fold increase in the energy cost of a given commute.[39] Some authors have questioned how far patients can understand the concept of brisk walking.[42] This is certainly a problem when offering a simple leisure prescription, but since the commuting distance is known rather precisely,[43] it is easy to recommend a travel time corresponding to the desired briskness of pace. The ability to maintain a conversation while walking provides a useful subjective check to avoid an excessive intensity of effort in the face of variables such as a heavy snowfall.

Physical demands of cycling

Energy expenditures are more difficult to predict for cycling than for walking. On urban streets, a comfortable riding speed of 16 km/h might be anticipated, with an energy cost of about 7 METs (24.5 ml/[kg.min], or 36 kJ/min.[44] An energy expenditure of 4 MJ per week is then accumulated with a commute of only 11 minutes (2.9 km) in each direction (110 minutes per week). Moreover, the intensity of effort seems likely to reach the training zone, even for a young adult, and some older individuals may even need to ride at less than 16 km/h in order to remain within a safe and comfortable training zone.

Several empirical studies support these theoretical estimates of speed and effectiveness. One report examined the intensity of effort developed by individuals who, for the first time, had begun cycling a minimum of 2 km to work. By the end of the study, the energy expenditure in a trial ride averaged 6.8 METs, or 75% of the individuals' maximal aerobic power; however, the authors commented that subjects rode somewhat faster than their normal pace during this trial.[45] A second study from the Netherlands found that six months of commuter cycling over an average distance of 8.5 km augmented the peak power output of the workers involved by 13% relative to a control group; in those individuals who were initially unfit, benefit was seen from daily rides as short as 3 km.[46] An investigation from Norway noted an average 15.8% increase of maximal oxygen intake in people who were persuaded to cycle to work for one year.[47] A controlled trial on the island of Funen involved participants who had not cycled during the previous 3 months; after 8 weeks of cycling (20 min/day at a speed of 15 km/h) the maximal oxygen intake of the experimental subjects increased by 12.5%, although that of the controls also showed a gain of some 4.6%.[48] Finally, a six-year prospective study of Danish children noted that normal daily cycling was effective in improving cardiorespiratory fitness; by the end of the trial, students initially aged 9.7 years who began to cycle to school had a peak power output that was 9% higher than that of their peers who still did not engage in active commuting.[49]

The physical demands of cycling plainly vary relative to these estimates, depending on the design of the bicycle, the speed of riding, the terrain, and any headwinds that are encountered. However, in most circumstances energy expenditures are greater than for walking. Thus, from the standpoint of cardiovascular health, cycling is the preferred option for young commuters. On the other hand, older patients can obtain adequate amounts of physical activity by walking all or part of the way to work.

The Commuter's Choice Between Walking and Cycling

Ardent active commuters have contemplated many forms of transportation, including canoes, row-boats and skateboards. Such choices may sometimes be both practicable and enjoyable. But for most patients, the choice lies essentially between walking and cycling. The preferred option depends in part on the age of the individual and the distance to be covered. The size of many modern cities precludes walking the entire distance to and from work, although even in a vast metropolis, some part of the journey can be covered on foot, for instance, by walking one or two subway or bus stops. Children and adolescents commonly enjoy cycling to school, but adults who work in the central business district may face heavy traffic, narrow streets and a lack of facilities to store their cycles on arrival; the risk of theft of an expensive bicycle is an important disincentive to many urban cyclists.[50,51] Cyclists may also find difficulty in meeting office dress codes, unless the employer provides on-site shower and changing facilities. Since active commuters reduce the need for parking space, companies should be encouraged to allocate some of the resulting financial savings[52] to the construction of cycle lockers and shower facilities. In cities with continental climates, the icing of streets is a further concern during the winter months, more so for the cyclist than the pedestrian.

Cycling to work is still relatively common in Holland, Denmark, and parts of Sweden and Finland where the terrain is relatively flat. It was also the normal mode of transportation in less-developed countries until recently, but now ownership of a moped has become a third-world status symbol. Questionnaire responses suggest that deliberate walking is the most popular form of leisure physical activity for most North American adults.[53] When the average patient is asked "what do you do for exercise?" the commonest response is "walking."[53,54] Morris once argued that walking was a "near perfect" form of exercise.[55] It required no special equipment or facilities, saved rather than spent money, and required no special training. Given a pleasant route, it could be a very agreeable part of the working day, and the risk of injury was low relative to most other forms of physical activity.[56] In the U.S., encouragement of walking has been seen as the most effective tactic to enhance the physical activity of sedentary populations.[57] The main danger comes from fast-moving traffic. Although reports of vehicle-related injuries have become less frequent in recent years, part of the apparent decline in injury rate could reflect a smaller number of walkers rather than improved road safety.[55] Sidewalk exposure to carbon monoxide[58] and oxidant smog[59] remain important issues for active commuters in many large cities. Street crime is unlikely to be a major problem during normal working hours, but walkers can sustain injuries from tripping on curbs and broken pavement, slipping on ice or wet leaves, and colliding with sidewalk furniture such as lamp standards.[60,61]

Despite these specific concerns, walking remains a very safe physical activity that can be continued throughout a person's working career. Moreover, the intensity of activity can readily be adjusted to accommodate both increasing age and any short-term deterioration in an individual's health.

Secular Trends in Commuting Behavior

In many countries, the percentage of adults who walk or cycle to work is currently very small, and seems to be decreasing further. However, the continuing surge in gasoline prices may well reverse this trend in the near future.

Perhaps because of flat terrain, Denmark and Holland have an above-average proportion of cyclists. During the late 1980s, 25% of trips in Holland were made by cycle,[62] compared with only 11% in neighboring Germany,[63] and only 2% in England.[64] Some 12 years ago, 46% of 25-year-old Danish men and women traveled to work by bicycle throughout the year, and 70% did so during the summer.[65] Figures were somewhat smaller in Copenhagen, with 20-30% of adults spending an average of 3 hours per week cycling to work; moreover, the Copenhagen data showed a socio-economic gradient, with cycling decreasing from 28% among the least educated to 20% among the most educated workers.[65] In the same era, 19% of Dutch workers walked and 27% cycled to work, and in Sweden the corresponding figures were 39% and 10%.[20] Many Londoners still include some walking in their daily commute. Short walks were quite popular among British adults in 1992-94, with 81% of the population making journeys of under 1.6 km on foot. However, the distance to be covered is critical; in 1992-1994, walking accounted for only 24% of journeys of 1.6 to 3.2 km, substantially less than the 32% of people who walked this distance in 1985-86.[66] Perhaps because of a high traffic density and narrow streets, only 7% of adults cycle to work in central London.[67]

In North America, there are very few active commuters. Only 6.6% of Canadians walk to work, and a mere 1.2 % are cyclists.[20] Weather conditions are an important factor in Central Canada, and in the more temperate climate of Victoria, B.C., 10.4% of commuters are walkers and 4.8% are cyclists.[20] Those who practice active transportation during their working lives are apt to continue this practice into their retirement years. A report from small-town Japan showed that those aged 65-74 years spent 10.8 Met-hours per week on active transportation (corresponding to about 3 hours of moderate paced walking per week).[68]

Many children live at an optimal commuting distance from their place of schooling,[69] and in some countries this is an important source of physical activity. In Switzerland, 78% of children still traveled actively to school in 2004-2005,[70] and a recent Swedish national survey of 11-15-year-old students found 63% still engaged in active commuting.[4] Nevertheless, in other countries, the proportion of students who walk or cycle to school has decreased markedly as parents have had greater access to cars, and the perceived hazards of active commuting have increased. In the U.K., the number of children walking to school decreased by 20% between 1970 and 1991,[71] and the average distance walked decreased by 28% between 1975-76 and 1992-94.[66] By 1993, half of British primary school children were being driven over distances of less than 1.6 km.[72] In Ireland, the most recent data found only 36% of students aged 9-11 years were walking to school.[7] In the U.S., likewise, personal chauffeuring of schoolchildren has become the population norm. One study showed that cycling to school had decreased from 48% of students aged 5-15 years in 1968 to 1% in 2001, and in 2001 only 15% of the remaining students were making the journey on foot.[73] A second report from the U.S. noted a 37% decrease in active travel between 1977 and 1995.[74,75] In the province of Quebec, walking to school is less frequent among girls, recent immigrants and children from high-income homes.[76] In New South Wales, Australia, 55.7% and 44.2% of children aged 5-9 and 10-14 years, respectively, walked to school in 1971, but by 1999-2003, the corresponding figures were only 25.5% and 21.1%, with at least corresponding increases in the percentages traveling by car.[77]

Persuading More Patients to Become Active Commuters

Both positive and negative reinforcement have been used in attempts to increase the proportion of the population who are active commuters. Surveys of travel patterns at the University of Bristol found that in contrast to national trends for the U.K., the proportion of staff walking to work increased from 19% in 1998 to 30% in 2007; this was attributed primarily to an increase in parking restrictions at the university.[1] Several authors have urged that positive changes in the "built environment" could encourage an increase of walking and cycling,[78-81] although a person's built environment may be a somewhat less critical issue for active commuters than for those who engage in leisure-time walking and cycling.[79-82] Walking is likely to be encouraged by well-maintained sidewalks and pedestrian crossings, improved street lighting, the development of greenways and connections between streets,[83] pedestrian precincts, and the proximity of the desired destinations; one gloomy report suggested that currently, most people in the U.S. were unlikely to walk farther than 400 m, a 5-minute journey.[81-84] Attempts to increase the proximity of common destinations often rely on high-density development of houses and offices, but this can also reduce the aesthetics of walking. Despite a relatively low incidence of injuries in some studies,[85] the safety of active commuting is an important pre-occupation, particularly in the case of women and children.[86,87] The safety of cycling can be increased by traffic-calming devices, appropriately marked cycle lanes, and specific traffic signals for bicycles at busy intersections; bicycle traffic on one street in New Orleans increased by 57% immediately subsequent to the simple tactic of painting cycle lanes.[9] In Auckland, a program to encourage active commuting by primary school students included education, more rigid enforcement of parking restrictions near schools and changes in urban form; by the third year, there had been a very modest gain in active commuters (from 40.5% to 42.2%).[3] In the long-term, a radical redesign of cities could allow schools and workplaces to be built close to residential areas, with inter-connections by attractively landscaped cycle and pedestrian paths, away from the noise, pollution and danger of motor traffic.[88-90] Other benefits that may help to motivate active commuting include the avoidance of parking problems, financial savings, improved personal health, and reduced environmental pollution.[91]

Safety is often said to be particularly critical when attempting to increase active commuting by younger children,[70,92,93] although a systematic review of 14 studies found that the only significant environmental correlate of active commuting was the distance to be covered.[10] Many students prefer to use their bicycles as the means of commuting, but walking is more easily controlled and is generally a safer option. An organized neighborhood walk or cycle trip to school may be a useful way both to reduce risks and to reassure anxious parents.[94]

Given the relative prevalence of walking and cycling in most countries, health planners have thought it more promising to promote walking than cycling, and many of the studies examining the response to an encouragement of active transportation have looked at walking rather than cycling. One meta-analysis[95] searched 25 databases, 12 Web sites, prior systematic reviews and the input of an international panel of experts, with a yield of 53 491 papers over the years 1990-2006. Only 441 of the original 53 491 papers were studied in detail, the primary inclusion criterion being the presentation of data on walking behavior before and after an intervention.

Nineteen randomized and 29 non-randomized controlled trials met this criterion. In the most promising of these studies, the immediate response was a 30-60 minutes per week increase in walking. However, there was no exploration of long-term adherence, possible reductions in other forms of voluntary activity, or adverse consequences (such as injuries), and few of the interventions involved active commuting. The increases of walking observed in even the most effective commuter studies were much smaller (15-30 minutes per week) than those seen in leisure walking programs. Investigations with a commuter focus were generally targeted to those considering such an option, and the intervention was personally tailored; for example, in children, there was a mapping of safe routes for active commuting to school.[69] Significant increases of walking were seen when interventions were addressed to individuals, households, or small groups, but evidence of gains from more broadly directed workplace, school or community-wide initiatives was less convincing. From a policy point of view, even an increase of 15-30 minutes *per week* is quite disappointing relative to published recommendations that adults should undertake at least 150 minutes of moderate physical activity per week. Moreover, most studies targeted interested individuals, and it seems likely that the response would have been even smaller if the intervention had been applied on a population-wide basis.

Impact of Active Commuting on Health Outcomes

Studies of adults

Controlled studies examining the impact of active commuting on health outcomes in adults have differed in their conclusions. This seems in part because investigators have neglected the influence of the individual's age on the relative intensity of activity.[37] We have noted above several reports showing that active commuting increases aerobic fitness. Other recent investigations suggest a decrease in obesity and other cardiac risk factors, and a reduced overall and disease specific mortality rate.

A public health survey of adults aged 18-80 years was conducted in southern Sweden; it found that the odds of being overweight or obese were significantly lower for those individuals who walked or cycled rather than used their car (odds ratios of 0.62 and 0.79 for men and women, respectively).[12] Likewise, a study from Atlanta, GA, found that the likelihood of being obese decreased by 4.8% for each km walked per day.[11] One early meta-analysis found no difference of health outcomes between controls and individuals who increased their walking by 30-60 minutes per week[95]; however, critics argued that inclusion criteria led to the omission of some important studies where an improvement of health had been demonstrated.[96,97] A second review analyzed five major cross-sectional studies.[98] It indicated that after statistical adjustments for age, body mass index, and other forms of physical activity, walking was associated with a 20-50% decrease in the risk of diabetes mellitus, and a 40-50% decrease in all-cause and cardiovascular deaths. A further meta-analysis based on 8 studies with a total of 173 146 participants found that walking or cycling to work was linked to a 11% reduction in overall cardiovascular risk. The end-points examined in this study included mortality, incident coronary heart disease, stroke, hypertension and diabetes. Benefits were seen more strongly in women than in men (and were statistically significant only for the women).[99] Cross-sectional comparisons have found greater aerobic fitness in adult active commuters than in their peers.[100] The U.S. CARDIA Study found favorable associations between commuting (irrespective of whether cycling or walking) and aerobic fitness in men and women. And in men (but not in women) there were also inverse associations with BMI, obesity, triglyceride levels, blood pressure, and insulin level.[101] A population-based study in Australia found an inverse relationship between cycling to work and overweight or obesity in men (although less clearly in women).[13] In Finland, walking or cycling to work reduced cardiovascular mortality in hypertensive women.[102] A study of 30 000 Copenhagen residents also noted that over 14.5 years, all-cause mortality was 40% lower in cyclists than in passive commuters, even after data had been adjusted for reported leisure-time activities.[65] In the U.K., the incidence of myocardial infarction among those cycling to work was half of that in the general population,[103] and in Finland [40] 15 minutes or more per day of walking or cycling to work was associated with reduced all-cause and cardiovascular mortality in women, but not in men. In Shanghai, all-cause mortality was inversely correlated with cycling to work after data adjustment for other forms of physical activity,[104] but the all-cause mortality of Chinese was less strongly associated with walking than with cycling to work.[104] Shanghai residents, Hou and associates[105] also showed a strong association between substantial commuting activity and a reduced risk of colon cancer, particularly if commuting had continued for 35 or more years (odds ratio 0.34 for men and 0.31 for women). Women in Shanghai who reported exercise from adolescence had a 37% reduction in the risk of endometrial cancer, although in this study the impact of commuting was not clearly delineated from the health benefits of other forms of exercise and heavy household chores.[106]

The above observations appear to support the health value of active commuting for adults. Moreover, some workers can be persuaded to commute over substantial daily distances without making compensatory reductions in their other activities, and when cycling they often exercise at a substantial fraction of their heart rate reserve and/or aerobic power.[45,107-109] However, the available information cannot establish cause and effect. Possibly, those who choose to cycle to work have a better initial health and/or lifestyle than the comparison group, and this could account for their more favorable health experience. As might be anticipated from our discussion above, trials that also show health benefits among those who walk to work have generally involved older or less fit workers.

Studies of children and adolescents

Most studies have shown that walking to school is associated with a greater overall physical activity. Among a small sample of Irish students aged 9-11 years, those who walked to school had a pedometer count that was almost 3000 steps/day greater than that of their peers who traveled by car or bus.[7] Likewise, the HELENA accelerometer study of 3112 European adolescents found that active commuting was associated with increased daily amounts of moderate and moderate-to-vigorous physical activity,[2] the 2003-2004 US National Health & Nutrition Examination Survey (NHANES) found a positive association between active commuting and total daily physical activity in 789 adolescents aged 12-19 years,[6] and the odds ratio of meeting the daily pedometer activity target was greater (1.48) in Australian students aged 10-12 years who were not driven to school.[5] The SPEEDY study of 9-10-year-old children found that the longer the distance to school, the greater the association between active commuting and the student's total daily physical activity.[8] One accelerometer study showed a sex difference in the overall weekly physical activity of active commuters; in boys, scores were greater with either walking or cycling to school, but only walking was associated with greater overall physical activity in the girls.[110] Unfortunately, such data is far from reliable, since pedometers and uniaxial accelerometers tend to record little of the energy expended in cycling.

Cross-sectional studies of both children and adolescents have found better health and possibly cognitive development[111] in active commuters. In Odense, children and adolescents who cycled to school were substantially more fit than those who walked or were driven.[112] In Brasil, passively commuting students were more likely to be obese than those who were active commuters.[113] However, one U.S. review noted a lower body mass index in only 3 of 18 active groups.[114] In this study, the active students possibly ate more, or the average distance traveled was insufficient for benefit.[115] A more recent analysis of the 2003-2004 NHANES data for students aged 12-19 years confirmed the general trend, BMI and skinfold readings being inversely associated with active commuting.[6]

Conclusions and Suggestions for Further Research

Depending on an individual's age, empirical data suggest that regular walking or cycling to work can enhance a variety of health outcomes. Quite brief journeys are enough to generate the weekly gross energy expenditure of 4 MJ that some epidemiologists have associated with enhanced health and reduced mortality rates. Moreover, the weekly time commitment needed to reach a 4 MJ expenditure (220 min of walking, 110 min of for cycling) seems in line with the most recent recommendations on the minimal duration of physical activity needed to maintain health. Most policy recommendations do not give a clear indication of the minimum intensity that is needed, but if for cardiovascular benefit this should reach the aerobic training zone. Cycling, with an energy cost >7 METs, is likely to satisfy this requirement at all ages, in agreement with the observed favorable health outcomes seen in both young and older adults. Level walking demands an energy expenditure of only about 3.5 METs; this intensity can reach the training zone of an elderly worker, but is insufficient for a young man. Observed age differences in health outcomes for walkers support this inference. If walking to work is to enhance the health of a young person, it is necessary to choose a hilly route or to adopt a rapid pace.

Although active commuting seems to have potential as a means of enhancing a patient's health, we need further studies relating physical activity patterns (duration and intensity of activity, typical number of journeys per week) and health outcomes in those who choose to cycle or walk to work. We also need studies such as that of Saksvig and associates[116] to clarify whether such active commuting discourages other forms of active leisure. Adults who are active commuters are often dedicated exercisers, but in the case of children we need to know whether the encouragement of active commuting at a young age will develop a love of walking or cycling that will continue into adulthood. Currently, few North Americans cycle or walk to work. This provides scope for health promotion, but we need much more information on effective methods of persuading patients to engage in active transportation. In particular, the merits of individual office counseling need to be weighed critically against the effectiveness of nation-wide promotional campaigns and changes in the built environment.[80-90] It is important not only to know that active commuting has the potential to make our patients more healthy, but also to understand how we can persuade them to engage regularly in such activity.

References

1. Brockman R, Fox KR. Physical activity by stealth? The potential health benefits of a workplace transport plan. *Public Health.* 2011;125:210-216.
2. Chillón P, Ortega FB, Ruiz JR, et al. Active commuting and physical activity in adolescents from Europe: results from the HELENA Study. *Pediatr Exerc Sci.* 2011;23:207-217.
3. Hinckson EA, Garrett N, Duncan S. Active commuting to school in New Zealand children (2004-2008): a quantitative analysis. *Prev Med.* 2011;52:332-336.
4. Johansson K, Laflamme L, Hasselberg M. Active commuting to and from school among Swedish children—a national and regional study. *Eur J Public Health.* 2012;22:209-214.
5. McCormack GR, Giles-Corti B, Timperio A, Wood G, Villanueva K. A cross-sectional study of the individual, social, and built environmental correlates of pedometer-based physical activity among elementary school children. *Int J Behav Nutr Phys Act.* 2011;8:30.
6. Mendoza JA, Watson K, Nguyen N, Cerin E, Baranowski T, Nicklas TA. Active commuting to school and association with physical activity and adiposity among US youth. *J Phys Act Health.* 2011;8:488-495.
7. Murtagh EM, Murphy MH. Active travel to school and physical activity levels of Irish primary school children. *Pediatr Exerc Sci.* 2011;23:230-236.
8. Panter J, Jones A, Van Sluijs E, Griffin S. The influence of distance to school on the associations between active commuting and physical activity. *Pediatr Exerc Sci.* 2011;23:72-86.
9. Parker KM, Gustat J, Rice JC. Installation of bicycle lanes and increased ridership in an urban, mixed-income setting in New Orleans, Louisiana. *J Phys Act Health.* 2011;8:S98-S102.
10. Wong BY, Faulkner G, Buliung R. GIS measured environmental correlates of active school transport: a systematic review of 14 studies. *Int J Behav Nutr Phys Act.* 2011;8:39.
11. Frank LD, Andresen MA, Schmid TL. Obesity relationships with community design, physical activity, and time spent in cars. *Am J Prev Med.* 2004;27:87-96.

12. Lindström M. Means of transportation to work and overweight and obesity: a population-based study in southern Sweden. *Prev Med.* 2008;46:22-28.
13. Wen LM, Rissel C. Inverse associations between cycling to work, public transport, and overweight and obesity: findings from a population based study in Australia. *Prev Med.* 2008;46:29-32.
14. Zheng Y. The benefit of public transportation: physical activity to reduce obesity and ecological footprint. *Prev Med.* 2008;46:4-5.
15. Colley RC, Garriguet D, Janssen I, Craig CL, Clarke J, Tremblay MS. Physical activity of Canadian adults: accelerometer results from the 2007 to 2009 Canadian Health Measures Survey. *Health Rep.* 2011;22:7-14.
16. Shephard RJ. *Endurance Fitness.* 2nd ed. Toronto, Ontario: University of Toronto Press; 1977.
17. U.S. Department of Health and Human Services. *Healthy People 2010.* 2nd ed. Washington, DC: U.S. Government Printing Office; 2000.
18. Parks Victoria. *The Health Benefits of Contact with Nature in a Park Context: An Annotated Bibliography.* Victoria, British Columbia: Parks Victoria; 2002.
19. Shephard RJ. *Aerobic Fitness and Health.* Champaign, IL: Human Kinetics; 1994.
20. Campbell R, Wittgens M. *The Business Case for Active Transportation. The Economic Benefits of Walking and Cycling.* Gloucester, Ontario: Go for Green; 2004.
21. Edwards RD. Public transit, obesity, and medical costs: assessing the magnitudes. *Prev Med.* 2008;46:14-21.
22. Shephard RJ. What is an effective dose of physical activity? In: Shephard RJ, ed. *Year Book of Sports Medicine, 2004.* Philadelphia, PA: Elsevier; 2004:xvii-xxii.
23. Shephard RJ. Advancing physical activity measurements and guidelines in Canada: a scientific review and evidence-based foundations for the future of Canadian physical activity guideline. *Appl Physiol Nutr Metab.* 2007;32:S1-S224.
24. U.S. Department of Health and Human Services PHS, Centres for Disease Control and Prevention, National Centre for Chronic Disease Prevention and Health Promotion, Division of Nutrition and Physical Activity. *Physical Activity and Health: A Report of the Surgeon General.* Atlanta, GA: U.S. Department of Health and Human Services, Centers for Disease Control and Prevention, National Center for Chronic Disease Prevention and Health Promotion; 1996.
25. Andersen LB, Harro M, Sardinha LB, et al. Physical activity and clustered cardiovascular risk in children: a cross-sectional study (The European Youth Heart Study). *Lancet.* 2006;368:299-304.
26. Health Canada CSEP. *Handbook for Canada's Physical Activity Guide to Healthy Active Living.* Ottawa, Ontario: Health Canada; 1998.
27. Tremblay MS, Shephard RJ, Brawley LR. Research that informs Canada's Physical Activity Guides. *Appl Physiol Nutr Metab.* 2007;32:S1-S8.
28. World Health Organization. *Obesity. Preventing and Managing the Global Epidemic. Report of a WHO Consultation.* Geneva, Switzerland: World Health Organization; 1998.
29. Janssen I. Physical activity guidelines for children and youth. *Can J Public Health.* 2007;98:S109-S121.
30. Paffenbarger R, Hyde RT, Wing AL, et al. Some interrelations of physical activity, physiological fitness, health, and longevity. In: Bouchard C, Shephard RJ, Stephens T, eds. *Physical Activity, Fitness and Health.* Champaign, IL: Human Kinetics; 1994:119-133.
31. Shephard RJ. Limits to the measurement of habitual physical activity by questionnaires. *Br J Sports Med.* 2003;37:197-206.
32. Lee CD, Blair SN, Jackson AS. Cardiorespiratory fitness, body composition, and all-cause and cardiovascular disease mortality in men. *Am J Clin Nutr.* 1999;69:373-380.
33. Blair SN, Kampert JB, Kohl HW 3rd, et al. Influences of cardiorespiratory fitness and other precursors on cardiovascular disease and all-cause mortality in men and women. *JAMA.* 1996;276:205-210.

34. Warburton DE, Charlesworth S, Ivey A, Nettlefold L, Bredin SS. A systematic review of the evidence for Canada's Physical Activity Guidelines for Adults. *Int J Behav Nutr Phys Act.* 2010;7:39.

35. World Health Organization. *Global Recommendations on Physical Activity for Health. Geneva, World Health Organization.* Geneva, Switzerland: World Health Organization; 2010.

36. Pate RR, Pratt M, Blair SN, et al. Physical activity and public health. A recommendation from the Centers for Disease Control and Prevention and the American College of Sports Medicine. *JAMA.* 1995;273:402-407.

37. Bouchard C, Shephard RJ. Physical activity, fitness, and health: the model and key concepts. In: Bouchard C, Shephard RJ, Stephens T, eds. *Physical Activity, Fitness and Health.* Champaign, IL: Human Kinetics; 1994:77-88.

38. Shephard RJ. Intensity, duration and frequency of exercise as determinants of the response to a training regime. *Int Z Angew Physiol.* 1968;26:272-278.

39. Shephard RJ. *Physiology and Biochemistry of Exercise.* New York, NY: Praeger Publications; 1982.

40. Barengo NC, Hu G, Lakka TA, Pekkarinen H, Nissinen A, Tuomilehto J. Low physical activity as a predictor for total and cardiovascular disease mortality in middle-aged men and women in Finland. *Eur Heart J.* 2004;25:2204-2211.

41. Sutherland DH, Kaufman KR, Moitoza JR. Kinematics of normal walking. In: Rose J, Gamble JG, eds. *Human Walking.* Baltimore, MD: Williams and Wilkins; 1993:23-44.

42. Lee IM, Buchner DM. The importance of walking to public health. *Med Sci Sports Exerc.* 2008;40:S512-S518.

43. Schantz P, Stigell E. A criterion method for measuring route distance in physically active commuting. *Med Sci Sports Exerc.* 2009;41:472-478.

44. American College of Sports Medicine. *ACSM's Guidelines for Exercise Testing and Prescription.* 7th ed. Philadelphia, PA: Lippincott, Williams & Wilkins; 2006.

45. de Geus B, De Smet S, Nijs J, Meeusen R. Determining the intensity and energy expenditure during commuter cycling. *Br J Sports Med.* 2007;41:8-12.

46. Hendriksen IJ, Zuiderveld B, Kemper HC, Bezemer PD. Effect of commuter cycling on physical performance of male and female employees. *Med Sci Sports Exerc.* 2000;32:504-510.

47. Tjelta LI, Kvåle OH, Dyrstad SM. Health effects of cycling to and from work. *Tidsskr Nor Laegeforen.* 2010;130:1246-1249.

48. Møller NC, Østergaard L, Gade JR, et al. The effect on cardiorespiratory fitness after an 8-week period of commuter cycling—a randomized controlled study in adults. *Prev Med.* 2011;53:172-177.

49. Cooper AR, Wedderkopp N, Jago R, et al. Longitudinal associations of cycling to school with adolescent fitness. *Prev Med.* 2008;47:324-328.

50. Brunsing J. Public transport and cycling experience of modal integration in West Germany. In: Tolley R, ed. *The Greening of Urban Transport Planning for Walking and Cycling in Western Cities.* London, UK: Belhaven Press; 1990:309.

51. Unwin N. Cycling behavior and cycle helmet use: a study of university students. *Health Ed J.* 1992;51:184-188.

52. Shoup D. Evaluating the effects of cashing out employer-paid parking: eight case studies. *Transport Policy.* 1997;4:201-216.

53. Canada Fitness Survey. *Fitness and Lifestyle in Canada.* Ottawa, Ontario: Canadian Fitness and Lifestyle Research Institute; 1983.

54. Simpson ME, Serdula M, Galuska DA, et al. Walking trends among U.S. adults: the Behavioral Risk Factor Surveillance System, 1987-2000. *Am J Prev Med.* 2003;25:95-100.

55. Morris JN, Hardman AE. Walking to Health. *Sports Med.* 1997;23:306-332.

56. Hootman JM, Macera CA, Ainsworth BE, Addy CL, Martin M, Blair SN. Epidemiology of musculoskeletal injuries among sedentary and physically active adults. *Med Sci Sports Exerc.* 2002;34:838-844.

57. Hillsdon M, Thorogood M. A systematic review of physical activity promotion strategies. *Br J Sports Med.* 1996;30:84-89.
58. Shephard RJ. *Carbon Monoxide-the Silent Killer.* Springfield, IL: C.C. Thomas; 1983.
59. Folinsbee LA. Exercise and air pollution. In: Torg J, Shephard RJ, eds. *Current Therapy in Sports Medicine.* 3rd ed. St. Louis, MO: Mosby; 1995:574-578.
60. David HG, Freedman LS. Injuries caused by tripping over paving stones: an unappreciated problem. *BMJ.* 1990;300:784-785.
61. U.K. National Consumer Council. *What's Wrong with Walking?.* London, UK: Her Majesty's Stationery Office; 1987.
62. Netherland Central Bureau voor de Statistiek. Mobility of the Dutch population in 1989. In: Hillman M, British Medical Association, eds. *Cycling Towards Health and Safety.* Oxford, UK: Oxford University Press; 1992:168.
63. Monheim R. Policy issues in promoting the green modes. In: Tolley R, ed. *The Greening of Urban Transport Planning for Walking and Cycling.* London, UK: Belhaven Press; 1990:309.
64. U.K. Department of Transport. *Department of Transport National Travel Survey 1985/86 Report, Part 1 An Analysis of Personal Travel.* London, UK: Her Majesty's Stationery Office; 1988.
65. Andersen LB, Schnohr P, Schroll M, Hein HO. All-cause mortality associated with physical activity during leisure time, work, sports, and cycling to work. *Arch Intern Med.* 2000;160:1621-1628.
66. U.K. Department of Transport. *National Travel Survey.* London, UK: Her Majesty's Stationery Office; 1995.
67. Cycling and Health. *Friends of the Earth Conference, London.* London, UK: Friends of the Earth; 1990.
68. Yasunaga A, Park H, Watanabe E, et al. Development and evaluation of the physical activity questionnaire for elderly Japanese: the Nakanojo Study. *J Aging Phys Act.* 2007;15:398-411.
69. Tudor-Locke C, Ainsworth BE, Popkin BM. Active commuting to school: an overlooked source of childrens' physical activity? *Sports Med.* 2001;31: 309-313.
70. Bringolf-Isler B, Grize L, Mäder U, Ruch N, Sennhauser FH, Braun-Fahrländer C. Personal and environmental factors associated with active commuting to school in Switzerland. *Prev Med.* 2008;46:67-73.
71. Hillman M. *Children, Transport and the Quality of Life.* London, UK: Policy Studies Institute; 1993.
72. Sleap M, Warburton P. Are primary school children gaining heart health benefits from their journeys to school? *Child Care Health Dev.* 1993;19:99-108.
73. U.S. Environmental Protection Agency. Travel and Environmental Implications of School Siting. Washington, DC: 2003.
74. U.S. Department of Transportation. *National Personal Transportation Symposium, October, 1997.* Bethesda, MD: U.S. Federal Highway Administration; 1999.
75. McCann B, DeLille B. *Mean Streets 2000: Pedestrian Safety, Health and Federal Transportation Spending.* Columbia, SC: Surface transportation policy project; 2000.
76. Pabayo R, Gauvin L. Proportions of students who use various modes of transportation to and from school in a representative population-based sample of children and adolescents, 1999. *Prev Med.* 2008;46:63-66.
77. van der Ploeg HP, Merom D, Corpuz G, Bauman AE. Trends in Australian children traveling to school 1971-2003: burning petrol or carbohydrates? *Prev Med.* 2008;46:60-62.
78. Giles-Corti B, Knuiman M, Timperio A, et al. Evaluation of the implementation of a state government community design policy aimed at increasing local walking: design issues and baseline results from RESIDE, Perth Western Australia. *Prev Med.* 2008;46:46-54.

79. Owen N, Humpel N, Leslie E, Bauman A, Sallis JF. Understanding environmental influences on walking: review and research agenda. *Am J Prev Med.* 2004; 27:67-76.

80. Sallis JF, Kerr J. Physical activity and the built environment. *Res Digest.* 2006;7.

81. Sallis JF. Angels in the details: comment on "The relationship between destination proximity, destination mix and physical activity behaviors." *Prev Med.* 2008;46:6-7.

82. Saelens BE, Handy SL. Built environment correlates of walking: a review. *Med Sci Sports Exerc.* 2008;40:S550-S566.

83. Chin GK, Van Niel KP, Giles-Corti B, Knuiman M. Accessibility and connectivity in physical activity studies: the impact of missing pedestrian data. *Prev Med.* 2008;46:41-45.

84. McCormack GR, Giles-Corti B, Bulsara M. The relationship between destination proximity, destination mix and physical activity behaviors. *Prev Med.* 2008;46:33-40.

85. Schofield GM, Gianotti S, Badland HM, Hinckson EA. The incidence of injuries traveling to and from school by travel mode. *Prev Med.* 2008;46:74-76.

86. Garrard J, Rose G, Lo SK. Promoting transportation cycling for women: the role of bicycle infrastructure. *Prev Med.* 2008;46:55-59.

87. Kayser B. Determinants of active commuting. *Prev Med.* 2008;46:8.

88. Anderson T. Safe routes to school in Odense, Denmark. In: Tolley R, ed. Chichester, UK: Wiley; 1997.

89. Boarnet M, Day K, Anderson C, et al. California's safe routes to school program - impacts on walking, bicycling and pedestrian safety. *J Am Plan Assoc.* 2005; 71:301-317.

90. Pikora TJ, Giles-Corti B, Knuiman MW, Bull FC, Jamrozik K, Donovan RJ. Neighborhood environmental factors correlated with walking near home: using SPACES. *Med Sci Sports Exerc.* 2006;38:708-714.

91. Merom D, Miller YD, van der Ploeg HP, Bauman A. Predictors of initiating and maintaining active commuting to work using transport and public health perspectives in Australia. *Prev Med.* 2008;47:342-346.

92. Hume C, Timperio A, Salmon J, Carver A, Giles-Corti B, Crawford D. Walking and cycling to school: predictors of increases among children and adolescents. *Am J Prev Med.* 2009;36:195-200.

93. Forman H, Kerr J, Norman GJ, et al. Reliability and validity of destination-specific barriers to walking and cycling for youth. *Prev Med.* 2008;46:311-316.

94. Kennedy J, Kowey B, Downey M. *How to Organize a Walking/Cycling School Bus (WSB/CSB).* Gloucester, Ontario: Go for Green; 1999.

95. Ogilvie D, Foster CE, Rothnie H, et al. Interventions to promote walking: systematic review. *BMJ.* 2007;334:1204.

96. Tully MA, Cupples ME, Chan WS, McGlade K, Young IS. Brisk walking, fitness, and cardiovascular risk: a randomized controlled trial in primary care. *Prev Med.* 2005;41:622-628.

97. Tully MA, Cupples ME. The effects of walking on health. *BMJ.* 2007;334:1204.

98. Caspersen CJ, Fulton JE. Epidemiology of walking and type 2 diabetes. *Med Sci Sports Exerc.* 2008;40:S519-S528.

99. Hamer M, Chida Y. Active commuting and cardiovascular risk: a meta-analytic review. *Prev Med.* 2008;46:9-13.

100. de Geus B, Joncheere J, Meeusen R. Commuter cycling: effect on physical performance in untrained men and women in Flanders: minimum dose to improve indexes of fitness. *Scand J Med Sci Sports.* 2009;19:179-187.

101. Gordon-Larsen P, Boone-Heinonen J, Sidney S, Sternfeld B, Jacobs DR Jr, Lewis CE. Active commuting and cardiovascular disease risk: the CARDIA study. *Arch Intern Med.* 2009;169:1216-1223.

102. Hu G, Jousilahti P, Antikainen R, Tuomilehto J. Occupational, commuting, and leisure-time physical activity in relation to cardiovascular mortality among Finnish subjects with hypertension. *Am J Hypertens.* 2007;20:1242-1250.

103. Morris JN, Clayton DG, Everitt MG, Semmence AM, Burgess EH. Exercise in leisure time: coronary attack and death rates. *Br Heart J*. 1990;63:325-334.
104. Matthews CE, Jurj AL, Shu XO, et al. Influence of exercise, walking, cycling, and overall nonexercise physical activity on mortality in Chinese women. *Am J Epidemiol*. 2007;165:1343-1350.
105. Hou L, Ji BT, Blair A, Dai Q, Gao YT, Chow WH. Commuting physical activity and risk of colon cancer in Shanghai, China. *Am J Epidemiol*. 2004;160: 860-867.
106. Matthews CE, Xu WH, Zheng W, et al. Physical activity and risk of endometrial cancer: a report from the Shanghai endometrial cancer study. *Cancer Epidemiol Biomarkers Prev*. 2005;14:779-785.
107. Asikainen TM, Miilunpalo S, Oja P, et al. Randomised, controlled walking trials in postmenopausal women: the minimum dose to improve aerobic fitness? *Br J Sports Med*. 2002;36:189-194.
108. Moreau KL, Degarmo R, Langley J, et al. Increasing daily walking lowers blood pressure in postmenopausal women. *Med Sci Sports Exerc*. 2001;33: 1825-1831.
109. Murphy MH, Nevill AM, Murtagh EM, Holder RL. The effect of walking on fitness, fatness and resting blood pressure: a meta-analysis of randomised, controlled trials. *Prev Med*. 2007;44:377-385.
110. Cooper AR, Andersen LB, Wedderkopp N, Page AS, Froberg K. Physical activity levels of children who walk, cycle, or are driven to school. *Am J Prev Med*. 2005;29:179-184.
111. Martínez-Gómez D, Ruiz JR, Gómez-Martínez S, et al. Active commuting to school and cognitive performance in adolescents: the AVENA study. *Arch Pediatr Adolesc Med*. 2011;165:300-305.
112. Cooper AR, Wedderkopp N, Wang H, Andersen LB, Froberg K, Page AS. Active travel to school and cardiovascular fitness in Danish children and adolescents. *Med Sci Sports Exerc*. 2006;38:1724-1731.
113. Silva KS, Lopes AS. Excess weight, arterial pressure and physical activity in commuting to school: correlations. *Arq Bras Cardiol*. 2008;91:84-91.
114. Lee MC, Orenstein MR, Richardson MJ. Systematic review of active commuting to school and childrens physical activity and weight. *J Phys Act Health*. 2008;5:930-949.
115. Landsberg B, Plachta-Danielzik S, Much D, Johannsen M, Lange D, Müller MJ. Associations between active commuting to school, fat mass and lifestyle factors in adolescents: the Kiel Obesity Prevention Study (KOPS). *Eur J Clin Nutr*. 2008;62:739-747.
116. Saksvig BI, Catellier DJ, Pfeiffer K, et al. Travel by walking before and after school and physical activity among adolescent girls. *Arch Pediatr Adolesc Med*. 2007;161:153-158.

1 Epidemiology, Prevention of Injuries, Lesions of Head and Neck

Physical Exercise, Body Mass Index, and Risk of Chronic Pain in the Low Back and Neck/Shoulders: Longitudinal Data From the Nord-Trøndelag Health Study
Nilsen TIL, Holtermann A, Mork PJ (Norwegian Univ of Science and Technology, Trondheim; Natl Res Centre for the Working Environment, Copenhagen, Denmark)
Am J Epidemiol 174:267-273, 2011

Chronic musculoskeletal pain constitutes a large socioeconomic challenge, and preventive measures with documented effects are warranted. The authors' aim in this study was to prospectively investigate the association between physical exercise, body mass index (BMI), and risk of chronic pain in the low back and neck/shoulders. The study comprised data on approximately 30,000 women and men in the Nord-Trøndelag Health Study (Norway) who reported no pain or physical impairment at baseline in 1984–1986. Occurrence of chronic musculoskeletal pain was assessed at follow-up in 1995–1997. A generalized linear model was used to calculate adjusted risk ratios. For both females and males, hours of physical exercise per week were linearly and inversely associated with risk of chronic pain in the low back (women: P-trend $= 0.02$; men: P-trend < 0.001) and neck/shoulders (women: P-trend $= 0.002$; men: P-trend < 0.001). Obese women and men had an approximately 20% increased risk of chronic pain in both the low back and the neck/shoulders. Exercising for 1 or more hours per week compensated, to some extent, for the adverse effect of high BMI on risk of chronic pain. The authors conclude that physical inactivity and high BMI are associated with an increased risk of chronic pain in the low back and neck/shoulders in the general adult population.

▶ In this large epidemiologic study, a relatively small amount of physical exercise predicted a lower risk of chronic pain in the low back and neck and shoulders in both men and women. In contrast, overweight or obesity was linked to a higher risk that could be attenuated by physical exercise. Lumbar disc disease is a common musculoskeletal disease affecting about 5% of all individuals.[1] It is characterized by lumbar disc herniation, which causes nerve root irritation, either mechanically or via inflammatory mediators, and results in radiating pain, known as sciatica. Lumbar disc degeneration often coexists with low back pain. Before the last decade, disc degeneration was often attributed to cumulative trauma from work-related physical activities, such as heavy materials handling, postural loading, and vehicular vibration. However, the best evidence now shows that genetic influences are strongly related to disc degeneration, not wear and tear trauma.[2] Moreover, more recent findings suggest that greater routine physical loading, as confirmed in this study, may actually have beneficial effects on spinal discs and chronic back pain.

D. C. Nieman, DrPH

References

1. Ala-Kokko L. Genetic risk factors for lumbar disc disease. *Ann Med.* 2002;34: 42-47.
2. Battié MC, Videman T, Kaprio J. The Twin Spine Study: contributions to a changing view of disc degeneration. *Spine J.* 2009;9:47-59.

Review: Exercise/physical therapy and vitamin D each reduce risk for falls in older community-dwelling adults
Kiel DP (Hebrew SeniorLife and Harvard Med School, Boston, MA)
Ann Intern Med 154:JC4-JC5, 2011

Questions.—Do primary care interventions reduce risk for falls in older adults living in the community? What are the adverse effects?

Review Scope.—Included studies compared fall-prevention interventions with a control group in community-dwelling, older adults (mean age ≥ 65 y); were conducted in primary care or similar settings; assessed falling or falls as primary or secondary outcomes; and were good or fair quality (US Preventive Services Task Force quality criteria). Outcomes were number of participants who fell and harms.

Review Methods.—MEDLINE, Cochrane Database of Systematic Reviews, Database of Abstracts of Reviews of Effects, Health Technology Assessments, and Web sites (1991 to Oct 2007) were searched for good-quality systematic reviews; 1 was selected. MEDLINE, CINAHL, Cochrane Central Register of Controlled Trials, and Cochrane Database of Systematic Reviews (2002 to Feb 2010) were searched for English-language, randomized, controlled trials (RCTs) published after the selected systematic review and reporting intervention efficacy. MEDLINE and CINAHL (1992 to Feb 2010) were searched for trials reporting harms. 54 RCTs ($n = 26\ 102$) met the selection criteria: 19 ($n = 7099$) assessed multifactorial assessment and management programs, 18 ($n = 3986$) assessed exercise or physical therapy, 9 ($n = 5809$) evaluated vitamin D (daily oral dose range, 10 IU to 1000 IU;

median, 800 IU), 4 ($n = 1437$) assessed vision correction procedures, 3 ($n = 2348$) assessed home-hazard modification, and 1 each assessed medication assessment and withdrawal ($n = 48$) or clinical education or behavioral counseling ($n = 310$).

Main Results.—The main results are shown in the Table. Vision correction procedures did not reduce falls (data not reported). Harms were not consistently reported.

Conclusion.—In older community-dwelling adults, exercise/physical therapy and vitamin D each reduce risk for falls; results for other primary care interventions are mixed.

▶ This meta-analysis highlights the efficacy of certain primary care interventions for senior community-dwelling persons who are at risk of falling. Among the various interventions, the authors reviewed multifactorial assessment and management strategies (including case management, management of identified fall-related risk factors), exercise and physical therapy, vitamin D supplementation, vision correction, medication assessment and withdrawal, home-hazard modification, clinical education, or behavioral counseling. Although their analysis provided evidence for the efficacy of physical therapy/activity and vitamin D supplementation, they also discuss the possible efficacy of comprehensive multifactorial assessment and management interventions in view of more recent research subsequent to their meta-analysis. The authors also documented adverse effects and found that there were no major clinical harms for these 2 effective interventions. They did, however, note a minor harm for vision correction (multifocal lens use), although vision correction was not one of the effective interventions for reducing risk of falls.

The evidence seems quite clear: there are interventions that can help reduce the risk of falling among the community-dwelling elderly. Wide-scale implementation of these programs now needs to be done.

D. E. Feldman, PT, PhD

Rib Stress Fractures Among Rowers: Definition, Epidemiology, Mechanisms, Risk Factors and Effectiveness of Injury Prevention Strategies
McDonnell LK, Hume PA, Nolte V (Auckland Univ of Technology, New Zealand; Univ of Western Ontario, London, Ontario, Canada)
Sports Med 41:883-901, 2011

Rib stress fractures (RSFs) can have serious effects on rowing training and performance and accordingly represent an important topic for sports medicine practitioners. Therefore, the aim of this review is to outline the definition, epidemiology, mechanisms, intrinsic and extrinsic risk factors, injury management and injury prevention strategies for RSF in rowers. To this end, nine relevant books, 140 journal articles, the proceedings of five conferences and two unpublished presentations were reviewed after searches of electronic databases using the keywords 'rowing', 'rib', 'stress fracture', 'injury', 'mechanics' and 'kinetics'. The review showed that RSF is an incomplete fracture occurring from an imbalance between the rate of bone resorption and the rate of bone formation. RSF occurs in 8.1−16.4% of elite rowers, 2% of university rowers and 1% of junior elite rowers. Approximately 86% of rowing RSF cases with known locations occur in ribs four to eight, mostly along the anterolateral/lateral rib cage. Elite rowers are more likely to experience RSF than nonelite rowers. Injury occurrence is equal among sweep rowers and scullers, but the regional location of the injury differs. The mechanism of injury is multifactorial with numerous intrinsic and extrinsic risk factors contributing. Posterior-directed resultant forces arising from the forward directed force vector through the arms to the oar handle in combination with the force vector induced by the scapula retractors during mid-drive, or repetitive stress from the external obliques and rectus abdominis in the 'finish' position, may be responsible for RSF. Joint hypomobility, vertebral malalignment or low bone mineral density may be associated with RSF. Case studies have shown increased risk associated with amenorrhoea, low bone density or poor technique, in combination with increases in training volume. Training volume alone may have less effect on injury than other factors. Large differences in seat and handle velocity, sequential movement patterns, higher elbow-flexion to knee-extension strength ratios, higher seat-to-handle velocity during the initial drive, or higher shoulder angle excursion may result in RSF. Gearing may indirectly affect rib loading. Increased risk may be due to low calcium, low vitamin D, eating disorders, low testosterone or use of depot medroxy-progesterone injections. Injury management involves 1−2 weeks cessation of rowing with analgesic modalities followed by a slow return to rowing with low-impact intensity and modified pain-free training. Some evidence shows injury prevention strategies should focus on strengthening the serratus anterior, strengthening leg extensors, stretching the lumbar spine, increasing hip joint flexibility, reducing excessive protraction, training with ergometers on slides or floating-head ergometers, and calcium and vitamin D supplementation. Future research should focus on the epidemiology of RSF over 4-year Olympic cycles in elite rowers, the aetiology of the condition, and the effectiveness of RSF prevention strategies for injury incidence and performance in rowing.

▶ Rib stress fractures in rowers are the most common cause of time loss from training and competition, not only at the elite level but also in university and junior elite rowers. The incidence in Masters' level rowers is not really well known, most likely because of the lack of reporting. However, I have either personally diagnosed or known at least 3 Masters' athletes (1 man and 2 women) in our local rowing club who have sustained rib stress fractures over the past 2 years! Increases in training load, larger blades that transmit greater forces through the arms to the thorax, and other intrinsic and extrinsic risk factors have been explored but not in a systematic fashion. This review summarizes the current knowledge gleaned from a thorough literature search, including 9 relevant books, 140 journal articles, proceedings from 5 conferences, and 2 unpublished presentations. It elaborates on the regional location and multifactorial mechanisms of injury.

Training volume may have less effect than previously thought, while rowing technique and rigging, equipment, and underlying medical risk factors (such as low calcium level, low vitamin D level, eating disorders/low energy availability and/or menstrual dysfunction, low testosterone level, or use of depot medroxyprogesterone injections) are now being implicated in the etiology of this condition. There has been a fair amount of recent scientific investigation into biomechanics, anatomical factors, muscle strength, endurance and activation patterns, areas of maximal rib cage compression, and timing during the rowing stroke. Determination of the major causative contributions from the lists above can help lead treatment programs and preventative strategies.

C. Lebrun, MDCM, MPE, CCFP, Dip Sport Med, FACSM

Risk of injury associated with bodychecking experience among youth hockey players
Emery C, Kang J, Shrier I, et al (Univ of Calgary, Alberta, Canada; McGill Univ, Montréal, Quebec, Canada; et al)
CMAJ 183:1249-1256, 2011

Background.—In a previous prospective study, the risk of concussion and all injury was more than threefold higher among Pee Wee ice hockey players (ages 11—12 years) in a league that allows bodychecking than among those in a league that does not. We examined whether two years of bodychecking experience in Pee Wee influenced the risk of concussion and other injury among players in a Bantam league (ages 13—14) compared with Bantam players introduced to bodychecking for the first time at age 13.

Methods.—We conducted a prospective cohort study in volving hockey players aged 13—14 years in the top 30% of divisions of play in their leagues. Sixty-eight teams from the province of Alberta ($n = 995$), whose players had two years of bodychecking experience in Pee Wee, and 62 teams from the province of Quebec ($n = 976$), whose players had no bodychecking experience in Pee Wee, participated. We estimated incidence rate ratios (IRRs) for injury and for concussion.

Results.—There were 272 injuries (51 concussions) among the Bantam hockey players who had bodychecking experience in Pee Wee and 244 injuries (49 concussions) among those without such experience. The adjusted IRRs for game-related injuries and concussion overall between players with bodychecking experience in Pee Wee and those without it were as follows: injury overall 0.85 (95% confidence interval [CI] 0.63 to 1.16); concussion overall 0.84 (95% CI 0.48 to 1.48); and injury resulting in more than seven days of time loss (i.e., time between injury and return to play) 0.67 (95% CI 0.46 to 0.99). The unadjusted IRR for concussion resulting in more than 10 days of time loss was 0.60 (95% CI 0.26 to 1.41).

Interpretation.—The risk of injury resulting in more than seven days of time loss from play was reduced by 33% among Bantam hockey players in a league where bodychecking was allowed two years earlier in Pee Wee compared with Bantam players introduced to bodychecking for the first time at age 13. In light of the increased risk of concussion and other injury among Pee Wee players in a league where bodychecking is permitted, policy regarding the age at which hockey players are introduced to bodychecking requires further consideration.

▶ Canadians are very passionate about their hockey. For as long as I can remember, Canadians (myself included) have been debating the merits of bodychecking in youth hockey and the age at which it should be introduced into the game. Different provinces, such as Alberta and Quebec, introduce bodychecking at different ages. This allowed Emery and colleagues to examine whether 13- to 14-year-old hockey players (Bantam level) who were introduced to bodychecking at age 11 (Pee Wee level) were able to better cope with bodychecking than 13- to 14-year-olds who were just being introduced to bodychecking. The premise is that allowing youth to learn how to give and take a bodycheck at younger ages, when they are lighter and play the game at a slower speed, may allow them to adapt to the physicality of bodychecking at a more appropriate developmental stage. The main findings and conclusion of this report is that the risk of different types and severities of injury were reduced by 15%–40% among 13- to 14-year-old hockey players who were introduced to bodychecking at age 11 compared with 13- to 14-year-old hockey players who were introduced to bodychecking for the first time at age 13. This finding will provide more evidence that can be used by those in favor of introducing bodychecking to the game at younger ages and will undoubtedly lead to more debate and discussion on bodychecking within the hockey community.

I. Janssen, PhD

Risk of injury associated with bodychecking experience among youth hockey players
Emery C, Kang J, Shrier I, et al (Univ of Calgary, Alberta, Canada; McGill Univ, Montréal, Quebec, Canada)
CMAJ 183:1249-1256, 2011

Background.—In a previous prospective study, the risk of concussion and all injury was more than threefold higher among Pee Wee ice hockey players (ages 11–12 years) in a league that allows bodychecking than among those in a league that does not. We examined whether two years of bodychecking experience in Pee Wee influenced the risk of concussion and other injury among players in a Bantam league (ages 13–14) compared with Bantam players introduced to bodychecking for the first time at age 13.

Methods.—We conducted a prospective cohort study involving hockey players aged 13–14 years in the top 30% of divisions of play in their leagues. Sixty-eight teams from the province of Alberta ($n = 995$), whose players had two years of bodychecking experience in Pee Wee, and 62 teams from the province of Quebec ($n = 976$), whose players had no bodychecking experience in Pee Wee, participated. We estimated incidence rate ratios (IRRs) for injury and for concussion.

Results.—There were 272 injuries (51 concussions) among the Bantam hockey players who had bodychecking experience in Pee Wee and 244 injuries (49 concussions) among those without such experience. The adjusted IRRs for game-related injuries and concussion overall between players with bodychecking experience in Pee Wee and those without it were as follows: injury overall 0.85 (95% confidence interval [CI] 0.63 to 1.16); concussion overall 0.84 (95% CI 0.48 to 1.48); and injury resulting in more than seven days of time loss (i.e., time between injury and return to play) 0.67 (95% CI 0.46 to 0.99). The unadjusted IRR for concussion resulting in more than 10 days of time loss was 0.60 (95% CI 0.26 to 1.41).

Interpretation.—The risk of injury resulting in more than seven days of time loss from play was reduced by 33% among Bantam hockey players in a league where bodychecking was allowed two years earlier in Pee Wee compared with Bantam players introduced to bodychecking for the first time at age 13. In light of the increased risk of concussion and other injury among Pee Wee players in a league where bodychecking is permitted, policy regarding the age at which hockey players are introduced to bodychecking requires further consideration.

▶ This study builds on the already impressive body of work by this group of investigators, looking at risks of concussion and other injuries in youth hockey players. Similar to their previous publications, there is strong attention to detail in the conception and design of the research, meticulous documentation of player hours and athletic exposure, and sophisticated statistical interpretation of the results. The comparison groups included 68 teams in Alberta, who already had 2 years of bodychecking experience at the Pee Wee level (ages, 11-12 years), with 62 teams in Quebec, in a league that does not allow bodychecking until Bantam level of play (ages, 13-14 years). The conundrum now is that despite the fact their previous prospective study in these populations documented a risk of concussion and all injury more than 3-fold higher among Pee Wee players in a league that allows bodychecking in the younger age category,[1] it appears as if the 2 more years of experience in bodychecking that is gained by these youth hockey players (as opposed to the Quebec teams, in which bodychecking is not allowed until the Bantam level) do seem to have a protective effect, in terms of reducing by 33% the number of injuries resulting in more than 7 days of time loss. Advocates for allowing early bodychecking experience in these young hockey players will no doubt liberally quote the results of this study, while the more conservative proponents of waiting until Bantam level to introduce bodychecking will continue to promote the findings of the previous study. However, as pointed out by the authors themselves, further research and consideration of policy is warranted.

C. Lebrun, MDCM, MPE, CCFP, Dip Sport Med, FACSM

Reference

1. Emery CA, Kang J, Shrier I, et al. Risk of injury associated with body checking among youth ice hockey players. *JAMA.* 2010;303:2265-2272.

The Chronic Effects of Concussion on Gait

Martini DN, Sabin MJ, Depesa SA, et al (Univ of Illinois at Urbana-Champaign)
Arch Phys Med Rehabil 92:585-589, 2011

Objective.—To examine the effects of concussion on gait patterns of young adults with and without a history of concussion during single- and dual-task paradigms.

Design.—Cross-sectional evaluation.

Setting.—A research laboratory.

Participants.—Persons with (n = 28; mean, 6.32y postinjury) and without (n = 40) a concussion history.

Intervention.—Not applicable.

Main Outcome Measures.—A battery of gait analyses during single- and dual-task conditions. Normalized velocity, step length, stride width, number correct from cognitive task, time in single-leg stance, and time in double-leg stance were the variables of interest. Gait was analyzed using an electronic walkway system, and the Brooks visuospatial cognitive task was used to index cognition.

Results.—Data analyses using multiple 2-way repeated-measures analyses of variance and correlations indicated that participants with a history of concussion spent significantly more time in a double-leg stance and significantly decreased time in a single-leg stance and had slower gait velocity. There also was a significant negative correlation between number of concussions and time in single-leg stance and positive correlations between number of concussions and time in double-leg stance and double-stance percent.

Conclusion.—These findings suggest that persons with a history of concussion adopt a more conservative gait strategy.

▶ Headache is the most common postconcussion symptom, and the next 2 most common are arguably dizziness and instability, both reflective of motor control of balance issues. The usefulness of a detailed balance assessment has long been known to be crucial in making the diagnosis of an acute concussion, but it has generally been thought that these symptoms are only sensitive in the first several days after sustaining a concussion.

Literature has been accumulating, however, on individuals with balance deficits that have lasted a protracted period of time after a concussion, and I can attest that many of my postconcussion syndrome patients still have balance issues.

Other researchers have reported that previously concussed patients may have alterations in gait such that when carrying out cognitive tasks, there is a slower walking velocity in the concussed group, and the strides, in addition to being slower, are shorter in length.

These researchers found in their cohort of 28 concussed individuals and 40 without a concussion that those who had sustained a concussion showed a slower walking velocity and greater time spent in double-leg stance support and less time spent in single-leg stance support throughout the gait cycle.

This suggested a more conservative gait pattern in the group that had sustained a concussion.

This is an interesting study and certainly one that, it is hoped, will be replicated by other observers.

One weakness of the study is that the severity of the concussion was not scored, and it would be of interest to this researcher if the severity of the gait abnormalities could be correlated with the severity of the concussion as defined by the length of concussion symptoms. It could be theorized that the group of individuals with the more severe concussions defined as symptoms that lasted the longest period of time such as weeks or months may well have more profound gait abnormalities than those who had symptoms that lasted a shorter period of time. Also by doing this assessment one could better determine whether a few individuals skewed the concussion group to be significantly different from the control group or whether the concussion group consistently tested differently from the control group.

R. C. Cantu, MD, MA

A prospective study of concussions among National Hockey League players during regular season games: the NHL-NHLPA Concussion Program
Benson BW, Meeuwisse WH, Rizos J, et al (Univ of Calgary, Alberta, Canada; Univ of Toronto, Ontario, Canada; et al)
CMAJ 183:905-911, 2011

Background.—In 1997, the National Hockey League (NHL) and NHL Players' Association (NHLPA) launched a concussion program to improve the understanding of this injury. We explored initial postconcussion signs, symptoms, physical examination findings and time loss (i.e., time between the injury and medical clearance by the physician to return to competitive play), experienced by male professional ice-hockey players, and assessed the utility of initial postconcussion clinical manifestations in predicting time loss among hockey players.

Methods.—We conducted a prospective case series of concussions over seven NHL regular seasons (1997–2004) using an inclusive cohort of players. The primary outcome was concussion and the secondary outcome was time loss. NHL team physicians documented postconcussion clinical manifestations and recorded the date when a player was medically cleared to return to play.

Results.—Team physicians reported 559 concussions during regular season games. The estimated incidence was 1.8 concussions per 1000 player-hours. The most common postconcussion symptom was headache (71%). On average, time loss (in days) increased 2.25 times (95% confidence interval [CI] 1.41–3.62) for every subsequent (i.e., recurrent) concussion sustained during the study period. Controlling for age and position, significant predictors of time loss were postconcussion headache $(p < 0.001)$, low energy or fatigue $(p = 0.01)$, amnesia $(p = 0.02)$ and abnormal neurologic examination $(p = 0.01)$. Using a previously suggested time loss cut-point of 10 days, headache (odds ratio [OR] 2.17, 95% CI 1.33−3.54) and low energy or fatigue (OR 1.72, 95% CI 1.04−2.85) were significant predictors of time loss of more than 10 days.

Interpretation.—Postconcussion headache, low energy or fatigue, amnesia and abnormal neurologic examination were significant predictors of time loss among professional hockey players.

▶ Concussion, particularly in the sport of hockey, is a hot topic these days. Continued focus on the progress (or lack thereof) of professional players such as Sidney Crosby has driven home the message that the art and science of managing sport-related concussion is still evolving. This study prospectively followed and analyzed the concussions sustained by players in the National Hockey League (NHL) over 7 consecutive regular seasons. Strengths of the study include accurate player and game data and utilization of a standardized definition of concussion, albeit the official definition was altered slightly midway through this period, because of the changes suggested by the International Consensus Group on Concussion in the Vienna Concussion in Sport Agreement Statement.[1] A common injury reporting form was used, and evaluations were done by trained NHL physicians. This prospective case series provides useful information on the yearly and position-specific incidence and outcomes (including time loss) of the 559 physician-diagnosed, regular-season, in-game concussions. (Concussions sustained during practice, exhibition, and play-off games were not included.) Most importantly, this is one of the first studies to be able to relate the frequency of initial post concussion clinical manifestations to the time loss experienced by male professional ice hockey players. Using modeling techniques for multiple regressions, 4 initial postconcussion clinical manifestations (headache, low energy or fatigue, amnesia, and abnormal neurologic examination) were found to be significant predictors of time loss in this cohort of male professional ice hockey players. On average, time loss increased 2.25% (95% confidence interval, 1.41-3.62) for every subsequent (ie, recurrent) concussion sustained during the study period. It is unknown whether similar results would be observed for children or women or athletes in other sports and levels of play. Another limitation of this investigation is that the NHL Players' Association Concussion Program evolved over the 7-year period of the study, perhaps skewing the management toward more conservative management of these injuries over this time frame (Fig 1 in the original article). It would also have been interesting if the authors had included data on any concurrent neuropsychological testing. Nevertheless, the results are helpful for the practicing clinician, in terms of suggesting the type of immediate postconcussion symptoms that presage a longer recovery period before return to play.

C. Lebrun, MDCM, MPE, CCFP, Dip Sport Med, FACSM

Reference

1. Aubry M, Cantu R, Dvorak J, et al. Summary and agreement statement of the 1st International Symposium on Concussion in Sport, Vienna 2001. *Clin J Sport Med.* 2002;12:6-11.

Diagnosing Mild Traumatic Brain Injury: Where Are We Now?

Dutton RP, Prior K, Cohen R, et al (Univ of Maryland School of Medicine, Baltimore)
J Trauma 70:554-559, 2011

Background.—The brain acoustic monitor (BAM), an indicator of cerebral autoregulation, has previously shown high sensitivity but low specificity for computed tomographic (CT) abnormality in patients following the clinical diagnosis of traumatic brain injury. We assessed the utility of the BAM in diagnosing mild TBI (mTBI) in patients with and without normal findings of CT scan, a population for which there are a few objective markers of disease.

Methods.—We prospectively studied 369 patients with mechanism of injury consistent with TBI. The diagnosis was evaluated by five methods: (a) study enrollment (i.e., mechanism of injury), (b) signs of head trauma, (c) expert physician assessment, (d) presence of initial symptoms (loss of consciousness [LOC]; amnesia), and (e) BAM. All patients had a head CT scan. We compared the BAM screen results with the diagnosis of mTBI and BAM data from 50 normal volunteers and 49 trauma control patients not thought to have TBI.

Results.—None of the diagnostic methods correlated well with the others. Correlation between the methods ranged from 21% to 71%. BAM discriminated between patients with mTBI versus without TBI ($p < 0.01$) and patients with mTBI versus normal subjects ($p < 0.001$). There were 14 patients with new abnormal findings of CT scans. A history of LOC and physical signs of head injury were associated with a new abnormality on head CT ($p < 0.05$ and $p < 0.01$, respectively), whereas an abnormal BAM signal was suggestive ($p = 0.08$). The sensitivity of BAM abnormality for head CT abnormality was 100%, with a specificity of 30.14%.

Conclusion.—There is no gold standard for the diagnosis of mTBI. BAM screening is a useful diagnostic adjunct in patients with mTBI and may facilitate decision making. An abnormal BAM reading adds significance to LOC as a predictor of a new abnormality on head CT. In our study, opting not to CT scan patients with a normal BAM signal would have missed no new CT findings and no patients who required medical intervention for TBI, at a cost savings of $202,950.

▶ The brain acoustic monitor (BAM) is a noninvasive device that assesses global cerebral perfusion and is sensitive to abnormalities in traumatic brain injury that will show abnormalities on a CT scan, such as a subdural hematoma or hemorrhagic contusion. This device has not been found to be highly sensitive in diagnosing concussion where the CT scan is normal. This study essentially supports those facts. What is intriguing to me, however, is that increasingly, especially in pediatrics, we are becoming concerned about the amount of radiation a child receives from a head CT scan. A head CT is roughly equivalent to 100 chest x-rays, not only in assessing head injuries but even acute abdomens suspected of having appendicitis. We are getting away from using the CT scan because of concern for the amount of radiation a child receives. Although this article clearly makes the point that use of the BAM, just like any other stand-alone test, has low sensitivity in diagnosing mild traumatic brain injury, it is highly sensitive in predicting abnormalities that would show up on a head CT. Therefore, the authors make the point that the use of the BAM could eliminate many head CTs performed for mild traumatic brain injuries, affording not only a significant cost savings but avoidance of a substantial radiation dose.

R. C. Cantu, MD, MA

The National Football League and Concussion: Leading a Culture Change in Contact Sports
Ellenbogen RG, Berger MS, Batjer HH (Univ of Washington, Seattle; Univ of California, San Francisco; Northwestern Univ Med Ctr, Chicago, IL)
World Neurosurg 74:560-565, 2010

Background.—The National Football League (NFL) has responded to concern over traumatic brain injury (TBI) or concussion injuries in professional sports with a plan to make games safer. Included in the plan are rule changes on and off the field and the appointment of a scientific advisory committee to study the neurologic issues associated with concussions in NFL athletes. The Centers for Disease Control and Prevention (CDC) is also seeking to educate involved persons on how to reduce risks of TBI in sports at all levels and in both genders. The NFL Head, Neck and Spine (HNS) Committee comprises members of the National Institutes of Health, CDC, Department of Defense, NFL team physicians, retired NFL athletes, professional athletic trainers, and clinicians and scientists, as well as members of the NFL Players Association. The goal is to make the NFL as safe as possible for all active athletes and study the neurologic issues that affect former athletes. There will be a substantial trickle-down effect to all sports and athletes of all ages and both genders as well as military applications. The NFL seeks to lead the way in TBI/concussion research, education, and advocacy.

NFL TBI/Concussion Approaches.—Subcommittees of the HNS Committee report on the development and management of a prospective database of NFL players, safety equipment, former players' experiences with brain and spinal injury issues, brain and spine research, advocacy and education, and return-to-play issues. Of particular interest are questions related to the long-term effects of concussions, such as whether brain structure and function decrease faster in former NFL players compared to the general population, whether dementia and mild cognitive impairment are more common in former players than nonathletes, and if brain structure, function, and biomarkers are related to the length and severity of a concussive history. Multidisciplinary assessments are conducted at baseline and over several years of study and include neurologic examinations, extensive histories, and measures of daily function, neuropsychological assessments, sleep and mood inventories, brain imaging, and blood markers. Scientists will also seek to model and measure the forces that impact headgear and transfer energy through the skull and into the brain after collisions. Engineers can use the data to assess and improve helmet design, perhaps using newer materials that better absorb and dissipate the energy, reducing risks for athletes and soldiers. Examinations of the brains of professional athletes show neuronal loss and atrophy and tauopathy with intraneural and extracellular neurofibrillary tangles in persons with traumatic-related dementia. In addition, NFL rules about hits that could produce concussion now extend to all players, rather than just receivers. A second opinion by an outside independent neurologic consultant is also required before an athlete with concussion can return to participation. As a result of the NFL efforts, players more willingly report concussions to team medical staff than previously.

Youth Sports.—The "Zachary Lystedt" law sets uniform guidelines for concussion management designed to protect youth athletes and includes education regarding informed consent, immediate removal of athletes who have concussion or might have one from competition and practice, and the requirement for clearance by a licensed health care professional trained in concussions before the athlete can return to participation. The HSN Committee has also prepared informational materials that emphasize the importance of recognizing concussion and seeking treatment and/or rest until full recovery, which have been adapted by the CDC for youth athletes.

Conclusions.—The HNS Committee of the NFL has brought together persons from sports, medicine, and science who are interested in TBI research, treatment, and prevention. It is the NFL's mission to make all sports safer at all levels of play for both genders while preserving the positive attributes of organized team athletics. A significant educational and cultural transformation among the athletes themselves and among spectators will be critical to a successful outcome.

▶ Since 2010, no professional sports organization has better promoted concussion awareness, changed rules to make their sport safer, and thrown their considerable political and public clout behind state legislation enacting concussion laws along the Lystedt Law format than the National Football League.

At the time of dictating this comment, 30 states have enacted laws incorporating the basic concepts of concussion education for players, their parents, and coaches, such as any player suspected of or diagnosed with a concussion being removed from practice or game play, and only an authorized medical professional being allowed to return a suspected concussion athlete to play after sustaining a suspected concussion.

In their article, the cochairs of the newly constituted National Football League's Head, Neck and Spine committee, Dr. Richard Ellenbogen and Dr. Hunt Batjer, along with committee member, Dr. Mitchel Berger, all chairmen of departments of Neurosurgery at the University of Seattle, Northwestern University Medical Center, and the University of California at San Francisco, respectively, chronicle the National Football League's role in leading the culture change with regard to concussion.

I highly recommend this article for all interested in this subject.

R. C. Cantu, MD, MA

Do Somatic and Cognitive Symptoms of Traumatic Brain Injury Confound Depression Screening?
Cook KF, Bombardier CH, Bamer AM, et al (Univ of Washington School of Medicine, Seattle; et al)
Arch Phys Med Rehabil 92:818-823, 2011

Objective.—To evaluate whether items of the Patient Health Questionnaire 9 (PHQ-9) function differently in persons with traumatic brain injury (TBI) than in persons from a primary care sample.

Design.—This study was a retrospective analysis of responses to the PHQ-9 collected in 2 previous studies. Responses to the PHQ-9 were modeled using item response theory, and the presence of DIF was evaluated using ordinal logistic regression.

Setting.—Eight primary care sites and a single trauma center in Washington state.

Participants.—Participants (N = 3365) were persons from 8 primary care sites (n = 3000) and a consecutive sample of persons with complicated mild to severe TBI from a trauma center who were 1 year postinjury (n = 365).

Interventions.—Not applicable.

Main Outcome Measure.—PHQ-9.

Results.—No PHQ-9 item demonstrated statistically significant or meaningful DIF attributable to TBI. A sensitivity analysis failed to show that the cumulative effects of nonsignificant DIF resulted in a systematic inflation of PHQ-9 total scores. Therefore, the results also do not support the hypothesis that cumulative DIF for PHQ-9 items spuriously inflates the numbers of persons with TBI screened as potentially having major depressive disorder.

Conclusions.—The PHQ-9 is a valid screener of major depressive disorder in people with complicated mild to severe TBI, and all symptoms can be counted toward the diagnosis of major depressive disorder without special concern about overdiagnosis or unnecessary treatment.

▶ This provocative article strongly supports using all symptoms in assessing for major depressive disorder, despite the fact that some symptoms, such as in the case of post—head injury patients, are cognitive and somatic symptoms of the head injury, such as reduced energy, impaired concentration, and poor sleep. These authors found that in comparing a primary care group of patients to a group after moderately severe brain injury, the Patient Health Questionnaire-9 is a reliable and valid screener of major depressive disorder in the traumatic brain injury group 1 year after injury and that all symptoms should be counted toward the diagnosis of major depressive disorder without concern about overdiagnosis. They strongly stress the many studies that show that major depressive disorders are frequently missed in the traumatic brain injury group, with less than half being diagnosed and treated in the first year after brain injury, and that awareness of this stresses the need for enhanced diagnosis and treatment of major depressive disorder after a traumatic brain injury. To that end, the authors strongly make the case for the Patient Health Questionnaire-9 as a valid screener of major depressive disorder in the traumatic brain-injured population.

R. C. Cantu, MD, MA

Concussive symptoms in emergency department patients diagnosed with minor head injury
Cunningham J, Brison RJ, Pickett W (Queen's Univ, Kingston, Ontario, Canada)
J Emerg Med 40:262-266, 2011

Background.—Evidence-based protocols exist for Emergency Department (ED) patients diagnosed with minor head injury. These protocols focus on the need for acute intervention or in-hospital management. The frequency and nature of concussive symptoms experienced by patients discharged from the ED are not well understood.

Objectives.—To examine the prevalence and nature of concussive symptoms, up to 1 month postpresentation, among ED patients diagnosed with minor head injury.

Methods.—Eligible and consenting patients presenting to Kingston EDs with minor head injury (n = 94) were recruited for study. The Rivermead Post-Concussion Symptoms Questionnaire was administered at baseline and at 1 month post-injury to assess concussive symptoms. This analysis focused upon acute and ongoing symptoms.

Results.—Proportions of patients reporting concussive symptoms were 68/94 (72%) at baseline and 59/94 (63%) at follow-up. Seventeen percent of patients (18/102) were investigated with computed tomography scanning during their ED encounter. The prevalence of somatic symptoms declined between baseline and follow-up, whereas some cognitive and emotional symptoms persisted.

Conclusion.—The majority of patients who present to the ED with minor head injuries suffer from concussive symptoms that do not resolve quickly. This information should be incorporated into discharge planning for these patients.

▶ Most individuals diagnosed with minor concussion, perhaps as many as 80%, have been shown to have symptoms clear within 7 to 10 days. This was not the experience of these researchers in their study of individuals who came to an emergency department in Kingston, Ontario, Canada and were followed for concussion symptoms up to 1 month after presentation. Although the somatic symptoms in this group declined significantly from baseline to follow-up at 1 month, the majority of the patients (63%) still had cognitive and/or emotional symptoms at the 1-month follow-up. This certainly gives pause for reflection, but the reasons the majority of these individuals were still symptomatic at 1 month may be reflective of the severity of "mild traumatic brain injury" that provoked these patients going to the emergency department in the first place. It is also true that the number of patients (94) was modest. Other factors include that patients were interviewed from up to 1 week postinjury, and this could lead to some inaccuracy in symptom reporting. Furthermore, the fact that patients were involved in a study could lead to overreporting of symptoms. Nonetheless, as patients with postconcussion syndrome now make up more than half my practice, I believe it is important to understand and look for persistent symptoms in individuals who have been diagnosed with minor traumatic brain injury.

R. C. Cantu, MD, MA

Sport-Related Concussions: Knowledge Translation Among Minor Hockey Coaches
Mrazik M, Bawani F, Krol AL (Univ of Alberta, Edmonton, Canada)
Clin J Sport Med 21:315-319, 2011

Objective.—The objective of this study was to investigate minor hockey coaches' knowledge base of sport-related concussions.

Design.—Cross-sectional survey.

Setting.—Subjects independently completed the written survey at preseason organizational meetings.

Participants.—One hundred seventy-eight active coaches spanning 5 age levels (ages 5-15 years). Coaches reported 2.62 ± 3.73 years of coaching experience.

Main Outcome Measures.—Resources where coaches obtained information about concussions, perceptions of variables associated with concussions, knowledge level of issues associated with concussions, and decision-making practices.

Results.—Newspapers and magazines were the most frequent source of information regarding concussions, yet were rated as not very helpful. Family physicians were less frequently sought but were rated as most helpful. A majority of coaches reported limited knowledge about concussions but rated this knowledge as being important. There was a significant relationship between head coaching experience and concussion knowledge [$R^2 = 0.09$, $F_{3,156} = 4.41$, $P = 0.005$]. Most coaches demonstrated a good knowledge base of common issues associated with concussions, and a majority of individuals correctly identified return-to-play practices.

Conclusions.—A majority of minor hockey coaches correctly recognized and understood issues related to sport-related concussions. Results suggested that knowledge translation through various formal and informal sources has had a positive effect. However, a majority of coaches reported having limited knowledge about concussions yet consider it an important topic.

▶ Behavior change is one of the next frontiers of evidence-based guidelines about specific conditions, such as sport-related concussion. At the professional, elite, and college levels, athletes have access to numerous resources, including trained physicians, to help manage their injuries. However, at the lower levels of recreational sport, the coach becomes paramount in terms of diagnosis and management. To make informed decisions in keeping with the existing guidelines, such individuals first need to receive the educational material in some way. This particular study is interesting because it assessed both the knowledge base of sport-related concussion as well as their methods of obtaining it. From here, it was possible to see how this has translated into return-to-play practices. It appears as if there are improvements in all these measures compared with similar surveys among coaches published several years ago.[1] The sources of information for coaches is very interesting, with the Internet and other print media (magazine/newspaper) being prominent. The role of the family physician as a resource for coaches working with youth sports was also evident, further reinforcing the fact that knowledge translation efforts need to be aimed at this population as well. Further investigations into the optimal forums and methods of education about concussion and management must be aimed at all the groups that may be involved with the athletes, including not only coaches but also parents, referees, therapists, and physicians.

C. Lebrun, MDCM, MPE, CCFP, Dip Sport Med, FACSM

Reference

1. Valovich McLeod TC, Schwartz C, Bay RC. Sport-related concussion misunderstandings among youth coaches. *Clin J Sport Med*. 2007;17:140-142.

Evidence-based Community Consultation for Traumatic Brain Injury
Lynch CA, Houry DE, Dai D, et al (Emory Univ School of Medicine, Atlanta, GA; Georgia State Univ, Atlanta)
Acad Emerg Med 18:972-976, 2011

Objectives.—The objective was to determine if geospatial techniques can be used to inform targeted community consultation (CC) and public disclosure (PD) for a clinical trial requiring emergency exception from informed consent (EFIC).

Methods.—Data from January 2007 to December 2009 were extracted from a Level I trauma center's trauma database using the National Trauma Registry of the American College of Surgeon (NTRACS). Injury details, demographics, geographic codes, and clinical data necessary to match core elements of the clinical trial inclusion criteria (Glasgow Coma Scale [GCS] 3–12 and blunt head injury) were collected on all patients. Patients' home zip codes were geocoded to compare with population density and clustering analysis.

Results.—Over a 2-year period, 179 patients presented with moderate to severe traumatic brain injury (TBI). Mapping the rate and frequency of TBI patients presenting to the trauma center delineated at-risk populations for moderate to severe head injury. Four zip codes had higher incidences of TBI than the rest, with one zip code having a very high rate of 80 per 100,000 population.

Conclusions.—Geospatial techniques and hospital data records can be used to characterize potential subjects and delineate a high-risk population to inform directed CC and public disclosure strategies.

▶ The current multicenter, randomized, double-blind, placebo-control, clinical trial of progesterone for the treatment of traumatic brain injury that the US Food and Drug Administration has given clearance to carry out is an example of a study made possible by the emergency exception from Informed Consent Act of 1996. In this somewhat smallish study of moderate and severe brain injury involving 179 patients extracted from a level-1 trauma center's experience in the state of Georgia, similar inclusion and exclusion criteria were used to determine if using geographic information systems and hospital data could better define the community of interest for focused community consultation and public disclosure information. The preliminary information from this somewhat limited study clearly pointed out that geographic information systems could be used to pinpoint geographic areas at highest risk of moderate and severe traumatic brain injury and therefore target where community consultation and public disclosure information could best be used. The authors point out that the next logical study is to carry out such a use of community consultation and public disclosure to the "hot spots" and see what the effectiveness is in reducing moderate and severe traumatic brain injury.

R. C. Cantu, MD, MA

Can a clinical test of reaction time predict a functional head-protective response?
Eckner JT, Lipps DB, Kim H, et al (Univ of Michigan, Ann Arbor)
Med Sci Sports Exerc 43:382-387, 2011

Purpose.—Reaction time is commonly prolonged after a sport-related concussion. Besides being a marker for injury, a rapid reaction time is necessary for protective maneuvers that can reduce the frequency and severity of additional head impacts. The purpose of this study was to determine whether a clinical test of simple visuomotor reaction time predicted the time taken to raise the hands to protect the head from a rapidly approaching ball.

Methods.—Twenty-six healthy adult participants recruited from campus and community recreation and exercise facilities completed two experimental protocols during a single session: a manual visuomotor simple reaction time test (RT(clin)) and a sport-related head-protective response (RT(sprt)). RT(clin) measured the time required to catch a thin vertically oriented device on its release by the tester and was calculated from the distance the device fell before being arrested. RT(sprt) measured the time required to raise the hands from waist level to block a foam tennis ball fired toward the subject's face from an air cannon and was determined using an optoelectronic camera system. A correlation coefficient was calculated between RT(clin) and RT(sprt), with linear regression used to assess for effect modification by other covariates.

Results.—A strong positive correlation was found between RT(clin) and RT(sprt) (r = 0.725, P < 0.001) independent of age, gender, height, or weight.

Conclusions.—RT(clin) is predictive of a functional sport-related head-protective response. To our knowledge, this is the first demonstration of a clinical test predicting the ability to protect the head in a simulated sport environment. This correlation with a functional head-protective response is a relevant consideration for the potential use of RT(clin) as part of a multifaceted concussion assessment program.

▶ It has long been known that reaction times are often slowed after a concussion and are predictive of a concussion that has not completely recovered. Indeed, this fact has often been cited as one of the major advantages of computer-based neuropsychological tests over paper-and-pencil tests because the computer-based tests allow for and often include reaction times as part of the score of the test battery. Such reaction times can be measured in a variety of ways, one of the simplest being to hold a yardstick level with one's open hand and then, upon releasing the yardstick, seeing how many inches go by before the individual can squeeze the yardstick to a stop. Although it would seem to be intuitive and also has been cited that slowed reaction time could certainly place the athlete at risk of injury, especially in sports involving high speeds such as automobile racing, this study to my knowledge is the first that actually demonstrates in a prospective way how reaction time is indeed highly correlated to a functional head protective response. This study makes the case that reaction times should be a part of the concussion battery tests that are used to assess an athlete before coming to the conclusion that the athlete is ready to return to competition. Thus, this is yet one more tool that medical personnel making concussion return-to-play decisions should use.

R. C. Cantu, MD, MA

Impact of Pharmacological Treatments on Cognitive and Behavioral Outcome in the Postacute Stages of Adult Traumatic Brain Injury: A Meta-Analysis
Wheaton P, Mathias JL, Vink R (Univ of Adelaide, South Australia, Australia)
J Clin Psychopharmacol 31:745-757, 2011

Pharmacological treatments that are administered to adults in the postacute stage after a traumatic brain injury (TBI) (≥4 weeks after injury) have the potential to reduce persistent cognitive and behavioral problems. While a variety of treatments have been examined, the findings have yet to be consolidated, hampering advances in the treatment of TBI. A meta-analysis of research that has investigated the cognitive and behavioral effects of pharmacological treatments administered in the later stage after TBI was therefore conducted. The PubMed and PsycINFO databases were searched, and Cohen *d* effect sizes, percent overlap, and failsafe N statistics were calculated for each treatment. Both randomized controlled trials and open-label studies (prospective and retrospective) were included. Nineteen treatments were investigated by 30 independent studies, comprising 395 participants with TBI in the treatment groups and 137 control subjects. When treated in the postacute period, 1 dopaminergic agent (methylphenidate) improved behavior (anger/aggression, psychosocial function) and 1 cholinergic agent (donepezil) improved cognition (memory, attention). In addition, when the injury-to-treatment interval was broadened to include studies that administered treatment just before the postacute period, 2 dopaminergic agents (methylphenidate, amantadine) showed clinically useful treatment benefits for behavior, whereas 1 serotonergic agent (sertraline) markedly impaired cognition and psychomotor speed.

▶ Apparently, posttraumatic syndrome and even acute concussions have not been shown to be positively affected by pharmacologic interventions. The symptoms of postconcussion syndrome, however, have been treated successfully pharmacologically. The literature in this area, however, is confusing and often conflicting. These authors performed a meta-analysis of 30 independent studies comprising 395 participants with traumatic brain injury in the treatment group and 137 controls. They try to make sense for us out of what is very conflicting literature. Their findings are that treatment for postconcussion syndrome is positively affected for the symptoms of anger/aggression, psychosocial function, and memory cognition by the dopamine agents in the methylphenidate group, Ritalin. For treatment of memory and attention, the cholinergic agent, donepezil, was found to be useful. Serotonergic agents, while improving depression symptoms, exacerbated other postconcussion symptoms and reduced psychomotor speed, and therefore, overall, was detrimental. In addition, methylphenidate was found to be useful for depression and amantadine for global outcome. This article suffered these limitations: there was a range of traumatic brain injuries far exceeding concussion; many of the studies involved in the meta-analysis did not report all the necessary data; there was considerable variability between the studies with respect to the time after the injury and the treatment intervention; and the studies did not consistently report adverse events. This is nonetheless a very useful document for all of us treating postconcussion syndrome and possible early chronic traumatic encephalopathy patients.

This reviewer, who has more than half his clinical practice with concussion patients in the postconcussion syndrome, contrary to the findings of the meta-analysis, has found cognitive symptoms to be improved more consistently with methylphenidate medications than with donepezil.

R. C. Cantu, MD, MA

Boxing Injuries Presenting to U.S. Emergency Departments, 1990-2008
Potter MR, Snyder AJ, Smith GA (The Res Inst at Nationwide Children's Hosp, Columbus, OH)
Am J Prev Med 40:462-467, 2011

Background.—Boxing injuries can have serious consequences.

Purpose.—To examine the epidemiology of boxing injuries in the U.S. with attention to head injuries and children.

Methods.—National estimates of boxing injuries were calculated using data from the National Electronic Injury Surveillance System. Injury rates per 1000 participants for the year 2003 were calculated using boxing participation data. Data analysis was conducted in 2009—2010.

Results.—An estimated 165,602 individuals (95% CI = 134891, 196313) sustained boxing injuries that resulted in a visit to a U.S. hospital emergency department from 1990 through 2008. An average of 8716 (95% CI = 7078, 10354) injuries occurred annually, and there was a statistically significant increase in the annual number of injuries during the 19-year study period (slope = 610, $p<0.001$). The rate of injury was 12.7 per 1000 participants. Those injured were predominately male (90.9%). The most common diagnosis was fracture (27.5%), and the most common body regions injured were the hand (33.0%) and head and neck (22.5%). Punching bag—related injuries accounted for 36.8% of boxing injuries. The percentage of injuries that were concussions/closed head injuries in the group aged 12—17 years (8.9%) was similar to that in the group aged 18—24 years (8.1%) and the group aged 25—34 years (8.5%).

Conclusions.—These findings, based on a nationally representative sample, indicate that injuries related to boxing are increasing in number. Increased efforts are needed to prevent boxing injuries.

▶ These authors conclude that boxing injuries presenting to US Emergency Departments between 1990 and 2008 showed a substantial improvement. All injuries incurred were included, and the most common injury was a fracture of a hand followed by head and neck injuries. Unfortunately, this study's limitations are significant. Many individuals receiving boxing injuries do not present themselves to emergency departments; therefore, the number of injuries in this study is grossly underestimated. It would not have captured boxing injuries that may have been treated in other health care settings, such as school health services or physician offices. Another major limitation is that the recognition of head injuries, and concussion in particular, has dramatically increased during this time. It is the increased recognition and resulting diagnosis of concussion that is believed to be responsible for the increased numbers seen in football, and I suspect the same is true of this study in boxing.

R. C. Cantu, MD, MA

Evaluation of pituitary function after traumatic brain injury in childhood

Khadr SN, Crofton PM, Jones PA, et al (Univ of Edinburgh Royal Hosp for Sick Children, UK)
Clin Endocrinol (Oxf) 73:637-643, 2010

Objectives.—Post-traumatic hypopituitarism is well described amongst adult traumatic brain injury (TBI) survivors. We aimed to determine the prevalence and clinical significance of pituitary dysfunction after head injury in childhood.

Design.—Retrospective exploratory study.

Patients.—33 survivors of accidental head injury (27 boys). Mean (range) age at study was 13·4 years (5·4-21·7 years) and median (range) interval since injury 4·3 years (1·4-7·8 years). Functional outcome at study: 15 good recovery, 16 moderate disability, two severe disability.

Measurements.—Early morning urine osmolality and basal hormone evaluation were followed by the gonadotrophin releasing hormone (GnRH) and insulin tolerance (n = 25) or glucagon tests (if previous seizures, n = 8). Subjects were not primed. Head injury details were extracted from patient records.

Results.—No subject had short stature (mean height SD score +0·50, range −1·57 to +3·00). Suboptimal GH responses (<5 μg/l) occurred in six peri-pubertal boys (one with slow growth on follow-up) and one post-pubertal adolescent (peak GH 3·2 μg/l). Median peak cortisol responses to insulin tolerance or glucagon tests were 538 and 562 nm. Nine of twenty-five and two of eight subjects had suboptimal responses, respectively, two with high basal cortisol levels. None required routine glucocorticoid replacement. In three, steroid cover was recommended for moderate/severe illness or injury. One boy was prolactin deficient. Other basal endocrine results and GnRH-stimulated LH and FSH were appropriate for age, sex and pubertal stage. Abnormal endocrine findings were unrelated to the severity or other characteristics of TBI or functional outcome.

Conclusions.—No clinically significant endocrinopathy was identified amongst survivors of accidental childhood TBI, although minor pituitary hormone abnormalities were observed.

▶ A number of publications have associated hypopituitarism in adults following traumatic brain injury. These studies have generally shown that with greater severity of brain injury, there is a higher likelihood of pituitary dysfunction. Of the various pituitary hormones, growth hormone is the most frequently reported to be affected. It has not been shown as clearly in pediatric head injury.

These authors assessed pituitary dysfunction in 33 survivors of accidental head injury, 15 of whom ultimately made a good recovery, 16 had moderate disability, and 2 had severe disability. All were assessed with regard to possible pituitary hormone abnormalities. The authors found no significant difference between normal and abnormal endocrine groups in terms of age at injury, age at the time of the study, or severity of head injury. They were thus unable to substantiate any link between head injury characteristics and endocrine outcome. In other words, they did not find that injuries with basal skull fractures, diffuse axonal injury, raised intracranial pressure, or prolonged intensive care admissions were necessarily risk factors for posttraumatic hypopituitarism.

Most importantly, clinical endocrinopathy was not identified among survivors of accidental childhood brain injury in the 1-year postinjury follow-up period of this study. Although some minor abnormalities of pituitary function were observed, none required hormone replacement.

These findings will certainly have to be corroborated by other studies because it would be expected that the same type of pituitary dysfunction as seen in adult moderate and severe head injuries would have been anticipated in the pediatric population.

R. C. Cantu, MD, MA

Trends in Concussion Incidence in High School Sports: A Prospective 11-Year Study
Lincoln AE, Caswell SV, Almquist JL, et al (MedStar Health Res Inst, Baltimore, MD; George Mason Univ, Manassas, VA; Fairfax County Public Schools, VA; et al)
Am J Sports Med 39:958-963, 2011

Background.—Understanding the risk and trends of sports-related concussion among 12 scholastic sports may contribute to concussion detection, treatment, and prevention.

Purpose.—To examine the incidence and relative risk of concussion in 12 high school boys' and girls' sports between academic years 1997-1998 and 2007-2008.

Study Design.—Descriptive epidemiology study.

Methods.—Data were prospectively gathered for 25 schools in a large public high school system. All schools used an electronic medical record-keeping program. A certified athletic trainer was on-site for games and practices and electronically recorded all injuries daily.

Results.—In sum, 2651 concussions were observed in 10 926 892 athlete-exposures, with an incidence rate of 0.24 per 1000. Boys' sports accounted for 53% of athlete-exposures and 75% of all concussions. Football accounted for more than half of all concussions, and it had the highest incidence rate (0.60). Girls' soccer had the most concussions among the girls' sports and the second-highest incidence rate of all 12 sports (0.35). Concussion rate increased 4.2-fold (95% confidence interval, 3.4-5.2) over the 11 years (15.5% annual increase). In similar boys' and girls' sports (baseball/softball, basketball, and soccer), girls had roughly twice the concussion risk of boys. Concussion rate increased over time in all 12 sports.

Conclusion.—Although the collision sports of football and boys' lacrosse had the highest number of concussions and football the highest concussion rate, concussion occurred in all other sports and was observed in girls' sports at rates similar to or higher than those of boys' sports. The increase over time in all sports may reflect actual increased occurrence or greater coding sensitivity with widely disseminated guidance on concussion detection and treatment. The high-participation collision sports of football and boys' lacrosse warrant continued vigilance, but the findings suggest that focus on concussion detection, treatment, and prevention should not be limited to those sports traditionally associated with concussion risk.

▶ This is an interesting 11-year prospective study on concussion incidence in high school sports. Perhaps the most interesting finding to this researcher is that in sports played by women and men (baseball/softball, basketball, soccer), women once again had higher incidences of concussion than their male counterparts. Although football had the highest incidences of concussion of any sport (0.6 per 1000 athletic exposures), the true incidence of concussion in football is probably 6 to 8 times higher than that figure. So, too, are the figures for other collision sports. I would suggest that these authors therefore might amend their use of the word concussion to "recognized concussion" because "unrecognized concussions" exceed recognized concussions in many of the sports they were following. To this researcher, the reason there was an increase in concussion incidence over the course of the study was clearly because of the better recognition of what were previously unrecognized concussions. Although we have a long way to go, significant strides have been made in concussion recognition, and with better education of not only the medical team and coaches but the athletes and their parents about concussion symptoms, it is hoped that there will be fewer unrecognized concussions in the future.

R. C. Cantu, MD, MA

Which On-field Signs/Symptoms Predict Protracted Recovery From Sport-Related Concussion Among High School Football Players?
Lau BC, Kontos AP, Collins MW, et al (Univ of Pittsburgh Med Ctr, PA)
Am J Sports Med 39:2311-2318, 2011

Background.—There has been increasing attention and understanding of sport-related concussions. Recent studies show that neurocognitive testing and symptom clusters may predict protracted recovery in concussed athletes. On-field signs and symptoms have not been examined empirically as possible predictors of protracted recovery.

Purpose.—This study was undertaken to determine which on-field signs and symptoms were predictive of a protracted (≥21 days) versus rapid (≤7 days) recovery after a sports-related concussion. On-field signs and symptoms included confusion, loss of consciousness, posttraumatic amnesia, retrograde amnesia, imbalance, dizziness, visual problems, personality changes, fatigue, sensitivity to light/noise, numbness, and vomiting.

Study Design.—Cohort study (prognosis); Level of evidence, 2.

Methods.—The sample included 107 male high school football athletes who completed computerized neurocognitive testing within an average

2.4 days after injury, and who were followed until returned to play as determined by neuropsychologists using international clinical concussion management guidelines. Athletes were then grouped into rapid ($\leq$7 days, n = 62) or protracted ($\geq$21 days, n = 36) recovery time groups. The presence of on-field signs and symptoms was determined at the time of injury by trained sports medicine professionals (ie, ATC [certified athletic trainer], team physician). A series of odds ratios with χ^2 analyses and subsequent logistic regression were used to determine which on-field signs and symptoms were associated with an increased risk for a protracted recovery.

Results.—Dizziness at the time of injury was associated with a 6.34 odds ratio (95% confidence interval = 1.34-29.91, $\chi^2 = 5.44$, $P = .02$) of a protracted recovery from concussion. Surprisingly, the remaining on-field signs and symptoms were not associated with an increased risk of protracted recovery in the current study.

Conclusion.—Assessment of on-field dizziness may help identify high school athletes at risk for a protracted recovery. Such information will improve prognostic information and allow clinicians to manage and treat concussion more effectively in these at-risk athletes.

▶ This study involving high school football players looked at the various on-field presenting signs and symptoms to determine if they could be used as predictors for the athletes making a rapid (defined as 7 days or less) return to play versus a more protracted (defined as $\geq$21 days) return to play. Previous studies have suggested that on the field, posttraumatic amnesia and retrograde amnesia were predictive of concussion severity. Balance in this study was not determined by using the Balance Error Scoring System (BESS) or other sophisticated testing, but was determined by using the Rhomberg test, tandem walking, and heel toe testing. The authors' finding that abnormality of balance was not predictive of delayed return or delayed clearance of symptoms, therefore, may have been due to the lack of more sophisticated testing of balance. In this study, on-field dizziness was correlated with the delayed recovery group by a factor of 6 and no other on-field symptoms were found to be predictors of delayed recovery.

This researcher and clinician found a high correlation between imbalance and symptoms of dizziness; therefore, it is likely that it is the way balance was tested that did not find a correlation in this study. I believe that to test balance with anything less sophisticated than the BESS system is an imprecise measurement. Because this was a study of high school football players only, its findings should not be generalized to other sports, women, or older athletes. The authors suggest that it is certainly a study that should be repeated by other investigators to see if their findings are the same, and when those other studies are done this reviewer would suggest the use of the best testing method to detect balance. These authors make a strong plea that dizziness assessment be carried out using a formal questionnaire, such as the dizziness beliefs scale or dizziness handicap inventory.

R. C. Cantu, MD, MA

Traumatic Brain Injury in Children and Adolescents: Surveillance for Pituitary Dysfunction

Norwood KW, DeBoer MD, Gurka MJ, et al (Univ of Virginia, Charlottesville)
Clin Pediatr (Phila) 49:1044-1049, 2010

Background.—Children who sustain traumatic brain injury (TBI) are at risk for developing hypopituitarism, of which growth hormone deficiency (GHD) is the most common manifestation.

Objective.—To determine the prevalence of GHD and associated features following TBI among children and adolescents.

Study Design.—A total of 32 children and adolescents were recruited from a pediatric TBI clinic. Participants were diagnosed with GHD based on insufficient growth hormone release during both spontaneous overnight testing and following arginine/glucagon administration.

Results.—GHD was diagnosed in 5/32 participants (16%). Those with GHD exhibited more rapid weight gain following injury than those without GHD and had lower levels of free thyroxine and follicle-stimulating hormone. Males with GHD had lower testosterone levels.

Conclusions.—GHD following TBI is common in children and adolescents, underscoring the importance of assessing for GHD, including evaluating height and weight velocities after TBI. Children and adolescents with GHD may further exhibit absence or intermediate function for other pituitary hormones.

▶ Pituitary dysfunction has been shown to occur in both children and adults who undergo a traumatic brain injury. The incidence of the occurrence of the pituitary dysfunction has been shown to be much more prevalent with severe traumatic brain injury compared with the mild end of the spectrum, often called concussion. In most studies, growth hormone deficiency has been the most common pituitary dysfunction, and in this study of 32 children, it was found to be abnormally low in 16%. Although this study shows that such deficiencies can be found in children, it is important to realize that the arginine/glucagon growth hormone stimulation test was used to determine low levels of growth hormone, and this provocative test is not one that is commonly administered. It is also important that the traumatic brain injuries studied in this group of children were in the moderate to severe range and did not include the mild traumatic brain injury. Therefore, this data cannot be extrapolated to concussion.

R. C. Cantu, MD, MA

Physician Concussion Knowledge and the Effect of Mailing the CDC's "Heads Up" Toolkit

Chrisman SP, Schiff MA, Rivara FP (Univ of Washington, Seattle)
Clin Pediatr 50:1031-1039, 2011

Background.—The Centers for Disease Control and Prevention's (CDC) "Heads Up" toolkit was designed to educate physicians about concussion, but it has not been well studied. This study proposed to evaluate the effect of receiving the toolkit on physician concussion knowledge.

Methods.—The authors obtained a sample of physicians from the American Medical Association masterfile and randomly selected half to be mailed the CDC's "Heads Up" toolkit. All physicians were then sent a survey on concussion knowledge. Data were analyzed to evaluate the effect of the toolkit on concussion knowledge.

Results.—The survey was completed by 414 physicians (183 intervention, 231 control). There were no differences in general concussion knowledge between intervention and control groups, but physicians in the intervention group were significantly less likely to recommend next day return to play after a concussion (adjusted odds ratio = 0.31, 95% confidence interval = 0.12-0.76).

Conclusions.—Mailing the CDC's "Heads Up" toolkit appears to affect physicians' recommendations regarding returning to play after a concussion.

▶ One of the biggest hurdles in knowledge transfer and exchange is implementation and behavior change in the affected end users. With the ever-increasing information available (in print and electronically) regarding sport-related concussion, it is critical to evaluate whether or not the messages are getting through to the appropriate groups—athletes, parents, coaches, referees, or treating health care professionals. This study evaluates the effect of a multimedia campaign about concussion done by the Centers for Disease Control and Prevention (CDC), specifically the "Heads Up" toolkit that was designed for physicians. A good-sized sample of pediatricians, family physicians, and internists was selected, with half of them receiving the kit by mail. A subsequent survey about concussion knowledge and management was mailed to participating physicians, with appropriate follow-up techniques designed to enhance participation, giving a final response rate of 27.2% (414/1469). The only significant finding was that mailing the toolkit was associated with a decreased likelihood of recommending next day return to play, consistent with current concussion guidelines. A limitation of this study was that although there were data on specialty, years of clinical practice, number of concussions seen per year, and other factors, there was no information on what type of education (besides the CDC toolkit) these physicians had received regarding concussion. Specifically, if any of the respondents had completed sport medicine fellowships, they may have had more baseline knowledge in this area. There are substantial challenges not only in altering practice patterns to keep up with current evidence-based guidelines, but also in evaluating the effects of targeted educational interventions. This is an area for much future research.

C. Lebrun, MDCM, MPE, CCFP, Dip Sport Med, FACSM

Assessment and Management of Sport-Related Concussions in United States High Schools
Meehan WP, d'Hemecourt P, Collins CL, et al (Children's Hosp Boston, MA; Nationwide Children's Hosp, Columbus, OH)
Am J Sports Med 39:2304-2310, 2011

Background.—Little existing data describe which medical professionals and which medical studies are used to assess sport-related concussions in high school athletes.

Purpose.—To describe the medical providers and medical studies used when assessing sport-related concussions. To determine the effects of medical provider type on timing of return to play, frequency of imaging, and frequency of neuropsychological testing.

Study Design.—Descriptive epidemiology study.

Methods.—All concussions recorded by the High School Reporting Information Online (HS RIO) injury surveillance system during the 2009 to 2010 academic year were included. χ^2 analyses were conducted for categorical variables. Fisher exact test was used for nonparametric data. Logistic regression analyses were used when adjusting for potential confounders. Statistical significance was considered for $P < .05$.

Results.—The HS RIO recorded 1056 sport-related concussions, representing 14.6% of all injuries. Most (94.4%) concussions were assessed by athletic trainers (ATs), 58.8% by a primary care physician. Few concussions were managed by specialists. The assessment of 21.2% included computed tomography. Computerized neuropsychological testing was used for 41.2%. For 50.1%, a physician decided when to return the athlete to play; for 46.2%, the decision was made by an AT. After adjusting for potential confounders, no associations between timing of return to play and the type of provider (physician vs AT) deciding to return the athlete to play were found.

Conclusion.—Concussions account for nearly 15% of all sport-related injuries in high school athletes. The timing of return to play after a sport-related concussion is similar regardless of whether the decision to return the athlete to play is made by a physician or an AT. When a medical doctor is involved, most concussions are assessed by primary care physicians as opposed to subspecialists. Computed tomography is obtained during the assessment of 1 of every 5 concussions occurring in high school athletes (Table 1).

▶ This prospective cohort study of a large national sample of US high schools provides some extremely interesting descriptive epidemiological information regarding number of concussive injuries, type of sport, and the medical and

TABLE 1.—Number of Sport-Related Concussions Per 100 000 Athletic Exposures[a]

Sport	Concussions Per 100 000 Athletic Exposures, n (95% CI)
Boys' football	76.8 (74.1-79.5)
Boys' ice hockey	61.9 (59.4-64.4)
Boys' lacrosse	46.6 (44.5-48.7)
Girls' soccer	33.0 (31.2-34.8)
Girls' lacrosse	31.0 (29.3-32.7)
Girls' field hockey	24.9 (23.3-26.5)
Boys' wrestling	23.9 (22.4-25.4)
Boys' basketball	21.2 (19.8-22.6)
Boys' soccer	19.2 (17.8-20.6)
Girls' basketball	18.6 (17.2-20.0)
Girls' softball	16.3 (15.0-17.6)
Cheerleading	11.5 (10.4-12.6)
Girls' volleyball	8.6 (7.7-9.5)
Girls' gymnastics	8.2 (7.3-9.1)
Boys' baseball	4.6 (3.9-5.3)
Boys' track and field	3.5 (2.9-4.1)
Girls' track and field	1.4 (1.2-1.6)
Girls' swimming	1.0 (0.8-1.2)
Boys' volleyball	0.0 (N/A)
Boys' swimming	0.0 (N/A)

[a]CI, confidence interval; N/A, not applicable.

paramedical professionals involved in assessment and management. The fact that concussions account for nearly 15% of all sport-related injuries in this population of high school athletes is disturbing. The use of the online High School Reporting Information Online injury surveillance system, in schools in which the high school had at least one athletic therapist affiliated with the National Athletic Trainer's Association, allowed for reasonably accurate data capture regarding injuries and athletic exposures, for 192 US high schools, with athletes participating in 20 different sports (Table 1). With a total of 1056 reported concussions (14.6% of the total recorded 7257 sport-related injuries), the authors were able to ascertain which medical professionals were primarily involved in the initial assessment, subsequent evaluations, and return-to-play decisions, as well as the increasing use of computerized neurocognitive testing. Athletic therapists were the most commonly involved, but approximately 60% of concussions in this study were assessed by primary care physicians, as opposed to sport medicine subspecialists. Orthopedic surgeons and midlevel providers, such as nurse practitioners and physician assistants, were caring for an additional 8.2% of concussions. These findings have important implications, in terms of the need to target these particular clinicians and professionals, when communicating evidence-based concussion management recommendations. Strategies to improve this type of knowledge transfer and exchange have the potential to improve the quality of care for individual athletes sustaining sport-related concussions.

C. Lebrun, MDCM, MPE, CCFP, Dip Sport Med, FACSM

Cognitive impairment 3 months after moderate and severe traumatic brain injury: a prospective follow-up study

Skandsen T, Finnanger TG, Andersson S, et al (Norwegian Univ of Science and Technology, Trondheim, Norway)
Arch Phys Med Rehabil 91:1904-1913, 2010

Objective.—To explore the magnitude and frequency of cognitive impairment 3 months after moderate to severe traumatic brain injury (TBI), and to evaluate its relationship to disability at 1-year follow-up.

Design.—Prospective follow-up study.

Setting.—Regional level I trauma center.

Participants.—Patients aged 15 to 65 years with definite TBI, defined as Glasgow Coma Scale score of 3 to 13 and injury documented by magnetic resonance imaging (n=59) or computed tomography (n=2); healthy volunteers (n=47) served as controls.

Interventions.—Not applicable.

Main Outcome Measures.—Neuropsychological assessment 3 months postinjury and Glasgow Outcome Scale Extended (GOSE) at 3 and 12 months postinjury.

Results.—Patients with TBI performed worse than controls, most consistently in terms of information processing speed and verbal memory. However, a maximum of only 43% of patients with TBI had impaired test scores (defined as <1.5 SD below mean of normative data) on any one measure. Based on a selection of 9 tests, a 0 or 1 impaired score was seen in 46 (98%) of 47 controls, in 20 (57%) of 35 patients with moderate TBI, and in 9 (35%) of 26 patients with severe TBI. At 1 year postinjury, disability (defined as GOSE score ≤6) was present in 57% of those with 2 or more impaired test scores and in 21% of those with 0 or 1 impaired score ($P = .005$).

Conclusions.—In this sample of patients with recent, definite TBI and healthy volunteers, we found that TBI affected cognition in moderate as well as severe cases. The presence of cognitive impairment was associated with future disability. However, half of the patients with moderate TBI and even one third of those with severe TBI had a normal cognitive assessment 3 months postinjury.

▶ This study compared individuals with moderate or severe traumatic brain injury defined as a Glasgow Coma Scale score between 3 and 13 and abnormalities seen on magnetic resonance imaging (MRI) or computed tomography (CT), which represented either contusion or diffuse axonal injury. The Glasgow Outcome Scale Extended (GOSE) was also used at 3 and 12 months in this group, and then this group was compared with controls that had not sustained brain injury.

It is no surprise that the authors found that individuals with traumatic brain injury performed worse than controls on cognitive tasks involving information processing speed and verbal memory. It was also found that individuals who had abnormalities affecting cognition 3 months after injury were more likely to have disability at 1 year as scored by the GOSE method. The study found that half of the patients with moderate traumatic brain injury and one-third with severe traumatic brain injury had normal cognitive assessments 3 months after injury. The study also found that a significant proportion (43%) of individuals in the traumatic brain-injured group that had an early normal assessment complained of deficits at the 1-year mark on the GOSE score.

This study suffers from the fact that many of the individuals in it were involved in automobile accidents. It is possible that their complaints at 1 year—after not showing difficulties at 3 months—may have been influenced by litigation. It is also true that the most severely injured individuals in the severe group were excluded from being involved in the study by the fact that they were incapable of undergoing the neuropsychological testing assessment. It is also possible that there were IQ differences involved in the traumatic brain-injured group and control groups prior to the traumatic brain injury group's injuries.

Even with these limitations, it is interesting that the authors found a lower-than-expected cognitive impairment in the injured group at 3 months and found many individuals at the 1-year mark reporting a significant number of complaints affecting quality of life despite having tested cognitively normal at 3 months.

This reviewer would like to see this study repeated with symptom validity verified.

R. C. Cantu, MD, MA

The King-Devick test as a determinant of head trauma and concussion in boxers and MMA fighters
Galetta KM, Barrett J, Allen M, et al (Univ of Pennsylvania School of Medicine, Philadelphia)
Neurology 76:1456-1462, 2011

Objective.—Sports-related concussion has received increasing attention as a cause of short- and long-term neurologic symptoms among athletes. The King—Devick (K—D) test is based on measurement of the speed of rapid number naming (reading aloud single-digit numbers from 3 test cards), and captures impairment of eye movements, attention, language, and other correlates of suboptimal brain function. We investigated the K—D test as a potential rapid sideline screening for concussion in a cohort of boxers and mixed martial arts fighters.

Methods.—The K—D test was administered prefight and postfight. The Military Acute Concussion Evaluation (MACE) was administered as a more comprehensive but longer test for concussion. Differences in postfight K—D scores and changes in scores from prefight to postfight were compared for athletes with head trauma during the fight vs those without.

Results.—Postfight K—D scores (n = 39 participants) were significantly higher (worse) for those with head trauma during the match (59.1 ± 7.4 vs 41.0 ± 6.7 seconds, p < 0.0001, Wilcoxon rank sum test). Those with loss of consciousness showed the greatest worsening from prefight to postfight. Worse postfight K−D scores (r(s) = −0.79, p = 0.0001) and greater worsening of scores (r(s) = 0.90, p < 0.0001) correlated well with postfight MACE scores. Worsening of K−D scores by ≥5 seconds was a distinguishing characteristic noted only among participants with head trauma. High levels of test−retest reliability were observed (intraclass correlation coefficient 0.97 [95% confidence interval 0.90−1.0]).

Conclusions.—The K−D test is an accurate and reliable method for identifying athletes with head trauma, and is a strong candidate for rapid sideline screening test for concussion.

▶ Because it is well recognized that most mild concussions are missed on the sidelines at collision sports such as football and ice hockey, a rapid, accurate sideline assessment tool would be particularly valuable. This is especially true at the youth level where there are rarely medically trained personnel such as certified athletic trainers, emergency medical technicians, or physicians on the sideline.

One such test that has been proposed as a determinant of head trauma and concussion in particular is the King-Devick Test. This test has particular appeal because its use simply requires participants to read numbers on a card from left to right as quickly as possible without making errors. This is, therefore, a test that does not require sophisticated medical personnel to administer. It measures impairment of eye movement, attention, language, and other areas that correlate with suboptimal brain function. It has particular appeal because it uses visual and eye movement pathways that involve multiple areas of the brain.

In this article, use of a King-Devick Test was compared with the military acute concussion evaluation (MACE) in following boxers and mixed martial arts participants before and after contests. There was a significant difference both on the King-Devick Test and the MACE in those combatants who incurred significant head trauma, especially to the point of loss of consciousness. There was high correlation between the King-Devick Test and the MACE results. These preliminary findings suggest that the King-Devick Test may be an accurate and reliable method for identifying athletes with head trauma and could be used as a sideline screening tool for concussion.

Although additional studies need to be done, such as comparing the King-Devick Test with a neurologic examination, including detailed balance studies such as the BESS as well as other neuropsychological tests, these findings are certainly encouraging. It is probable that no single test will ever completely and accurately identify all concussions, and therefore to have passed this test does not necessarily mean that one has not had a concussion; however, failing to pass this test would most probably cause individuals to be removed from play and save them from further brain injury.

R. C. Cantu, MD, MA

The King-Devick test and sports-related concussion: Study of a rapid visual screening tool in a collegiate cohort

Galetta KM, Brandes LE, Maki K, et al (Univ of Pennsylvania School of Medicine, Philadelphia; et al)

J Neurol Sci 309:34-39, 2011

Objective.—Concussion, defined as an impulse blow to the head or body resulting in transient neurologic signs or symptoms, has received increasing attention in sports at all levels. The King—Devick (K—D) test is based on the time to perform rapid number naming and captures eye movements and other correlates of suboptimal brain function. In a study of boxers and mixed martial arts (MMA) fighters, the K—D test was shown to have high degrees of test—retest and inter-rater reliability and to be an accurate method for rapidly identifying boxers and mixed martial arts fighters with concussion. We performed a study of the K—D test as a rapid sideline screening tool in collegiate athletes to determine the effect of concussion on K—D scores compared to a pre-season baseline.

Methods.—In this longitudinal study, athletes from the University of Pennsylvania varsity football, sprint football, and women's and men's soccer and basketball teams underwent baseline K—D testing prior to the start of the 2010—11 playing season. Post-season testing was also performed. For athletes who had concussions during the season, K—D testing was administered immediately on the sidelines and changes in score from baseline were determined.

Results.—Among 219 athletes tested at baseline, post-season K—D scores were lower (better) than the best pre-season scores (35.1 vs. 37.9 s, P = 0.03, Wilcoxon signed-rank test), reflecting mild learning effects in the absence of concussion. For the 10 athletes who had concussions, K—D testing on the sidelines showed significant worsening from baseline (46.9 vs. 37.0 s, P = 0.009), with all except one athlete demonstrating worsening from baseline (median 5.9 s).

Conclusion.—This study of collegiate athletes provides initial evidence in support of the K—D test as a strong candidate for a rapid sideline visual screening tool for concussion. Data show worsening of scores following concussion, and ongoing follow-up in this study with additional concussion events and different athlete populations will further examine the effectiveness of the K—D test.

▶ In an attempt to enhance concussion assessment on the sideline, a number of new tools have recently been brought forward. This includes a single strip on the field recording of electroencephalograms called BrainScope as well as electrophysiologic recordings of evoked potentials. For several decades, there have been simplified neuropsychological tests, the most widely used being the sideline assessment of concussion, or SAC. The King-Devick test uses impairment of eye movements and attention and language to assess suboptimal brain function. It is based on the measurement of the speed of the individual being able to assess rapid number naming and in this study was found to be reliable for identifying postconcussion symptoms compared with athletes who did not sustain head trauma. This test is being promoted as one that does not require sophisticated medical background to administer and therefore one that may be helpful for coaches and trainers making game decisions. I believe it is important that this test be regarded as an additional tool in the toolbox of concussion assessment rather than the toolbox itself. If anyone is suspected of having a concussion or is diagnosed with one because of alterations in level of consciousness or showing signs or symptoms of concussion, the individual should be immediately removed from play. Passing this test should never allow such an individual to be allowed to return to play. Rather, this test could be used in situations in which a coach did not think one was showing signs or was not admitting to symptoms of a concussion but just wanted further assurance; failing this test would be a reason to remove the individual from game play. Therefore, properly used, I believe that this is a positive tool for sideline concussion assessment, although further studies will need to be done to better define its sensitivity and specificity.

R. C. Cantu, MD, MA

Early Indicators of Enduring Symptoms in High School Athletes With Multiple Previous Concussions

Schatz P, Moser RS, Covassin T, et al (Saint Joseph's Univ, Philadelphia, PA; International Brain Res Foundation, Edison, NJ; Michigan State Univ, East Lansing; et al)
Neurosurgery 68:1562-1567, 2011

Background.—Despite recent findings of cognitive, emotional, physical, and behavioral symptomatology in retired professional athletes with a history of multiple concussions, there is little systematic research examining these symptoms in high school athletes with a history of concussion.

Objective.—To identify cognitive, emotional, and physical symptoms at baseline in nonconcussed high school athletes based on concussion history.

Methods.—A multicenter sample of 616 high school athletes who completed baseline evaluations were assigned to groups based on history of concussion (none, 1, 2, or more previous concussions). The Post-Concussion Symptom Scale was administered as part of a computerized neuropsychological test battery during athletes' preseason baseline evaluations. Cross-sectional analyses were used to examine symptoms reported at the time of baseline neuropsychological testing.

Results.—High school athletes with a history of 2 or more concussions showed significantly higher ratings of concussion-related symptoms (cognitive, physical, sleep difficulties) than athletes with a history of one or no previous concussions.

Conclusion.—It appears that youth athletes who sustain multiple concussions experience a variety of subtle effects, which may be possible precursors of the future onset of concussion-related difficulties.

▶ This was a somewhat alarming study to this reviewer in that it found that athletes who had sustained two or more prior concussions experienced a statistically higher number of postconcussive physical, cognitive, emotional, or sleep symptoms than a group of athletes who had no or one concussion. This study purported to sample 2,557 athletes from high schools in Michigan, New Jersey, and Pennsylvania who were actively practicing and/or competing in athletic seasons. My concern is why or how the group with postconcussion symptoms was cleared and allowed to participate in sport activities. The research was done with a self-report questionnaire, which of course has the limitations of such reporting, but I am very concerned about the number of postconcussive symptoms that these athletes experienced in this study and why they may have been cleared to be in their respective sports.

R. C. Cantu, MD, MA

Concussion (Mild Traumatic Brain Injury) and the Team Physician: A Consensus Statement—2011 Update
Herring SA, Cantu RC, Guskiewicz KM, et al
Med Sci Sports Exerc 43:2412-2422, 2011

This document provides an overview of select medical issues that are important to team physicians who are responsible for athletes with concussion. It is not intended as a standard of care and should not be interpreted as such. This document is only a guide and, as such, is of a general nature, consistent with the reasonable, objective practice of the healthcare professional. Individual treatment will turn on the specific facts and circumstances presented to the physician. Adequate insurance should be in place to help protect the physician, the athlete, and the sponsoring organization. This statement was developed by a collaboration of six major professional associations concerned about clinical sports medicine issues; they have committed to forming an ongoing project-based alliance to bring together sports medicine organizations to best serve active people and athletes. These organizations are the American Academy of Family Physicians, the American Academy of Orthopaedic Surgeons, the American College of Sports Medicine, the American Medical Society for Sports Medicine, the American Orthopaedic Society for Sports Medicine, and the American Osteopathic Academy of Sports Medicine.

▶ The American College of Sports Medicine in 2006 published an article on concussion and mild traumatic brain injury for the team physician. This 2011 publication reflects an update of that original article and I believe should be mandatory reading for all team physicians. The publication represents collaboration among 6 major professional associations concerned with clinical sports medicine issues and was spearheaded as it originally was by the American College of Sports Medicine. The article presents in bullet format the major points the team physician should be familiar with, such as concussion epidemiology, biomechanics and pathophysiology, preseason planning and assessment, same-day evaluation and treatment, post–same day evaluation and treatment, diagnostic testing complications, prevention, and legislature and government issues. I believe this is a very valuable resource, especially for all sideline team physicians. It is clearly stated that while this document is very comprehensive, it is not intended as a standard of care and should be interpreted only as a guide, as each concussion requires individual treatment specific to the facts and circumstances presented to the treating physician.

R. C. Cantu, MD, MA

Traumatic Brain Injury: Is the Pituitary Out of Harm's Way?
Heather N, Cutfield W (Univ of Auckland, New Zealand)
J Pediatr 159:686-690, 2011

Background.—Hypopituitarism after childhood traumatic brain injury (TBI) may cause treatable morbidity in survivors. Over 25% of adults develop subclinical hypopituitarism after TBI, and the risk for children is believed to be similar. However, few children with head injuries are seen in endocrine clinics, so either cases are not being identified or data are misinterpreted. Growth hormone (GH) is the hormone most commonly affected, but seldom is head injury identified as the cause of GH deficiency. The relationship between TBI and hypopituitarism was explored.

Facts About TBI.—Retrospective studies of hospital admissions show TBI is common but underreported. Prospective studies find its incidence may be 10-fold higher than assumed. Most cases are mild and not seen in the hospital. Factors altering TBI reports are case definition, geographic location, variable hospital coding, and lost notes.

Current ways of grading TBI, such as the Glasgow Coma Scale (GCS), poorly predict possible effects on pituitary function. GCS assessment is altered by increased use of pre-hospital intubation and paralyzing or sedating agents, highly variable time between injury and grading, weak inter-observer reliability, and poor usefulness in pre-verbal subjects. Alternatively, imaging studies permit structural classification of TBI and may better predict pituitary damage. Magnetic resonance imaging (MRI) is the gold standard for pituitary imaging, but computed tomography (CT) scans are usually obtained acutely and may have predictive value. However, techniques focused on pituitary injury offer the best indicators of hypopituitarism.

There is a high rate of TBI in late adolescence and abusive head trauma in infancy. Causes in late adolescence are usually contact sports, motor vehicle accidents, and assaults. Children are more likely to suffer falls, be struck by objects, or suffer pedestrian road accidents. Abusive head trauma can lead to severe TBI and is conservatively estimated to affect 15 to 25 children per

100,000 annually. Low socioeconomic groups and minority populations are at higher risk. Male persons have higher risk at all ages.

Relationships to Hypopituitarism.—Rates of subclinical pituitary deficiency vary greatly (5% to 61%), but the overall rate is about 20% in children. Biochemical abnormalities are noted without definite endocrine disease. Most TBIs produce GH deficiency, but adrenocorticotropin (ACTH) and thyrotropin can also be deficient. Gonadotropin status is hard to assess but precocious puberty occurs in up to 12% of cases. The course of post-traumatic hypopituitarism involves early abnormalities that resolve completely in 3 to 6 months. New pituitary deficiencies are uncommon after 6 months, but transient deficiencies can affect recovery from TBI. Hypopituitarism after 6 to 12 months is likely to persist, but may resolve in half of subjects in 1 to 3 years.

Vascular and traumatic hypotheses may explain the mechanisms by which hypopituitarism develops after TBI. The pituitary gland's anatomy makes it vulnerable to vascular injury. Pituitary edema in the first week after TBI, atrophy, and perfusion defects support a vascular mechanism of injury. However, pituitary and hypothalamic lesions can accompany basal skull fractures and reflect higher impact forces. Post-mortem studies often show hypothalamic lesions in patients after TBI. Anti-pituitary antibodies are common after TBI and are also associated with hypopituitarism.

Reports of hypopituitarism after TBI are limited by several factors. Essentially, they tend to come from small cross-sectional studies and involve highly selected populations who have undergone nonstandardized assessments.

Recommendations.—Evidence suggests that comprehensive endocrine assessment should be used only for children with poor growth or other symptoms of hypopituitarism. An alternative is for family doctors or outpatient care providers to measure growth routinely after TBI, including height, weight, pubertal status, and height velocity.

Conclusions.—The incidence of post-traumatic hypopituitarism associated with TBI in children appears to be overestimated, although large prospective studies using rigorous diagnostic criteria are needed to better guide clinical practice. The best approach to early assessment of risk after TBI is likely to rely on pituitary swelling on MRI or levels of anti-pituitary antibodies. Transient GH deficiency may contribute to post-concussion syndrome as well.

▶ This is a very provocative and insightful article coming from researchers at the University of Auckland New Zealand. Because the Christchurch Berth cohort study was both prospective and population-based, these researchers have a unique insight into childhood traumatic brain injury and the subsequent incidence of pituitary dysfunction. The authors based their conclusion on their own experience and on a very careful assessment of the literature, which is predominantly cross-sectional and involves relatively small numbers of individuals whose pituitary dysfunction was diagnosed only on abnormal laboratory data rather than confirmatory clinical findings; much of the laboratory data involved provocative tests that have a high rate of false-positive results. This led these authors to conclude that the rate of pituitary dysfunction after moderate and severe head injury in the world's literature is grossly overstated. The authors further concluded that it is not cost-effective to work up children after a traumatic brain injury for pituitary dysfunction and that this should be reserved for children with poor growth or other symptoms suggestive of hypopituitarism. Two exceptions to this group might be individuals who are demonstrated to show swelling of the pituitary gland on MRI or increased levels of antipituitary antibodies after traumatic brain injury.

I believe these authors' suggestions are extremely cogent and certainly explain why there is such a wide variability in reported pituitary dysfunction after traumatic brain injury in adults, but even more so in children.

R. C. Cantu, MD, MA

S100b immunoassay: an assessment of diagnostic utility in minor head trauma
Kotlyar S, Larkin GL, Moore CL, et al (Yale Univ, School of Medicine, New Haven, CT)
J Emerg Med 41:285-293, 2011

Background.—Over 1.4 million patients present annually to United States (US) emergency departments with minor head trauma. Many undergo unnecessary head computed tomography (HCT).

Objectives.—We sought to determine the diagnostic accuracy of S100B, a central nervous system peptide, to screen for HCT+ head injury.

Methods.—This study was a prospective observational study of adults with minor head trauma. Patients presenting within 6 h of injury and undergoing HCT for evaluation were eligible. All HCTs were blindly reviewed for presence of a priori defined intracranial injury (HCT+). Quantitative S100B levels were determined by enzyme-linked immunosorbent assay.

Results.—A total of 346 patients were enrolled over 12 months, mean age 48 years ($\pm$ 23 years), 62% male. Twenty-two (6.4%) were HCT+. Vomiting, headache, anterograde amnesia, Glasgow Coma Scale score < 15, nausea, and loss of consciousness were associated with HCT+ results. Median S100B levels were significantly elevated in HCT+ (115 ng/dL) vs. HCT− (56.0 ng/dL) patients ($p = 0.032$). Receiver operator characteristic analysis demonstrated an area under the curve of 0.643. Sensitivity and specificity were 86% (95% confidence interval [CI] 67−96) and 37% (95% CI 29−45%) at 42 ng/dL, 91% (95% CI 72−98%) and 24% (95% CI 17−31%) at 32 ng/dL, and 96% (95% CI 78−100%) and 13% (95% CI 9−20%) at 24 ng/dL, respectively.

Conclusion.—The study demonstrates that S100B may be a sensitive but non-specific marker of HCT+ injury.

▶ Biomarkers of brain injury as well as other neurologic conditions have long been the focus of intense research effort. With regard to mild traumatic brain injury, a number of biomarkers, including S100B protein in the spinal fluid, has been the subject of many prior publications. Generally it has not been found to be specific enough to be useful in the diagnosis of mild traumatic brain injury, and most articles have been negative with regard to its diagnostic merits. This study, which is one of the largest trials involving S100B, suggests that serum S100B may be a sensitive marker of intracranial injury. Although this is encouraging, its specificity is poor, and its utility as an independent tool for the evaluation of minor head trauma is extremely limited. Nonetheless, in this study, patients who had subarachnoid and intraparenchymal brain bleeding had the highest median S100B levels. This study suggests that a larger, more robust study is warranted to determine the effectiveness of S100B protein in minor head trauma. Although muscle breakdown and fractures make this a nonspecific marker of intracranial injury, it is speculated that larger studies and an assessment of optimal cutoff values may make this a useful clinical tool.

R. C. Cantu, MD, MA

The Influence of Musculoskeletal Injury on Cognition: Implications for Concussion Research

Hutchison M, Comper P, Mainwaring L, et al (Univ of Toronto, Ontario, Canada)

Am J Sports Med 39:2331-2337, 2011

Background.—Safe return-to-play decisions after concussion can be challenging for sports medicine specialists. Neuropsychological testing is recommended to objectively measure concussion-related cognitive impairments.

Purpose.—The objective of this study was to measure cognitive functioning among 3 specific athletic groups: (1) athletes with no injuries (n = 36), (2) athletes with musculoskeletal injuries (n = 18), and (3) athletes with concussion (n = 18).

Study Design.—Case-control study; Level of evidence, 3.

Methods.—Seventy-two intercollegiate athletes completed preseason baseline cognitive testing and follow-up assessment using the Automated Neuropsychological Assessment Metrics (ANAM) test battery. Injured athletes were tested within 72 hours of injury. A 1-way analysis of covariance adjusted for baseline scores was performed to determine if differences existed in cognitive test scores among the 3 groups.

Results.—A group of athletes with concussion performed significantly worse than a group of athletes with no injuries on the following subtests of the ANAM at follow-up: Code Substitution Learning, Match to Sample, and Simple Reaction. Athletes with musculoskeletal injuries performed significantly worse than those with no injury on the Match to Sample subtest. No significant differences between athletes with concussion and athletes with musculoskeletal injuries were found on all ANAM subtests.

Conclusion.—Concussion produces cognitive impairment in the acute recovery period. Interestingly, athletes with musculoskeletal injuries also display a degree of cognitive impairment as measured by computerized tests.

Clinical Relevance.—Although these findings support previous research that neuropsychological tests can effectively measure concussion-related cognitive impairment, this study provides evidence that athletic injury, in general, also may produce a degree of cognitive disruption. Therefore, a narrow interpretation of scores of neuropsychological tests in a sports concussion context should be avoided.

▶ Current diagnosis and management of concussion, including return-to-play decisions, are based on a combination of clinical assessment, some type of neuropsychological (NP) testing, and assessment of balance. Another relatively recent area of investigation is the importance of the oculovestibular system, particularly for screening purposes and for rehabilitation of concussed athletes. There are several well-known computerized NP batteries available for concussion assessment. The test battery described here, Automated Neuropsychological Assessment Metrics (ANAM), is somewhat less frequently used than the more commonly known Immediate Postconcussion Assessment and Cognitive Testing (ImPACT) and CogSport. Domains of testing in ANAM include working memory, attention, concentration, information processing, reaction time, and short-term verbal and nonverbal memory abilities. Multiple test versions help limit practice effects. But for all these tools, baseline testing and serial retesting after injury and during recovery yield the best information.

There is much current interest in the metrics of these various tests, particularly in terms of the self-report symptoms, which are by their very nature, more subjective. The ANAM measures symptom intensities in 36 items grouped into 5 core categories: (1) functional, (2) cognitive, (3) physical, (4) sensory/perceptual, and (5) mood. The ImPACT test, on the other hand, uses 22 items, in similar categories. Research has shown that normal people, without concussion, can report symptoms and that various conditions, including gender, state of nutrition and hydration, fatigue, and so forth, can have an influence on how a person scores these symptoms. Specific groups of symptoms may be more predictive of a prolonged recovery and might even be used at baseline testing to help screen and identify athletes at risk of sustaining a concussion during the season. This well-designed study followed cognitive functioning among 3 specific athletic groups and found that athletes with other musculoskeletal injuries had scores intermediate between the scores of concussed athletes and healthy controls on some of the components of the test. This provides further evidence that such NP assessment tools should definitely not be used in isolation and that results should be interpreted with caution because of the numerous factors that may alter cognitive impairment. It also underscores the importance of clinical evaluation of injured and concussed athletes by a suitably trained and experienced physician.

C. Lebrun, MDCM, MPE, CCFP, Dip Sport Med, FACSM

Mechanisms of Anterior Cruciate Ligament Injury in World Cup Alpine Skiing: A Systematic Video Analysis of 20 Cases

Bere T, Flørenes TW, Krosshaug T, et al (Norwegian School of Sport Sciences, Oslo, Norway; et al)
Am J Sports Med 39:1421-1429, 2011

Background.—There is limited insight into the mechanisms of anterior cruciate ligament injuries in alpine skiing, particularly among professional ski racers.

Purpose.—This study was undertaken to qualitatively describe the mechanisms of anterior cruciate ligament injury in World Cup alpine skiing.

Study Design.—Case series; Level of evidence, 4.

Methods.—Twenty cases of anterior cruciate ligament injuries reported through the International Ski Federation Injury Surveillance System for 3 consecutive World Cup seasons (2006-2009) were obtained on video. Seven international experts in the field of skiing biomechanics and sports medicine related to alpine skiing performed visual analyses of each case to describe the injury mechanisms in detail (skiing situation, skier behavior, biomechanical characteristics).

Results.—Three main categories of injury mechanisms were identified: slip-catch, landing back-weighted, and dynamic snowplow. The slip-catch mechanism accounted for half of the cases (n = 10), and all these injuries occurred during turning, without or before falling. The skier lost pressure on the outer ski, and while extending the outer knee to regain grip, the inside edge of the outer ski caught abruptly in the snow, forcing the knee into internal rotation and valgus. The same loading pattern was observed for the dynamic snowplow (n = 3). The landing back-weighted category included cases (n = 4) where the skier was out of balance backward in flight after a jump and landed on the ski tails with nearly extended knees. The suggested loading mechanism was a combination of tibiofemoral compression, boot-induced anterior drawer, and quadriceps anterior drawer.

Conclusion.—Based on this video analysis of 20 injury situations, the main mechanism of anterior cruciate ligament injury in World Cup alpine skiing appeared to be a slip-catch situation where the outer ski catches the inside edge, forcing the outer knee into internal rotation and valgus. A similar loading pattern was observed for the dynamic snowplow. Injury prevention efforts should focus on the slip-catch mechanism and the dynamic snowplow.

▶ Anterior cruciate ligament (ACL) injury is common among both recreational and professional competitive skiers. While there have been substantive improvements in equipment, such as the boots and bindings, and some work done on preventative measures,[1] this injury continues to decimate the ranks of professional World Cup (WC) alpine skiers. The International Ski Federation (FIS), in partnership with the scientists and clinicians at the Oslo Sports Trauma

Research Center at the Norwegian School of Sport Sciences in Oslo, Norway, with their Injury Surveillance System is making a concerted effort to scientifically investigate the incidence and causes of ACL injury. Their thorough research to date has documented that during the 5-month FIS WC season, 1 in every 3 skiers sustains a time-loss injury, with an incidence rate during competition of 9.8 injuries per 1000 runs. Knee injuries, in particular, ACL ruptures, are the most common.

This study gathered together a group of international experts in skiing biomechanics and sports medicine related to alpine skiing to do systematic qualitative analyses of video recordings of 20 cases of documented ACL injuries. Further information about the exact methods of analysis is available as Appendices in the online version of this article at http://ajs.sagepub.com/supplemental/. With sophisticated video editing, it was possible to identify the index moment of injury (as agreed upon by consensus decision of at least 4 of the 7 experts), as well as the causative mechanism. Other variables, such as characteristics of the ACL injury, weather and snow conditions, and skiing situation, were recorded on the injury reporting forms used by FIS at the time of the injury. Based on the video analysis, injury mechanisms were classified into 3 main categories: slip-catch and dynamic snowplow, both of which involve internal rotation and valgus loading of the knee, and landing back-weighted. Landing back-weighted is somewhat similar to the boot-induced anterior drawer (BIAD) mechanism, previously reported for recreational skiers. Other postulated dynamics, including the phantom foot in recreational skiers and the eccentric quadriceps contraction following BIAD, were not identified by video analysis in this more elite group. These findings are of extreme importance, in that they represent the first step toward developing prevention programs for these devastating injuries.

C. Lebrun, MDCM, MPE, CCFP, Dip Sport Med, FACSM

Reference

1. Ettlinger CF, Johnson RJ, Shealy JE. A method to help reduce the risk of serious knee sprains incurred in alpine skiing. *Am J Sports Med*. 1995;23:531-537.

2 Other Musculoskeletal Injuries

Functional assessment of proximal arm muscles by target-reaching movements in patients with cervical myelopathy
Igarashi K, Shibuya S, Sano H, et al (Kyorin Univ School of Medicine, Mitaka, Tokyo, Japan)
Spine J 11:270-280, 2011

Background Context.—In animal studies, distal and proximal arm movements are differently affected by spinal pyramidotomy because of the contributions of spinal interneuronal systems. In animals, interneuronal systems are also suggested to contribute to the recovery of dexterous hand movements. However, no clinical tests to evaluate proximal arm movements and functions of interneuronal systems have been described.

Purpose.—To compare parameters from proximal arm movements between patients and controls and in patients before and after decompression surgery.

Study Design.—A cross-sectional and longitudinal study performed at Kyorin University School of Medicine, Japan.

Patient Sample.—Patients with clinical features of cervical spondylotic myelopathy, without coexisting neurological abnormality.

Methods.—Twenty-eight patients and 15 age-matched controls performed reach-to-touch movements. Analysis of these movements identified several parameters, including time for online correction (correction time) induced by sudden target jump. Parameters were compared with scores from conventional tests, such as Japanese Orthopedic Association (JOA) score, 10-second grip-and-release test, manual muscle testing, and motor-evoked potential.

Results.—Preoperatively, patients showed long correction time and variable touch position, neither of which correlated with any scores from conventional tests. Reaching parameters recovered markedly immediately after decompression surgery, whereas conventional scores, which mainly assess hand functions, recovered much more slowly. Correction time and JOA score showed correlations when postoperative data were included,

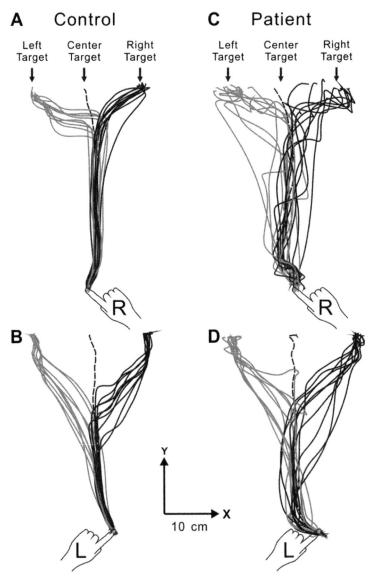

A   Control

Left Target   Center Target   Right Target

C   Patient

Left Target   Center Target   Right Target

B

D

Y

X

10 cm

R

L

R

L

FIGURE 2.—Finger trajectories of (gray lines) left-jump trials and (black lines) right-jump trials in (A, B) two typical control subjects and (C, D) two typical patients. For no-jump trials, (dashed lines) single typical trajectories are shown. (Reprinted from The Spine Journal. Igarashi K, Shibuya S, Sano H, et al. Functional assessment of proximal arm muscles by target-reaching movements in patients with cervical myelopathy. *Spine J.* 2011;11:270-280, Copyright 2011, with permission from Elsevier.)

and long-term recovery of JOA score was more predictable with the inclusion of data for correction times from before and immediately after surgery.

Conclusion.—Analysis of arm movements is useful to evaluate symptoms and predict recovery of hand functions after surgery in patients

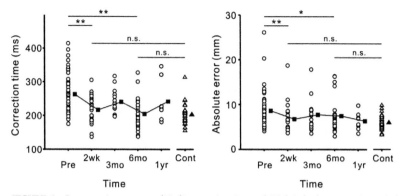

FIGURE 6.—Postoperative recovery of (Left) correction time and (Right) absolute error. Open circles show data from single patients at different times relative to the operation, whereas triangles indicate data from control subjects. Filled symbols represent averages. (Reprinted from The Spine Journal. Igarashi K, Shibuya S, Sano H, et al. Functional assessment of proximal arm muscles by target-reaching movements in patients with cervical myelopathy. *Spine J.* 2011;11:270-280, Copyright 2011, with permission from Elsevier.)

with cervical myelopathy. These results suggest the importance of interneuronal systems, in addition to the pyramidal tract, for motor control even in humans (Figs 2 and 6).

▶ Patients with cervical myelopathy often present with variable impairments but most commonly complain of motor and sensory symptoms in their hands. Cervical myelopathy occurs because of compression of the cervical spinal cord and is often resolved through surgical decompression. The fact that this condition is often seen in the elderly and that variable amounts of time may elapse before decompression is performed results in variable restoration of function. This very good study with well-designed protocols asks the question of whether proximal arm movements are affected differently from distal arm movements given the contribution of spinal interneuronal systems to both. Clinical tests used with this population do not evaluate proximal arm movements nor do they evaluate segmental or multisegmental interneuronal systems, so functional tests are therefore necessary. Igarashi and coworkers developed a novel functional (reach and point) task in which participants were cued to point to 1 of 3 light-emitting diode targets, surrounded by an electrostatic touch sensor, upon a sound cue. In a number of the trials, the target would "jump" 25 milliseconds after the onset of the movement. This paradigm allowed for the collection of 3 temporal aspects of reaching reaction time, movement time, and correction time. A fourth parameter chosen was accuracy measured as the absolute error in millimeters between the actual target and the location of the finger touch by the participants. Fig 2 represents the right and left finger trajectories from 1 age-matched control and 1 patient pre-decompression. Although no differences were found between reaction time and movement time, there were clear deficits in the patients' ability to make smooth corrections during the jump trials. Interestingly, both correction time and absolute error improved significantly by 2 weeks postoperative and were similar to the control group values by 6 months postoperative (see Fig 6). This early recovery was not reflected in the clinical manual muscle tests for either proximal or distal muscles or in the 10-second handgrip test. The inability of ordinary clinical tests to detect the deficits in online adjustments or the improvements postsurgery is noteworthy because proximal reach is obviously missed and is clearly impaired in these patients. This publication is rich in information regarding the state of the human spinal cord and condition of interneuronal circuits. Included are acquisition of motor-evoked potentials using single-pulse transcranial magnetic stimulation of hand and upper arm muscles. Coupled with the evidence from animal studies, it is clear that interneuronal circuits in the spinal cord support both proximal and distal motor control, and recovery of such systems is vital to postoperative recovery following decompression.

V. Galea, PhD

Self-Management of Persistent Neck Pain: Two-Year Follow-up of a Randomized Controlled Trial of a Multicomponent Group Intervention in Primary Health Care

Gustavsson C, Denison E, von Koch L (Ctr for Clinical Res Dalarna, Falun, Sweden; Uppsala Univ, Sweden)
Spine 36:2105-2115, 2011

Study Design.—A 2-year follow-up of a randomized controlled trial.

Objective.—To compare long-term effects of (a) a multicomponent pain and stress self-management group intervention (PASS) and (b) individually administered physical therapy (IAPT) on patients with persistent tension—type neck pain in a primary health care (PHC) setting.

Summary of Background Data.—In a previously reported short-term follow-up, PASS had better effects on pain control, pain-related self-efficacy, disability, and catastrophizing than IAPT. Long-term effects of self-management interventions for persistent neck pain, for example, maintenance of improvement and adherence to coping skills are sparsely investigated.

Methods.—Persons with persistent tension—type neck pain seeking physical therapy treatment at nine PHC centers in Sweden were randomly assigned to either PASS or IAPT. Before intervention, at 10 and 20 weeks and at 1 and 2 years after the intervention, the participants completed a self-assessment questionnaire comprising: the Self-Efficacy Scale, the Neck Disability Index, the Coping Strategies Questionnaire, the Hospital Anxiety and Depression Scale, and questions regarding neck pain and analgesics. Analyses were performed using linear mixed models for repeated measures.

Results.—The study included 156 participants (PASS n = 77, IAPT n = 79). Between baseline, 10-week, 20-week, 1-year, and 2-year follow-up, significant time-by-group interaction effects were found in favor of PASS regarding the primary outcomes ability to control pain ($P < 0.001$)

and self-efficacy for performing activities in spite of pain ($P = 0.002$), and the secondary outcome catastrophic thinking ($P < 0.001$) but not in neck pain—related disability.

Conclusion.—The initial treatment effects of a self-management group intervention were largely maintained over a 2-year follow-up period and with a tendency to have superior long-term effects as compared to individually-administered physical therapy, in the treatment of persistent tension—type neck pain with regard to coping with pain, in terms of pain control, self-efficacy, and catastrophizing (Fig 2).

▶ Self-management is important for persons with any chronic disease or condition. Although there are reports of self-management programs for persons with musculoskeletal conditions, few have assessed long-term effects on outcomes. This randomized, controlled trial evaluates a pain and stress self-management group intervention and compares it with individualized physical therapy sessions for persistent tension-type neck pain (duration > 3 months) with respect to several outcomes 1 and 2 years after intervention. The self-management intervention consisted of 7 weekly group sessions and a booster session at 20 weeks. The individualized physical therapy sessions were left to the judgment of the treating physical therapists. Outcomes assessed were pain intensity, pain control, self-efficacy, disability, catastrophization, depression, and anxiety. The results

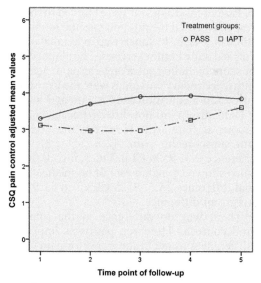

FIGURE 2.—Estimated marginal means for the Coping Strategies Questionnaire, the pain control question (CSQ pain control) adjusted for baseline differences in Neck Disability Index at each point of follow-up: 1 = baseline, 2 = 10 weeks, 3 = 20 weeks, 4 = 1 year, 5 = 2 years. IAPT indicates individually administered physical therapy; PASS, pain and stress self-management group treatment. (Reprinted from the Spine Journal. Gustavsson C, Denison E, von Koch L. Self-management of persistent neck pain: Two-year follow-up of a randomized controlled trial of a multicomponent group intervention in primary health care. *Spine.* 2011;36:2105-2115, Copyright 2011, with permission from North American Spine Society.)

indicated that both groups improved over time; however, the group that received the self-management intervention improved to a greater extent with respect to pain control (Fig 2), self-efficacy, and catastrophization. Withdrawal rate was 35%, and the authors excluded participants with signs of depression—factors that may limit generalizability of the study. Nevertheless, the research underscores that this particular self-management program succeeded in maintaining improvement over time—a vital goal of all self-management programs, to sustain self-management skills over time.

D. E. Feldman, PT, PhD

Assessment of dynamic humeral centering in shoulder pain with impingement syndrome: a randomised clinical trial
Beaudreuil J, Lasbleiz S, Richette P, et al (Université Paris, France)
Ann Rheum Dis 70:1613-1618, 2011

Objectives.—Treatment for degenerative rotator cuff disease of the shoulder includes physiotherapy. Dynamic humeral centering (DHC) aims at preventing subacromial impingement, which contributes to the disease. The goal of this study was to assess the effectiveness of DHC.

Method.—69 patients with shoulder pain and impingement syndrome were prospectively included in a single-centre randomised trial with a 12-month follow-up. Patients and assessor were blinded to the study hypothesis and treatment, respectively. DHC and non-specific mobilisation as control were performed for 6 weeks, in 15 supervised individual outpatient sessions, and patients performed daily home exercises. The planned primary outcome was the Constant score including subscores for pain, activity, mobility and strength at 3 months. Secondary outcomes were the Constant score and subscores at 12 months, and medication use for pain at 3 and 12 months.

Results.—The DHC group did not differ from the control group in the total Constant score at 3 months. However, the DHC group showed a higher Constant subscore for pain (12.2 (SD 2.8) vs 9.9 (2.9), least square means difference 2.1, 95% CI 0.7 to 3.5, p=0.004). At 3 months, the DHC group also showed a higher rate of no medication use (96.7% vs 71%, proportional difference 25.7, 95% CI 3.7 to 51.9, p=0.012). There was no other intergroup difference.

Conclusions.—There was no difference in the total Constant score between DHC and controls. However, pain was improved at 3 months after DHC. The differences found in subscores for pain should be explored in future studies.

Trial registration clinicaltrials.gov Identifier: NCT01022775.

▶ Shoulder disorders such as degenerative rotator cuff disease (which often involves tendon impingement) are common conditions treated by physical therapists. Techniques used by physical therapists include shoulder mobilization and exercises to stretch and to strengthen shoulder musculature. One technique that may be promising in the treatment of shoulder pain with impingement syndrome is dynamic humeral centering. This technique consists of lowering the humeral head during passive shoulder abduction as well as actively lowering the humeral head by cocontraction of pectoralis major and latissimus dorsi during active shoulder abduction. The current study was a randomized, controlled trial to compare this technique with a control program of physical therapy exercises. Although there were no significant differences between groups at 3 months with respect to the Constant total score (a score that measures shoulder function, with subscores for pain, activity, mobility, and strength) the total score was higher (indicating better function) in the experimental group. Further, the experimental group had significantly lower pain than the control group, and they used significantly less medication than those in the conventional shoulder physical therapy group. It is important to note that both groups improved over time. Although it is possible that with time they may have improved regardless of treatment, this is improbable because most of the patients had pain for more than 3 months (25 of 34 and 30 of 35, respectively, in the experimental and control groups). The study was likely underpowered but nevertheless, the results indicate that dynamic humeral centering is a promising technique to treat shoulder pain in impingement syndrome and should be included in physical therapy programs that manage these conditions.

D. E. Feldman, PT, PhD

Comparison of High-Power Pain Threshold Ultrasound Therapy With Local Injection in the Treatment of Active Myofascial Trigger Points of the Upper Trapezius Muscle

Unalan H, Majlesi J, Aydin FY, et al (Istanbul Univ, Turkey; Medicana International Hosp, Istanbul, Turkey)
Arch Phys Med Rehabil 92:657-662, 2011

Objective.—To compare the effects of high-power pain threshold ultrasound (HPPTUS) therapy and local anesthetic injection on pain and active cervical lateral bending in patients with active myofascial trigger points (MTrPs) of the upper trapezius muscle.

Design.—Randomized single-blinded controlled trial.

Setting.—Physical medicine and rehabilitation department of university hospital.

Participants.—Subjects (N = 49) who had active MTrPs of the upper trapezius muscle.

Interventions.—HPPTUS or trigger point injection (TrP).

Main Outcome Measures.—Visual analog scale, range of motion (ROM) of the cervical spine, and total length of treatments.

Results.—All patients in both groups improved significantly in terms of pain and ROM, but there was no statistically significant difference between groups. Mean numbers of therapy sessions were 1 and 1.5 in the local injection and HPPTUS groups, respectively.

Conclusions.—We failed to show differences between the HPPTUS technique and TrP injection in the treatment of active MTrPs of the upper trapezius muscle. The HPPTUS technique can be used as an effective alternative to TrP injection in the treatment of myofascial pain syndrome.

▶ This randomized controlled trial compared a technique called high-power pain threshold ultrasound with lidocaine injection for myofascial trigger points of the upper trapezius in patients with neck pain. The high-power pain threshold ultrasound consists of a technique in which continuous mode ultrasound is applied at a high intensity (to elicit threshold pain) and kept on for 3 to 4 seconds after which the intensity is reduced to half for 15 seconds; this procedure is repeated 3 times. There were no differences between the 2 groups regarding change in pain (as measured on a visual analog scale) or range of motion of the neck. On average, the ultrasound group received 1.5 sessions versus 1 treatment for the injection group. The authors conclude that there were no differences between the 2 groups and that ultrasound, being less invasive, is a possible option to treat this type of pain. However, as noted by the authors, there is no indication of whether there was long-term improvement (the outcomes were measured after treatment, at 1 week after treatment, and a telephone follow-up was done at 4 weeks after treatment). In addition to comparisons with other techniques, including exercise, longer-term follow-up is needed.

D. E. Feldman, PT, PhD

Clavicular Fracture in a Collegiate Football Player: A Case Report of Rapid Return to Play
Rabe SB, Oliver GD (Univ of Arkansas, Fayetteville)
J Athl Train 46:107-111, 2011

Objective.—To present the case of surgical treatment and rehabilitation of a midshaft clavicular fracture in a National Collegiate Athletic Association Division I football athlete.

Background.—While attempting to catch a pass during practice, the athlete jumped up and then landed on the tip of his shoulder. On-the-field evaluation was inconclusive, with a sideline evaluation diagnosis of clavicular fracture. Postinjury radiographs revealed a midshaft clavicular fracture.

Differential Diagnosis.—Spiral oblique midshaft clavicular fracture.

Treatment.—The sports medicine staff discussed surgical and nonsurgical options. A surgical procedure of internal fixation with an 8-hole plate was performed.

Uniqueness.—Surgical treatment for clavicular fractures is becoming increasingly common. This is the first report of an advanced rehabilitation protocol for surgical repair. We suggest that new rehabilitation protocols for clavicular repairs be investigated now that surgical treatment is being pursued more frequently.

Conclusions.—More aggressive treatment procedures and rehabilitation protocols for clavicular fractures have evolved in recent years. With these medical advancements, athletes are able to return to play much more quickly without compromising their health and safety.

▶ This is a case report of surgical treatment of a midshaft clavicular fracture, with early aggressive rehabilitation, which allowed this National Collegiate Athletic Association Division I football athlete to return to active competition (starting line-up) within 6 weeks. This is akin to surgical fixation of a Jones fracture (fracture of the base of the fifth metatarsal bone), in order to allow earlier return-to-play in running and jumping sports. Even though this type of injury has traditionally been treated nonoperatively, increasingly, early plate fixation has been used to allow athletes to return to sport activity. The literature is a bit divided on this point, with results of randomized controlled clinical trials just beginning to emerge. More studies are presently underway. This article provides some background to current orthopedic opinion but, more importantly, details an accelerated rehabilitation program for clavicle fracture. Future research should include standardization of the rehabilitation treatment program for both operative and nonoperative groups in order to more accurately document important differences in healing and recovery.

C. Lebrun, MDCM, MPE, CCFP, Dip Sport Med, FACSM

Does Platelet-Rich Plasma Accelerate Recovery After Rotator Cuff Repair? A Prospective Cohort Study
Jo CH, Kim JE, Yoon KS, et al (Seoul Natl Univ College of Medicine, Korea)
Am J Sports Med 39:2082-2090, 2011

Background.—Platelet-rich plasma (PRP) has been recently used to enhance and accelerate the healing of musculoskeletal injuries and diseases, but evidence is still lacking, especially on its effects after rotator cuff repair.

Hypothesis.—Platelet-rich plasma accelerates recovery after arthroscopic rotator cuff repair in pain relief, functional outcome, overall satisfaction, and enhanced structural integrity of repaired tendon.

Study Design.—Cohort study; Level of evidence, 2.

Methods.—Forty-two patients with full-thickness rotator cuff tears were included. Patients were informed about the use of PRP before surgery and decided themselves whether to have PRP placed at the time of surgery. Nineteen patients underwent arthroscopic rotator cuff repair with PRP and 23 without. Platelet-rich plasma was prepared via plateletpheresis and applied in the form of a gel threaded to a suture and placed at the interface between tendon and bone. Outcomes were assessed preoperatively and at 3, 6, 12, and finally at a minimum of 16 months after surgery (at an average of 19.7 ± 1.9 months) with respect to pain, range of motion, strength, and overall satisfaction, and with respect to functional scores as determined using the following scoring systems: the American Shoulder and Elbow Surgeon (ASES) system, the Constant system, the University of California at Los Angeles (UCLA) system, the Disabilities of the Arm, Shoulder and Hand (DASH) system, the Simple Shoulder Test (SST) system, and the Shoulder Pain and Disability Index (SPADI) system. At a minimum of 9 months after surgery, repaired tendon structural integrities were assessed by magnetic resonance imaging.

Results.—Platelet-rich plasma gel application to arthroscopic rotator cuff repairs did not accelerate recovery with respect to pain, range of motion, strength, functional scores, or overall satisfaction as compared with conventional repair at any time point. Whereas magnetic resonance imaging demonstrated a retear rate of 26.7% in the PRP group and 41.2% in the conventional group, there was no statistical significance between the groups ($P = .388$).

Conclusion.—The results suggest that PRP application during arthroscopic rotator cuff repair did not clearly demonstrate accelerated recovery clinically or anatomically except for an improvement in internal rotation. Nevertheless, as the study may have been underpowered to detect clinically important differences in the structural integrity, additional investigations, including the optimization of PRP preparation and a larger randomized study powered for healing rate, are necessary to further determine the effect of PRP (Fig 1).

▶ The use of platelet-rich plasma (PRP) is increasingly touted as a strategy to enhance repair and regeneration of tendon, ligament, and muscle. This is thought to occur via the release of a myriad of different growth factors. However, depending on the commercial kit utilized to prepare the PRP, there is wide variation in the amount of platelets obtained and contamination of the final product with leukocytes. The optimal platelet concentration has not yet been scientifically determined. In addition, the mode of delivery of the PRP concentrate to the correct anatomical site is critical. The strengths of this study, even though patients were not randomized and the outcomes were not assessed in a blinded fashion, revolve around the standardization of PRP production and the reproducible application of PRP. The investigators used a fully automated plasmapheresis system to obtain a final product with a consistent platelet count. They were able to ensure placement at the appropriate site through producing a gel, which was threaded onto a suture and interposed between tendon and bone under direct vision through the arthroscope (Fig 1). The theoretical risks of infection (because of introducing something into the joint that was prepared ex vivo) and arthrofibrosis (because of the potential effects of PRP) did not occur. Postoperatively, structural integrity of the repair was assessed by MRI, done approximately 1 year later. Although there were no significant differences found between the 2 groups (PRP or no PRP) on any of the outcome measures, the authors do suggest that this study may have been underpowered to detect statistically significant differences in the measures of interest. Further research is warranted, especially using randomized double blind designs, to build more knowledge about this theoretically beneficial treatment. However, practically, most users of this new technology would not have access in their offices to a fully automated platelet-pheresis system, but at least the mode of delivery of the PRP product should be

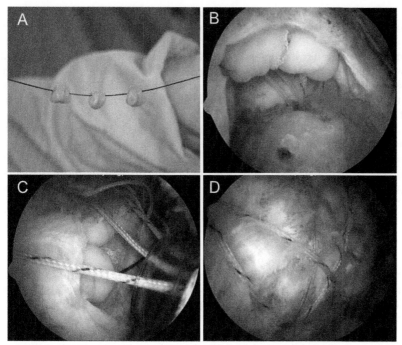

FIGURE 1.—The arthroscopic procedure applying platelet-rich plasma (PRP) gels. A, 3 PRP gels of 3 mL each are threaded to a No. 1 PDS (polydioxanone) II suture. B, after sutures were placed in the medial row through torn rotator cuff, the 3 PRP gels are placed in the repair site, viewed from the postero-lateral viewing portal. C, just before sutures of the lateral row were tightened using a suture bridge technique, PRP gels are interposed between the tendon-bone interface. D, the final appearance of the repaired rotator cuff tendon. The PRP gels are not visible because they are snuggled between the repaired tendon and the bone insertion. (Reprinted from Jo CH, Kim JE, Yoon KS, et al. Does platelet-rich plasma accelerate recovery after rotator cuff repair? A prospective cohort study. *Am J Sports Med.* 2011;39:2082-2090, with permission from The Author(s).)

as accurate as possible. Outside the operating room, the use of diagnostic ultrasound can aid in optimal visualization of the specific site to be treated.

C. Lebrun, MDCM, MPE, CCFP, Dip Sport Med, FACSM

Matched-Cohort Study of Body Composition, Physical Function, and Quality of Life in Men With Idiopathic Vertebral Fracture
Macdonald JH, Evans SF, Davies HL, et al (Bangor Univ, Gwynedd, UK; Robert Jones & Agnes Hunt Orthopaedic Hosp NHS Foundation Trust, Gobowen, Shropshire, UK)
Arthritis Care Res (Hoboken) 64:92-100, 2012

Objective.—To determine the effect of 6 years of routine management on body composition, physical functioning, and quality of life, and their interrelationships, in men with idiopathic vertebral fracture.

Methods.—Twenty men with idiopathic vertebral fracture (patients: mean ± SD age 58 ± 6 years) were age and height matched to 28 healthy controls with no known disease. The primary outcome was skeletal muscle mass (appendicular lean mass by dual x-ray absorptiometry) assessed at 2 visits (0 and 6 years). Physical functioning and quality of life domains were assessed by the Senior Fitness Test and Short Form 36 (SF-36) questionnaire at visit 2 only. Data were analyzed by repeated-measures analysis of variance, independent *t*-tests, and correlation.

Results.—At visit 1, appendicular lean mass was 9% lower in patients than controls. Although patients better maintained appendicular lean mass between visits (interaction $P = 0.016$), at visit 2 appendicular lean mass remained 5% lower in patients than controls. Furthermore, patients' appendicular lean mass change was correlated with femoral neck bone density change (r = 0.507, $P = 0.023$). Physical function tests were 13–27% lower in patients compared with controls ($P = 0.056$ to 0.003), as were SF-36 quality of life physical domains (13–26% lower; $P = 0.028$ to <0.001).

Conclusion.—Despite an association between changes in muscle mass and bone density, routine management of men with idiopathic vertebral fracture does not address muscle loss. Combined with the observation of reduced physical functioning and quality of life, this study identifies novel targets for intervention in men with idiopathic vertebral fracture.

▶ The importance of this study rests on the underappreciated fact that the incidence of vertebral (thoracic and lumbar) fracture in men equals that of women, even though fewer men have osteoporosis. Treatment of men with osteoporosis addresses mitigation of bone loss and fracture prevention but does not encompass comorbidities that could impact quality of life and physical function. This is the first longitudinal study of body composition changes in men with idiopathic vertebral fracture. At study entry, appendicular lean mass, lumbar spine and femoral neck bone mineral density (BMD), and total body bone mineral content were significantly lower in men with fractures compared with controls matched on age and height. Over the 6-year follow-up period, appendicular lean mass remained stable, and lumbar spine increased 11% in the men with fractures. The 2% decrease in appendicular lean mass found in the control group suggests age-related changes, although it is not clear why the fracture group was spared this change. In contrast, femoral neck BMD was stable over time in both groups. Notably, in men with fractures, the changes in femoral neck BMD and appendicular lean mass were positively correlated (r = 0.51, $P = .023$). Muscle and bone mass may be synchronized by mechanical strain, anabolic hormonal interactions, or other mechanisms. The changes in lumbar spine BMD and appendicular lean mass were not significantly correlated, suggesting perhaps more potent, local interactions between leg lean mass and femoral bone than lumbar vertebral bone. Nearly all of the objective and subjective measures of physical function were significantly lower in men with fracture compared with controls at the follow-up visit (no longitudinal measures). Greater body pain was strongly related to poorer upper and lower extremity function in the fracture patients.

Better pain management may help men with vertebral fracture to improve physical function. It is not known if exercise interventions could reduce pain, among other benefits, in this population who has increased risk of another fracture.

C. M. Jankowski, PhD

Safety of "pain exposure" physical therapy in patients with complex regional pain syndrome type 1
van de Meent H, Oerlemans M, Bruggeman A, et al (Radboud Univ Nijmegen Med Centre, The Netherlands)
Pain 152:1431-1438, 2011

"Pain exposure" physical therapy (PEPT) is a new treatment for patients with complex regional pain syndrome type 1 (CRPS-1) that consists of a progressive-loading exercise program and management of pain-avoidance behavior without the use of specific CRPS-1 medication or analgesics. The aim of this study was to investigate primarily whether PEPT could be applied safely in patients with CRPS-1. Twenty patients with CRPS-1 were consecutively enrolled in the study after giving informed consent. The diagnosis of CRPS-1 was defined using the Bruehl and Harden/IASP diagnostic criteria. CRPS-1 was diagnosed between 3 and 18 months after the inciting event (trauma). According to a multiple single-case design (baseline [A1], treatment [B], follow-up [A2]), multiple baseline and follow-up measurements were performed to evaluate changes in CRPS signs and symptoms and to assess functional parameters. When comparing the baseline with the follow-up phase, patients improved significantly with respect to pain on the visual analogue scale (57%), pain intensity (48%), muscle strength (52%), arm/shoulder/hand disability (36%), 10-meter walking speed (29%), pain disability index (60%), kinesiophobia (18%), and the domains of perceived health change in the SF-36 survey (269%). Three patients initially showed increased vegetative signs but improved in all other CRPS parameters and showed good functional recovery at follow-up. We conclude that PEPT is a safe and effective treatment for patients with CRPS-1.

▶ A randomized controlled trial would be necessary to show whether pain exposure physical therapy (PEPT) is beneficial in patients with complex regional pain syndrome type I (CRPS I); however, the researchers are able to make a strong case for the use of these techniques using a prospective observational study on patients with long-standing CRPS I. PEPT consists of a progressive loading exercise program and desensitization beyond patients' pain limits. Along with cognitive behavioral elements (which include reassurance of patients that pain is not a sign of tissue damage), medications are gradually stopped. The investigators monitored multiple outcomes over time on 20 patients who were undergoing PEPT treatment and found improvement with respect to pain, joint mobility, muscle strength, function, kinesiophobia, and perceived health change. The conclusion is that PEPT is safe and can be used safely to treat this difficult condition. Further proof of the efficacy of PEPT (and its superiority to current treatment techniques) will require a randomized trial design.

D. E. Feldman, PT, PhD

The efficacy, safety, effectiveness, and cost-effectiveness of ultrasound and shock wave therapies for low back pain: a systematic review
Seco J, Kovacs FM, Urrutia G (Univ of León, Ponferrada, Spain; Spanish Back Pain Res Network, Palma de Mallorca)
Spine J 11:966-977, 2011

Background Context.—Shock wave and especially ultrasound are commonly used to treat low back pain (LBP) in routine practice.

Purpose.—To assess the evidence on the efficacy, effectiveness, cost-effectiveness, and safety of ultrasound and shock wave to treat LBP.

Study Design.—Systematic review.

Methods.—An electronic search was performed in MEDLINE, EMBASE, and the Cochrane Library databases up to July 2009 to identify randomized controlled trials (RCTs) comparing vibro-therapy with placebo or with other treatments for LBP. No language restrictions were applied. Additional data were requested from the authors of the original studies. The risk of bias of each study was assessed following the criteria recommended by the Cochrane Back Review Group.

Results.—Thirteen studies were identified. The four RCTs complying with the inclusion criteria included 252 patients. Two of the three RCTs on ultrasound had a high risk of bias. For acute patients with LBP and leg pain attributed to disc herniation, ultrasound, traction, and low-power laser obtained similar results. For chronic LBP patients without leg pain, ultrasound was less effective than spinal manipulation, whereas a shock wave device and transcutaneous electrical nerve stimulation led to similar results. Results from the only study comparing ultrasound versus a sham procedure are unreliable because of the inappropriateness of the sham procedure, low sample size, and lack of adjustment for potential confounders. No study assessed cost-effectiveness. No adverse events were reported.

Conclusion.—The available evidence does not support the effectiveness of ultrasound or shock wave for treating LBP. High-quality RCTs are needed to assess their efficacy versus appropriate sham procedures, and their effectiveness and cost-effectiveness versus other procedures shown to be effective for LBP. In the absence of such evidence, the clinical use of these forms of treatment is not justified and should be discouraged.

▶ The 2007 guidelines for diagnosis and treatment of low back pain[1] support the following treatments for nonspecific low back pain (strong recommendation, moderate level of evidence): exercise, remaining active, patient education, and pain-relieving medication such as acetaminophen or nonsteroidal anti-inflammatory drugs. Weaker recommendations regarding other types of interventions include spinal manipulation, intensive interdisciplinary rehabilitation, acupuncture, massage, yoga, and cognitive behavioral therapy. However, neither ultrasound nor shockwave therapy are currently recommended for low back pain treatment. This study examines these 2 types of treatment, in view of their popularity and possible efficacy in treating other musculoskeletal conditions. The authors performed a systematic review to analyze the efficacy and safety of these modalities in the treatment of low back pain. Although their search did result in 13 studies on the subject, only 4 were deemed of sufficiently high quality: 3 on ultrasound and 1 on shockwave. Neither ultrasound nor shockwave resulted in better outcomes for patients. The conclusions are sound: there is no evidence to support the effectiveness of ultrasound or shockwave for low back pain. However, this study also highlights the need for high-quality research studies in the area of low back pain, an extremely common and costly problem in our society.

D. E. Feldman, PT, PhD

Reference

1. Chou R, Qaseem A, Snow V, et al; Clinical Efficacy Assessment Subcommittee of the American College of Physicians. Diagnosis and treatment of low back pain: a joint clinical practice guideline from the American College of Physicians and the American Pain Society. *Ann Intern Med.* 2007;147:478-491.

Aerobic Exercise Training in Addition to Conventional Physiotherapy for Chronic Low Back Pain: A Randomized Controlled Trial
Chan CW, Mok NW, Yeung EW (The Hong Kong Polytechnic Univ, Kowloon)
Arch Phys Med Rehabil 92:1681-1685, 2011

Objective.—To examine the effect of adding aerobic exercise to conventional physiotherapy treatment for patients with chronic low back pain (LBP) in reducing pain and disability.

Design.—Randomized controlled trial.

Setting.—A physiotherapy outpatient setting in Hong Kong.

Participants.—Patients with chronic LBP (N = 46) were recruited and randomly assigned to either a control (n = 22) or an intervention (n = 24) group.

Interventions.—An 8-week intervention; both groups received conventional physiotherapy with additional individually tailored aerobic exercise prescribed only to the intervention group.

Main Outcome Measures.—Visual analog pain scale, Aberdeen Low Back Pain Disability Scale, and physical fitness measurements were taken at baseline, 8 weeks, and 12 months from the commencement of the intervention. Multivariate analysis of variance was performed to examine between-group differences.

Results.—Both groups demonstrated a significant reduction in pain ($P<.001$) and an improvement in disability ($P<.001$) at 8 weeks and 12 months; however, no differences were observed between groups. There was no significant difference in LBP relapse at 12 months between the 2 groups (χ^2=2.30, P=.13).

Conclusions.—The addition of aerobic training to conventional physiotherapy treatment did not enhance either short- or long-term improvement of pain and disability in patients with chronic LBP.

▶ There have been numerous studies related to low back pain with respect to the various treatment approaches that may be beneficial. This randomized controlled trial assessed whether the addition of aerobic training improves outcomes in patients who receive conventional physical therapy for low back pain over an 8-week period compared with conventional therapy alone. Conventional treatment was up to the discretion of the treating physical therapist and included electrical modalities, passive mobilization, back care advice, and exercise (back mobilization, abdominal stabilization). Aerobic training consisted of 2 training sessions under the supervision of a physical therapist and instruction to perform at least 1 more training session at home per week. Both groups improved at both the 8-week evaluation (posttreatment) and at 12 weeks, although there were no differences between the 2 groups. The authors conclude that the addition of aerobic exercise to conventional physical therapy does not appear to improve pain (at the 8-week time point) or disability (at 8- and 12-week time points) in patients with chronic low back pain. Although the conclusion is sound based on the study results, the authors did not measure pain at the 12-week assessment (claiming that "fluctuation in pain level seems to be one of the characteristic features in low back pain"). This explanation would hold as well for the 8-week assessment. Furthermore, the 12-week assessment was done over the phone; pain level could be assessed by numerical rating scales with relative ease. Finally, as the authors point out, the aerobic exercise training improved physical fitness parameters in the intervention group. Possibly the magnitude of change was small, and a more intense or longer program is needed.

D. E. Feldman, PT, PhD

The McKenzie Method Compared With Manipulation When Used Adjunctive to Information and Advice in Low Back Pain Patients Presenting With Centralization or Peripheralization: A Randomized Controlled Trial
Petersen T, Larsen K, Nordsteen J, et al (Back Ctr Copenhagen, Denmark; Holstebro Univ Hosp, Denmark; Copenhagen Univ Hosp, Denmark)
Spine 36:1999-2010, 2011

Study Design.—Randomized controlled trial.

Objective.—To compare the effects of the McKenzie method performed by certified therapists with spinal manipulation performed by chiropractors when used adjunctive to information and advice.

Summary of Background Data.—Recent guidelines recommend a structured exercise program tailored to the individual patient as well as manual therapy for the treatment of persistent low back pain. There is presently insufficient evidence to recommend the use of specific decision methods tailoring specific therapies to clinical subgroups of patients in primary care.

Methods.—A total of 350 patients suffering from low back pain with a duration of more than 6 weeks who presented with centralization or peripheralization of symptoms with or without signs of nerve root involvement, were enrolled in the trial. Main outcome was number of patients with treatment success defined as a reduction of at least 5 points or an absolute score below 5 points on the Roland Morris Questionnaire. Secondary outcomes were reduction in disability and pain, global perceived effect, general health, mental health, lost work time, and medical care utilization.

Results.—Both treatment groups showed clinically meaningful improvements in this study. At 2 months follow-up, the McKenzie treatment was superior to manipulation with respect to the number of patients who reported success after treatment (71% and 59%, respectively) (odds ratio 0.58, 95% confidence interval [CI] 0.36 to 0.91, $P = 0.018$). The number needed to treat with the McKenzie method was 7 (95% CI 4 to 47). The McKenzie group showed improvement in level of disability compared to the manipulation group reaching a statistical significance at 2 and 12 months follow-up (mean difference 1.5, 95% CI 0.2 to 2.8, $P = 0.022$ and 1.5, 95% CI 0.2 to 2.9, $P = 0.030$, respectively). There was also a significant difference of 13% in number of patients reporting global perceived effect at end of treatment ($P = 0.016$). None of the other secondary outcomes showed statistically significant differences.

Conclusion.—In patients with low back pain for more than 6 weeks presenting with centralization or peripheralization of symptoms, we found the McKenzie method to be slightly more effective than manipulation when used adjunctive to information and advice.

▶ Among current recommendations for management of low back pain are providing evidence-based information regarding expected course of the problem, advising patients to stay active, self-management information, use of medications if needed, and nonpharmacologic treatments, such as rehabilitation, exercise, and spinal manipulation. Many studies have compared various types of interventions for persons with low back pain. This study aimed to compare the effects of the McKenzie method with that of spinal manipulation in patients with low back pain lasting longer than 6 weeks. The McKenzie method utilizes assessment, treatment, and prevention strategies and aims at reducing pain (especially for those with pain in the extremities). The study was a randomized, controlled trial. The 2 groups consisted of those treated via the McKenzie method (delivered by McKenzie method—trained physical therapists, using no manual vertebral mobilization techniques) and those treated with spinal manipulation (delivered by experienced chiropractors using any type of manual technique). Both groups also received advice and guidance on back care and the importance of remaining active. The main outcome measure was treatment success, defined as a reduction of at least 5 points on the Roland Morris Disability Questionnaire. Other outcomes were also assessed (eg, change in the disability score, pain, global perceived effect, quality of life, days with reduced activity, return to work, satisfaction, and use of health care following treatment completion). In both groups there was a reduction in mean disability greater than 50%. Global perceived effect was significantly higher in the McKenzie group as was reported treatment success at 2 months follow-up, although the differences were not large. The authors conclude that the McKenzie method is slightly more effective than manipulation. However, there were more patients who withdrew from the trial in the manipulation group. As the authors point out, future research should focus on identifying which patients respond better to each treatment or perhaps even a combination of the 2.

D. E. Feldman, PT, PhD

Rapid Enlargement of Elastofibroma Dorsi After Physical Therapy
Tokat AO, Karasu S, Turan A, et al (Ministry of Health Ankara Education and Res Hosp, Turkey)
Ann Thorac Surg 91:1622-1624, 2011

Elastofibroma dorsi is an uncommon, slow-growing, ill-defined soft tissue tumor. Its most prominent symptom is back and shoulder pain. Elastofibroma dorsi is usually located beneath the scapula and bilateral involvement occurs in only 10% of patients. We report herein a case of bilateral elastofibroma dorsi who underwent physical therapy for treatment of shoulder pain. Elastofibroma was misdiagnosed and rapidly progressed after physical therapy. We conclude that elastofibroma should be kept in mind for patients with shoulder or back pain, and the patient should be evaluated carefully before initiating physical therapy.

▶ This article describes a case of elastofibroma that, although rare, may be responsible for certain types of shoulder pain. This tumor, characterized by a proliferation of fibrous tissue with elastin, usually arises between the lower angle of the scapula and the thoracic wall. In the case described, the tumor was not initially detected and the patient underwent physical therapy that included application of heat. The patient did not improve and actually noticed some swelling after the physical therapy treatment. Upon further investigation, the tumor was diagnosed and subsequently excised. The authors suggest that perhaps heat treatment increased tumor growth by enhancing blood flow. Although there is no direct evidence to support this contention, patients who have persistent upper back and shoulder pain should be thoroughly evaluated prior to initiating heat treatment.

D. E. Feldman, PT, PhD

Physiotherapy Rehabilitation Post First Lumbar Discectomy: A Systematic Review and Meta-Analysis of Randomized Controlled Trials

Rushton A, Wright C, Goodwin P, et al (Univ of Birmingham, Edgbaston, UK; Manchester Metropolitan Univ, UK; et al)
Spine 36:E961-E972, 2011

Study Design.—Systematic review and meta-analysis.

Objective.—To evaluate effectiveness of physiotherapy intervention in patients post first lumbar discectomy on clinically relevant outcomes short (3 months) and longer term (12 months).

Summary of Background Data.—Physiotherapy intervention is recommended post discectomy, although the most beneficial intervention and the effectiveness of physiotherapy management is unclear.

Methods.—Randomized Controlled Trials (RCTs) published in English before December 31, 2009 investigating physiotherapy outpatient management of patients (>16 years), post first single level lumbar discectomy were included. Measurements reported on ≥1 outcome of disability, function, and health were included. Two reviewers independently searched information sources, assessed studies for inclusion, and evaluated risk of bias. Quantitative synthesis was conducted on comparable outcomes across studies with similar interventions and no clearly identified overall risk of bias.

Results.—Sixteen RCTs (1336 participants) from 11 countries were included. Interventions were categorized as intervention *versus* control/ sham, and less *versus* more intensive comparisons. Eight of 16 trials were evaluated as high risk of bias, 7 as unclear and 1 as low. Six hundred and thirty-five participants were incorporated in the meta-analysis on eight trials. Although evidence from two trials suggested that intervention might reduce disability short-term, and more intensive intervention may be more beneficial than less intensive, the pooled effects (−0.89, 95% CI −1.84 to 0.06 for intervention *vs.* control/sham; −0.27, 95% CI −0.80 to 0.25 for more *vs.* less intensive) did not show statistically significant effects. There was no evidence that intervention changes range of movement flexion (ROM) or overall impairment short term, or disability or back pain longer term. There was no evidence that intensity of intervention affects back pain short or longer term, ROM short term, or patients' satisfaction with outcome longer term. Substantial heterogeneity was evident.

Conclusion.—Inconclusive evidence exists for the effectiveness of outpatient physiotherapy post first lumbar discectomy. Best practice remains unclear.

▶ This meta-analysis and systematic review underscores the lack of high-quality (low risk of bias) randomized controlled trials regarding physiotherapy interventions after lumbar discectomy surgery. Although a few studies indicated short-term benefits, pooled analysis did not uphold these results. In addition, there was no evidence of long-term benefits for physiotherapy interventions, although there was some suggestion that more intensive intervention may be beneficial. It must be emphasized that there was heterogeneity in the studies, with some investigating group interventions and some evaluating individualized management. Moreover, these interventions may have included exercise, behavioral rehabilitation, back school, and other treatments. The authors discuss that the lack of evidence regarding benefits of physiotherapy (especially long-term benefits) may explain the large variation in practice regarding routine treatment after spinal surgery with respect to physiotherapy referral, functional restrictions advised by the surgeons, and types of physiotherapy interventions. There is a clear need for further research in this area.

D. E. Feldman, PT, PhD

Change in Psychosocial Distress Associated With Pain and Functional Status Outcomes in Patients With Lumbar Impairments Referred to Physical Therapy Services
Werneke MW, Hart DL, George SZ, et al (CentraState Med Ctr, Freehold, NJ; Focus on Therapeutic Outcomes Inc, White Stone, VA; Univ of Florida, Gainesville; et al)
J Orthop Sports Phys Ther 41:969-980, 2011

Study Design.—Prospective, longitudinal, observational cohort design.

Objective.—The primary aim was to examine the association between changes in psychosocial distress (PD), and functional status (FS) and pain intensity at discharge from physical therapy.

Background.—Patients with lumbar impairments seeking physical therapy commonly demonstrate elevated PD. However, it is not clear if PD changes that occur during physical therapy management are associated with improved clinical outcomes.

Methods.—Data from adults (n = 692) with lumbar impairment were analyzed. Patients were screened using the Symptom Checklist Back Pain Prediction Model questionnaire (SCL BPPM) to identify patients at intake and discharge into 3 levels of risk for persistent disability (high, intermediate, or low). SCL BPPM classifications allowed for 5 patterns of change in PD during therapy (decreased, stable low, stable intermediate, stable high, or increased). Associations between PD change patterns and discharge FS and pain intensity were assessed using multivariable linear regression models, controlling for selected risk-adjustment variables.

Results.—Proportions of patients classified by patterns of PD change for decreased, stable low, stable intermediate, stable high, and increased were 0.34, 0.52, 0.05, 0.06, and 0.03, respectively. Compared to the decreased PD group, (1) increased, stable high, and stable intermediate PD patterns were associated with worse discharge FS scores (-7.9 [95% CI: -13.5, -2.21], -10.9 [95% CI: -15.25, -6.49], and -8.9 [95% CI: -13.65, -4.21] units, respectively), and (2) stable high and stable intermediate PD patterns were associated with higher pain intensity (2.59 [95% CI: 1.81, 3.56] and 2.14 [95% CI: 1.25, 3.04] units, respectively).

Conclusions.—Lower FS and higher pain intensity outcomes were associated in similar but not identical patterns with patients whose SCL BPPM classification of PD increased, or remained at high or intermediate levels during physical therapy. Serial assessments of change in PD during rehabilitation are recommended as a possible treatment-monitoring tool.

▶ Many studies have identified psychosocial distress as a prognostic factor for chronic disability in persons with low back pain. This cohort study examines whether there is an association between changes in psychosocial distress over the course of physical therapy treatment and outcomes (function and pain) in persons who were followed up in physical therapy for low back pain. All patients were followed up by physical therapists skilled in McKenzie mechanical diagnosis and treatment method in 8 different clinics. Change in psychosocial distress was classified using the System Checklist Back Pain Predictive Model by using intake and discharge scores to categorize patients in 5 risk categories (decreased risk, increased risk, stable low risk, stable intermediate risk, and stable high risk). Pain intensity was measured on the 11-point numeric pain scale, and functional status was evaluated using computerized adaptive testing that used items from various scales to assign a score per patient corresponding to a person's perception of the ability to perform daily functional tasks. Almost half of the patients had intermediate to high levels of psychosocial distress at intake; however, approximately 75% of these had less distress and improved functional outcomes at discharge. Further, those patients whose distress increased or remained unchanged at high or intermediate levels had fewer improvements in function and higher pain compared with those whose psychosocial distress level was low or decreased. Almost one-fifth of patients remained at intermediate or high risk for persistent functional limitations and higher pain. These findings have implications for practice: monitoring psychosocial distress over time may be important to monitor distress and refer those patients who maintain a high level of distress over time.

D. E. Feldman, PT, PhD

Bone Quality and Muscle Strength in Female Athletes with Lower Limb Stress Fractures
Schnackenburg KE, MacDonald HM, Ferber R, et al (Univ of Calgary, Alberta, Canada; Univ of British Columbia, Vancouver, Canada)
Med Sci Sports Exerc 43:2110-2119, 2011

Purpose.—Lower limb stress fractures (SF) have a high prevalence in female athletes of running-related sports. The purpose of this study was to investigate bone quality, including bone microarchitecture and strength, and muscle strength in athletes diagnosed with SF.

Methods.—Female athletes with lower limb SF (SF subjects, $n = 19$, 18−45 yr, premenopausal) and healthy female athletes (NSF subjects, $n = 19$) matched according to age, sport, and weekly training volume were recruited. Bone microarchitecture of all participants was assessed using high-resolution peripheral quantitative computed tomography at two skeletal sites along the distal tibia of the dominant leg. Bone strength and load distribution between cortical and trabecular bone was estimated by finite element analysis. Using dual-energy X-ray absorptiometry, areal bone mineral density (aBMD) at the hip, femoral neck, and spine was measured. Muscle torque (knee extension, plantarflexion, eversion/inversion) was assessed (Biodex dynamometer) as a measure of lower leg muscle strength.

Results.—SF subjects, after adjusting for body weight, had thinner tibia compared with NSF subjects as indicated by a lower tibial cross-sectional area (-7.8%, $P = 0.02$) and higher load carried by the cortex as indicated by finite element analysis (4.1%, $P = 0.02$). Further site-specific regional analysis revealed that, in the posterior region of the tibia, SF subjects had lower trabecular BMD (-19.8%, $P = 0.02$) and less cortical area (-5.2%, $P = 0.02$). The SF group exhibited reduced knee extension strength (-18.3%, $P = 0.03$) compared with NSF subjects.

Conclusions.—These data suggest an association of impaired bone quality, particularly in the posterior region of the distal tibia, and decreased muscle strength with lower limb SF in female athletes (Fig 2).

▶ In this study, 2 new technologies, high-resolution peripheral quantitative computed tomography (HR-pQCT) and finite element analysis (FEA), were used to compare bone qualities in female athletes aged 18 to 45 years with a radiologically confirmed history of stress fractures (SF) with age- and training-matched control athletes with no SF (NSF). HR-pQCT provides measures of volumetric bone mineral density (BMD) and morphological outcomes such as trabecular number and cortical thickness (Fig 2). FEA estimates bone strength

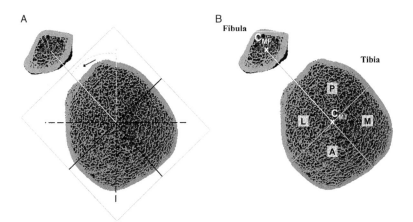

FIGURE 2.—A, HR-pQCT scan of a human distal tibia illustrating the alignment of the quadrant template with the center of mass of the fibula (C_{MF}) and tibia (C_{MT}). B, Regions of the left tibia that were analyzed separately using the customized regional analysis method. A, anterior; L, lateral; M, medial; P, posterior. (Reprinted from Schnackenburg KE, MacDonald HM, Ferber R, et al. Bone quality and muscle strength in female athletes with lower limb stress fractures. *Med Sci Sports Exerc.* 2011;43:2110-2119, with permission from the American College of Sports Medicine.)

and load distribution between the cortical and trabecular compartments. The analyses were performed at ultra-distal and distal sites on the tibia; the distal site was selected to represent the distal one-third of the tibia, a common site of tibial SF in runner-athletes. Athletes with SF had significantly lower areal BMD (measured by dual-energy x-ray absorptiometry) of the hip and spine compared with control subjects; tibial volumetric BMD was not significantly different between groups. The posterior quadrant of the distal tibia had significantly lower trabecular BMD, trends for lower trabecular thickness and number, and significantly lower cortical area in the SF group compared with control subjects. The cortex of the distal region carried 4% more load in the SF group, and the failure load was 13% lower compared with the NSF group. Muscle strength was also considered a contributing factor to SF. Theoretically, muscle weakness would result in the transfer of greater shear stress to the underlying bone than would occur with stronger muscles. Indeed, quadriceps peak isometric strength was 18% lower in the SF group compared with NSF. The authors provided a musculo-skeletal profile of a site in women that is prone to SF. HR-pQCT and FEA hold promise for better understanding of how SFs occur and how to prevent and/or repair this injury.

C. M. Jankowski, PhD

The Effects of Isolated Hip Abductor and External Rotator Muscle Strengthening on Pain, Health Status, and Hip Strength in Females With Patellofemoral Pain: A Randomized Controlled Trial
Khayambashi K, Mohammadkhani Z, Ghaznavi K, et al (Univ of Isfahan, Iran; Rheumatology Res Ctr of Univ of Tehran, Iran; et al)
J Orthop Sports Phys Ther 42:22-29, 2012

Study Design.—Randomized controlled trial.

Objectives.—To examine the effectiveness of isolated hip abductor and external rotator strengthening on pain, health status, and hip strength in females with patellofemoral pain (PFP).

Background.—Altered hip kinematics resulting from hip muscle weakness has been proposed as a contributing factor in the development of PFP. To date, no study has examined clinical outcomes associated with isolated hip muscle strengthening in those with PFP.

Methods.—Twenty-eight females with PFP were sequentially assigned to an exercise (n = 14) or a no-exercise control group (n = 14). The exercise group completed bilateral hip abductor and external rotator strengthening 3 times per week for 8 weeks. Pain (visual analog scale), health status (WOMAC), and hip strength (handheld dynamometer) were assessed at baseline and postintervention. Pain and health status were also evaluated at 6 months postintervention in the exercise group. Two-factor mixed-model analyses of variance were used to determine the effects of the intervention on each outcome variable.

Results.—Significant group-by-time interactions were observed for each variable of interest. Post hoc testing revealed that pain, health status, and

TABLE 1.—Standardized Exercise Progression Using Elastic Tubing

Weeks	Set 1*	Set 2*	Set 3*	Frequency per Week
1-2	Red (20)	Green (20)	Blue (20)	3
3-4	Red (25)	Green (25)	Blue (25)	3
5-6	Green (20)	Blue (20)	Black (20)	3
7-8	Green (25)	Blue (25)	Black (25)	3

*Value are band color, indicating resistance, with repetitions in parentheses. resistance designation: red, medium; green, heavy; blue, extra heavy; black, special heavy.

bilateral hip strength improved in the exercise group following the 8-week intervention but did not change in the control group. Improvements in pain and health status were sustained at 6-month follow-up in the exercise group.

Conclusion.—A program of isolated hip abductor and external rotator strengthening was effective in improving pain and health status in females with PFP compared to a no-exercise control group. The incorporation of hip-strengthening exercises should be considered when designing a rehabilitation program for females with PFP.

Level of Evidence.—Therapy, level 2b (Table 1).

▶ There is growing evidence that impaired muscular control of the hip can contribute to patellofemoral pain (PFP), leading these investigators to determine the effects of a training program of isolated hip exercises on PFP and hip strength. Twenty-eight sedentary women with clinically confirmed bilateral PFP of at least 6 months' duration were randomly allocated to training and control groups. Women with other potential causes of knee pain (eg, patellar tendinitis, iliotibial band syndrome) were excluded from the study. The training comprised 8 weeks of progressive bilateral hip abduction and external rotation exercises using Thera-Band elastic tubing (Table 1). All participants were instructed not to increase their daily activities. Pain was assessed by a visual analog scale (VAS) and the Western Ontario and McMaster Universities (WOMAC) questionnaire. Women in the training group had statistically and clinically significant lower VAS and WOMAC pain scores after 8 weeks of training compared with the control group; the training effect on pain was retained 6 months later. Hip abduction and external rotation strength increased significantly in the training group at the 8-week time point. Participants in both groups were allowed to take pain-relieving medications during the study, but the use of pain relievers was not monitored. Although the study included only a small number of women, isolated hip strengthening focused on abduction and external rotation appears to be a reasonable approach to PFP rehabilitation.

C. M. Jankowski, PhD

Platelet-Rich Plasma Treatment for Ligament and Tendon Injuries

Paoloni J, De Vos RJ, Hamilton B, et al (Sports Medicine, Aspetar, Doha, Qatar; The Hague Med Centre, the Netherlands; et al)
Clin J Sport Med 21:37-45, 2011

Platelet-rich plasma (PRP) is derived from centrifuging whole blood, has a platelet concentration higher than that of the whole blood, is the cellular component of plasma that settles after centrifugation, and contains numerous growth factors. There is increasing interest in the sports medicine and athletic community about providing endogenous growth factors directly to the injury site, using autologous blood products such as PRP, to potentially facilitate healing and earlier return to sport after musculoskeletal injury. Despite this interest, and apparent widespread use, there is a lack of high-level evidence regarding randomized clinical trials assessing the efficacy of PRP in treating ligament and tendon injuries. Basic science and animal studies and small case series reports on PRP injections for ligament or tendon injuries, but few randomized controlled clinical trials have assessed the efficacy of PRP injections and none have demonstrated scientific evidence of efficacy. Scientific studies should be performed to assess clinical indications, efficacy, and safety of PRP, and this will require appropriately powered randomized controlled trials with adequate and validated clinical and functional outcome measures and sound statistical analysis. Other aspects of PRP use that need to be determined are (1) volume of injection/application, (2) most effective preparation, (3) buffering/activation, (4) injection technique (1 depot vs multiple depots), (5) timing of injection to injury, (6) single application versus series of injections, and (7) the most effective rehabilitation protocol to use after PRP injection. With all proposed treatments, the doctor and the patient should weigh up potential benefits of treatment, potential risks, and costs. Based on the limited publications to date and theoretical considerations, the potential risks involved with PRP are fortunately very low. However, benefits remain unproven to date, particularly when comparing PRP with other injections for ligament and tendon injuries.

▶ The use of platelet-rich plasma (PRP) treatment for either acute or chronic ligament and tendon injuries continues to be controversial, and adequate scientific trials are lacking. Multiple aspects of this popularized therapy, such as the preparation of PRP, optimal concentration of platelets, buffering/activation, timing and placement of injections, and others, remain unclear. This article reviews the results to that date of all the related studies on PRP in human subjects and presents the details in table form (Table 2 in the original article), including the level of evidence of each (as determined by the Oxford Centre for Evidence-Based Medicine). Thus the reader can easily view the existing evidence and types of trials that have been conducted. Obviously there have been more publications in this area since the time this manuscript was written, and other larger randomized clinical trials are presently underway, but this review does provide a better understanding of the limitations of the investigations to date as well as the future areas that need to be researched further. The authors conclude that there is currently no reason to consider PRP a more efficacious injection option than other treatments being used, including polidocanol, autologous blood, normal saline, or glucose prolotherapy. Although the potential risks associated with PRP are fortunately very low, it is important to emphasize to patients considering this treatment the paucity of scientific evidence, at least at this point in time, to support its use.

C. Lebrun, MDCM, MPE, CCFP, Dip Sport Med, FACSM

Treatment of Proximal Hamstring Ruptures — A Systematic Review
Harris JD, Griesser MJ, Best TM, et al (The Ohio State Univ, Columbus)
Int J Sports Med 32:490-495, 2011

Proximal hamstring ruptures are increasingly treated surgically, despite little high-level supporting evidence. We sought to determine whether there are differences in clinical outcome after surgical vs. non-surgical treatment of proximal hamstring tendinous avulsions/ruptures and acute vs. chronic surgical repair of tendinous avulsions. Multiple medical databases were searched for Level I–IV evidence. 18 studies were included. 298 subjects (300 proximal hamstring injuries) were analyzed with mean age of 39.7 years. 286 injuries were managed with surgical repair vs. 14 non-operative. 95 surgical cases were performed within 4 weeks of the injury (acute), while 191 were performed beyond 4 weeks (chronic). 292 injuries were tendinous avulsions while 8 were bony tuberosity avulsions. Surgical repair resulted in significantly (p < 0.05) better subjective outcomes, greater rate of return to pre-injury level of sport, and greater strength/endurance than non-surgical management. Similarly, acute surgical repair had significantly better patient satisfaction, subjective outcomes, pain relief, strength/endurance, and higher rate of return to pre-injury level of sport than chronic repair (p < 0.001) with reduced risk of complications and re-rupture (p < 0.05). Chronic surgical repair also improves outcomes, strength and endurance, and return-to-sport, but not as well as acute repair. Non-operative treatment results in reduced patient satisfaction, with significantly lower rates of return to pre-injury level of sport and reduced hamstring muscle strength.

▶ Proximal hamstring ruptures can lead to significant long-term disability, in terms of muscle weakness and sciatic nerve symptoms and, therefore, are increasingly being treated with surgical repair, even in chronic cases (> 4 weeks). However, there is little high-level evidence to support the premise that operative management is better than conservative therapy. This systematic review of 18 studies used a very good search strategy and selection criteria, which are well documented. Some of the clinical outcomes analyzed after injury in these studies were return to sport, patient satisfaction, Harris Hip Score, Proximal Hamstring Injury Questionnaire, isokinetic strength testing, and variable study-specific subjective questionnaires. Since this article was published, there have been 2 additional series published,[1,2] but, overall, there is little homogeneity among the different subject populations. Note that reference 25 is an incorrect citation by the same authors, which describes a surgical technique. The correct citation is noted below.[3] Other limitations of the literature to date include level IV evidence with small patient numbers, retrospective series designs, heterogeneous outcomes measures, variable surgical techniques, and short-term and midterm follow-up. No randomization was performed in these case series, resulting in significant selection bias. Chronic surgical repair also improves outcomes, strength and endurance, and return to sport but obviously not as well as acute repair. Nevertheless, the take-home message is that it may never be too late for surgical repair if indicated, and the effect of patient age on outcome following surgical treatment was not significant. More prospective randomized controlled trials are warranted.

C. Lebrun, MDCM, MPE, CCFP, Dip Sport Med, FACSM

References

1. Kwak HY, Bae SW, Choi YS, Jang MS. Early surgical repair of acute complete rupture of the proximal hamstring tendons. *Clin Orthop Surg*. 2011;3:249-253.
2. Birmingham P, Muller M, Wickiewicz T, Cavanaugh J, Rodeo S, Warren R. Functional outcome after repair of proximal hamstring avulsions. *J Bone Joint Surg Am*. 2011;93:1819-1826.
3. Lempainen L, Sarimo J, Heikkilä J, Mattila K, Orava S. Surgical treatment of partial tears of the proximal origin of the hamstring muscles. *Br J Sports Med*. 2006;40:688-691.

Single-Legged Hop Tests as Predictors of Self-Reported Knee Function in Nonoperatively Treated Individuals With Anterior Cruciate Ligament Injury
Grindem H, Logerstedt D, Eitzen I, et al (Norwegian Res Ctr for Active Rehabilitation (NAR), Oslo, Norway; Univ of Delaware, Newark; et al)
Am J Sports Med 39:2347-2354, 2011

Background.—Previous studies have found significant predictors for functional outcome after anterior cruciate ligament (ACL) reconstruction; however, studies examining predictors for functional outcome in nonoperatively treated individuals are lacking.

Hypothesis.—Single-legged hop tests predict self-reported knee function (International Knee Documentation Committee [IKDC] 2000) in nonoperatively treated ACL-injured individuals 1 year after baseline testing.

Study Design.—Cohort study (prognosis); Level of evidence, 2.

Methods.—Ninety-one nonoperatively treated patients with an ACL injury were tested using 4 single-legged hop tests on average 74 ± 30 days after injury in a prospective cohort study. Eighty-one patients (89%) completed the IKDC 2000 1 year later. Patients with an IKDC 2000 score equal to or higher than the age- and gender-specific 15th percentile score from previously published data on an uninjured population were classified as having self-reported function within normal ranges. Logistic regression analyses were performed to identify predictors of self-reported knee function. The area under the curve (AUC) from receiver operating characteristic curves was used as a measure of discriminative accuracy. Optimal limb symmetry index (LSI) cutoff for the best single-legged hop test was defined as the LSI with the highest product of sensitivity and specificity.

Results.—Single hop for distance symmetry indexes predicted self-reported knee function at the 1-year follow-up ($P = .036$). Combinations of any 2 hop tests (AUC = 0.64-0.71) did not give a higher discriminative accuracy than the single hop alone (AUC = 0.71). A cutoff of 88% (LSI) for the single hop revealed a sensitivity of 71.4% and a specificity of 71.7%.

Conclusion.—The single hop for distance (LSI) significantly predicted self-reported knee function after 1 year in nonoperatively treated ACL-injured patients. Combinations of 2 single-legged hop tests did not lead to higher discriminative accuracy than the single hop alone (Fig 2).

▶ Although traditionally operative management of tears of the anterior cruciate ligament (ACL) has been recommended as the preferred treatment in highly active individuals, there is increasing interest in the role of nonoperative treatment. A recently published randomized trial comparing structured rehabilitation and early surgery with structured rehabilitation and optional delayed surgery did not find any significant differences in patients' self-reported knee function 2 years after inclusion.[1] Clinicians are beginning to use quality-of-life questionnaires, such as the International Knee Documentation Committee Subjective

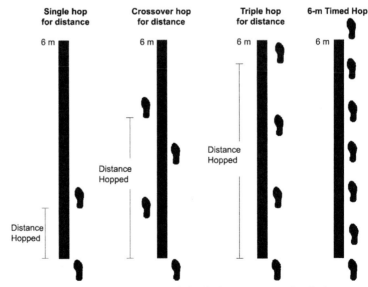

FIGURE 2.—The 4 single-legged hop tests: single hop for distance, crossover hop for distance, triple hop for distance, and 6-m timed hop. (Reprinted from Grindem H, Logerstedt D, Eitzen I, et al. Single-legged Hop tests as predictors of self-reported knee function in nonoperatively treated individuals with anterior cruciate ligament injury. *Am J Sports Med.* 2011;39:2347-2354, with permission from The Author(s).)

Knee Form (IKDC 2000), quantitative measurement of knee laxity and anterior tibial translation (KT-1000 or KT-2000 arthrometry), and/or functional tests, such as the single-legged hop tests (Fig 2), to help differentiate patients who might do well with nonoperative treatment. However, these have not been evaluated in a systematic fashion to determine the discriminatory accuracy and predictive value of these measures, whether conducted at baseline, or at some interval thereafter. This well-designed study evaluated the results from 81 subjects (40 women and 41 men, with a mean age of 29.2 ± 8.8 years) 1 year out from an ACL injury treated nonoperatively, who had undergone specific functional rehabilitation programs designed to prepare them for return to their desired activity level. Baseline testing was performed after initial rehabilitation, so that the subjects had no knee effusion, had no limitations in knee range of motion, and were able to hop on the involved limb without subsequent effusion or pain. This included the single hop for distance, crossover hop for distance, triple hop for distance and 6-m timed hop (in that order), and the IKDC-2000. An optimal limb symmetry index (LSI) was defined, and multiple logistic regression analyses were used. Results showed that single hop for distance symmetry indexes predicted self-reported knee function in these patients that was greater than the age- and gender-specific 15th percentile scores from previously published data on an uninjured population. A cutoff of 88% (LSI) for the single hop revealed a sensitivity of 71.4% and a specificity of 71.7%, and the addition of a second single-legged hop test did not increase the accuracy.

Such studies are important to give some guidance to clinicians and patients alike in the selection of nonoperative versus operative management of ACL injuries, particularly in a younger more active population who have expectations of returning to a higher level of sport. It would also have been interesting to have seen the results of comparisons between the IKDC 2000 scores at baseline and at the 1-year testing point, but they were not mentioned in this article. Ideally, some combination of quality-of-life questionnaires, physical assessment parameters and measurement of knee laxity, and functional tests should be developed and validated as an ACL Knee Index score to use in a predictive fashion to determine those patients most suited to a nonoperative course of treatment. However, to be the most useful, such a battery of tests would need to be practical for the clinical setting in terms of time, expense, ease of use, and the need for special equipment, training, or space for testing.

C. Lebrun, MDCM, MPE, CCFP, Dip Sport Med, FACSM

Reference

1. Frobell RB, Roos EM, Roos HP, Ranstam J, Lohmander LS. A randomized trial of treatment for acute anterior cruciate ligament tears. *N Engl J Med*. 2010;363: 331-342.

3 Biomechanics, Muscle Strength and Training

Effects of an Age-Specific Anterior Cruciate Ligament Injury Prevention Program on Lower Extremity Biomechanics in Children
DiStefano LJ, Blackburn JT, Marshall SW, et al (Univ of Connecticut, Storrs; Univ of North Carolina at Chapel Hill; et al)
Am J Sports Med 39:949-957, 2011

Background.—Implementing an anterior cruciate ligament injury prevention program to athletes before the age at which the greatest injury risk occurs (15-17 years) is important from a prevention standpoint. However, it is unknown whether standard programs can modify lower extremity biomechanics in pediatric populations or if specialized training is required.

Hypothesis/Purpose.—To compare the effects of traditional and age-specific pediatric anterior cruciate ligament injury prevention programs on lower extremity biomechanics during a cutting task in youth athletes. The authors hypothesized that the age-specific pediatric program would result in greater sagittal plane motion (ie, hip and knee flexion) and less motion in the transverse and frontal plane (ie, knee valgus, knee and hip rotation) as compared with the traditional program.

Study Design.—Randomized controlled trial; Level of evidence, 1.

Methods.—Sixty-five youth soccer athletes (38 boys, 27 girls) volunteered to participate. The mean age of participants was 10 ± 1 years. Teams (n, 7) were cluster randomized to a pediatric injury prevention program, a traditional injury prevention program, or a control group. The pediatric program was modified from the traditional program to include more feedback, progressions, and variety. Teams performed their programs as part of their normal warm-up routine. Three-dimensional lower extremity biomechanics were assessed during a sidestep cutting task before and after completion of the 9-week intervention period.

Results.—The pediatric program reduced the amount of knee external rotation at initial ground contact during the cutting task, $F_{(2,62)} = 3.79$, $P = .03$ (change: pediatric, 7.73° ± 10.71°; control, −0.35° ± 7.76°), as compared with the control group after the intervention period. No other changes were observed.

Conclusion.—The injury prevention program designed for a pediatric population modified only knee rotation during the cutting task, whereas

TABLE 1.—Comparison of Injury Prevention Programs: Traditional vs Pediatric

Exercises	Traditional Program Nonprogressive	Pediatric Program Phase 1	Phase 2	Phase 3
Time/duration				
Minutes	12-14	12-14	12-14	12-14
Days/week	3	2	3	3
Weeks	9	3	3	3
Lower extremity strengthening	Forward lunge	Forward lunge	Sideways lunge	Twisting lunge
	Broad jump	Double-leg squat	Double- to single-leg squat	
	Single-leg squat	Toe walk	Broad jump	
		Double-leg heel raise		
Repetitions	1 × 5 each leg	1 × 15	1 × 15	1 × 15
Core strengthening	Hip bridge	Hip bridge	Human arrow	Sideways plank
Repetitions	1 × 10; hold 3 seconds	1 × 10; hold 3 seconds	1 × 10; hold 3 seconds	1 × 10; hold 3 seconds
Flexibility type	*Static*	*Dynamic*	*Dynamic*	*Dynamic*
	Calf	Straight leg march	Straight leg skip	Straight leg skip
	Hip flexor	Hand walk	Walking calf stretch	Leg cradle
	Adductor	Walking butt kicks	Hip flexor walk	Twisting hip flexor walk
		Walking quad stretch	Knee to chest	Running butt kicks
				High knee run
Repetitions	30 seconds each	30 seconds each	30 seconds each	30 seconds each
Plyometric	Squat jumps	Double-leg forward line hops	Single-leg forward line hops	Single-leg sideways line hops
	Double-leg forward hops (single leg)		Double-leg sideways line hops	Squat jumps
	Double-leg sideways hops (single leg)		Up and down hops	Tuck jumps
Repetitions	10	20	20	20
Balance	180° jump to balance	180° jump to balance	Sideways hop to balance	Twisting hop to balance
	Single-leg forward hop to balance	Forward hop to balance	Single-leg ball toss	Single-leg balance perturbations
	Single-leg ball toss			
Repetitions	1 × 10 each leg	1 × 10	1 × 10	1 × 10
Agility	Toe-heel walk	Forward skipping	Forward and back skipping	Unanticipated side cuts
	High knee run	Sideways shuffle	Side cuts	
	Sideways shuffle			
	Z cuts			
Repetitions	30 seconds each	30 seconds each	30 seconds each	30 seconds each

the traditional program did not result in any changes in cutting biomechanics. These findings suggest limited effectiveness of both programs for athletes younger than 12 years of age in terms of biomechanics during a cutting task (Table 1).

▶ Individuals aged between 16 and 18 years appear to be at the highest risk for injuries to the anterior cruciate ligament (ACL), but the frequency increases steadily starting in late childhood or between the ages of 10 and 12 years. There is already a large body of literature investigating the effects of various specific preventative programs for ACL injury in the adolescent and young adult population but none in the pediatric age group. This study builds on previous work by this same research group on lower extremity biomechanics during movement patterns associated with injury risk during sport-related movements, such as landing or cutting. Specifically, these include decreased knee flexion, knee valgus, and excessive leg rotation. What is unique about this study, however, is that it also incorporates the tenets of motor learning, stages of development, and physical abilities of children. A progressive pediatric injury prevention program (Table 1) was designed with these in mind and administered to a group of youth soccer athletes (boys and girls; ages, 9-10 years). This was compared with a group completing a more traditional program and a control group using a cluster-randomized controlled trial study design (with 1 boys team and 1 girls team for each program). Sophisticated laboratory analyses of lower extremity biomechanics, focusing on a sidestep cutting task and movement in the transverse plane, were performed prior to and after the 9-week intervention program. There was excellent compliance with the ACL injury prevention programs, with participants attending greater than 80% of all program sessions.

The pediatric injury prevention program had limited effect, with reduction in knee external rotation only, and no change in movements or forces in the frontal or sagittal plane during the sidestep cutting tasks. The results show that further research in this area is needed.

C. Lebrun, MDCM, MPE, CCFP, Dip Sport Med, FACSM

Exercise Dosing to Retain Resistance Training Adaptations in Young and Older Adults

Bickel CS, Cross JM, Bamman MM (Univ of Alabama at Birmingham)
Med Sci Sports Exerc 43:1177-1187, 2011

Resistance training (RT) is a proven sarcopenia countermeasure with a high degree of potency. However, sustainability remains a major issue that could limit the appeal of RT as a therapeutic approach without well-defined dosing requirements to maintain gains.

Purpose.—To test the efficacy of two maintenance prescriptions on muscle mass, myofiber size and type distribution, and strength. We hypothesized the minimum dose required to maintain RT-induced adaptations would be greater in the old (60—75 yr) versus young (20—35 yr).

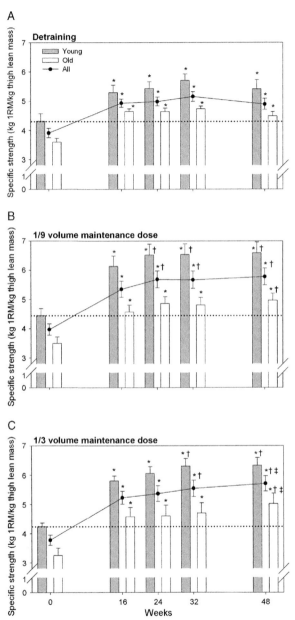

FIGURE 4.—Specific strength estimates by phase 2 group determined by ratio of 1RM knee extension (kg) to TLM (kg). *Different from baseline ($P < 0.05$). †Different from week 16 ($P < 0.05$). ‡Different from week 24. *Dotted line* indicates pretraining specific strength of the untrained young. (Reprinted from Bickel CS, Cross JM, Bamman MM. Exercise dosing to retain resistance training adaptations in young and older adults. *Med Sci Sports Exerc.* 2011;43:1177-1187, with permission from the American College of Sports Medicine.)

Methods.—Seventy adults participated in a two-phase exercise trial that consisted of RT 3 d·wk^{-1} for 16 wk (phase 1) followed by a 32-wk period (phase 2) with random assignment to detraining or one of two maintenance prescriptions (reducing the dose to one-third or one-ninth of that during phase 1).

Results.—Phase 1 resulted in expected gains in strength, myofiber size, and muscle mass along with the typical IIx-to-IIa shift in myofiber-type distribution. Both maintenance prescriptions preserved phase 1 muscle hypertrophy in the young but not the old. In fact, the one-third maintenance dose led to additional myofiber hypertrophy in the young. In both age groups, detraining reversed the phase 1 IIx-to-IIa myofiber-type shift, whereas a dose response was evident during maintenance training with the one-third dose better maintaining the shift. Strength gained during phase 1 was largely retained throughout detraining with only a slight reduction at the final time point.

Conclusions.—We conclude that older adults require a higher dose of weekly loading than the young to maintain myofiber hypertrophy attained during a progressive RT program, yet gains in specific strength among older adults were well preserved and remained at or above levels of the untrained young (Fig 4).

▶ The potency of resistance exercise training (RT) as a countermeasure for sarcopenia has been established. Less is known about the sustainability of the beneficial effects of exercise on muscle function, morphology, and histology in older adults. The minimum maintenance dose of exercise that prevents reversibility after RT is a relevant question given that even dedicated exercisers have lapses in training. Bickel and colleagues studied young and older adults (presumably women and men) during a 36-week detraining period that followed a 16-week RT intervention of lower extremity exercises. To determine the dose response for detraining, participants engaged in training that was reduced to one-third, one-ninth, or complete cessation of RT. The maintenance exercise was performed at the same intensity as during RT. The dose response for maintenance and effects of age differed by the outcome of interest. Thigh lean mass was better preserved in the one-third than one-ninth exercise dose compared with complete detraining, regardless of age. Maximal voluntary knee extensor strength was preserved with both maintenance doses of exercise compared with nonexercise controls in the young and old. Muscle fiber area continued to increase in the young group during the first 16 weeks of detraining, whereas myofiber area began to decline in the older group in the same time frame. The shift in the distribution of type IIx to IIa fibers (a marker of fatigue resistance) exhibited a full reversal of training-induced changes by the 16th week of complete detraining but was partially maintained with the one-third training dose, regardless of age. Specific strength of the knee extensors (strength/thigh lean mass) was preserved up to 48 weeks with both detraining doses (Fig 4). Overall, this study supports the notion that older adults can maintain multiple RT effects with a reduced training volume (3 sets of exercises once weekly).

C. M. Jankowski, PhD

Anatomy, Function, Injuries, and Treatment of the Long Head of the Biceps Brachii Tendon

Elser F, Braun S, Dewing CB, et al (Steadman Philippon Res Inst, Vail, CO)
Arthroscopy 27:581-592, 2011

Lesions of the long head biceps tendon (LHB) are frequent causes of shoulder pain and disability. Biceps tenotomy and tenodesis have gained widespread acceptance as effective procedures to manage both isolated LHB pathology and combined lesions of the rotator cuff and biceps-labral complex. The function of the LHB tendon and its role in glenohumeral kinematics presently remain only partially understood because of the difficulty of cadaveric and in vivo biomechanical studies. The purpose of this article is to offer an up-to-date review of the anatomy and biomechanical properties of the LHB and to provide an evidence-based approach to current treatment strategies for LHB disorders.

▶ The function of the long head of biceps (LHB) in glenohumeral joint stability remains somewhat controversial. Cadaveric biomechanical studies maintain the importance of the LHB in limiting anterior and superior translation of the humeral head with abduction and external rotation of the glenohumeral (GH) joint. However, this does depend on the amount and application of truly physiologic loads on this structure. Elser and coauthors conclude in this excellent article that biomechanical cadaveric studies fail to apply physiologic loads to the LHB, resulting in an overestimation of its role in GH stability and function. This is important because of the tendency of the LHB as a source of shoulder pain and dysfunction. For young active individuals involved in throwing sports, persistent shoulder dysfunction due to LHB pathologies can be life altering and compromising to continuation in their sport. This article provides an excellent review of the anatomic, cadaveric, biomechanical, and in vivo studies of the actual function of this structure. They provide excellent clinical information as to the best management of chronic pain due to LHB pathology; for example, they recommend surgical repair such as a tenodesis for the young active individual who wants to continue in sport activity but conservative management for middle-aged and older individuals with LHB tendon rupture. A very good case is made for research into the actual function of the LHB using application of physiologic loads in cadaveric studies; however, they do recommend more emphasis on in vivo studies in individuals in which the articular portion of the LHB tendon has been removed. Considerable potential exists in studies of this nature to unearth the physiologic function of the LHB in shoulder stability.

V. Galea, PhD

Interactive Processes Link the Multiple Symptoms of Fatigue in Sport Competition

Knicker AJ, Renshaw I, Oldham ARH, et al (German Sport Univ Cologne, Germany; Queensland Univ of Technology, Brisbane, Australia; AUT Univ, Auckland, New Zealand)
Sports Med 41:307-328, 2011

Muscle physiologists often describe fatigue simply as a decline of muscle force and infer this causes an athlete to slow down. In contrast, exercise scientists describe fatigue during sport competition more holistically as an exercise induced impairment of performance. The aim of this review is to reconcile the different views by evaluating the many performance symptoms/measures and mechanisms of fatigue. We describe how fatigue is assessed with muscle, exercise or competition performance measures. Muscle performance (single muscle test measures) declines due to peripheral fatigue (reduced muscle cell force) and/or central fatigue (reduced motor drive from the CNS). Peak muscle force seldom falls by >30% during sport but is often exacerbated during electrical stimulation and laboratory exercise tasks. Exercise performance (whole body exercise test measures) reveals impaired physical/technical abilities and subjective fatigue sensations. Exercise intensity is initially sustained by recruitment of new motor units and help from synergistic muscles before it declines. Technique/motor skill execution deviates as exercise proceeds to maintain outcomes before they deteriorate, e.g. reduced accuracy or velocity. The sensation of fatigue incorporates an elevated rating of perceived exertion (RPE) during submaximal tasks, due to a combination of peripheral and higher CNS inputs. Competition performance (sport symptoms) is affected more by decision-making and psychological aspects, since there are opponents and a greater importance on the result. Laboratory based decision making is generally faster or unimpaired. Motivation, self-efficacy and anxiety can change during exercise to modify RPE and, hence, alter physical performance.

Symptoms of fatigue during racing, team-game or racquet sports are largely anecdotal, but sometimes assessed with time-motion analysis. Fatigue during brief all-out racing is described biomechanically as a decline of peak velocity, along with altered kinematic components. Longer sport events involve pacing strategies, central and peripheral fatigue contributions and elevated RPE. During match play, the work rate can decline late in a match (or tournament) and/or transiently after intense exercise bursts. Repeated sprint ability, agility and leg strength become slightly impaired. Technique outcomes, such as velocity and accuracy for throwing, passing, hitting and kicking, can deteriorate. Physical and subjective changes are both less severe in real rather than simulated sport activities. Little objective evidence exists to support exercise-induced mental lapses during sport.

A model depicting mind-body interactions during sport competition shows that the RPE centre-motor cortex-working muscle sequence drives overall performance levels and, hence, fatigue symptoms. The sporting outputs from this sequence can be modulated by interactions with muscle afferent and circulatory feedback, psychological and decision-making inputs. Importantly, compensatory processes exist at many levels to protect against performance decrements. Small changes of putative fatigue factors can also be protective. We show that individual fatigue factors including diminished carbohydrate availability, elevated serotonin, hypoxia, acidosis, hyperkalaemia, hyperthermia, dehydration and reactive oxygen species, each contribute to several fatigue symptoms. Thus, multiple symptoms of fatigue can occur simultaneously and the underlying mechanisms overlap and interact. Based on this understanding, we reinforce the proposal that fatigue is best described globally as an exercise induced decline of performance as this is inclusive of all viewpoints.

▶ In this excellent review, the authors make the case for a global definition of fatigue to be "An exercise-induced decline of performance." The nature of fatigue as a multifactorial, interactive process that does lead to a decline in performance is supported by an extensive review of the literature on not only physical, technical, and subjective fatigue but also an excellent section on effects of fatigue during competition performance in terms of impact on decision making and anticipatory capacity. Also of interest to the readers of this volume are the sections on sports-specific symptoms and measures of fatigue. Interestingly, the elite athlete will obviate the effects of declines in muscle force and power by using different motor strategies and a reorganization of the system so that performance does not suffer. Not so with the novice or recreational athlete. Evidence for the plausibility of this strategy comes from studies using dynamical systems theory and the concept of abundance of motor strategies for performance of the same task. This is an excellent demonstration of the capacity of the highly trained athlete who is able to make use of the abundance within the sensory motor system. The last section is of particular use to professionals who work with athletes and the linkage of fatigue factors to multiple fatigue symptoms. For example, hypoglycemia (decreased blood glucose) will affect peripheral fatigue, afferent feedback, and central fatigue symptoms such as decreased motor drive will decrease time to exhaustion, increase ratings of perceived exertion, decrease motor skill outcome/performance, and will impair decision making. Management of elite athletes will benefit from this knowledge because their decline in performance would not only be due to single factors but likely this multifactorial interaction of fatigue factors with fatigue symptoms.

V. Galea, PhD

ISSLS Prize Winner: Smudging the Motor Brain in Young Adults With Recurrent Low Back Pain
Tsao H, Danneels LA, Hodges PW (The Univ of Queensland, Brisbane, Australia; Ghent Univ, Belgium)
Spine 36:1721-1727, 2011

Study Design.—Cross-sectional design.

Objective.—To investigate whether recurrent low back pain (LBP) is associated with changes in motor cortical representation of different paraspinal muscle fascicles.

Summary of Background Data.—Fascicles of the lumbar paraspinal muscles are differentially activated during function. Human studies indicate this may be associated with a spatially separate array of neuronal networks at the motor cortex. Loss of discrete control of paraspinal muscle fascicles in LBP may be because of changes in cortical organization.

Methods.—Data were collected from 9 individuals with recurrent unilateral LBP and compared with 11 healthy participants from an earlier study. Fine-wire electrodes selectively recorded myoelectric activity from short/deep fascicles of deep multifidus (DM) and long/superficial fascicles of *longissimus erector spinae* (LES), bilaterally. Motor cortical organization was investigated using transcranial magnetic stimulation at different scalp sites to evoke responses in paraspinal muscles. Location of cortical representation (center of gravity; CoG) and motor excitability (map volume) were compared between healthy and LBP groups.

Results.—Individuals with LBP had a more posterior location of LES center of gravity, which overlapped with that for DM on both hemispheres. In healthy individuals, LES center of gravity was located separately at a more anterior location to that for DM. Map volume was reduced in LBP compared to healthy individuals across muscles.

Conclusion.—The findings highlight that LBP is associated with a loss of discrete cortical organization of inputs to back muscles. Increased overlap in motor cortical representation of DM and LES may underpin loss of differential activation in this group. The results further unravel the neurophysiological mechanisms of motor changes in recurrent LBP and suggest motor rehabilitation that includes training of differential activation of the paraspinal muscles may be required to restore optimal control in LBP.

▶ Considerable evidence now exists that chronic pain induces plastic changes in the brain and spinal cord. In this article by Tsao and colleagues,[1,2] indices of change in brain maps of the deep multifidus muscles (DM) and the longissimus erector spinae (LES) were observed via changes in brain mapping using transcranial magnetic stimulation (TMS) of the motor-evoked potential. The human primary motor cortex is highly somatotopically organized to represent specific areas of the body. While areas of motor cortex dedicated to the trunk are not as extensive as those to the hand, for example, localized projections, as discrete cortical networks, to muscles of the back have been identified by and published in other publications from the laboratory of Paul Hodges and collaborators.[3]

Cortical reorganization was observed as a decrease in the map volume of both right and left cortical areas to DM and LES in individuals with low back pain compared with healthy controls. In addition, the center of gravity as calculated by the mediolateral and anteroposterior locations divided by the normalized amplitude of the evoked motor potentials for the LES was overlapped with that of DM. In other words, there was a shift of the representation of this muscle backwards from the location identified in the healthy controls. The authors refer to this phenomena as cortical "smudging" and propose that this occurs in individuals with low back pain as a compensatory response intended to reduce pain by a global splinting or more global activation of these paraspinal muscles. Unfortunately, this also reflects a reduction in the discrete activation of different fascicles of paraspinal muscles. What this implies to function still remains to be determined, but these observations do imply that this compromise of segmental control alters the loading on spinal soft tissue and may open these individuals to a recurrence of low back pain. The authors do suggest that consideration be given to motor training to potentially restore cortical reorganization to reduce the risk of recurrence of low back pain in susceptible individuals.

V. Galea, PhD

References

1. Tsao H, Danneels L, Hodges PW. Individual fascicles of the paraspinal muscles are activated by discrete cortical networks in humans. *Clin Neurophysiol.* 2011;122: 1580-1587.
2. Tsao H, Galea MP, Hodges PW. Driving plasticity in the motor cortex in recurrent low back pain. *Eur J Pain.* 2010;14:832-839.
3. Hodges PW. Changes in motor planning of feed forward postural responses of the trunk muscles in low back pain. *Exp Brain Res.* 2001;141:261-266.

Effects of Strength Training on Motor Performance Skills in Children and Adolescents: A Meta-Analysis
Behringer M, vom Heede A, Matthews M, et al (German Sport Univ Cologne, Germany; East Stroudsburg Univ, PA)
Pediatr Exerc Sci 23:186-206, 2011

The recent literature delineates resistance training in children and adolescents to be effective and safe. However, only little is known about the transfer of achieved strength gains to athletic performance. The present meta-analysis revealed a combined mean effect size for motor skill types jumping, running, and throwing of 0.52 (95% CI: 0.33−0.71). Effect sizes for each of aforementioned skill types separately were 0.54 (95% CI: 0.34−0.74), 0.53 (95% CI: 0.23−0.83), and 0.99 (95% CI: 0.19−1.79) respectively. Furthermore, it could be shown that younger subjects and nonathletes showed higher gains in motor performance following resistance training than their counterparts and that specific resistance training regimes were not advantageous over traditional resistance training programs. Finally, a positive dose response relationship for "intensity" could be found in subgroups using traditional training regimens. These results emphasize that resistance training provides an effective way for enhancing motor performance in children and adolescents.

▶ If appropriately prescribed and supervised, resistance training is an effective and safe way to enhance muscle strength in youth. Resistance training can also improve bone strength and density, thereby decreasing the long-term risk of fractures and osteoporosis. Surprisingly little is known about the effects of resistance training on sport and athletic performance in youth. In fact, this meta-analysis was only able to identify 34 published studies that addressed this question. There were 1432 research participants included in these 34 studies, and most (71%) of these participants were male. The meta-analysis found significant effect sizes of strength training on jumping and sprinting test results. These effect sizes were moderate in size. Conversely, the effect sizes for throwing tests were strong. This led the authors to conclude that because motor performance skills are known to be essential components in different types of sports, it can be assumed that there is a positive transfer of resistance training effects to sport-specific performance in young athletes. These findings also support a recent position statement of the National Strength and Conditioning Association, which reports that resistance training is an effective method for improving sports performance in youth.[1]

I. Janssen, PhD

Reference

1. Faigenbaum AD, Kraemer WJ, Blimkie CJ, et al. Youth resistance training: updated position statement paper from the national strength and conditioning association. *J Strength Cond Res.* 2009;23:S60-S79.

Antioxidant Supplementation Reduces Skeletal Muscle Mitochondrial Biogenesis
Strobel NA, Peake JM, Matsumoto A, et al (The Univ of Queensland, St Lucia, Australia; et al)
Med Sci Sports Exerc 43:1017-1024, 2011

Purpose.—Exercise increases the production of reactive oxygen species (ROS) in skeletal muscle, and athletes often consume antioxidant supplements in the belief they will attenuate ROS-related muscle damage and fatigue during exercise. However, exercise-induced ROS may regulate beneficial skeletal muscle adaptations, such as increased mitochondrial biogenesis. We therefore investigated the effects of long-term antioxidant supplementation with vitamin E and α-lipoic acid on changes in markers of mitochondrial biogenesis in the skeletal muscle of exercise-trained and sedentary rats.
Methods.—Male Wistar rats were divided into four groups: 1) sedentary control diet, 2) sedentary antioxidant diet, 3) exercise control diet, and

4) exercise antioxidant diet. Animals ran on a treadmill $4 \, d \cdot wk^{-1}$ at $\sim 70\%$ $\dot{V}O_{2max}$ for up to $90 \, min \cdot d^{-1}$ for 14 wk.

Results.—Consistent with the augmentation of skeletal muscle mitochondrial biogenesis and antioxidant defenses, after training there were significant increases in peroxisome proliferator—activated receptor γ coactivator 1α (PGC-1α) messenger RNA (mRNA) and protein, cytochrome C oxidase subunit IV (COX IV) and cytochrome C protein abundance, citrate synthase activity, Nfe2l2, and SOD2 protein ($P < 0.05$). Antioxidant supplementation reduced PGC-1α mRNA, PGC-1α and COX IV protein, and citrate synthase enzyme activity ($P < 0.05$) in both sedentary and exercise-trained rats.

Conclusions.—Vitamin E and α-lipoic acid supplementation suppresses skeletal muscle mitochondrial biogenesis, regardless of training status (Fig 1).

▶ The idea that supplements of vitamin E or wheat germ oil might enhance athletic performance dates back to the time of Dr Tom Cureton.[1] We carried out a double-blind, placebo-controlled trial of this supposed ergogenic aid in a sample of university swimmers, and we found no gains of performance in those individuals who received the supplements[2]; however, perhaps in keeping with earlier findings of benefit in vitamin-depleted animals,[3] the experimental group showed somewhat less loss of muscular strength over the course of 3 months of rigorous endurance training. Others[4] continue to maintain that vitamin E supplements help in the recovery of function by elderly patients following hip fracture. One possible explanation of any benefit is that vitamin E serves as an antioxidant, countering the reactive oxygen species (ROS) that are released during vigorous training. However, this may not always help training in the endurance competitor; a growing number of reports suggest that ROS may indeed be needed to stimulate mitochondrial biogenesis, via its action on peroxisome proliferator—activated

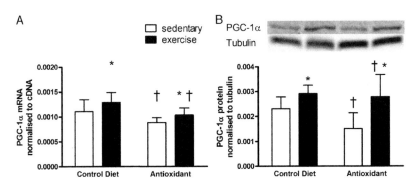

FIGURE 1.—Effects of antioxidant supplementation and exercise training on PGC-1α mRNA (A) and PGC-1α protein content (B) in the skeletal muscle. Western blots are representative from one rat from each group. Values for PGC-1α mRNA and protein are geometric mean (95% confidence interval); sample sizes for each variable ranged from $n = 7$ to 10 for all groups. *$P < 0.05$, main effect for exercise. †$P < 0.05$, main effect for antioxidant. (Reprinted from Strobel NA, Peake JM, Matsumoto A, et al. Antioxidant supplementation reduces skeletal muscle mitochondrial biogenesis. *Med Sci Sports Exerc.* 2011;43:1017-1024, with permission from the American College of Sports Medicine.)

receptor γ coactivator 1α (PGC- 1α).[5-8] The study of Strobel and associates, conducted in rats, confirms that 3 months of vitamin E supplementation (1000 U/kg added to standard rat chow) reduced but did not totally suppress the enzyme chain responsible for muscle hypertrophy. This effect was seen in both exercised and sedentary animals, starting with decreases in PGC-1α mRNA (Fig 1). One previous human study found no effect of vitamin E on resting mitochondrial biogenesis, but the antioxidant supplement was given for a much shorter period (only 8 days) than in the study by Strobel et al.[8] Further studies of the benefits and dangers of antioxidant supplements seem warranted, both in endurance and resistance athletes, and in patients with various types of muscular dystrophy.

R. J. Shephard, MD (Lond), PhD, DPE

References

1. Cureton TK. *The Physiological Effects of Wheat Germ Oil on Humans in Exercise.* Springfield, IL: CC Thomas; 1972.
2. Shephard RJ, Campbell R, Pimm P, Stuart D, Wright GR. Vitamin E, exercise, and the recovery from physical activity. *Eur J Appl Physiol Occup Physiol.* 1974;33: 119-126.
3. Garton GA, Duncan WR, Blaxter KL, Mcgill RF, Sharman GA, Hutcheson MK. Muscular dystrophy of beef cattle and unsaturated fats. *Nature.* 1956;177:792-793.
4. D'Adamo CR, Miller RR, Hicks GE, et al. Serum vitamin E concentrations and recovery of physical function during the year after hip fracture. *J Gerontol A Biol Sci Med Sci.* 2011;66:784-793.
5. Gomez-Cabrera MC, Domenech E, Romagnoli M, et al. Oral administration of vitamin C decreases muscle mitochondrial biogenesis and hampers training-induced adaptations in endurance performance. *Am J Clin Nutr.* 2008;87:142-149.
6. Hood DA. Mechanisms of exercise-induced mitochondrial biogenesis in skeletal muscle. *Appl Physiol Nutr Metab.* 2009;34:465-472.
7. Pilegaard H, Saltin B, Neufer PD. Exercise induces transient transcriptional activation of the PGC-1α gene in human skeletal muscle. *J Physiol.* 2003;546:851-858.
8. Ristow M, Zarse K, Oberbach A, et al. Antioxidants prevent health-promoting effects of physical exercise in humans. *Proc Natl Acad Sci U S A.* 2009;106: 8665-8670.

Metabolic muscle damage and oxidative stress markers in an America's Cup yachting crew

Barrios C, Hadala M, Almansa I, et al (Valencia Univ Med School, Spain; Universidad Cardenal Herrera-CEU, Valencia, Spain)
Eur J Appl Physiol 111:1341-1350, 2011

Activities of enzymes involved in muscle damage [creatine kinase (CK) and aspartate aminotransferase (AST)] and levels of malondialdehyde (MDA) as a marker of oxidative stress were monitored in the plasma of 27 members of an America's Cup yachting crew. The preventive benefits of allopurinol on muscle damage were also tested. In racing period A, the crew was divided into two groups according to their tasks on board. Blood samples from all 27 sailors were obtained before the start of a 5-day fleet race, after the last race, and after the ten match races. In period

B, crew members were divided at random into two groups. One group (13 participants) received 300 mg/day of allopurinol 3 h before racing. The other ten members received placebo. Blood samples were collected just before and after the second round of the Louis Vuitton Cup. All participants showed increased CK and AST activities after the racing period A. The increase in CK activity was highest in sailors involved in strenuous physical work. At the end of period A, plasma MDA levels were higher in all participants as compared with non-participant athletes. In period B, a significant decrease in CK activity, but not in AST, appeared among participants receiving allopurinol. Plasma MDA decreased in sailors treated with allopurinol, but this reduction did not reach statistical significance. America's Cup is a sailing sport with high physical demands, as

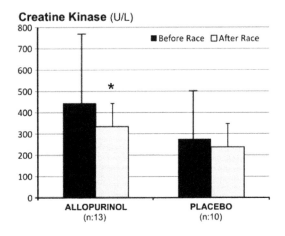

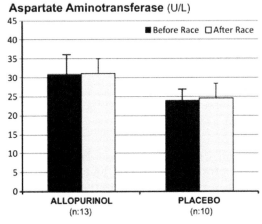

FIGURE 4.—CK activity and AST levels in sailors treated with allopurinol and in those receiving a placebo (racing period B). *$p < 0.05$ versus pre-treatment values. (Reprinted from Barrios C, Hadala M, Almansa I, et al. Metabolic muscle damage and oxidative stress markers in an America's Cup yachting crew. *Eur J Appl Physiol.* 2011;111:1341-1350, with kind permission of Springer Science+Business Media.)

shown by the increase in muscle-damage markers. Treatment with allopurinol appeared to decrease the levels of muscle damage markers (Fig 4).

▶ Allopurinol (Zyloprim) is a naturally occurring purine analog that inhibits the enzyme, xanthine oxidase. It is used primarily for the treatment of gout but is also effective in countering the oxidative stress associated with prolonged and strenuous exercise. The America's Cup event is one form of very strenuous physical activity that has had relatively little previous study. Barrios and associates noted 13 consecutive competitions, each consisting of 5 to 7 days of racing (once or twice per day for 1-2 hours), culminating in the final event, the Louis Vuitton Cup. Thirteen of the 27-member crew had assignments that required prolonged and high-intensity physical activity, and these individuals showed a doubling of basal creatine kinase levels 3 hours after the end of the racing (unfortunately, data were not collected 1-3 days postexercise, when creatine kinase levels normally peak). The leakage of creatine kinase from the damaged muscles was substantially reduced by taking the maximal daily dose of allopurinol (300 mg, 3 hours before racing; Fig 4). The findings confirm those of earlier studies in which allopurinol was administered to participants in the Tour de France[1] and marathoners.[2] There remains a need for further study of possible adverse effects from the inhibition of xanthine oxidase; the up-regulation of antioxidant defenses is likely reduced by allopurinol, and some degree of membrane leakage may also play a significant role in muscle hypertrophy.

R. J. Shephard, MD (Lond), PhD, DPE

References

1. Gómez-Cabrera MC, Pallardó FV, Sastre J, Viña J, García-del-Moral L. Allopurinol and markers of muscle damage among participants in the Tour de France. *JAMA*. 2003;289:2503-2504.
2. Gomez-Cabrera MC, Martinez A, Santangelo G, Pallardó FV, Sastre J, Viña J. Oxidative stress in marathon runners: interest of antioxidant supplementation. *Br J Nutr*. 2006;96:S31-S33.

Training in the fasted state facilitates re-activation of eEF2 activity during recovery from endurance exercise
Van Proeyen K, De Bock K, Hespel P (Res Centre for Exercise and Health, Leuven, Belgium)
Eur J Appl Physiol 111:1297-1305, 2011

Nutrition is an important co-factor in exercise-induced training adaptations in muscle. We compared the effect of 6 weeks endurance training (3 days/week, 1–2 h at 75% VO_{2peak}) in either the fasted state (F; $n = 10$) or in the high carbohydrate state (CHO, $n = 10$), on Ca^{2+}-dependent intramyocellular signalling in young male volunteers. Subjects in CHO received a carbohydrate-rich breakfast before each training session, as well as ingested carbohydrates during exercise. Before (*pretest*) and after (*posttest*) the training period, subjects performed a 2 h constant-load exercise bout

($\sim$70% of *pretest* VO_{2peak}) while ingesting carbohydrates (1 g/kg h^{-1}). A muscle biopsy was taken from m. vastus lateralis immediately before and after the test, and after 4 h of recovery. Compared with *pretest*, in the posttest basal eukaryotic elongation factor 2 (eEF2) phosphorylation was elevated in CHO ($P < 0.05$), but not in F. In the *pretest*, exercise increased the degree of eEF2 phosphorylation about twofold ($P < 0.05$), and values returned to baseline within the 4 h recovery period in each group. However, in the *posttest* dephosphorylation of eEF2 was negated after recovery in CHO, but not in F. Independent of the dietary condition training enhanced the basal phosphorylation status of Phospholamban at Thr^{17}, 5'-AMP-activated protein kinase α (AMPKα), and Acetyl CoA carboxylase β (ACCβ), and abolished the exercise-induced increase of AMPKα and ACCβ ($P < 0.05$). In conclusion, training in the fasted state, compared with identical training with ample carbohydrate intake, facilitates post-exercise dephosphorylation of eEF2. This may contribute to rapid re-activation of muscle protein translation following endurance exercise.

▶ The effects of endurance training and fasting on eukaryotic elongation factor 2 (eEF2) may seem a rather esoteric topic for the *Year Book of Sports Medicine*, but the article of Van Proeyen and colleagues points to an important practical application. During muscle contraction, the rising intramyocellular Ca^{2+} level initiates a signaling cascade that activates protein kinases, such as eEF2 kinase, that are important to the metabolic adaptations of skeletal muscle during endurance training. Fasting appears to facilitate further the postexercise dephosphorylation of eEF2, and thus encourages the rapid reactivation of muscle protein translation via eEF2 during the recovery period.[1] Although carbohydrate loading may be important to maximizing peak performance during competition, the present observations suggest that muscle protein translation may be enhanced if normal training is performed when glycogen stores are low.

R. J. Shephard, MD (Lond), PhD, DPE

Reference

1. Dreyer HC, Fujita S, Cadenas JG, Chinkes DL, Volpi E, Rasmussen BB. Resistance exercise increases AMPK activity and reduces 4E-BP1 phosphorylation and protein synthesis in human skeletal muscle. *J Physiol.* 2006;576:613-624.

Changes in Functional Magnetic Resonance Imaging Cortical Activation with Cross Education to an Immobilized Limb
Farthing JP, Krentz JR, Magnus CRA, et al (Univ of Saskatchewan, Saskatoon, Canada)
Med Sci Sports Exerc 43:1394-1405, 2011

Purpose.—The purpose of this study was to assess cortical activation associated with the cross-education effect to an immobilized limb, using functional magnetic resonance imaging.

Methods.—Fourteen right-handed participants were assigned to two groups. One group ($n = 7$) wore a cast and strength trained the free arm (CAST—TRAIN). The second group ($n = 7$) wore a cast and did not strength train (CAST). Casts were applied to the nondominant (left) wrist and hand. Strength training was maximal isometric handgrip contractions (right hand) 5 d·wk^{-1}. Peak force (handgrip dynamometer), muscle thickness (ultrasound), EMG, and cortical activation (functional magnetic resonance imaging) were assessed before and after the intervention.

Results.—CAST—TRAIN improved right handgrip strength by 10.7% ($P < 0.01$) with no change in muscle thickness. There was a significant group × time interaction for strength of the immobilized arm ($P < 0.05$). Handgrip strength of the immobilized arm of CAST—TRAIN was maintained, whereas the immobilized arm of CAST significantly decreased by 11% ($P < 0.05$). Muscle thickness of the immobilized arm decreased by an average of 3.3% ($P < 0.05$) for all participants and was not different between groups after adjusting for baseline differences. There was a significant group × time interaction for EMG activation ($P < 0.05$), where CAST—TRAIN showed an increasing trend and CAST showed a decreasing trend, pooled across arms. For the immobilized arm of CAST—TRAIN, there was a significant increase in contralateral motor cortex activation after training ($P < 0.05$). For the immobilized arm of CAST, there was no change in motor cortex activation.

Conclusions.—Handgrip strength training of the free limb attenuated strength loss during unilateral immobilization. The maintenance of strength

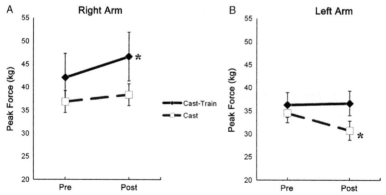

FIGURE 1.—Peak force generated during an isometric handgrip contraction before and after the intervention period for the right (A) and left (B) arms. Note that the left arm was immobilized for 21 d for both groups. For the CAST—TRAIN group, strength was clearly increased in the training right arm and was maintained in the immobilized left arm. For the CAST group, who did not train, strength was unchanged in the right arm and significantly decreased in the immobilized left arm. Note that the "control arm" comparison can be the right arm of CAST group because it did not receive an intervention. *Significantly different from pre value, $P < 0.05$. (Reprinted from Farthing JP, Krentz JR, Magnus CRA, et al. Changes in functional magnetic resonance imaging cortical activation with cross education to an immobilized limb. *Med Sci Sports Exerc.* 2011;43:1394-1405, with permission from the American College of Sports Medicine.)

in the immobilized limb via the cross-education effect may be associated with increased motor cortex activation (Fig 1).

▶ Loss of limb function during immobilization in a plaster cast is a common practical problem. Various options have been attempted to avert this, including electrical stimulation of the muscles within the plaster and voluntary isometric contractions of the affected limb. However, the article by Farthing and associates suggests that because of contralateral cortical activation, a program of training for the uninjured limb can in itself have beneficial consequences for the injured limb, and functional magnetic resonance imaging of the motor cortex supports the hypothesis that contralateral activation is the mechanism. Previous studies in uninjured limbs have suggested that about half of the gains from unilateral strength training are transferred to the opposite limb.[1-3] The results of this 3-week intervention seem of this order (Fig 1), although it will be important to verify this in a group of patients whose limbs have actually been injured. It is also important to underline that the loss of muscle mass was similar in experimental and control groups. The gains were realized mainly by an improvement in neuromuscular control; further, the method of training throughout the study consisted of repeated handgrip contractions, as used in assessing response. Again, the proof would have been more convincing if the measurement and training procedures had differed.

R. J. Shephard, MD (Lond), PhD, DPE

References

1. Carroll TJ, Herbert RD, Munn J, Lee M, Gandevia SC. Contralateral effects of unilateral strength training: evidence and possible mechanisms. *J Appl Physiol.* 2006;101:1514-1522.
2. Farthing JP. Cross-education of strength depends on limb dominance: implications for theory and application. *Exerc Sport Sci Rev.* 2009;37:179-187.
3. Lee M, Carroll TJ. Cross education: possible mechanisms for the contralateral effects of unilateral resistance training. *Sports Med.* 2007;37:1-14.

Extracellular Matrix and Myofibrils During Unloading and Reloading of Skeletal Muscle

Kaasik P, Riso E-M, Seene T (Univ of Tartu, Estonia)
Int J Sports Med 32:247-253, 2011

The aim of the study was to elucidate the effect of unloading and reloading on the collagen expression and synthesis rate of myofibrillar proteins in fast-twitch (FT) muscle in relation to changes in muscle strength and motor activity. Northern blot analysis was used for testing the specificity of cDNA probes and protein synthesis rate was measured according to incorporation of radioactive leucine into different protein fractions. Unloading depresses collagen type I and III ($p < 0.001$), type IV ($p < 0.05$) and reloading enhances collagen expression in fast-twitch skeletal muscle in comparison with unloading. Enhanced expression of matrix metalloproteinase-2 continued

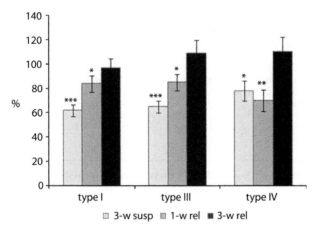

FIGURE 4.—Changes in mRNA levels of type I, type III, and type IV in *gastrocnemius* muscle during unloading and following reloading in comparison with control group (100%). Values are mean ± standard error. 3 w susp – after 3 weeks of hindlimb suspension. 1 w rel – after 1 week of reloading. 3 w rel – after 3 weeks of reloading. * – $p < 0.05$ in comparison with control group. ** – $p < 0.01$ in comparison with control group. *** – $p < 0.001$ in comparison with control group. (Reprinted from Kaasik P, Riso E-M, Seene T. Extracellular matrix and myofibrils during unloading and reloading of skeletal muscle. *Int J Sports Med.* 2011;32:247-253, with permission from Georg Thieme Verlag KG Stuttgart.)

during the first week of reloading ($p < 0.01$) and tissue inhibitor of metalloproteinase-2 during reloading ($p < 0.05$). Changes in collagen expression in FT muscle are in good agreement with changes in myofibrillar protein synthesis during unloading and reloading. In conclusion alterations in extracellular matrix and myofibrillar apparatus in FT skeletal muscle are related to changes in muscle strength and motor activity, and are significant in exercise training and determination of recovery periods in the training process as well as in athletes' rehabilitation (Fig 4).

▶ Those concerned with either the adverse effects of both loss of gravitational stimulation during space flight or immobilization by bed rest have tended to focus on deteriorations in muscle strength and cardiovascular function. Muscles show a decrease in cross section, a loss of myofibrillar protein, and an increase in the proportion of fast-twitch fibers.[1,2] Because of the nature of the observations to be made, the article by Kaasik and associates is based on small groups of rats subjected to 3 weeks of unloading by suspension of the hind limbs, followed by 3 weeks of free cage activity. The article offers a useful reminder that although the tendons seem to be affected relatively little by unloading,[3] a lack of gravitational stimulation leads to a decreased synthesis of several of the collagenous components of muscle (fibrillar collagens I and III and network forming collagen IV), as estimated by the rate of incorporation of radioactive leucine (Fig 4). Normal values were restored over a period of 3 weeks, which offers a useful guide to the necessary period of rehabilitation.

R. J. Shephard, MD (Lond), PhD, DPE

References

1. Roy RR, Baldwin KM, Edgerton VR. Response of the neuromuscular unit to spaceflight: what has been learned from the rat model. *Exerc Sport Sci Rev.* 1996;24:399-425.
2. Trappe T. Influence of aging and long-term unloading on the structure and function of human skeletal muscle. *Appl Physiol Nutr Metab.* 2009;34:459-464.
3. Heinemeier KM, Olesen JL, Haddad F, Schjerling P, Baldwin KM, Kjaer M. Effect of unloading followed by reloading on expression of collagen and related growth factors in rat tendon and muscle. *J Appl Physiol.* 2009;106:178-186.

Strength Training with Blood Flow Restriction Diminishes Myostatin Gene Expression
Laurentino GC, Ugrinowitsch C, Roschel H, et al (Univ of São Paulo, Brazil; et al)
Med Sci Sports Exerc 44:406-412, 2012

Purpose.—The aim of the study was to determine whether the similar muscle strength and hypertrophy responses observed after either low-intensity resistance exercise associated with moderate blood flow restriction or high-intensity resistance exercise are associated with similar changes in messenger RNA (mRNA) expression of selected genes involved in myostatin (*MSTN*) signaling.

Methods.—Twenty-nine physically active male subjects were divided into three groups: low-intensity (20% one-repetition maximum (1RM)) resistance training (LI) ($n = 10$), low-intensity resistance exercise associated with moderate blood flow restriction (LIR) ($n = 10$), and high-intensity (80% 1RM) resistance exercise (HI) ($n = 9$). All of the groups underwent an 8-wk training program. Maximal dynamic knee extension strength (1RM), quadriceps cross-sectional area (CSA), *MSTN*, follistatin-like related genes (follistatin (*FLST*), follistatin-like 3 (*FLST-3*)), activin IIb, growth and differentiation factor—associated serum protein 1 (*GASP-1*), and MAD-related protein (*SMAD-7*) mRNA gene expression were assessed before and after training.

Results.—Knee extension 1RM significantly increased in all groups (LI = 20.7%, LIR = 40.1%, and HI = 36.2%). CSA increased in both the LIR and HI groups (6.3% and 6.1%, respectively). *MSTN* mRNA expression decreased in the LIR and HI groups (45% and 41%, respectively). There were no significant changes in activin IIb ($P > 0.05$). *FLST* and *FLST-3* mRNA expression increased in all groups from pre- to posttest ($P < 0.001$). *FLST-3* expression was significantly greater in the HI when compared with the LIR and LI groups at posttest ($P = 0.024$ and $P = 0.018$, respectively). *GASP-1* and *SMAD-7* gene expression significantly increased in both the LIR and HI groups.

Conclusions.—We concluded that LIR was able to induce gains in 1RM and quadriceps CSA similar to those observed after traditional HI. These responses may be related to the concomitant decrease in *MSTN* and increase in *FLST* isoforms, *GASP-1*, and *SMAD-7* mRNA gene expression.

▶ There is growing evidence that low-resistance exercise coupled with blood-flow restriction is able to induce similar gains of muscle mass to those seen with high-resistance exercise.[1,2] The study of Laurentino and associates aimed to examine whether the 2 methods of training induced similar changes in the mRNA associated with myostatin signaling, the transforming growth factor-β family member that regulates muscle mass.[3-5] Overexpression of myostatin reduces muscle mass, fiber count, and the number of myonuclei. Their small-scale comparison among 3 groups of active young men suggested that relative to low-resistance training alone, a combination of low-resistance training (3 sets of 15 repetitions at 20% 1 repetition maximum, 1 RM) with moderate flow restriction (80% of the pressure needed to cause complete obstruction of blood flow through the inguinal region) produced the same changes in myostatin signaling as 3 sets of 8 repetitions at 80% of 1 RM. Gains of dynamic strength and quadriceps cross-section were also comparable with the low-intensity, flow-restricted training regimen. The practical significance of such findings for training and rehabilitation remains to be resolved. Less motivation is required from the patient for a 20% 1 RM contraction, but presumably to generate an equivalent signal for muscle hypertrophy, the combination of a weak muscle contraction plus flow obstruction induces at least as large an increase of systemic blood pressure as a stronger contraction with free blood flow.

R. J. Shephard, MD (Lond), PhD, DPE

References

1. Karabulut M, Abe T, Sato Y, Bemben MG. The effects of low-intensity resistance training with vascular restriction on leg muscle strength in older men. *Eur J Appl Physiol*. 2010;108:147-155.
2. Kubo K, Komuro T, Ishiguro N, et al. Effects of low-load resistance training with vascular occlusion on the mechanical properties of muscle and tendon. *J Appl Biomech*. 2006;22:112-119.
3. Jespersen JG, Nedergaard A, Andersen LL, Schjerling P, Andersen JL. Myostatin expression during human muscle hypertrophy and subsequent atrophy: increased myostatin with detraining. *Scand J Med Sci Sports*. 2011;21:215-223.
4. Lee SJ. Regulation of muscle mass by myostatin. *Annu Rev Cell Dev Biol*. 2004; 20:61-86.
5. Lee SJ, McPherron AC. Regulation of myostatin activity and muscle growth. *Proc Natl Acad Sci U S A*. 2001;98:9306-9311.

Single-leg cycle training is superior to double-leg cycling in improving the oxidative potential and metabolic profile of trained skeletal muscle
Abbiss CR, Karagounis LG, Laursen PB, et al (Edith Cowan Univ, Joondalup, Western Australia, Australia; Royal Melbourne Inst of Technology, Melbourne, Victoria, Australia; et al)
J Appl Physiol 110:1248-1255, 2011

Single-leg cycling may enhance the peripheral adaptations of skeletal muscle to a greater extent than double-leg cycling. The purpose of the current study was to determine the influence of 3 wk of high-intensity single-and double-leg cycle training on markers of oxidative potential and muscle metabolism and exercise performance. In a crossover design, nine trained cyclists (78 ± 7 kg body wt, 59 ± 5 ml·kg^{-1}·min^{-1} maximal O_2 consumption) performed an incremental cycling test and a 16-km cycling time trial before and after 3 wk of double-leg and counterweighted single-leg cycle training (2 training sessions per week). Training involved three (double) or six (single) maximal 4-min intervals with 6 min of recovery. Mean power output during the single-leg intervals was more than half that during the double-leg intervals (198 ± 29 vs. 344 ± 38 W, $P < 0.05$). Skeletal muscle biopsy samples from the vastus lateralis revealed a training-induced increase in Thr^{172}-phosphorylated 5'-AMP-activated protein kinase α-subunit for both groups ($P < 0.05$). However, the increase in cytochrome c oxidase subunits II and IV and GLUT-4 protein concentration was greater following single-than double-leg cycling ($P < 0.05$). Training-induced improvements in maximal O_2 consumption (3.9 ± 6.2% vs. 0.6 ± 3.6%) and time-trial performance (1.3 ± 0.5% vs. 2.3 ± 4.2%) were similar following both interventions. We conclude that short-term high-intensity single-leg cycle training can elicit greater enhancement in the metabolic and oxidative potential of skeletal muscle than traditional double-leg cycling. Single-leg cycling may therefore provide a valuable training stimulus for trained and clinical populations (Fig 3).

▶ When interval training is performed using the large muscles of the leg, it is likely that the peak intensity of effort will be limited as much by cardiac performance as by muscular activity.[1-3] To circumvent this problem of a circulatory limitation, other investigators have trained subjects in a hyperbaric environment, or to breathe oxygen during training.[4,5] However, a simpler alternative might be to exercise a single leg; this would then allow the body to receive more than 50% of the maximal cardiac output (although not the entire 100%, because a considerable amount of energy is spent in stabilizing body posture when exercising a single leg). This study used a simple randomized crossover design to test the advantages of single versus 2-leg training in a group of 9 fairly fit trained cyclists (maximal oxygen intake, 59 mL/[kg.min]). The single leg was able to develop an additional power output of 10% when the second leg was resting. The result was a greater increase in key biochemical constituents of the muscle, such as cytochrome c subunits II and IV and GLUT-4 protein (Fig 3), indicative of an enhanced mitochondrial oxidative capacity and glucose

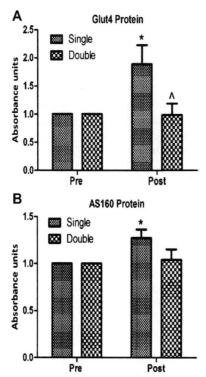

FIGURE 3.—Total protein content of GLUT-4 (*A*) and AS160 (*B*) in muscle samples from vastus lateralis prior to (Pre) and following (Post) 3 wk of single- and double-leg cycle training. Values are means ± SE. *$P < 0.05$ vs. Pre-single. ^$P < 0.05$ vs. Post-single. (Reprinted from Abbiss CR, Karagounis LG, Laursen PB, et al. Single-leg cycle training is superior to double-leg cycling in improving the oxidative potential and metabolic profile of trained skeletal muscle. *J Appl Physiol.* 2011;110:1248-1255, used with permission from the American Physiological Society.)

transport potential. Surprisingly, the single-leg training yielded no measurable advantages in terms of maximal oxygen intake, cycling efficiency, or time trial performance. Possibly, this reflects the crossover design of the study and thus the limited duration of each type of training; a significant advantage of performance might have emerged with more prolonged training. However, the current evidence is insufficient to warrant commending the unilateral training approach to athletes.

R. J. Shephard, MD (Lond), PhD, DPE

References

1. Davies CT, Sargeant AJ. Effects of training on the physiological responses to one- and two-leg work. *J Appl Physiol.* 1975;38:375-377.
2. Neary JP, McKenzie DC, Bhambhani YN. Effects of short-term endurance training on muscle deoxygenation trends using NIRS. *Med Sci Sports Exerc.* 2002;34:1725-1732.
3. Richardson RS, Grassi B, Gavin TP, et al. Evidence of O2 supply-dependent VO2 max in the exercise-trained human quadriceps. *J Appl Physiol.* 1999;86:1048-1053.

4. Perry CGR, Reid J, Perry W, Wilson BA. Effects of hyperoxic training on performance and cardiorespiratory response to exercise. *Med Sci Sports Exerc.* 2005;37: 1175-1179.
5. Perry CGR, Talanian JL, Heigenhauser GJ, Spriet LL. The effects of training in hyperoxia vs. normoxia on skeletal muscle enzyme activities and exercise performance. *J Appl Physiol.* 2007;102:1022-1027.

Relations of Meeting National Public Health Recommendations for Muscular Strengthening Activities With Strength, Body Composition, and Obesity: The Women's Injury Study

Trudelle-Jackson E, Jackson AW, Morrow JR Jr (Texas Woman's Univ, Dallas; Univ of North Texas, Denton; Cooper Inst, Dallas,TX)
Am J Public Health 101:1930-1935, 2011

Objectives.—We examined the relations of meeting or not meeting the 2008 *Physical Activity Guidelines for Americans* recommendations for muscular strengthening activities with percentage of body fat, body mass index (BMI; defined as weight in kilograms divided by height in meters, squared), muscular strength, and obesity classification in women.

Methods.—We analyzed data on 918 women aged 20 to 83 years in the Women's Injury Study from 2007 to 2009. A baseline orthopedic examination included measurement of height, body weight, skinfolds, and muscle strength.

Results.—Women who met muscle strengthening activity recommendations had significantly lower BMI and percentage of body fat and higher muscle strength. Women not meeting those recommendations were more likely to be obese (BMI≥30) compared with women who met the recommendations after we adjusted for age, race, and aerobic physical activity (odds ratio = 2.28; 95% confidence interval = 1.61, 3.23).

Conclusions.—There was a small but significant positive association between meeting muscle strengthening activity recommendations and muscular strength, a moderate inverse association with body fat percentage, and a strong inverse association with obesity classification, providing preliminary support for the muscle strengthening activity recommendation for women.

▶ The backdrop for this study is that only 14% to 17% of women reported participating in muscle strengthening activity in a 1998 to 2004 survey.[1] Evidence supporting the health benefits of muscle strength led to the 2008 Physical Activity Guidelines for Americans[2] to perform muscle strengthening exercise on 2 or more days per week. It is not known whether women are meeting this recommendation and whether they are healthier for having done so. In this observational study of baseline data (collected from 2007 to 2009) from the Women's Injury Study, women who did not meet the 2008 Guidelines for muscle strengthening exercise had a 128% greater prevalence of obesity (body mass index ≥ 30 kg/m^2) compared with women who met the recommendations. The participants reported whether they had performed "resistance exercises (using free weights or weight machines, calisthenics, power yoga, pilates, etc.)" They also reported on participation in moderate and vigorous aerobic physical activity and were classified as accumulating at least 150 min or less than 150 min of these activities per week. Participants who met neither recommendation had the highest prevalence of obesity at 40% whereas the lowest prevalence, at 14%, was in women meeting the strength and aerobic exercise recommendations. Of the 905 women in the survey, 42% reported meeting the 2008 Guidelines for muscle strength, which is a substantial jump from the 1998 to 2004 survey. This change may be partially explained by the inclusion of activities such as yoga and pilates in the Women's Injury Study survey. A dose-response of muscle strengthening exercise and health benefits has yet to be determined and will require carefully constructed assessments of exercise type (eg, free weights, yoga), loads, and training volume. Notably, women in this study were aged approximately 50 years and had a similar overweight/obese profile (61%) as the general US population (63%). The study cohort represents a population that has increased risk of developing sarcopenia, sarcopenic obesity, and osteoporosis.

C. M. Jankowski, PhD

References

1. Centers for Disease Control and Prevention (CDC). Trends in strength training—United States, 1998-2004. *MMWR Morb Mortal Wkly Rep.* 2006;55:769-772.
2. *2008 Physical Activity Guidelines for Americans.* Washington, DC: US Department of Health and Human Services; 2008.

Conditioning of the Achilles tendon via ankle exercise improves correlations between sonographic measures of tendon thickness and body anthropometry

Wearing SC, Grigg NL, Hooper SL, et al (Bond Univ, Queensland, Australia; Queensland Univ of Technology, Kelvin Grove, Australia; Queensland Academy of Sport, Sunnybank, Australia)

J Appl Physiol 110:1384-1389, 2011

Although conditioning is routinely used in mechanical tests of tendon in vitro, previous in vivo research evaluating the influence of body anthropometry on Achilles tendon thickness has not considered its potential effects on tendon structure. This study evaluated the relationship between Achilles tendon thickness and body anthropometry in healthy adults both before and after resistive ankle plantarflexion exercise. A convenience sample of 30 healthy male adults underwent sonographic examination of the Achilles tendon in addition to standard anthropometric measures of stature and body weight. A 10—5 MHz linear array transducer was used to acquire longitudinal sonograms of the Achilles tendon, 20 mm proximal to the tendon insertion. Participants then completed a series (90—100 repetitions) of conditioning exercises against an effective resistance between 100% and 150% body weight. Longitudinal sonograms were repeated immediately on completion of the exercise intervention, and anteroposterior Achilles tendon thickness was determined. Achilles tendon thickness was significantly reduced immediately following conditioning exercise ($t = 9.71$, $P < 0.001$), resulting in an average transverse strain of -18.8%. In contrast to preexercise measures, Achilles tendon thickness was significantly correlated with body weight ($r = 0.72$, $P < 0.001$) and to a lesser extent height ($r = 0.45$, $P < 0.01$) and body mass index ($r = 0.63$, $P < 0.001$) after exercise. Conditioning of the Achilles tendon via resistive ankle exercises induces alterations in tendon structure that substantially improve correlations between Achilles tendon thickness and body anthropometry. It is recommended that conditioning exercises, which standardize the load history of tendon, are employed before measurements of sonographic tendon thickness in vivo (Fig 2).

▶ Sonographic measurements of the thickness of the Achilles tendon are sometimes used to identify local pathologies,[1,2] although normal thicknesses vary widely, from about 4 to 7 mm.[3,4] Moreover, attempts to standardize data using various more general anthropometric measurements have accounted for only 6% to 30% of the total variance in the data.[3,5] One factor that could facilitate more accurate measurements is recent conditioning exercise, because this tends to express fluid from the tendon, reducing its dimensions to more stable values.[6] This study by Wearing and associates was based on a convenience sample of 30 healthy middle-aged men. Repeated (90-100) ankle plantar flexions were performed against 100% to 150% of body mass; this reduced thickness by 17.5% in subjects with a normal body mass index (BMI) and by about 9% in those who were overweight (BMI > 27 kg/m^2). Others who have failed to observe this may have included the paratenon in their estimates;

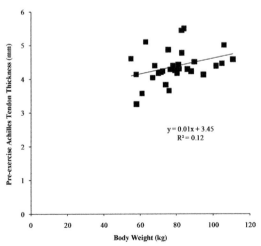

FIGURE 2.—Scatter plot of preexercise Achilles tendon thickness and body weight. (Reprinted from Wearing SC, Grigg NL, Hooper SL, et al. Conditioning of the Achilles tendon via ankle exercise improves correlations between sonographic measures of tendon thickness and body anthropometry. *J Appl Physiol.* 2011;110:1384-1389, used with permission from the American Physiological Society.)

the blood flow to this region is increased by exercise, canceling out any decrease in thickness of the tendon proper. Following conditioning, thickness became significantly correlated with body mass, height, and BMI, although the scatter remained such that the relationships were still not of great help in standardizing data; the closest relationship is with body mass, which accounts for about 50% of the variance in thickness (Fig 2).

R. J. Shephard, MD (Lond), PhD, DPE

References

1. Kainberger FM, Engel A, Barton P, Huebsch P, Neuhold A, Salomonowitz E. Injury of the Achilles tendon: diagnosis with sonography. *AJR Am J Roentgenol.* 1990;155:1031-1036.
2. Mathieson JR, Connell DG, Cooperberg PL, Lloyd-Smith DR. Sonography of the Achilles tendon and adjacent bursae. *AJR Am J Roentgenol.* 1988;151:127-131.
3. Koivunen-Niemelä T, Parkkola K. Anatomy of the Achilles tendon (tendo calcaneus) with respect to tendon thickness measurements. *Surg Radiol Anat.* 1995; 17:263-268.
4. Yuzawa K, Yamakawa K, Tohno E, et al. An ultrasonographic method for detection of Achilles tendon xanthomas in familial hypercholesterolemia. *Atherosclerosis.* 1989;75:211-218.
5. Akturk M, Ozdemir A, Maral I, Yetkin I, Arslan M. Evaluation of Achilles tendon thickening in type 2 diabetes mellitus. *Exp Clin Endocrinol Diabetes.* 2007;115: 92-96.
6. Wearing SC, Smeathers JE, Urry SR, et al. The time-course of acute changes in Achilles tendon morphology following exercise. In: Fuss FK, Subic A, Ujihashi S, eds. *The Impact of Technology on Sport II.* Singapore: Taylor and Francis; 2008:65-68.

Stretching before or after exercise does not reduce delayed-onset muscle soreness

Henschke N, Lin CC (The Univ of Sydney, Australia)
Br J Sports Med 45:1249-1250, 2011

Our aim was to determine the effect of stretching before or after exercise on the development of postexercise muscle soreness.

The search retrieved 43 potentially eligible studies of which 12 were eligible for inclusion in the review. Two of these studies (including one study involving 2377 participants) were added to the previous version of the review. The overall quality of evidence was low to moderate.

The pooled estimates indicated that pre-exercise and postexercise stretching reduces soreness, on average, by one point on a 100-point scale at one day (mean difference (MD) −0.9, 95% CI −6.1 to 4.2; seven studies; figure 1), increases soreness by one point on a 100-point scale at 2 days (MD 1.0, 95% CI −4.1 to 6.2; seven studies) and has no effect on soreness at 3 days (MD −0.3; 95% CI −6.8 to 6.2; five studies). None of these findings were statistically significant. The only large study 4 found that stretching reduced the intensity of the worst soreness experienced over a week by, on average, four points on a 100-point scale (MD −3.8; 95% CI −5.2 to −2.4). Although this result is statistically significant, the size of the treatment effect is small (ie, 3.8/100) and is unlikely to be clinically worthwhile. Hence, this review found that stretching pre or postexercise did not have important effects on muscle soreness.

▶ These data, pooled from 12 studies of 2597 participants, do not support the common belief that stretching reduces muscle soreness. This finding was consistent across settings (laboratory vs field studies), types and intensity of stretching, populations (athletic or untrained adults of both genders), and study quality. Many claims have been made for the performance-, fitness-, and health-related benefits of regular flexibility exercise. Some sports and physical activities require unique types of flexibility that enhance performance, including Olympic weight lifting, ballet dancing, gymnastics, swimming, baseball pitching, and wrestling. However, no consistent link has been shown between regular flexibility exercise and prevention of low back pain, injury, or, as supported by this review, delayed onset of muscle soreness.[1] Nonetheless, flexibility exercise is a valuable component of rehabilitation programs from injury. Of all age groups, the elderly have the most to gain through regular flexibility exercise, with several studies showing improved range of motion and capacity for daily activities of living.[1]

D. C. Nieman, DrPH

Reference

1. Garber CE, Blissmer B, Deschenes MR, et al; American College of Sports Medicine. American College of Sports Medicine position stand. Quantity and quality of exercise for developing and maintaining cardiorespiratory, musculoskeletal, and neuromotor fitness in apparently healthy adults: guidance for prescribing exercise. *Med Sci Sports Exerc*. 2011;43:1334-1359.

Effects of physiotherapy treatment on knee osteoarthritis gait data using principal component analysis
Gaudreault N, Mezghani N, Turcot K, et al (Centre de recherche du Centre hospitalier de l'Université de Montréal, Quebec City, Canada)
Clin Biomech 26:284-291, 2011

Background.—Interpreting gait data is challenging due to intersubject variability observed in the gait pattern of both normal and pathological populations. The objective of this study was to investigate the impact of using principal component analysis for grouping knee osteoarthritis (OA) patients' gait data in more homogeneous groups when studying the effect of a physiotherapy treatment.

Methods.—Three-dimensional (3D) knee kinematic and kinetic data were recorded during the gait of 29 participants diagnosed with knee OA before and after they received 12 weeks of physiotherapy treatment. Principal component analysis was applied to extract groups of knee flexion/extension, adduction/abduction and internal/external rotation angle and moment data. The treatment's effect on parameters of interest was assessed using paired *t*-tests performed before and after grouping the knee kinematic data.

Findings.—Increased quadriceps and hamstring strength was observed following treatment ($P<0.05$). Except for the knee flexion/extension angle, two different groups (G_1 and G_2) were extracted from the angle and moment data. When pre- and post-treatment analyses were performed considering the groups, participants exhibiting a G_2 knee moment pattern demonstrated a greater first peak flexion moment, lower adduction moment impulse and smaller rotation angle range post-treatment ($P<0.05$). When pre- and post-treatment comparisons were performed without grouping, the data showed no treatment effect.

Interpretation.—The results of the present study suggest that the effect of physiotherapy on gait mechanics of knee osteoarthritis patients may be masked or underestimated if kinematic data are not separated into more homogeneous groups when performing pre- and post-treatment comparisons.

▶ Exercise is considered beneficial for managing osteoarthritis of the knee in terms of decreasing pain and improving function. However, the effects on gait data have not been as conclusive. The authors use principal component analysis to divide their sample of 29 patients with knee osteoarthritis into 2 groups that are more homogeneous in terms of gait cycle data. Their analysis of pre-post physiotherapy exercise intervention demonstrated improvement in clinical evaluation measures (pain, stiffness, and function on the Western Ontario McMaster Universities Osteoarthritis Index; isometric muscle strength; locomotor function tests). Moreover, they found improvements in gait patterns after physiotherapy when grouping the patients. Although the sample is small, the authors were still able to show that grouping patients into homogeneous groups is important to demonstrate differences for pre- and posttest comparisons of kinematic data. The authors state that this method of grouping may be important in future research evaluating effectiveness of different types of rehabilitation strategies on the biomechanics of the knee. It is unfortunate that the clinical implications of kinematic data were not addressed much in the article.

D. E. Feldman, PT, PhD

Efficacy of physiotherapy interventions late after stroke: a meta-analysis
Ferrarello F, Baccini M, Rinaldi LA, et al (Unit of Functional Rehabilitation, Prato, Italy; Piero Palagi Hosp, Florence, Italy; University of Florence and Azienda Ospedaliero-Universitaria Careggi, Italy)
J Neurol Neurosurg Psychiatry 82:136-143, 2011

Objective.—Physiotherapy is usually provided only in the first few months after stroke, while its effectiveness and appropriateness in the chronic phase are uncertain. The authors conducted a systematic review and meta-analysis of randomised clinical trials (RCT) to evaluate the efficacy of physiotherapy interventions on motor and functional outcomes late after stroke.

Methods.—The authors searched published studies where participants were randomised to an active physiotherapy intervention, compared with placebo or no intervention, at least 6 months after stroke. The outcome was a change in mobility and activities of daily living (ADL) independence. The quality of the trials was evaluated using the PEDro scale. Findings were summarised across studies as effect size (ES) or, whenever possible, weighted mean difference (WMD) with 95% CI in random effects models.

Results.—Fifteen RCT were included, enrolling 700 participants with follow-up data. The meta-analysis of primary outcomes from the original studies showed a significant effect of the intervention (ES 0.29, 95% CI 0.14 to 0.45). The efficacy of the intervention was particularly evident when short- and long-distance walking were considered as separate outcomes, with WMD of 0.05 m/s (95% CI 0.008 to 0.088) and 20 m (95% CI 3.6 to 36.0), respectively. Also, ADL improvement was greater,

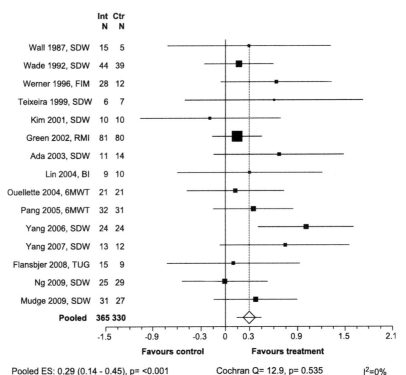

FIGURE 2.—Plot of random effects meta-analysis of effect size for all the outcomes considered. 6MWT, 6 min walking test; BI, Barthel Index; Ctr N, Control group sample size; ES, effect size; FIM, functional independence measure; Int N, intervention group sample size; RMI, Rivermead Mobility Index; SDW, short-distance walk; TUG, timed up-and-go test. (Republished with permission of BMJ Publishing Group Ltd, from the Journal of Neurology, Neurosurgery, and Psychiatry. Ferrarello F, Baccini M, Rinaldi LA, et al. Efficacy of physiotherapy interventions late after stroke: a meta-analysis. *J Neurol Neurosurg Psychiatry.* 2011;82:136-143, with permission from Copyright Clearance Center, Inc.)

though non-significantly, in the intervention group. No significant heterogeneity was found.

Interpretation.—A variety of physiotherapy interventions improve functional outcomes, even when applied late after stroke. These findings challenge the concept of a plateau in functional recovery of patients who had experienced stroke and should be valued in planning community rehabilitation services (Fig 2).

▶ The results of this meta-analysis indicate that physiotherapy is effective for improving certain outcomes for stroke patients even 6 months or more after stroke. As shown in Fig 2, the majority of the interventions improved function (eg, short distance walking, functional independence measure, 6-minute walk test). The authors call for further study in terms of the extent and frequency of treatment to optimize outcomes. However, there are economic implications; the authors do state that most health care systems would not be able to afford additional physiotherapy services later on after stroke. Thus, cost-effectiveness studies are also needed. In the meantime, the information in the study indicates that there are benefits to physiotherapy later on after stroke. How policy makers, administrators, clinicians, and patients deal with this evidence remains to be seen.

D. E. Feldman, PT, PhD

Extra Physical Therapy Reduces Patient Length of Stay and Improves Functional Outcomes and Quality of Life in People With Acute or Subacute Conditions: A Systematic Review
Peiris CL, Taylor NF, Shields N (La Trobe Univ, Victoria, Australia)
Arch Phys Med Rehabil 92:1490-1500, 2011

Objectives.—To investigate whether extra physical therapy intervention reduces length of stay and improves patient outcomes in people with acute or subacute conditions.

Data Sources.—Electronic databases CINAHL, MEDLINE, AMED, PEDro, PubMed, and EMBASE were searched from the earliest date possible through May 2010. Additional trials were identified by scanning reference lists and citation tracking.

Study Selection.—Randomized controlled trials evaluating the effect of extra physical therapy on patient outcomes were included for review. Two reviewers independently applied the inclusion and exclusion criteria, and any disagreements were discussed until consensus could be reached. Searching identified 2826 potentially relevant articles, of which 16 randomized controlled trials with 1699 participants met inclusion criteria.

Data Extraction.—Data were extracted using a predefined data extraction form by 1 reviewer and checked for accuracy by another. Methodological quality of trials was assessed independently by 2 reviewers using the PEDro scale.

Data Synthesis.—Pooled analyses with random effects model to calculate standardized mean differences (SMDs) and 95% confidence intervals (CIs) were used in meta-analyses. When compared with standard physical therapy, extra physical therapy reduced length of stay (SMD=−.22; 95% CI, −.39 to −.05) (mean difference of 1d [95% CI, 0−1] in acute settings and mean difference of 4d [95% CI, 0−7] in rehabilitation settings) and improved mobility (SMD=.37; 95% CI, .05−.69), activity (SMD=.22; 95% CI, .07−.37), and quality of life (SMD=.48; 95% CI, .29−.68). There were no significant changes in self-care (SMD=.35; 95% CI, −.06−.77).

Conclusions.—Extra physical therapy decreases length of stay and significantly improves mobility, activity, and quality of life. Future research could address the possible benefits of providing extra services from other allied health disciplines in addition to physical therapy.

▶ This systematic review of 16 randomized, controlled trials supports the contention that extra physical therapy reduces length of stay in the hospital or rehabilitation center and improves rate of improvement (ie, the results are more rapid) for walking ability, activity, and quality of life for persons with a variety of acute or subacute conditions. These conditions included stroke, multiple sclerosis, traumatic brain injury, post–coronary artery bypass surgery, total hip joint replacement, total knee joint replacement, and hip fracture. The authors do address the important question of just how much extra physical therapy is necessary to achieve these improvements. They state that an extra 19 minutes of physical therapy per day was needed: this could be achieved by having longer sessions, more sessions in a day, or extra sessions. The reduction in length of hospital stay was 1 day in the acute setting and 4 days in a rehabilitation setting. A formal cost analysis would be needed, but it appears that extra physical therapy may reduce costs due to the higher costs of hospital stay versus the cost of extra physical therapy. Further, there are benefits for the patient in terms of returning to the community sooner.

D. E. Feldman, PT, PhD

Clinical features and outcome of physiotherapy in early presenting congenital muscular torticollis with severe fibrosis on ultrasonography: a prospective study
Lee Y-T, Yoon K, Kim Y-B, et al (Sungkyunkwan Univ, Seoul, South Korea; et al)
J Pediatr Surg 46:1526-1531, 2011

Background.—It has been reported that ultrasonography (US) can detect the severity of congenital muscular torticollis (CMT), and severe fibrosis of the sternocleidomastoid (SCM) muscle noted on US is irreversible and likely to require surgery. Clinical outcome of CMT depends mainly on the patient's age, which is also associated with the severity of fibrosis as determined by US. However, there has been no well-designed study to elucidate the true relationship among these factors nor a definite consensus on treatment of young infants with severe fibrosis in the SCM compared with well-documented reports that late cases require surgery.

Purpose.—The purpose of the current study was to investigate whether severity of SCM fibrosis on US is correlated with clinical severity and outcome of standardized physiotherapy in early presenting CMT.

Methods.—Fifty patients with a palpable neck mass, initial deficit of passive neck rotation (ΔROT) more than 10°, and age less than 3 months were classified into 4 US types according to the severity of fibrosis in the SCM and underwent standardized physiotherapy and regular assessment. Relationship between US types and 2 variables (ΔROT and treatment duration) and success rate of physiotherapy was assessed.

Results.—None of the cases was classified as type 4. Type 3 showed greatest ΔROT and longest mean treatment duration. Both variables showed a significant linear trend of association with US types by P for trend $(P=.003, P<.001,$ respectively). Treatment was "successful" in 49 patients (98%).

Conclusion.—In young infants with CMT, US can document severity; and an early and adequate physiotherapy is a good treatment option, particularly even in those with severe fibrosis (Fig 3).

▶ Pediatric physical therapists are seeing more and more infants with torticollis. Infants with congenital muscular torticollis typically present with reduced neck

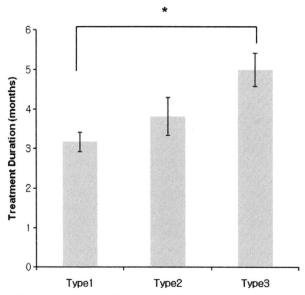

FIGURE 3.—Treatment duration according to severity of fibrosis on US. Mean duration of treatment was gradually lengthened as the severity of fibrosis on US increased from type 1 to 3. This showed a significant linear trend of association. *P for trend < .001. Values represent mean ± SEM. (Reprinted from Lee Y-T, Yoon K, Kim Y-B, et al. Clinical features and outcome of physiotherapy in early presenting congenital muscular torticollis with severe fibrosis on ultrasonography: a prospective study. *J Pediatr Surg*. 2011;46: 1526-1531, Copyright 2011, with permission from Elsevier.)

rotation and lateral neck tilt, and there may also be a palpable mass caused by fibrous contracture of the sterno-cleido-mastoid muscle. The theory is that fibrosis occurs during the intrauterine period and that those presenting with more severe fibrosis will have a poorer outcome with conservative physical therapy treatment (which typically consists of stretching exercises and positioning). This study used ultrasound scan to assess severity of the fibrosis according to 4 categories (1 being the most mild). Outcomes were difference in neck rotation between the affected and unaffected side and duration of physical therapy treatment (censored at 10 months of age if there was a difference of more than 6° in neck rotation or if no further improvement occurred after more than 6 months of successive treatment). Although the sample was small (50 infants), the results indicated that the ultrasound-diagnosed categories predicted outcomes. Interestingly, 49 of 50 patients were deemed to have been a success following physiotherapy treatment, even though the 17 patients (34%) with category 3 fibrosis had longer duration of treatment (Fig 3). This good result is encouraging and according to the authors may indicate that early intensive physical therapy is especially important for those with more severe fibrosis. The clinical implication is that patients with congenital muscular torticollis should be treated early with physical therapy.

D. E. Feldman, PT, PhD

Comparison of adaptive pacing therapy, cognitive behaviour therapy, graded exercise therapy, and specialist medical care for chronic fatigue syndrome (PACE): a randomised trial

White PD, on behalf of the PACE trial management group (Queen Mary Univ of London, UK; et al)

Lancet 377:823-836, 2011

Background.—Trial findings show cognitive behaviour therapy (CBT) and graded exercise therapy (GET) can be effective treatments for chronic fatigue syndrome, but patients' organisations have reported that these treatments can be harmful and favour pacing and specialist health care. We aimed to assess effectiveness and safety of all four treatments.

Methods.—In our parallel-group randomised trial, patients meeting Oxford criteria for chronic fatigue syndrome were recruited from six secondary-care clinics in the UK and randomly allocated by computer-generated sequence to receive specialist medical care (SMC) alone or with adaptive pacing therapy (APT), CBT, or GET. Primary outcomes were fatigue (measured by Chalder fatigue questionnaire score) and physical function (measured by short form-36 subscale score) up to 52 weeks after randomisation, and safety was assessed primarily by recording all serious adverse events, including serious adverse reactions to trial treatments. Primary outcomes were rated by participants, who were necessarily unmasked to treatment assignment; the statistician was masked to treatment assignment for the analysis of primary outcomes. We used longitudinal regression models to compare SMC alone with other treatments,

TABLE 3.—Primary Outcomes of Fatigue and Physical Function

	Fatigue*				Physical Function†			
	Adaptive Pacing Therapy	Cognitive Behaviour Therapy	Graded Exercise Therapy	Specialist Medical Care Alone	Adaptive Pacing Therapy	Cognitive Behaviour Therapy	Graded Exercise Therapy	Specialist Medical Care Alone
Baseline	28·5 (4·0); n=159	27·7 (3·7); n=161	28·2 (3·8); n=160	28·3 (3·6); n=160	37·2 (16·9); n=159	39·0 (15·3); n=161	36·7 (15·4); n=160	39·2 (15·4); n=160
12 weeks	24·2 (6·4); n=153	23·6 (6·5); n=153	22·8 (7·5); n=153	24·3 (6·5); n=154	41·7 (19·9); n=153	51·0 (20·7); n=153	48·1 (21·6); n=153	46·6 (20·4); n=154
24 weeks	23·7 (6·9); n=155	21·5 (7·8); n=148	21·7 (7·1); n=150	24·0 (6·9); n=152	43·2 (21·4); n=155	54·2 (21·6); n=148	55·4 (23·3); n=150	48·4 (23·1); n=152
52 weeks	23·1 (7·3); n=153	20·3 (8·0); n=148	20·6 (7·5); n=154	23·8 (6·6); n=152	45·9 (24·9); n=153	58·2 (24·1); n=148	57·7 (26·5); n=154	50·8 (24·7); n=152
Mean difference (95% CI) from SMC (52 weeks)	-0·7 (-2·3 to 0·9)	-3·4 (-5·0 to -1·8)	-3·2 (-4·8 to -1·7)	··	-3·4 (-8·4 to 1·6)	7·1 (2·0 to 12·1)	9·4 (4·4 to 14·4)	··
Unadjusted p values	0·38	0·0001	0·0003	··	0·18	0·0068	0·0005	··
Bonferroni adjusted p values	0·99	0·0006	0·0013	··	0·89	0·0342	0·0025	··
Mean difference (95% CI) from APT (52 weeks)	··	-2·7 (-4·4 to -1·1)	-2·5 (-4·2 to -0·9)	··	··	10·5 (5·4 to 15·6)	12·8 (7·7 to 17·9)	··
Unadjusted p values	··	0·0027	0·0059	··	··	0·0002	<0·0001	··
Bonferroni adjusted p values	··	0·0136	0·0294	··	··	0·0012	0·0002	··
Number improved from baseline‡	99 (65%)	113 (76%)	123 (80%)	98 (65%)	75 (49%)	105 (71%)	108 (70%)	88 (58%)

Data are mean scores (SD) or n (%), unless otherwise stated. Comparisons of differences across groups made at 52 weeks are from the final adjusted models, so are slightly different from unadjusted values. p values for comparisons are unadjusted, with Bonferroni values adjusted for five comparisons for every primary outcome.

Editor's Note: Please refer to original journal article for full references.

*Chalder fatigue questionnaire (range 0–33, 0=best).[15]

†Short form-36 physical function subscale score (range 0–100, 100=best).[16]

‡Participants improved from baseline by two or more points for fatigue and eight or more for physical function.

APT with CBT, and APT with GET. The final analysis included all participants for whom we had data for primary outcomes. This trial is registered at http://isrctn.org, number ISRCTN54285094.

Findings.—We recruited 641 eligible patients, of whom 160 were assigned to the APT group, 161 to the CBT group, 160 to the GET group, and 160 to the SMC-alone group. Compared with SMC alone, mean fatigue scores at 52 weeks were 3·4 (95% CI 1·8 to 5·0) points lower for CBT (p= 0·0001) and 3·2 (1·7 to 4·8) points lower for GET (p=0·0003), but did not differ for APT (0·7 [−0·9 to 2·3] points lower; p=0·38). Compared with SMC alone, mean physical function scores were 7·1 (2·0 to 12·1) points higher for CBT (p=0·0068) and 9·4 (4·4 to 14·4) points higher for GET (p=0·0005), but did not differ for APT (3·4 [−1·6 to 8·4] points lower; p=0·18). Compared with APT, CBT and GET were associated with less fatigue (CBT p=0·0027; GET p=0·0059) and better physical function (CBT p=0·0002; GET p<0·0001). Subgroup analysis of 427 participants meeting international criteria for chronic fatigue syndrome and 329 participants meeting London criteria for myalgic encephalomyelitis yielded equivalent results. Serious adverse reactions were recorded in two (1%) of 159 participants in the APT group, three (2%) of 161 in the CBT group, two (1%) of 160 in the GET group, and two (1%) of 160 in the SMC-alone group.

Interpretation.—CBT and GET can safely be added to SMC to moderately improve outcomes for chronic fatigue syndrome, but APT is not an effective addition (Table 3).

▶ Although a number of relatively small trials have previously indicated the effectiveness of progressive exercise in the treatment of chronic fatigue syndrome,[1-5] patients' organizations continue to argue that such treatment can be harmful, and they recommend as an alternative either adaptive pacing of physical activity to avoid fatigue or specialized medical care. White and associates here make a careful randomized comparison of exercise with cognitive therapy, pacing, and specialized medical care, using a substantial sample of carefully defined cases of chronic fatigue syndrome (the Oxford criteria were adopted, in which fatigue is the dominant symptom). The exercise program was negotiated with the individual patient and was based on the extent of initial deconditioning; the objective was a progression to light exercise performed for at least 30 minutes 5 times per week. The alternative of cognitive therapy aimed at reducing patients' fears of engaging in physical activity. The exercise and cognitive therapy groups showed much greater improvement in both fatigue and physical function scores than the other 2 treatment modalities, where little response was seen (Table 3). Complications were rare for any of the 4 treatments and clearly were no more likely in the exercise or cognitive therapy groups than with the other 2 treatment options. This study suggests that fears of exercise in chronic fatigue syndrome are unwarranted, and insistence on adopting alternative forms of treatment may be delaying a cure for the patient.

R. J. Shephard, MD (Lond), PhD, DPE

References

1. Shephard RJ. Chronic fatigue syndrome: an update. *Sports Med.* 2001;31: 167-194.
2. Shephard RJ. Chronic fatigue syndrome. A brief review of functional disturbances and potential therapy. *J Sports Med Phys Fitness.* 2005;45:381-392.
3. Edmonds M, McGuire H, Price JR. Exercise therapy for chronic fatigue syndrome. *Cochrane Database Syst Rev.* 2004;(3):CD003200.
4. Malouff JM, Thorsteinsson EB, Rooke SE, Bhullar N, Schutte NS. Efficacy of cognitive behavioral therapy for chronic fatigue syndrome: a meta-analysis. *Clin Psychol Rev.* 2008;28:736-745.
5. Price JR, Mitchell E, Tidy E, Hunot V. Cognitive behaviour therapy for chronic fatigue syndrome in adults. *Cochrane Database Syst Rev.* 2008;(3):CD001027.

Use of weekly, low dose, high frequency ultrasound for hard to heal venous leg ulcers: the VenUS III randomised controlled trial
Watson JM, on behalf of the VenUS III Team (Univ of York, UK; et al)
BMJ 342:d1092, 2011

Objective.—To assess the clinical effectiveness of weekly delivery of low dose, high frequency therapeutic ultrasound in conjunction with standard care for hard to heal venous leg ulcers.

Design.—Multicentre, pragmatic, two arm randomised controlled trial.

Setting.—Community and district nurse led services, community leg ulcer clinics, and hospital outpatient leg ulcer clinics in 12 urban and rural settings (11 in the United Kingdom and one in the Republic of Ireland).

Participants.—337 patients with at least one venous leg ulcer of >6 months' duration or >5 cm^2 area and an ankle brachial pressure index of ≥0.8.

Interventions.—Weekly administration of low dose, high frequency ultrasound therapy (0.5 W/cm^2, 1 MHz, pulsed pattern of 1:4) for up to 12 weeks plus standard care compared with standard care alone.

Main Outcome Measures.—Primary outcome was time to healing of the largest eligible leg ulcer. Secondary outcomes were proportion of patients healed by 12 months, percentage and absolute change in ulcer size, proportion of time participants were ulcer-free, health related quality of life, and adverse events.

Results.—The two groups showed no significant difference in the time to healing of the reference leg ulcer (log rank test, P=0.61). After adjustment for baseline ulcer area, baseline ulcer duration, use of compression bandaging, and study centre, there was still no evidence of a difference in time to healing (hazard ratio 0.99 (95% confidence interval 0.70 to 1.40), P=0.97). The median time to healing of the reference leg ulcer was inestimable. There was no significant difference between groups in the proportion of participants with all ulcers healed by 12 months (72/168 in ultrasound group *v* 78/169 in standard care group, P=0.39 for Fisher's exact test) nor in the change in ulcer size at four weeks by treatment group (model estimate 0.05 (95% CI −0.09 to 0.19)). There was no difference in time to complete healing of all ulcers (log rank test, P=0.61), with median time to healing of 328 days (95% CI 235 to inestimable) with standard care and 365 days (224 days to inestimable) with ultrasound. There was no evidence of a difference in rates of recurrence of healed ulcers (17/31 with ultrasound v 14/31 with standard care, P=0.68 for Fisher's exact test). There was no difference between the two groups in health related quality of life, both for the physical component score (model estimate 0.69 (-1.79 to 3.08)) and the mental component score (model estimate -0.93 (-3.30 to 1.44)), but there were significantly more adverse events in the ultrasound group (model estimate 0.30 (0.01 to 0.60)). There was a significant relation between time to ulcer healing and baseline ulcer area (hazard ratio 0.64 (0.55 to 0.75)) and baseline ulcer duration (hazard ratio 0.59 (0.50 to 0.71)), with larger and older ulcers taking longer to heal. In addition, those centres with high recruitment rates had the highest healing rates.

Conclusions.—Low dose, high frequency ultrasound administered weekly for 12 weeks during dressing changes in addition to standard care did not increase ulcer healing rates, affect quality of life, or reduce ulcer recurrence.

Trial Registration.—ISRCTN21175670 and National Research Register N0484162339 (Fig 2).

▶ This is a well-designed randomized clinical trial. The investigators provide a detailed description of their study (eg, inclusion and exclusion criteria, outcome measurement, analysis) and the ultrasound intervention (0.5 watts/cm^2, once a week for up to 12 weeks). As shown in Fig 2, there were no differences between the groups (standard care vs ultrasound + standard care) in terms of time to complete healing of the reference ulcer. Adjusting for several covariates did not change this. The investigators concluded that this particular regimen of ultrasound treatment did not produce additional benefits over standard treatment. They do caution that the results correspond to this particular treatment regimen. Others have recommended a higher treatment frequency for therapeutic

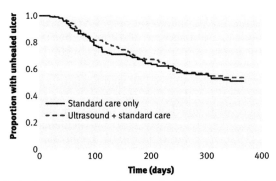

FIGURE 2.—Kaplan-Meier survival curve for time to healing of reference ulcers among 337 patients with venous leg ulcers randomised to standard care alone or to ultrasound plus standard care. (Reprinted from Watson JM, on behalf of the VenUS III Team. Use of weekly, low dose, high frequency ultrasound for hard to heal venous leg ulcers: the VenUS III randomised controlled trial. *BMJ.* 2011;342:d1092, with permission from the BMJ Publishing Group Ltd.)

ultrasound for wound healing (eg, 3 times a week instead of once a week used in this study). Even if the higher frequency of treatment sessions per week is shown to be beneficial, the cost-benefits of a more intensive treatment would have to be assessed.

D. E. Feldman, PT, PhD

4 Physical Activity, Cardiorespiratory Physiology and Immune Function

Effects of an 8-Month Exercise Training Program on Off-Exercise Physical Activity

Rangan VV, Willis LH, Slentz CA, et al (Duke Univ Med Ctr, Durham, NC; et al)

Med Sci Sports Exerc 43:1744-1751, 2011

Purpose.—An active lifestyle is widely recognized as having a beneficial effect on cardiovascular health. However, no clear consensus exists as to whether exercise training increases overall physical activity energy expenditure (PAEE) or whether individuals participating in regular exercise compensate by reducing their off-exercise physical activity. The purpose of this study was to evaluate changes in PAEE in response to aerobic training (AT), resistance training (RT), or combined aerobic and resistance training (AT/RT).

Methods.—Data are from 82 participants in the Studies of Targeted Risk Reduction Interventions through Defined Exercise—Aerobic Training versus Resistance Training study, a randomized trial of overweight (body mass index = 25–35 kg·m^{-2}) adults, in which participants were randomized to receive 8 months of AT, RT, or AT/RT. All subjects completed a 4-month control period before randomization. PAEE was measured using triaxial RT3 accelerometers, which subjects wore for a 5- to 7-d period before and after the exercise intervention. Data reduction was performed with a previously published computer-based algorithm.

Results.—There was no significant change in off-exercise PAEE in any of the exercise training groups. We observed a significant increase in total PAEE that included the exercise training, in both AT and AT/RT but not in RT.

Conclusions.—Eight months of exercise training was not associated with a compensatory reduction in off-exercise physical activity, regardless of exercise modality. The absence of compensation is particularly notable for AT/RT subjects, who performed a larger volume of exercise than did AT or RT subjects. We believe that the extended duration of our exercise training program was the key factor in allowing subjects to reach a new steady-state level of physical activity within their daily lives (Fig 2).

▶ This study addressed the controversial topic of whether prescribed exercise sessions cause reduced energy expenditure outside of exercise in previously sedentary adults. Because total energy expenditure is inversely associated with mortality risk, a reduction in spontaneous daily energy expenditure would offset the energy expenditure of each exercise session and overestimate the health benefits of regular exercise. As part of the Studies of Targeted Risk Reduction Interventions through Defined Exercise (STRRIDE) study, Rangan and colleagues estimated total daily energy expenditure in adults aged 18 to 70 years over an 8-month training intervention comprising resistance exercise (RT), aerobic exercise (AT), or both (AT/RT). Total physical activity energy expenditure (PAEE) and off-exercise PAEE were determined by the use of accelerometers during a run-in control period and after 8 months of training. The participants were overweight to obese and had other cardiovascular health risk factors, so they were the type of people who would be encouraged to exercise regularly for health benefits. The study team found that total PAEE increased significantly in the AT and AT/RT groups but not in the RT group (Fig 2A). Off-exercise PAEE was not significantly different among groups, although the AT/RT group had a tendency for greater off-exercise PAEE (Fig 2B). In contrast

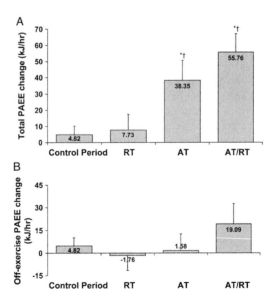

FIGURE 2.—Change score by group for total PAEE (A) and off-exercise PAEE (B). Error *bars* indicate SE. Although the control period (which includes the change that occurred during the run-in period in all 82 subjects) has been included in this figure for visual comparison only, there were no statistical comparisons between the control period data and the exercise groups. The only statistical comparisons were between the three independent exercise training groups. [†]Significant difference from RT ($P < 0.05$). (Reprinted from Rangan VV, Willis LH, Slentz CA, et al. Effects of an 8-month exercise training program on off-exercise physical activity. *Med Sci Sports Exerc.* 2011;43:1744-1751, with permission from the American College of Sports Medicine.)

to previous studies, the authors proposed that the longer duration of training (8 months) allowed for a new steady-state of total PAEE to be achieved. It is not known whether the STRRIDE participants had an early temporary compensation phase with reduced total PAEE that was reversed by the end of training. In previous exercise training studies of older adults, a compensatory decrease in off-exercise PAEE was found. In the study by Rangan and colleagues, age was not significantly associated with changes in off-exercise PAEE among individuals or by exercise type. The investigators were careful to exclude accelerometer data that appeared to show extreme changes in energy expenditure and acknowledged that accelerometers may more accurately measure energy expenditure during aerobic exercise than with resistance exercise. This study demonstrated that a combination of resistance and aerobic exercise induced the greatest increase in total PAEE and did not diminish off-exercise PAEE in adults.

C. M. Jankowski, PhD

Physical activity in Ontario preschoolers: prevalence and measurement issues
Obeid J, Nguyen T, Gabel L, et al (McMaster Univ and McMaster Children's Hosp, Hamilton, Ontario, Canada)
Appl Physiol Nutr Metab 36:291-297, 2011

Early childhood is a critical period for the development of active living behaviours; however, very little is known about the physical activity levels of preschoolers from Canada. The objectives of this study were to (*i*) examine physical activity in a sample of Ontario preschoolers by using high-frequency accelerometry to determine activity and step counts; (*ii*) assess the relationship between step counts and physical activity; (*iii*) examine the influence of epoch length or sampling interval on physical activity; and (*iv*) compare measured physical activity to existing recommendations. Thirty 3- to 5-year-old children wore accelerometers to monitor habitual physical activity in 3-s epochs over a 7-day period. Preschoolers engaged in an average of 220 min of daily physical activity, 75 min of which were spent in moderate-to-vigorous physical activity (MVPA), and they accumulated 7529 ± 1539 steps·day^{-1}. Preschoolers who engaged in more MVPA also took more steps on a daily basis ($r = 0.81$, $p < 0.001$). Compared with a 3-s epoch, sampling intervals of 15, 30, and 60 s resulted in an average of 2.9, 9.0, and 16.7 missed minutes of MVPA per day, respectively. All 30 preschoolers met the National Association for Sport and Physical Education recommendation of at least 120 min of total physical activity per day for preschool-age children. Our data highlight important methodological considerations when measuring physical activity in preschoolers and the need for preschool-specific physical activity guidelines for Canadian children.

▶ Preschool children are not exempt from developing unhealthy body weight. Overweight and obesity in Canadian preschool children are estimated at between 8% and 15%, but is also evident in children as young as 2 years.[1] Measuring physical activity (PA) in preschool children is challenging and, therefore, the data are sparse, making the connection between the contribution of low levels of PA and overweight and obesity difficult. In this study, Obeid and coworkers seek to address this gap in our knowledge of PA in preschoolers by examining PA using high-frequency accelerometry. One of the objectives of interest was to examine the influence of epoch length on PA level given the propensity of most accelerometer-based studies to use epoch of > 15 s. So as not to mask short intermittent bouts of vigorous activity, these investigators used epochs of 3 s but did study the effect of epoch length on PA. Although the sample size of only 30 children (only 10 were girls) is a definite limitation of this study, it is the first comprehensive study of habitual PA in preschoolers using accelerometry. The use of shorter epochs more correctly identified bouts of activity as moderate to vigorous PA, representing an accumulation of at least 60 min/d in this sample of preschoolers. They found no sex-related differences, possibly due to only 10 participants being girls; however, all children met the 120-min/d recommendation of the National Association for Sport and Physical Education and Active Health Kids Canada 2010 Report Card. This study makes an important contribution to the determination of PA in preschool children. A sedentary lifestyle puts children at high risk for unhealthy weight gain, and establishing active living behavior early in life is thought to be protective. It remains to be determined whether PA recommendations for school-age children are sufficient for preschoolers. Perhaps it is time, as proposed by the study's investigators, to implement specific guidelines for this age group using data from thorough, well-conducted studies such as this one.

V. Galea, PhD

Reference

1. Canning P, Courage ML, Frizzell LM, Seifert T. Obesity in a provincial population of Canadian preschool children: differences between 1984 and 1997 birth cohorts. *Int J Pediatr Obes.* 2007;2:51-57.

Recommended aerobic fitness level for metabolic health in children and adolescents: a study of diagnostic accuracy
Adegboye ARA, Anderssen SA, Froberg K, et al (Copenhagen Univ Hosp, Denmark; Univ of Southern Denmark, Odense, Denmark; Norwegian School of Sport Sciences, Oslo, Norway; et al)
Br J Sports Med 45:722-728, 2011

Objective.—To define the optimal cut-off for low aerobic fitness and to evaluate its accuracy to predict clustering of risk factors for cardiovascular disease in children and adolescents.

Design.—Study of diagnostic accuracy using a cross-sectional database.

Setting.—European Youth Heart Study including Denmark, Portugal, Estonia and Norway.

Participants.—4500 schoolchildren aged 9 or 15 years.

Main Outcome Measure.—Aerobic fitness was expressed as peak oxygen consumption relative to bodyweight (mlO_2/min/kg).

Results.—Risk factors included in the composite risk score (mean of z-scores) were systolic blood pressure, triglyceride, total cholesterol/HDL-cholesterol ratio, insulin resistance and sum of four skinfolds. 14.5% of the sample, with a risk score above one SD, were defined as being at risk. Receiver operating characteristic analysis was used to define the optimal cut-off for sex and age-specific distribution. In girls, the optimal cut-offs for identifying individuals at risk were: 37.4 mlO_2/min/kg (9-year-old) and 33.0 mlO_2/min/kg (15-year-old). In boys, the optimal cut-offs were 43.6 mlO_2/min/kg (9-year-old) and 46.0 mlO_2/min/kg (15-year-old). Specificity (range 79.3–86.4%) was markedly higher than sensitivity (range 29.7–55.6%) for all cut-offs. Positive predictive values ranged from 19% to 41% and negative predictive values ranged from 88% to 90%. The diagnostic accuracy for identifying children at risk, measured by the area under the curve (AUC), was significantly higher than what would be expected by chance (AUC >0.5) for all cut-offs.

Conclusions.—Aerobic fitness is easy to measure, and is an accurate tool for screening children with clustering of cardiovascular risk factors. Promoting physical activity in children with aerobic fitness level lower than the suggested cut-points might improve their health (Table 2).

▶ Maximal oxygen intake is increasingly suggested as a better measure of habitual physical activity and, thus, of the risk of future disease than the use of either questionnaires or actometers, although peak oxygen transport is also vulnerable to genetic influences. In children, questionnaires are often difficult to administer, and most designs of actometer also fail to indicate accurately such important activities of childhood as cycling. However, if aerobic power is to be the criterion, there is less agreement on what is an appropriate minimal level of maximal oxygen consumption for a child or an adolescent. Adegboye and associates sought to answer this question by comparing maximal aerobic power with a composite Z score of cardiovascular risk (based on systolic blood pressure, triglycerides, high-density lipoprotein cholesterol ratio, insulin resistance, and skinfold thicknesses, with log-transformation of skewed variables). The subjects were a large and randomly selected sample of students from 4 European countries. Aerobic fitness was determined as the peak power output observed during a progressive cycle ergometer test, a measure with a test-retest variation in the range of 2.5% to 4.8%[1]; somewhat oddly, instead of using the actual measurements as their criteria, equations were used to convert the findings to estimated equivalent maximal oxygen intakes.[2] Various levels of aerobic performance were evaluated for their ability to detect children with a risk score more than 1 SD above the average for the sample; the optimal cutoff points were in the range that we would have predicted from our studies of a representative sample of Toronto schoolchildren many years ago[3]; in the case of the boys, these figures are somewhat higher than 1 set of lower limits for child health[4] but are close to other more recent proposals.[5-7] The optimal cutoff points

TABLE 2.—Diagnostic Characteristics of Cut-Offs for Aerobic Fitness According to Sex and Age Groups

Cut-Offs	9-Year-Old Children				15-Year-Old Children			
	10th	Optimal	25th	50th	10th	Optimal	25th	50th
Sensitivity (%)								
Girls	22.4 (16.6–29.1)	49.7 (42.3–57.2)	54.6 (47.1–62.0)	74.9 (67.9–81.0)	19.3 (13.2–26.7)	29.7 (22.4–37.8)	32.4 (24.9–40.7)	57.9 (49.5–66.1)
Boys	28.8 (22.4–35.9)	55.4 (47.9–62.7)	53.3 (45.8–60.6)	75.5 (68.7–81.6)	31.0 (23.5–39.3)	55.6 (47.1–64.0)	57.0 (48.5–65.3)	73.9 (65.9–80.9)
Specificity (%)								
Girls	92.3 (90.5–93.9)	85.9 (83.6–88.0)	80.5 (77.9–82.9)	54.6 (51.5–57.7)	91.5 (89.5–93.2)	79.9 (77.2–82.5)	76.2 (73.2–78.9)	51.3 (48.0–54.6)
Boys	93.3 (91.6–94.8)	79.3 (76.7–81.8)	80.1 (77.5–82.5)	54.6 (51.5–57.7)	93.4 (91.6–94.9)	86.4 (84.0–88.6)	80.0 (77.3–82.6)	53.7 (50.4–57.0)
PPV (%)								
Girls	34.7 (26.2–44.1)	39.2 (32.9–45.8)	33.9 (28.5–39.6)	23.2 (19.9–26.8)	26.7 (18.5–36.2)	19.1 (14.2–24.9)	17.9 (13.4–23.0)	16.0 (13.0–19.4)
Boys	43.4 (34.5–52.7)	32.3 (27.2–37.7)	32.2 (27.0–37.8)	22.8 (19.5–26.4)	42.3 (32.7–52.4)	41.5 (34.6–48.5)	30.9 (25.4–36.9)	20.0 (16.7–23.7)
NPV (%)								
Girls	86.6 (84.4–88.6)	90.3 (88.2–92.1)	90.6 (88.5–92.5)	92.2 (89.8–94.2)	87.6 (85.4–89.7)	87.7 (85.2–89.8)	87.6 (85.1–89.8)	88.4 (85.4–91.0)
Boys	88.1 (86.0–89.9)	90.2 (88.9–92.7)	90.6 (88.5–92.4)	92.6 (90.3–94.6)	89.6 (87.5–91.5)	90.5 (88.3–92.4)	92.2 (90.2–94.0)	92.9 (90.4–95.0)

10th, 25th and 50th percentiles for fitness.
Negative-predictive value (NPV), probability of a negative risk status given a negative test result; positive-predictive value (PPV), probability of a positive risk status given a positive test result; sensitivity, proportion of diseased individuals correctly identified (true-positive rate); specificity, proportion of healthy individuals correctly identified (1 − false-positive rate).

based on aerobic power have a relatively good specificity but a rather poor sensitivity in identifying cardiovascular risk (Table 2). Before endorsing this approach, it would be interesting to test its practicality and success in identifying risk relative to other possible measures of physical activity or fitness. It must also be underlined that although the stated levels of aerobic fitness minimize cardiovascular risk, they are not necessarily optimal for other aspects of long-term health.

R. J. Shephard, MD (Lond), PhD, DPE

References

1. Anderssen SA, Cooper AR, Riddoch C, et al. Low cardiorespiratory fitness is a strong predictor for clustering of cardiovascular disease risk factors in children independent of country, age and sex. *Eur J Cardiovasc Prev Rehabil.* 2007;14: 526-531.
2. Kolle E, Steene-Johannessen J, Andersen LB, Anderssen SA. Objectively assessed physical activity and aerobic fitness in a population-based sample of Norwegian 9- and 15-year-olds. *Scand J Med Sci Sports.* 2010;20:e41-e47.
3. Shephard RJ, Allen C, Bar-Or O, et al. The working capacity of Toronto schoolchildren. *Can Med Assoc J.* 1969;100:560-566. 705—714.
4. Bell RD, Macek M, Rutenfranz J, et al. Health indicators and risk factors of cardiovascular diseases during childhood and adolescence. In: Rutenfranz J, Mocelin R, Klimt F, eds. *Children and Exercise XII.* Champaign, IL: Human Kinetics; 1986:19-27.
5. The Cooper Institute for Aerobics Research. *FITNESSGRAM Test Administration Manual.* 3rd ed. Champaign, IL: Human Kinetics; 2004.
6. Lobelo F, Pate RR, Dowda M, Liese AD, Ruiz JR. Validity of cardiorespiratory fitness criterion-referenced standards for adolescents. *Med Sci Sports Exerc.* 2009;41:1222-1229.
7. Ruiz JR, Ortega FB, Rizzo NS, et al. High cardiovascular fitness is associated with low metabolic risk score in children: the European Youth Heart Study. *Pediatr Res.* 2007;61:350-355.

Improved physical function and physical activity in older adults following a community-based intervention: Relationships with a history of depression
Porter KN, Fischer JG, Johnson MA (The Univ of Georgia, Athens)
Maturitas 70:290-294, 2011

The purpose of this study was to explore the relationship of a history of depression with moderate physical activity and physical function before and after a physical activity intervention of congregate meal participants in senior centers from all 12 Georgia Area Agencies on Aging (AAA). Participants were a convenience sample of older adults ($n = 376$, mean age = 76 years, 82% female, 64% Caucasian, 36% African American, 22% a history of depression). The physical activity intervention included educator-led chair exercises that incorporated balls and bands. Pre- and post-tests assessed moderate physical activity and physical function. At the pre-test, a history of depression was not related to moderate physical activity or physical function. Following the intervention there were significant increases in both moderate physical activity and physical function, but a history of depression was a negative predictor of improvements in physical activity when controlled for site, demographics, and health-related conditions. These results provide an evidence base for the effectiveness of this intervention in improving moderate physical activity and physical function in a community setting, but additional efforts may be needed to improve the impact of this type of intervention among older adults with a history of depression.

▶ This is the first study to examine the effects of a history of depression on improvements in physical activity and physical function in older adults following a moderate-intensity exercise program. An estimated 20% of community-dwelling older adults are depressed, and the prevalence of a lifetime diagnosis of depression is 15.7% nationwide. Although physical activity may help alleviate depressive symptoms, being depressed can be a significant barrier to becoming more physically active and have a negative impact on physical function. A unique aspect of the intervention was its location at 12 municipal senior adult centers belonging to the Area Agencies on Aging in Georgia. The intervention comprised 12 standardized sessions covering nutrition, health, and physical activity topics. Each session had a physical activity component that included chair exercises, exercise balls, and resistance bands. The physical activity outcome was self-reported moderate physical activity from the BRFSS questionnaire, physical function was objectively measured using the Short Physical Performance Battery, and history of depression was self-reported before and after the intervention. There were no significant differences in moderate physical activity or physical function between the groups at baseline; physical activity and function increased significantly in the total group. However, a history of depression was associated with less change in physical activity after adjustment for covariates such as age. The participants with a history of depression achieved better physical function even though fewer of them met the recommended level of exercising 5 or more days per week. The authors suggested that older adults with a history of depression may need more encouragement or changes in exercise modalities to further increase their level of moderate physical activity. This was a pragmatic approach to delivering exercise and other health-related information to groups of older adults.

C. M. Jankowski, PhD

Elevators or stairs?

Shah S, O'Byrne M, Wilson M, et al (Univ of Saskatchewan, Saskatoon, Sask, Canada)
CMAJ 183:E1353-E1355, 2011

Background.—Staff in hospitals frequently travel between floors and choose between taking the stairs or elevator. We compared the time savings with these two options.

Methods.—Four people aged 26–67 years completed 14 trips ranging from one to six floors, both ascending and descending. We compared the amount of time per floor travelled by stairs and by two banks of elevators. Participants reported their fatigue levels using a modified Borg scale. We performed two—way analysis of variance to compare the log—transformed data, with participant and time of day as independent variables.

Results.—The mean time taken to travel between each floor was 13.1 (standard deviation [SD] 1.7) seconds by stairs and 37.5 (SD 19.0) and 35.6 (SD 23.1) seconds by the two elevators (F = 8.61, p < 0.001). The difference in time taken to travel by stairs and elevator equaled about 15 minutes a day. Self—reported fatigue was less than 13 (out of 20) on the Borg scale for all participants, and they all stated that they were able to continue their duties without resting. The extra time associated with elevator use was because of waiting for its arrival. There was a difference in the amount of time taken to travel by elevator depending on the time of day and day of the week.

Interpretation.—Taking the stairs rather than the elevator saved about 15 minutes each workday. This 3% savings per workday could translate into improved productivity as well as increased fitness.

▶ When a patient is asked why he or she does not exercise, commonly the excuse is lack of time. When I first assumed my role as Director of the Fitness Research Unit at the University of Toronto, I was summoned to Ottawa to discuss my research plans with Health Canada. After a lunch in the basement, a meeting was convened in the 12th floor conference room of the Brooke-Claxton building, and I remember my colleagues milling around the lobby complaining about the slowness of the elevators. However, I told them that the meeting had been convened to discuss fitness, and I proposed to use the stairs. I took them 2 at a time, and I arrived at the 12th floor a good minute ahead of those who had used the elevator. Shah and colleagues make a similar point—time is not an obstacle to fitness—indeed, if properly used, physical activity (as in stair climbing and active commuting) can save time that can be put to other productive endeavors.

R. J. Shephard, MD (Lond), PhD, DPE

Use of a New Public Bicycle Share Program in Montreal, Canada

Fuller D, Gauvin L, Kestens Y, et al (Research Center of the Université de Montréal Hospital Center, Québec, Canada; et al)
Am J Prev Med 41:80-83, 2011

Background.—Cycling contributes to physical activity and health. Public bicycle share programs (PBSPs) increase population access to bicycles by deploying bicycles at docking stations throughout a city. Minimal research has systematically examined the prevalence and correlates of PBSP use.

Purpose.—To determine the prevalence and correlates of use of a new public bicycle share program called BIXI (name merges the word BIcycle and taXI) implemented in May 2009 in Montreal, Canada.

Methods.—A total of 2502 adults were recruited to a telephone survey in autumn 2009 via random-digit dialing according to a stratified random sampling design. The prevalence of BIXI bicycle use was estimated. Multivariate logistic regression allowed for identification of correlates of use. Data analysis was conducted in spring and summer 2010.

Results.—The unweighted mean age of respondents was 47.4 (SD = 16.8) years and 61.4% were female. The weighted prevalence for use of BIXI bicycles at least once was 8.2%. Significant correlates of BIXI bicycle use were having a BIXI docking station within 250 m of home, being aged 18–24 years, being university educated, being on work leave, and using cycling as the primary mode of transportation to work.

Conclusions.—A newly implemented public bicycle share program attracts a substantial fraction of the population and is more likely to attract younger and more educated people who currently use cycling as a primary transportation mode.

▶ The use of public transit is widely seen as one step in counteracting the accumulation of "greenhouse gases" from automobile exhaust, but those who attempt to use the bus too often find that the route finishes far from their intended destination. A possible solution is to use a combination of bus and bicycle; this would offer the additional advantage of "active commuting," with a potential to enhance personal fitness. One rather cumbersome venture in our small community has been to fit a rack that will carry 2 bicycles on the front of our buses. Larger communities in Europe have long experimented with a large supply of free or low-rent bicycles in the city center and at train stations,[1,2] and more recently this same concept has been tried in North America. Montreal undertook an initiative of this type beginning in May of 2009, with 5000 sturdy bicycles available at 450 docking stations; the annual membership fee is Cdn $78.00, and there is a supplementary charge of $1.50 for loans of more than 30 minutes per day. The bicycles were available in the central part of the city, and were viewed as an alternative to transit, rather than as a supplement to buses. The question is how far users are attracted by such a program. A total of 2502 Montreal residents were recruited to a telephone survey via random-digit dialing. The proportion of people trying the option (about 8% of respondents) compares favorably with the normal usage of bicycles for transportation in Montreal (1.6%–8.0%).[3,4] It was particularly encouraging to see that usage was 14% when the bicycles were closely available, but 6% of people living in areas where the cycles were not readily available had also tried them. There remains a need for further observations exploring whether those who try the bicycles continue to use them.

R. J. Shephard, MD (Lond), PhD, DPE

References

1. deMaio P. Bike-sharing history, impacts, models of provision, and future. *J Publ Transportation.* 2010;12:41-56.
2. Shaheen S, Guzman S, Zhang H. Bike-sharing in Europe, the Americas and Asia; past, present and future. Transportation Research Board Annual Meeting; March 15th, 2010:159-167.

3. Statistics Canada. *Census of Canada: Profile of Census Divisions and Census Subdivisions.* Ottawa, Ontario: Statistics Canada; 2006.
4. Vélo Québec. *L'État du vélo au Québec en,* www.velo.qc.ca/velo_quebec/etatduvelo. php; 2005.

Electric Bicycles as a New Active Transportation Modality to Promote Health

Gojanovic B, Welker J, Iglesias K, et al (Univ Hosp Ctr, Lausanne, Switzerland; Univ of Lausanne, Switzerland)
Med Sci Sports Exerc 43:2204-2210, 2011

Electrically assisted bicycles (EAB) are an emerging transportation modality favored for environmental reasons. Some physical effort is required to activate the supporting engine, making it a potential active commuting option.

Purpose.—We hypothesized that using an EAB in a hilly city allows sedentary subjects to commute comfortably, while providing a sufficient effort for health-enhancing purposes.

Methods.—Sedentary subjects performed four different trips at a self-selected pace: walking 1.7 km uphill from the train station to the hospital (WALK), biking 5.1 km from the lower part of town to the hospital with a regular bike (BIKE), or EAB at two different power assistance settings (EAB$_{high}$, EAB$_{std}$). HR, oxygen consumption, and need to shower were recorded.

Results.—Eighteen sedentary subjects (12 female, 6 male) age 36 $\pm$ 10 yr were included, with $\dot{V}O_{2max}$ of 39.4 $\pm$ 5.4 mL·min^{-1}·kg^{-1}. Time to complete the course was 22 (WALK), 19 (EAB$_{high}$), 21 (EAB$_{std}$), and 30 (BIKE) min. Mean % $\dot{V}O_{2max}$ was 59.0%, 54.9%, 65.7%, and 72.8%. Mean % HRmax was 71.5%, 74.5%, 80.3%, and 84.0%. There was no significant difference between WALK and EAB$_{high}$, but all other comparisons were different ($P < 0.05$). Two subjects needed to shower after EAB$_{high}$, 3 needed to shower after WALK, 8 needed to shower after EAB$_{std}$, and all 18 needed to shower after BIKE. WALK and EAB$_{high}$ elicited 6.5 and 6.1 METs (no difference), whereas it was 7.3 and 8.2 for EAB$_{std}$ and BIKE.

Conclusions.—EAB is a comfortable and ecological transportation modality, helping sedentary people commute to work and meet physical activity guidelines. Subjects appreciated ease of use and mild effort needed to activate the engine support climbing hills, without the need to shower at work. EAB can be promoted in a challenging urban environment to promote physical activity and mitigate pollution issues (Fig 2).

▶ The introductory article to this edition of the Year Book of Sports Medicine points to the health value of active commuting, particularly if trips are taken on a bicycle (where energy expenditures are usually relatively high). Active commuting immediately negates one of the most common excuses for not exercising—a lack of time. But what about the health benefits from those electric

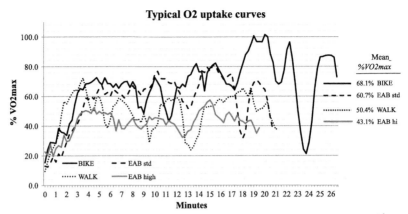

FIGURE 2.—Typical example of real-time oxygen consumption in one subject (as percentage of $\dot{V}O_{2max}$) for all four trials. On the *right*, mean % $\dot{V}O_{2max}$ for each modality. (Reprinted from Gojanovic B, Welker J, Iglesias K, et al. Electric bicycles as a new active transportation modality to promote health. *Med Sci Sports Exerc.* 2011;43:2204-2210, with permission from the American College of Sports Medicine.)

bicycles that are becoming ever more prevalent in our cities? Gojanovic and associates make the useful point that electric bicycles are not all the same—some have very small motors that give a little assistance on steep hills, some require only light effort from the user, and some are even a way of dodging regulations to enter areas restricted to pedestrians and cyclists. Gojanovic et al thus studied the energy cost of using standard bicycles and machines fitted with both average and large motors on a relatively hilly commuter route to the hospital in Lausanne. Their subjects were middle-aged and sedentary. Most reported a rate of perceived exertion of 15.5 (hard to very hard) when unassisted, and 2 were unable to complete their ride (Fig 2). One attraction of the assisted bicycle is that it is less necessary to shower on reaching one's place of employment, and with the standard electric bike, 10 of the 18 subjects were able to forego a shower. However, this reflects a lower intensity of average effort over the journey, and in terms of health, there may be no gain of cardiorespiratory fitness without inducing some sweating. The time needed to complete the commute also decreased from 29 minutes to 18 to 20 minutes with the support of the electric motors. In agreement with the earlier observations of Simons et al,[1] over a standard commute, the average oxygen consumption for an average electric bicycle was probably still sufficient to have some health benefit, 60.7% of maximal oxygen intake compared with 68.1% for a standard bicycle. However, expenditure dropped to 43.1% for the large motored bicycle, probably eliminating most of the health benefit of cycling.

R. J. Shephard, MD (Lond), PhD, DPE

Reference

1. Simons M, Van Es E, Hendriksen I. Electrically assisted cycling: a new mode for meeting physical activity guidelines? *Med Sci Sports Exerc.* 2009;41:2097-2102.

Sleep Duration or Bedtime? Exploring the Relationship between Sleep Habits and Weight Status and Activity Patterns

Olds TS, Maher CA, Matricciani L (Univ of South Australia, Adelaide)
Sleep 34:1299-1307, 2011

Study Objectives.—To assess the effects of early and late bedtimes and wake up times on use of time and weight status in Australian school-aged children.

Design.—Observational cross-sectional study involving use of time interviews and pedometers.

Setting.—Free-living Australian adolescents.

Participants.—2200 9- to 16-year-olds from all states of Australia.

Interventions.—NA.

Measurements and Results.—Bedtimes and wake times were adjusted for age and sex and classified as early or late using median splits. Adolescents were allocated into 4 sleep-wake pattern groups: Early-bed/Early-rise; Early-bed/Late-rise; Late-bed/Early-rise; Late-bed/Late-rise. The groups were compared for use of time (screen time, physical activity, and study-related time), sociodemographic characteristics, and weight status. Adolescents in the Late-bed/Late-rise category experienced 48 min/d more screen time and 27 min less moderate-to-vigorous physical activity (MVPA) ($P < 0.0001$) than adolescents in the Early-bed/Early-rise category, in spite of similar sleep durations. Late-bed/Late-rise adolescents had a higher BMI z-score (0.66 vs. 0.45, $P = 0.0015$). Late-bed/Late-rise adolescents were 1.47 times more likely to be overweight or obese than Early-bed/Early-rise adolescents, 2.16 times more likely to be obese, 1.77 times more likely to have low MVPA, and 2.92 times more likely to have high screen time. Late-bed/Late-rise adolescents were more likely to come from poorer households, to live in major cities, and have fewer siblings.

Conclusions.—Late bedtimes and late wake up times are associated with an unfavorable activity and weight status profile, independent of age, sex, household income, geographical remoteness, and sleep duration.

▶ While we all enjoy a good night's sleep, the amount of sleep we get often suffers as a consequence of busy work and personal schedules, stress, a loud and disruptive bedmate, and so forth. This is also the case with the current generation of children, who tend to sleep less than their parents did when they were the same age. A grouchy mood and poor attention span are obvious consequences of a sleep-deprived child. A short sleep duration has also been linked to obesity.[1]

In this study, Olds and colleagues explored the mechanisms by which a short sleep duration and different sleep cycle may be related to obesity within 9- to 16-year-old individuals. Specifically, they studied whether the time at which youth went to bed and woke up was related to their weight status, physical activity level, and time spent being sedentary. Compared with children who went to bed early and woke up early, children who went to bed late and woke up late were about 50% more likely to be obese, 80% more likely to engage in low levels of moderate to vigorous physical activity, and 190% more likely to have excessive screen time (television, computers, video games). These increased risks were apparent despite the fact that the early-bed/early-rise and late-bed/late-rise groups had approximately the same sleep duration. The findings suggest that an early bedtime is an important variable to target when trying to increase children's physical activity levels and decrease their body weight. As the idiom goes, the early bird catches the worm.

I. Janssen, PhD

Reference

1. Cappuccio FP, Taggart FM, Kandala NB, et al. Meta-analysis of short sleep duration and obesity in children and adults. *Sleep.* 2008;31:619-629.

2011 Compendium of Physical Activities: A Second Update of Codes and MET Values
Ainsworth BE, Haskell WL, Herrmann SD, et al (Arizona State Univ, Phoenix; Stanford Univ, Palo Alto, CA; et al)
Med Sci Sports Exerc 43:1575-1581, 2011

Purpose.—The Compendium of Physical Activities was developed to enhance the comparability of results across studies using self-report physical activity (PA) and is used to quantify the energy cost of a wide variety of PA. We provide the second update of the Compendium, called the 2011 Compendium.

Methods.—The 2011 Compendium retains the previous coding scheme to identify the major category headings and specific PA by their rate of energy expenditure in MET. Modifications in the 2011 Compendium include cataloging measured MET values and their source references, when available; addition of new codes and specific activities; an update of the Compendium tracking guide that links information in the 1993, 2000, and 2011 compendia versions; and the creation of a Web site to facilitate easy access and downloading of Compendium documents. Measured MET values were obtained from a systematic search of databases using defined key words.

Results.—The 2011 Compendium contains 821 codes for specific activities. Two hundred seventeen new codes were added, 68% (561/821) of which have measured MET values. Approximately half (317/604) of the codes from the 2000 Compendium were modified to improve the definitions and/or to consolidate specific activities and to update estimated MET values where measured values did not exist. Updated MET values accounted for 73% of all code changes.

Conclusions.—The Compendium is used globally to quantify the energy cost of PA in adults for surveillance activities, research studies, and, in clinical settings, to write PA recommendations and to assess energy expenditure in individuals. The 2011 Compendium is an update of a system for quantifying the energy cost of adult human PA and is a living document that is moving in the direction of being 100% evidence based.

▶ The first Compendium of Physical Activities was published in 1993,[1] updating painstakingly collected Scottish Kofranyi-Michaelis respirometer data from the long-used text of Durnin and Passmore.[2] The basic purpose of the compendium was to assign concrete and consistent estimates of intensity to the various activities identified on detailed North American physical activity questionnaires, although it was also recognized that such information could be important when prescribing exercise programs. The compendium was updated in 2000[3] and has now undergone a further revision, with the claim of moving toward evidence-based values; this last statement drew my attention because all the original figures provided by Durnin and Passmore were evidence based, although admittedly drawn from a single community (Glasgow) where people undertook quite a lot of activities that are now largely outdated (such as scrubbing their front steps). The changes in the third edition of the compendium are mainly of a second-order nature. For example, the energy cost of dancing has been changed from 6.5 to 7.3 METs. Precision is of course welcome in any estimate of energy costs, although when attempting to translate questionnaire data into total weekly energy expenditures, much of the error arises in identifying the duration and frequency of the various activities and in the use of gross rather than net energy costs. Moreover, the data are said to be relevant for people of all ages from 18 to 65 years, although one suspects that despite the updating of the compendium, an 18-year-old will still undertake many of the activities listed more vigorously than a 65-year-old. In terms of exercise prescription, I am also concerned that intensity is described without reference to the individual's age; for example, "bicycling, stationary" 30 to 50 W (I presume cycle ergometry) is described as very light to light effort. However, this assessment will certainly differ between an 18-year-old and a 65-year-old. The compendium may provide a start to an exercise prescription, but if the regulation of intensity is critical to safety of the program, it will remain necessary either for a clinical exercise physiologist to monitor this or for the patient to note ability to talk, perceptions of effort, and any critical symptoms.

R. J. Shephard, MD (Lond), PhD, DPE

References

1. Ainsworth BE, Haskell WL, Leon AS, et al. Compendium of physical activities: classification of energy costs of human physical activities. *Med Sci Sports Exerc.* 1993;25:71-80.
2. Durnin JVGA, Passmore R. *Energy, Work and Leisure.* London, UK: Heinemann; 1967.
3. Ainsworth BE, Haskell WL, Whitt MC, et al. Compendium of physical activities: an update of activity codes and MET intensities. *Med Sci Sports Exerc.* 2000;32: S498-S504.

Comparative Validity of Physical Activity Measures in Older Adults

Colbert LH, Matthews CE, Havighurst TC, et al (Univ of Wisconsin, Madison; Natl Cancer Inst, Bethesda, MD)

Med Sci Sports Exerc 43:867-876, 2011

Purpose.—To compare the validity of various physical activity measures with doubly labeled water (DLW)—measured physical activity energy expenditure (PAEE) in free-living older adults.

Methods.—Fifty-six adults aged ≥65 yr wore three activity monitors (New Lifestyles pedometer, ActiGraph accelerometer, and a SenseWear (SW) armband) during a 10-d free-living period and completed three different surveys (Yale Physical Activity Survey (YPAS), Community Health Activities Model Program for Seniors (CHAMPS), and a modified Physical Activity Scale for the Elderly (modPASE)). Total energy expenditure was measured using DLW, resting metabolic rate was measured with indirect calorimetry, the thermic effect of food was estimated, and from these, estimates of PAEE were calculated. The degree of linear association between the various measures and PAEE was assessed, as were differences in group PAEE, when estimable by a given measure.

Results.—All three monitors were significantly correlated with PAEE ($r = 0.48–0.60$, $P < 0.001$). Of the questionnaires, only CHAMPS was significantly correlated with PAEE ($r = 0.28$, $P = 0.04$). Statistical comparison of the correlations suggested that the monitors were superior to YPAS and modPASE. Mean squared errors for all correlations were high, and the median PAEE from the different tools was significantly different from DLW for all but the YPAS and regression-estimated PAEE from the ActiGraph.

Conclusions.—Objective devices more appropriately rank PAEE than self-reported instruments in older adults, but absolute estimates of PAEE are not accurate. Given the cost differential and ease of use, pedometers seem most useful in this population when ranking by physical activity level is adequate (Table 3).

▶ The problems in ascertaining habitual physical activity by the use of questionnaires have been recognized for a long time.[1] Often there is substantial overreporting of activity[2]; this difficulty is especially marked in older people, because much of their activity is taken at a relatively low intensity.[3] The search for more accurate information has thus turned to a variety of pedometers and actometers. These tend to be more accurate than questionnaires, particularly if the main daily activity of the individual is walking, although findings can still be biased by incidental movements recorded in a car on a bumpy road, the wearing of the instrument at an altered angle in the obese, and by movements that are insufficiently forceful to operate the recording mechanism. There has thus been interest in equipment that monitors other responses to physical activity such as sweat rate, heart rate, or body temperature.[4] The study of Colbert and colleagues compared 3 questionnaires that were designed specifically for the elderly, an electronic pedometer with a 7-day memory, an Actigraph uni-axial accelerometer, and a SenseWear armband

TABLE 3.—Spearman Correlation Coefficients Between Physical Activity Monitors, Questionnaire Measures, and Doubly Labeled Water-Derived Measures of PAEE.[a,b]

Measure	PAEE[a] (kcal·d⁻¹)				PAEE$_{adj}$[a]				PAI[a] (kcal·kg⁻¹·d⁻¹)			
	RMSE	MAPE	r	P	RMSE	MAPE	r	P	RMSE	MAPE	r	P
SenseWear armband												
PAEE[a] (kcal·d⁻¹)	210	26.8	0.479	<0.01	185	−75.2	0.604	<0.001	2.90	22.3	0.590	<0.001
Steps per day	212	26.3	0.564	<0.01								
ActiGraph												
Crouter EE (kcal·d⁻¹)	185	22.5	0.600	<0.01	185	−48.1	0.584	<0.001	2.97	23.1	0.561	<0.001
Freedson EE (kcal·d⁻¹)	202	24.4	0.489	<0.01	183	−103.4	0.618	<0.001	2.84	20.7	0.629	<0.001
Average counts per minute	206	25.2	0.559	<0.01								
Steps per day	212	26.0	0.585	<0.01								
Pedometer												
Steps per day	213	26.8	0.530	<0.01	182	−80.2	0.585	<0.001	2.82	21.3	0.597	<0.001
CHAMPS												
PAEE[a] (kcal·d⁻¹)	242	30.4	0.278	0.04	226	3.1	0.225	0.096				
PAI[a] (kcal·kg⁻¹·d⁻¹)									3.42	29.0	0.234	0.083
modPASE												
PAEE[a] (kcal·d⁻¹)	256	32.4	0.195	0.15	234	−20.6	0.111	0.412				
PAI (kcal·kg⁻¹·d⁻¹)									3.51	29.3	0.180	0.183
YPAS												
PAEE[a] (kcal·d⁻¹)	252	32.8	0.074	0.59	231	−15.6	0.093	0.496				
PAI[a] (kcal·kg⁻¹·d⁻¹)									3.45	29.4	0.182	0.179

[a]MAPE, mean absolute percent error (%); PAEE$_{adj}$, PAEE adjusted for body weight; PAI, physical activity index (= PAEE per body weight (kg)); RMSE, root mean squared error for univariate regression.
[b]Correlations are only presented for caloric expenditure when the units are equivalent (i.e., kcal·d⁻¹ or kcal·kg⁻¹·d⁻¹).

against what is generally considered the gold standard of long-term energy expenditure measurements (doubly labeled water estimates). Their subjects were fairly old (average age 75 years) but otherwise were healthy seniors. All of the methods tested showed substantial scatter and in most cases a substantial systematic error relative to the doubly labeled water data (Table 3). The Sense-Wear armband did not offer any advantage relative to the Actigraph, perhaps because most of the recorded activities were of low intensity, and the equations used in computing scores for the SenseWear device are not designed for an elderly population. Actigraph data showed a closer correlation with doubly labeled water scores than did values obtained from questionnaires. Scores from the pedometer also fared surprisingly well. Nevertheless, most people will prefer to use the Acti-graph type of device for scientific investigations, because it can also capture the frequency, intensity, and duration of bouts of activity.

R. J. Shephard, MD (Lond), PhD, DPE

References

1. Shephard RJ. Limits to the measurement of habitual physical activity by question-naires. *Br J Sports Med.* 2003;37:197-206.
2. Troiano RP, Berrigan D, Dodd KW, Mâsse LC, Tilert T, McDowell M. Physical activity in the United States measured by accelerometer. *Med Sci Sports Exerc.* 2008;40:181-188.
3. DiPietro L, Caspersen CJ, Ostfeld AM, Nadel ER. A survey for assessing physical activity among older adults. *Med Sci Sports Exerc.* 1993;25:628-642.
4. King GA, Torres N, Potter C, Brooks TJ, Coleman KJ. Comparison of activity monitors to estimate energy cost of treadmill exercise. *Med Sci Sports Exerc.* 2004;36:1244-1251.

Low-Risk Lifestyle Behaviors and All-Cause Mortality: Findings From the National Health and Nutrition Examination Survey III Mortality Study

Ford ES, Zhao G, Tsai J, et al (Ctrs for Disease Control and Prevention, Atlanta, GA)
Am J Public Health 101:1922-1929, 2011

Objectives.—We examined the relationship between 4 low-risk behaviors—never smoked, healthy diet, adequate physical activity, and moderate alcohol consumption—and mortality in a representative sample of people in the United States.

Methods.—We used data from 16958 participants aged 17 years and older in the National Health and Nutrition Examination Survey III Mortality Study from 1988 to 2006.

Results.—The number of low-risk behaviors was inversely related to the risk for mortality. Compared with participants who had no low-risk behaviors, those who had all 4 experienced reduced all-cause mortality (adjusted hazard ratio [AHR] = 0.37; 95% confidence interval [CI] = 0.28, 0.49), mortality from malignant neoplasms (AHR = 0.34; 95% CI = 0.20, 0.56), major cardiovascular disease (AHR = 0.35; 95% CI = 0.24, 0.50), and other causes (AHR = 0.43; 95% CI = 0.25, 0.74). The rate advancement periods, representing the equivalent risk from a certain number of years of chronological age, for participants who had all 4 high-risk behaviors compared with those who had none were 11.1 years for all-cause mortality, 14.4 years for malignant neoplasms, 9.9 years for major cardiovascular disease, and 10.6 years for other causes.

Conclusions.—Low-risk lifestyle factors exert a powerful and beneficial effect on mortality.

▶ This epidemiologic study of a large US population sample showed that 4 low-risk behaviors exerted a powerful protective effect on mortality. Compared with participants who had no low-risk lifestyle behaviors, those who had all 4 were 63% less likely to die (which translated to about 11 years of life). The 11-year differential is consistent with 2 other studies[1,2] and provides a powerful inducement for people to adopt healthy lifestyles. Having never smoked emerged as the most important lifestyle behavior, but healthy diet, adequate physical activity, and moderate alcohol consumption were each significantly related with a reduced risk of mortality.

D. C. Nieman, DrPH

References

1. Khaw KT, Wareham N, Bingham S, Welch A, Luben R, Day N. Combined impact of health behaviours and mortality in men and women: the EPIC-Norfolk prospective population study. *PLoS Med.* 2008;5:e12.
2. Kvaavik E, Batty GD, Ursin G, Huxley R, Gale CR. Influence of individual and combined health behaviors on total and cause-specific mortality in men and women: the United Kingdom health and lifestyle survey. *Arch Intern Med.* 2010;170:711-718.

The challenge of low physical activity during the school day: at recess, lunch and in physical education
Nettlefold L, McKay HA, Warburton DER, et al (Univ of British Columbia, Vancouver, Canada; et al)
Br J Sports Med 45:813-819, 2011

Purpose.—To describe physical activity (PA) intensity across a school day and assess the percentage of girls and boys achieving recommended guidelines.

Methods.—The authors measured PA via accelerometry in 380 children (8–11 years) and examined data representing (1) the whole school day, (2) regular class time, (3) recess, (4) lunch and (5) scheduled physical education (PE). Activity was categorised as sedentary (SED), light physical activity (LPA) or moderate to vigorous physical activity (MVPA) using age-specific thresholds. They examined sex differences across PA intensities during each time period and compliance with recommended guidelines.

Results.—Girls accumulated less MVPA and more SED than boys throughout the school day (MVPA −10.6 min; SED +13.9 min) recess

(MVPA −1.6 min; SED +1.7 min) and lunch (MVPA −3.1 min; SED +2.9 min). Girls accumulated less MVPA (−6.2 min), less LPA (−2.5 min) and more SED (+9.4 min) than boys during regular class time. Fewer girls than boys achieved PA guidelines during school (90.9% vs 96.2%), recess (15.7% vs 34.1%) and lunch (16.7% vs 37.4%). During PE, only 1.8% of girls and 2.9% of boys achieved the PA guidelines. Girls and boys accumulated similar amounts of MVPA, LPA and SED.

Conclusion.—The MVPA deficit in girls was due to their sedentary behaviour as opposed to LPA. Physical activity strategies that target girls are essential to overcome this deficit. Only a very small percentage of children met physical activity guidelines during PE. There is a great need for additional training and emphasis on PA during PE. In addition schools should complement PE with PA models that increase PA opportunities across the school day.

▶ A commonly held belief is that when children engage in play and sports, they are constantly active and, over the course of a day, will accumulate more than enough moderate to vigorous physical activity (MVPA) for optimal growth and health. This study by Nettlefold and colleagues used accelerometers to measure the physical activity across the school day in a group of 380 children aged 8 to 11 years. At recess, when allowed to play on their own with limited supervision and guidance by teachers, the girls spent 20% of their time participating in MVPA and the boys spent 28% of their time participating in MVPA. At lunchtime these values increased to 28% and 35%, respectively. During scheduled physical education classes, which were led by teachers and involved instruction time, children were participating in MVPA for only 12% of the class! In this study, MVPA was defined using metabolic equivalent (MET) threshold of 3.0 METs, which is lower than the 4.0 threshold typically used in children. Thus, the MVPA values may have been overrepresented. Nonetheless, these findings suggest that a third or less of the time children spend in play and organized physical education at school is spent in MVPA. Similar findings have been reported for organized sports that occur outside of school, such as soccer.[1] Thus, to accumulate the public health target of 60 minutes or more per day of MVPA, school-aged children will likely need to engage in several hours per day of play and sport. This is an important message that needs to be conveyed to children and their parents.

I. Janssen, PhD

Reference

1. Sacheck JM, Nelson T, Ficker L, Kafka T, Kuder J, Economos CD. Physical activity during soccer and its contribution to physical activity recommendations in normal weight and overweight children. *Pediatr Exerc Sci.* 2011;23:281-292.

Physical Activity During Youth Sports Practices

Leek D, Carlson JA, Cain KL, et al (San Diego State Univ/Univ of California; San Diego State Univ, CA; et al)
Arch Pediatr Adolesc Med 165:294-299, 2011

Objective.—To document physical activity (PA) during organized youth soccer and baseball/softball practices.

Design.—Cross-sectional study.

Setting.—Community sports leagues in San Diego County, California.

Participants.—Two hundred youth aged 7 to 14 years were recruited from 29 teams in 2 youth sports in middle-income cities with an approximately equal distribution across sports, sex, and age groups.

Main Exposure.—Youth sports practices.

Outcome Measures.—A sample of players wore accelerometers during practices. Minutes of PA at multiple intensity levels were calculated using established cutoff points. Participants were categorized as meeting or not meeting guidelines of at least 60 minutes of moderate to vigorous PA (MVPA) during practice.

Results.—The overall mean for MVPA was 45.1 minutes and 46.1% of practice time. Participants on soccer teams (+13.7 minutes, +10.6% of practice time), boys (+10.7 minutes, +7.8% of practice time), and those aged 7 to 10 years (+7.0 minutes, +5.8% of practice time) had significantly more MVPA than their counterparts. Participants on soccer teams spent an average of 17.0 more minutes and 15.9% more of practice time in vigorous-intensity PA than those on baseball/softball teams. Overall, 24% of participants met the 60-minute PA guideline during practice, but fewer than 10% of 11- to 14-year-olds and 2% of girl softball players met the guideline.

Conclusions.—Participation in organized sports does not ensure that youth meet PA recommendations on practice days. The health effects of youth sports could be improved by adopting policies that ensure participants obtain PA during practices.

▶ Children and adolescents should accumulate 60 minutes of moderate to vigorous physical activity (MVPA) each day, but less than 50% of children and 10% of adolescents meet these guidelines.[1] Parents expect that one benefit of organized youth sports participation is substantial amounts of physical activity, but this study showed that less than one-fourth of the youth obtained the recommended 60 minutes of MVPA during practice (Fig 2 in the original article). Soccer players spent about 17 more minutes per practice in vigorous physical activity than baseball/softball players, and girls were less active than boys by about 11 minutes overall. So even during sports training, coaches need to emphasize more physical activity drills and less standing around.

D. C. Nieman, DrPH

Reference

1. Troiano RP, Berrigan D, Dodd KW, Mâsse LC, Tilert T, McDowell M. Physical activity in the United States measured by accelerometer. *Med Sci Sports Exerc.* 2008;40:181-188.

Physical Activity and Other Health-Risk Behaviors During the Transition Into Early Adulthood: A Longitudinal Cohort Study

Kwan MY, Cairney J, Faulkner GE, et al (McMaster Univ, Hamilton, Ontario, Canada; Univ of Toronto, Ontario, Canada)
Am J Prev Med 42:14-20, 2012

Background.—Research consistently demonstrates that physical activity declines with age. However, such declines do not occur linearly. The transition into early adulthood is one period in which disproportionate declines in physical activity have been evident, but much of our understanding of such declines among young adults has been based on either cross-sectional data or prospective studies that focus exclusively on college/university students.

Purpose.—The purpose of the current study was to use multilevel modeling to discern patterns of physical activity based on gender and educational trajectory among a nationally representative cohort of Canadian adolescents (N = 640; ages at baseline, 12−15 years). Examinations of smoking and binge drinking also were conducted as a basis for comparison.

Methods.—Drawn from seven cycles of the National Population Health Survey (NPHS), participants were interviewed every 2 years from 1994−1995 to 2006−2007; data analysis was conducted in 2010.

Results.—Overall, there was a 24% decrease in physical activity (equivalent to 1 MET/day) across the 12-year period. A significant three-way time X gender X educational trajectory interaction (coefficient= −0.189, SE=0.09, $p<0.05$) emerged in the physical activity analysis; main effects in $time^2$ (coefficient= −0.114, SE=0.01, $p<0.01$) and $time^3$ (coefficient=0.028, SE=0.01, $p<0.01$) were significant for binge drinking and smoking, respectively.

Conclusion.—Physical activity decline was evident during young adults' transition into early adulthood, with declines being steepest among men who entered a college/university. Although there were increases in several health-risk behaviors during adolescence, individuals tend to grow out of binge drinking and smoking as they mature.

▶ Few adults exercise at appropriate levels, and most research has been directed at strategies to increase activity participation. Little work has focused on preventing physical activity declines. Children and youth are the most physically active segments of the population, but activity levels quickly decline during the transition from late adolescence to early adulthood, or when high school students go to higher levels of education.[1] Little research has focused on young adults who do not attend a college/university. Results from the current study highlight the steep declines in physical activity behaviors, especially for men entering colleges or universities, during the transition from adolescence to early adulthood. Physical activity decreased on average 24% across the 12-year transition period.

D. C. Nieman, DrPH

Reference

1. Caspersen CJ, Pereira MA, Curran KM. Changes in physical activity patterns in the United States, by sex and cross-sectional age. *Med Sci Sports Exerc.* 2000; 32:1601-1609.

Adherence to the 2008 Adult Physical Activity Guidelines and Mortality Risk

Schoenborn CA, Stommel M (Natl Ctr for Health Statistics/CDC, Hyattsville, MD; Michigan State Univ, East Lansing)
Am J Prev Med 40:514-521, 2011

Background.—Mortality differentials by level and intensity of physical activity have been widely documented. A comprehensive review of scientific evidence of the health benefits of physical activity led the USDHHS to issue new Federal Guidelines for physical activity in 2008. Reductions in mortality risk associated with adherence to these Guidelines among the general U.S. adult population have not yet been studied.

Purpose.—This study compared the relative mortality risks of U.S. adults who met the *2008 Guidelines* with adults who did not meet the recommendations.

Methods.—Cox proportional hazards models were used to examine the relative mortality risks of U.S. adults aged ≥ 18 years, using data from the 1997—2004 National Health Interview Survey and linked mortality records for deaths occurring in 1997—2006 (analyzed in 2010). Risks for adults with and without chronic health conditions were examined separately.

Results.—Meeting the recommendations for aerobic activity was associated with substantial survival benefits, especially among the population having chronic conditions, with estimated hazard ratios ranging from 0.65 to 0.75 ($p<0.05$). While strengthening activities by themselves did not appear to reduce mortality risks, they may provide added survival benefits to those already engaged in aerobic activities. The relative benefits of physical activity were greatest among adults who had at least one chronic condition.

Conclusions.—Adherence to the *2008 Physical Activity Guidelines* was associated with reduced all-cause mortality risks among U.S. adults, after controlling for sociodemographic characteristics, BMI, smoking, and alcohol use (Figs 1 and 2).

▶ The 2008 Adult Physical Activity Guidelines for Americans recommend that adults should accumulate 150 minutes of moderate- or 75 minutes of vigorous-intensity aerobic activity per week and complete muscle-strengthening exercise

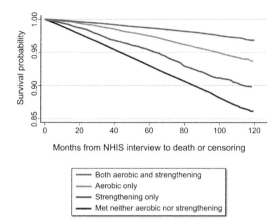

FIGURE 1.—Survival probabilities by levels of adherence to 2008 Physical Activity Guidelines. *Note*: U.S. adults aged ≥18 years (weighted); respondents not linked to death records were considered "censored," meaning they were presumed to be alive as of December 31, 2006. NHIS, National Health Interview Survey, 1997—2004. (Reprinted from Schoenborn CA, Stommel M. Adherence to the 2008 adult physical activity guidelines and mortality risk. *Am J Prev Med.* 2011;40:514-521, with permission from Elsevier.)

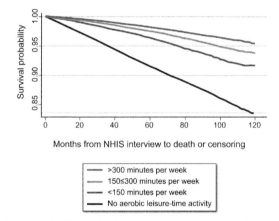

FIGURE 2.—Survival probabilities by levels of adherence to 2008 aerobic physical activity guidelines. *Note*: Respondents not linked to death records were considered "censored," meaning they were presumed to be alive as of December 31, 2006. NHIS, National Health Interview Survey, 1997—2004. (Reprinted from Schoenborn CA, Stommel M. Adherence to the 2008 adult physical activity guidelines and mortality risk. *Am J Prev Med.* 2011;40:514-521, with permission from Elsevier.)

2 days per week. Using the large database of the National Health Interview Survey, Schoenborn and Stommel found that these recommendations were associated with reduced all-cause mortality risk in adults, regardless of age. Perhaps the most important finding of this study was that mortality risk decreased to a greater extent in adults with 1 or more diagnosed comorbid chronic condition compared with those with no chronic conditions, regardless of age and other sociodemographic characteristics. In the full sample, aerobic activity alone was

associated with greater mortality risk reduction than strength exercise alone, but mortality risk was decreased the greatest in people who performed a combination of aerobic and muscle-strengthening exercise (Fig 1). This finding suggests a synergy between aerobic and muscle-strengthening exercise on overall health; however, this finding could also be due to less participation in strengthening compared with aerobic activity or less accurate recording of muscle-strengthening exercise. There was little evidence of a dose response between the amount of aerobic activity and survival (Fig 2). Survival was greatest in respondents who reported > 300 minutes of aerobic exercise per week and only slightly reduced with intermediate levels of activity. Performing < 150 minutes of aerobic activity per week conferred significantly greater survival than respondents reporting no aerobic activity. This study should arm clinicians with sufficient evidence to promote regular aerobic and muscle-strengthening activity to patients of all ages and regardless of comorbid conditions.

C. M. Jankowski, PhD

Adherence to the 2008 Adult Physical Activity Guidelines and Mortality Risk

Schoenborn CA, Stommel M (Natl Ctr for Health Statistics/CDC, Hyattsville, MD; Michigan State Univ, East Lansing)
Am J Prev Med 40:514-521, 2011

Background.—Mortality differentials by level and intensity of physical activity have been widely documented. A comprehensive review of scientific evidence of the health benefits of physical activity led the USDHHS to issue new Federal Guidelines for physical activity in 2008. Reductions in mortality risk associated with adherence to these Guidelines among the general U.S. adult population have not yet been studied.

Purpose.—This study compared the relative mortality risks of U.S. adults who met the *2008 Guidelines* with adults who did not meet the recommendations.

Methods.—Cox proportional hazards models were used to examine the relative mortality risks of U.S. adults aged ≥18 years, using data from the 1997–2004 National Health Interview Survey and linked mortality records for deaths occurring in 1997–2006 (analyzed in 2010). Risks for adults with and without chronic health conditions were examined separately.

Results.—Meeting the recommendations for aerobic activity was associated with substantial survival benefits, especially among the population having chronic conditions, with estimated hazard ratios ranging from 0.65 to 0.75 (*p*<0.05). While strengthening activities by themselves did not appear to reduce mortality risks, they may provide added survival benefits to those already engaged in aerobic activities. The relative benefits of physical activity were greatest among adults who had at least one chronic condition.

TABLE 2.—Adherence to the 2008 Physical Activity Guidelines for Adults, by Chronic Condition Status: 1997–2004

Characteristic	Total		No Conditions[a]		≥1 Conditions[a]	
	n	% (95% CI)	n	% (95% CI)	n	% (95% CI)
Physical activity guidelines met		100.0		100.0		100.0
Neither	132,613	52.5 (52.0, 53.0)	63,170	48.1 (47.5, 48.7)	69,443	57.7 (57.2, 58.2)
Strength only	8,173	3.4 (3.3, 3.5)	3947	3.2 (3.1, 3.3)	4,226	3.7 (3.6, 3.8)
Aerobic only	60,144	25.8 (25.5, 26.1)	33,842	27.4 (27.0, 27.8)	26,302	24.0 (23.6, 24.3)
Both	35,576	15.7 (15.4, 16.0)	22,776	18.7 (18.3, 19.1)	12,800	12.1 (11.8, 12.4)
Unknown	5,891	2.6 (2.4, 2.8)	3,128	2.6 (2.4, 2.8)	2,763	2.6 (2.3, 2.8)
Aerobic activity (minutes/week)						
0	96,416	37.2 (36.6, 37.7)	45,337	33.7 (33.1, 34.2)	51,079	41.3 (40.7, 41.9)
<150	44,502	18.8 (18.5, 19.1)	21,832	17.6 (17.3, 18.0)	22,670	20.2 (19.8, 20.5)
150–300	33,029	14.2 (14.0, 14.4)	18,558	15.1 (14.8, 15.4)	14,471	13.1 (12.8, 13.3)
>300	62,211	27.1 (26.7, 27.5)	37,794	30.8 (30.3, 31.3)	24,417	22.7 (22.4, 23.1)
Unknown	6,239	2.8 (2.6, 3.0)	3,342	2.8 (2.6, 3.0)	2,897	2.7 (2.5, 3.0)
Total	242,397		126,863		115,534	

Note: Table represents the civilian, non-institutionalized population aged ≥18 years. *n*, number of sample adult respondents; %, weighted percentage
[a]Chronic conditions include diabetes, hypertension, circulatory, respiratory (including chronic bronchitis), and one or more functional limitations.

Conclusions.—Adherence to the *2008 Physical Activity Guidelines* was associated with reduced all-cause mortality risks among U.S. adults, after controlling for sociodemographic characteristics, BMI, smoking, and alcohol use (Table 2).

▶ There is now general agreement that regular physical activity is associated with increased longevity.[1] However, the requisite amount of physical activity for benefit is more controversial, and frequent changes in the exercise recommendations from public health authorities have tended to leave the general public skeptical about the validity of the messages that are promulgated.[2,3] The prospective study of Schoenborn and Stommel shows a substantial association between the physical activity levels reported in several major US surveys and the individuals' subsequent mortality experiences (Fig 2 in the original article), with apparent benefit being seen among those people who have adhered to the US recommendations as formulated in 2008.[4] Interestingly, the association is limited to aerobic activity, with little apparent difference of prognosis among those who perceive themselves as conforming to recommendations for muscle-strengthening exercises. Further, although there seems some apparent benefit in exceeding the minimal recommendation of 150 minutes of aerobic activity per week, the added benefit is apparently fairly small. There remain a number of acknowledged limitations to the study. First, activity levels were determined by questionnaire, and such information is notoriously unreliable and at risk of exaggeration[5]; on the other hand, the questions that were posed corresponded closely with the recommendations. Second, the observed associations could have arisen because those who were unwell chose to take less exercise. There is some suggestion of this in the greater physical activity association for those with preexisting disease; the authors have attempted to circumvent this by discounting the first 2 years of data in those who were apparently initially healthy, but it would be helpful if the study were repeated with a longer initial period to sift out those with preexisting disease. Finally, the most important issue for many people is not their absolute longevity, but rather the quality of their lifespan, and this study has not addressed this question.

R. J. Shephard, MD (Lond), PhD, DPE

References

1. Bouchard C, Shephard RJ, Stephens T. *Physical Activity, Fitness & Health*. Champaign, IL: Humnan Kinetics; 1994.
2. Shephard RJ. Whistler 2001: a Health Canada/CDC conference on "Communicating physical activity and health messages: science into practice". *Am J Prev Med*. 2002;23:221-225.
3. Shephard RJ. What is the physical activity message, and how are we getting it across? In: Shephard RJ, et al., eds. *Year Book of Sports Medicine, 2003*. Philadelphia, PA: C.V. Mosby; 2003:xvii-xxxvi.
4. *Physical Activity Guidelines Advisory Committee Report, 2008*. Washington, DC: US DHHS; 2008.
5. Shephard RJ. Limits to the measurement of habitual physical activity by questionnaires. *Br J Sports Med*. 2003;37:197-206.

Adherence to the 2008 Adult Physical Activity Guidelines and Mortality Risk

Schoenborn CA, Stommel M (Natl Ctr for Health Statistics/CDC, Hyattsville, MD; Michigan State Univ, East Lansing)
Am J Prev Med 40:514-521, 2011

Background.—Mortality differentials by level and intensity of physical activity have been widely documented. A comprehensive review of scientific evidence of the health benefits of physical activity led the USDHHS to issue new Federal Guidelines for physical activity in 2008. Reductions in mortality risk associated with adherence to these Guidelines among the general U.S. adult population have not yet been studied.

Purpose.—This study compared the relative mortality risks of U.S. adults who met the *2008 Guidelines* with adults who did not meet the recommendations.

Methods.—Cox proportional hazards models were used to examine the relative mortality risks of U.S. adults aged ≥18 years, using data from the 1997–2004 National Health Interview Survey and linked mortality records for deaths occurring in 1997–2006 (analyzed in 2010). Risks for adults with and without chronic health conditions were examined separately.

Results.—Meeting the recommendations for aerobic activity was associated with substantial survival benefits, especially among the population having chronic conditions, with estimated hazard ratios ranging from

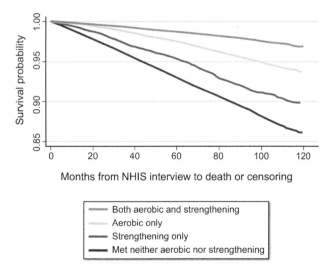

FIGURE 1.—Survival probabilities by levels of adherence to 2008 Physical Activity Guidelines. *Note*: U.S. adults aged ≥18 years (weighted); respondents not linked to death records were considered "censored," meaning they were presumed to be alive as of December 31, 2006. NHIS, National Health Interview Survey, 1997–2004. (Reprinted from Schoenborn CA, Stommel M. Adherence to the 2008 adult physical activity guidelines and mortality risk. *Am J Prev Med.* 2011;40:514-521, with permission from Elsevier.)

0.65 to 0.75 (*p*<0.05). While strengthening activities by themselves did not appear to reduce mortality risks, they may provide added survival benefits to those already engaged in aerobic activities. The relative benefits of physical activity were greatest among adults who had at least one chronic condition.

Conclusions.—Adherence to the *2008 Physical Activity Guidelines* was associated with reduced all-cause mortality risks among U.S. adults, after controlling for sociodemographic characteristics, BMI, smoking, and alcohol use (Fig 1).

▶ This study indicates that adherence to the levels of physical activity recommended in the 2008 Physical Activity Guidelines for Adults has substantial survival benefits (Fig 1). All-cause mortality risks were 27% lower in those without existing chronic comorbidities and by almost half among people with chronic comorbidities, regardless of age and obesity levels. Although recommendations set forth in the 2008 Physical Activity Guidelines for Adults may be met by non—leisure-time activities, for this analysis, adherence to recommended activity levels was assessed in terms of leisure-time physical activity (≥150 minutes of moderate or ≥75 minutes of vigorous aerobic activity per week or an equivalent combination) and muscle-strengthening activities 2 or more times per week.

D. C. Nieman, DrPH

Increase in sudden death from coronary artery disease in young adults
Arzamendi D, Benito B, Tizon-Marcos H, et al (Univ of Montreal, Canada; Université Laval, Quebec, Canada; et al)
Am Heart J 161:574-580, 2011

Background.—Sudden cardiac death (SCD) is the most common cause of death in adults aged <65 years, making it a major public health problem. A growing incidence in coronary artery disease (CAD) in young individuals has been predicted in developed countries, which could in turn be associated with an increase in SCD in this population. The aim of the study was to assess the prevalence of CAD among autopsies of young individuals (<40 years) who had sudden death (SD).

Methods.—We selected all the autopsies referred to the Montreal Heart Institute and Maisonneuve-Rosemont Hospital from January 2002 to December 2006 that corresponded to individuals <40 years old who had died suddenly. For each decedent, the following data were collected: cause of death, autopsy findings, available clinical history, toxicological findings, and cardiovascular risk factors.

Results.—From a total of 1,260 autopsies, 243 fulfilled the inclusion criteria. Coronary artery disease was the main cause of SCD from age 20 years, representing the 37% of deaths in the group of 21 to 30 years old, and up to 80% of deaths in the group of 31 to 40 years old. Among individuals who died of CAD, 3-vessel disease was observed in

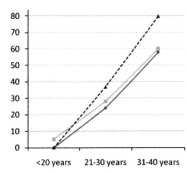

	Drory (1976-1985)	Virmani (1981-1988)	Arzamendi (2001-2007)
Age (years)	32	32	28
Male gender (%)	76	76	83
Race •White •Black •Asian	NA	56 46 1	93 4.5 2.5

FIGURE 3.—Evolution of SCD from CAD through different ranges of age in the 3 main studies. Age, gender, and race data about each series are represented in the table. (Reprinted from the American Journal of Emergency Medicine. Arzamendi D, Benito B, Tizon-Marcos H, et al. Increase in sudden death from coronary artery disease in young adults. *Am Heart J.* 2011;161:574-580, Copyright 2011, with permission from Elsevier.)

39.7% of cases. Moreover, among the whole population <40 years old, at least 1 significant coronary lesion was observed in 39.5% of cases, irrespective to the cause of death. In the multivariable analysis, an increased BMI (hazard ratio 1.1 for each kg/m^2, 95% CI 1.01-1.1) and hypercholesterolemia (hazard ratio 2.4, 95% CI 1.7-333.3) showed to be the modifiable factors related to an increased risk of SD from CAD.

Conclusions.—In our population, CAD was the main cause of SD from age 20 years. These data bring into question whether present prevention strategies are sufficient and reinforce the need to extend prevention to younger ages (Fig 3).

▶ Sports physicians tend to assume that sudden cardiac death in a young person reflects the presence of hypertrophic cardiomyopathy or some congenital abnormality of the coronary circulation. However, this postmortem study of sudden deaths from Montreal underlines the fact that in the general population, coronary vascular disease is the main culprit, even in the 20- to 40-year age group. Moreover, comparison with earlier studies suggests that the risk has increased substantially since the 1980s (Fig 3). Unfortunately, no information was obtained on what the subjects were doing when the catastrophe occurred, but it seems likely that many were related to a sudden and unexpected burst of exercise.

R. J. Shephard, MD (Lond), PhD, DPE

Increased Average Longevity among the "Tour de France" Cyclists
Sanchis-Gomar F, Olaso-Gonzalez G, Corella D, et al (Univ of Valencia, Spain)
Int J Sports Med 32:644-647, 2011

It is widely held among the general population and even among health professionals that moderate exercise is a healthy practice but long term high intensity exercise is not. The specific amount of physical activity necessary for good health remains unclear. To date, longevity studies of elite athletes have been relatively sparse and the results are somewhat conflicting. The Tour de France is among the most gruelling sport events in the world, during which highly trained professional cyclists undertake high intensity exercise for a full 3 weeks. Consequently we set out to determine the longevity of the participants in the Tour de France, compared with that of the general population. We studied the longevity of 834 cyclists from France (n = 465), Italy (n = 196) and Belgium (n = 173) who rode the Tour de France between the years 1930 and 1964. Dates of birth and death of the cyclists were obtained on December 31st 2007. We calculated the percentage of survivors for each age and compared them with the values for the pooled general population of France, Italy and Belgium for the appropriate age cohorts. We found a very significant increase in average longevity (17%) of the cyclists when compared with the general population. The age at which 50% of the general population died was 73.5 vs. 81.5 years in Tour de France participants. Our major finding is that repeated very intense exercise prolongs life span in well trained practitioners. Our findings underpin the importance of exercising without the fear that becoming exhausted might be bad for one's health (Fig 2).

▶ It has long been recognized that endurance athletes tend to live several years longer than their peers in the general population,[1,2] but it is has been less clear that this advantage was attributable to involvement in regular bouts of endurance exercise, because other aspects of lifestyle (particularly cigarette smoking) also differed between the athletes and the general population.[3] The Tour de

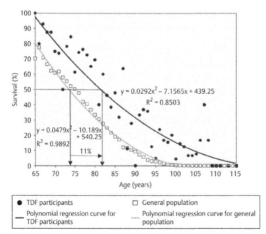

FIGURE 2.—Percentage of survival related to age in TdF participants and in the general population. Persons born between 1892 and 1942 have been studied. Average life span of TdF participants is higher (p = 0.004; 17.5 %) than the general population of the same country in which the cyclists were born. The age at which 50 % of the general population died was 73.5 vs. 81.5 years in TdF participants, i. e., 11 % increase. (Reprinted from Sanchis-Gomar F, Olaso-Gonzalez G, Corella D, et al. Increased average longevity among the "Tour de France" cyclists. *Int J Sports Med.* 2011;32:644-647, with permission from Georg Thieme Verlag KG Stuttgart, New York.)

France provides perhaps the ultimate example of endurance competition, with participants engaging in as much as 35 000 km of cycling per year. The future health prospects of competitors have sometimes been clouded by various forms of doping, although the period of competition (1930-1964) considered in this report was before recourse to some of the more serious abuses. The 8-year effect on the average age of death relative to the corresponding general populations (Fig 2) looks impressive, although it undoubtedly includes some benefit from not smoking. The study was also unable to confirm that the cyclists had maintained their vigorous activity as they aged. Nevertheless, these observations do seem to counter suspicions of long-term adverse consequences from the temporary derangements of cardiac function seen in the first few hours following ultra-endurance exercise.

R. J. Shephard, MD (Lond), PhD, DPE

References

1. Karvonen MJ, Klemola H, Virkajärvi J, Kekkonen A. Longevity of endurance skiers. *Med Sci Sports.* 1974;6:49-51.
2. Sarna S, Kaprio J. Life expectancy of former athletes. *Sports Med.* 1994;17:149-151.
3. Fogelholm M, Kaprio J, Sarna S. Healthy lifestyles of former Finnish world class athletes. *Med Sci Sports Exerc.* 1994;26:224-229.

Using the Tax System to Promote Physical Activity: Critical Analysis of Canadian Initiatives

von Tigerstrom B, Larre T, Sauder J (Univ of Saskatchewan, Saskatoon, Canada)
Am J Public Health 101:e10-e16, 2011

In Canada, tax incentives have been recently introduced to promote physical activity and reduce rates of obesity. The most prominent of these is the federal government's Children's Fitness Tax Credit, which came into effect in 2007. We critically assess the potential benefits and limitations of using tax measures to promote physical activity.

Careful design could make these measures more effective, but any tax-based measures have inherent limitations, and the costs of such programs are substantial.

Therefore, it is important to consider whether public funds are better spent on other strategies that could instead provide direct public funding to address environmental and systemic factors.

▶ Attempts to persuade urban populations to become more physically active through admonitions and policy statements seem to have had little effect on behavior; if anything, people in the United States and Canada have become even more inactive over the past 10 years.[1-5] There has thus been a growing interest in the possibility of government providing a financial carrot for those who wish to become more active or a stick to punish those who do not.

Such an approach has had demonstrated effectiveness in the fight against cigarette smoking and excessive alcohol consumption, both behaviors being sensitive to an increase in sales taxes. Canadian governments have recently been trying similar tactics to promote physical activity, allowing tax deductions (or in some provinces a cash grant) for enrollment of children in sports or organized physical activity programs and sales tax concessions on the purchase of some items of sports equipment, such as bicycles. Unfortunately, most of these measures have so far been introduced in a way that makes it difficult to assess their effectiveness, and the situation has been clouded by simplistic claims of benefit from those marketing expensive items of equipment. The article by Tigerstrom and associates argues that such initiatives have a substantial cost to government revenues, and the money might better have been invested in environmental initiatives that would favor physical activity. Nevertheless, there are some suggestions that tax policies can have an impact—most notably, the congestion tax imposed on central London[6]—and the loss of government revenue could well be recouped through a reduction of future costs for medical care. This approach thus merits further analysis and evaluation.

R. J. Shephard, MD (Lond), PhD, DPE

References

1. Troiano RP, Berrigan D, Dodd KW, Mâsse LC, Tilert T, McDowell M. Physical activity in the United States measured by accelerometer. *Med Sci Sports Exerc.* 2008;40:181-188.
2. Centers for Disease Control and Prevention. US Physical Activity Statistics. http://www.cdc.gov/nccdphp/dnpa/physical/stats/index.htm. Accessed June 28, 2010.
3. Canadian Fitness & Lifestyle Research Institute. Kids CAN PLAY! Activity Levels of Canadian Children and Youth. http://www.cflri.ca/eng/statistics/surveys/documents/CANPLAY2009_Bulletin01_PA_levelsEN.pdf. Accessed November 9th, 2011.
4. Canadian Fitness & Lifestyle Research Institute. Let's get active! Planning effective communication strategies, http://www.cflri.ca/eng/statistics/surveys/documents/PAM2008FactsFigures_Bulletin02_PA_among_CanadiansEN.pdf. Accessed November 9th, 2011.
5. Shields M, Tremblay MS, Laviolette M, et al. Fitness of Canadian adults: results from the 2007-2009 Canadian Health Measures Survey. *Health Rep.* 2010;21. http://www.statcan.gc.ca/pub/82-003-x/2010001/article/11064-eng.pdf. Accessed November 9th, 2011.
6. Bergman P, Grjibovski AM, Hagströmer M, Patterson E, Sjöström M. Congestion road tax and physical activity. *Am J Prev Med.* 2010;38:171-177.

Cost-effectiveness of exercise on prescription with telephone support among women in general practice over 2 years
Elley CR, Garrett S, Rose SB, et al (Univ of Auckland, New Zealand; Univ of Otago, Wellington, New Zealand)
Br J Sports Med 45:1223-1229, 2011

Aim.—To assess the cost-effectiveness of exercise on prescription with ongoing support in general practice.

Methods.—Prospective cost-effectiveness study undertaken as part of the 2-year Women's lifestyle study randomised controlled trial involving 1089 'less-active' women aged 40−74. The 'enhanced Green Prescription' intervention included written exercise prescription and brief advice from a primary care nurse, face-to-face follow-up at 6 months, and 9 months of telephone support. The primary outcome was incremental cost of moving one 'less-active' person into the 'active' category over 24 months. Direct costs of programme delivery were recorded. Other (indirect) costs covered in the analyses included participant costs of exercise, costs of primary and secondary healthcare utilisation, allied health therapies and time off work (lost productivity). Cost−effectiveness ratios were calculated with and without including indirect costs.

Results.—Follow-up rates were 93% at 12 months and 89% at 24 months. Significant improvements in physical activity were found at 12 and 24 months ($p<0.01$). The exercise programme cost was New Zealand dollars (NZ$) 93.68 (€45.90) per participant. There was no significant difference in indirect costs over the course of the trial between the two groups (rate ratios: 0.99 (95% CI 0.81 to 1.2) at 12 months and 1.01 (95% CI 0.83 to 1.23) at 24 months, p=0.9). Cost−effectiveness ratios using programme costs were NZ$687 (€331) per person made 'active' and sustained at 12 months and NZ$1407 (€678) per person made 'active' and sustained at 24 months.

Conclusions.—This nurse-delivered programme with ongoing support is very cost-effective and compares favourably with other primary care and community-based physical activity interventions internationally (Table 4).

▶ General practitioners are increasingly recognizing the wisdom of delegating details of exercise prescription and maintenance to exercise scientists and nurse practitioners associated with their practice. The study of Elley and colleagues examined the effectiveness of telephone support from a nurse on success in moving a group of older sedentary but otherwise healthy women from the "less active" to the "more active" category. Previous tests on a similar population, using physician advice and a shorter (3-month) period of telephone support, found limited maintenance of increased physical activity.[1,2] A longer period (five 10-minute phone calls over 9 months) of support with face-to-face nurse contact was thus evaluated in the present trial. Outcome measures were the cost of bringing 1 woman to undertake at least 150 min of moderate exercise per week, as assessed by questionnaire, and other costs (utilization of primary and secondary health care and time off work). It cost some NZ$687 to make a single woman active (a favorable cost relative to earlier trials[3,4] and the figure of NZ$1746 found for a physician-based trial on a different sample[5]), and a larger proportion of women were still active at 12 months, although there did not appear to be any change in immediate health care utilization (Table 4). Despite cost-effectiveness of the exercise stimulus, the proportion of subjects whose activity remained increased was fairly small (13% at 12 months, and only 6.7% at 24 months). Another possible limitation of the study is that there is no indication how far the reported increase in

TABLE 4.—Summary of Indirect Costs for Intervention and Control Groups at Baseline, 12 Months and 24 Months*

Cost	Baseline		12 Months		24 Months	
	Intervention	Control	Intervention	Control	Intervention	Control
N	544	545	488	497	482	480
Exercise costs (NZ$)	325.26 (578.28)	307.66 (546.01)	401.63 (2206.64)	279.14 (560.80)	262.30 (535.88)	268.56 (515.78)
GP cost to patient (NZ$)	181.30 (322.88)	153.77 (162.08)	109.68 (117.05)	109.20 (104.80)	99.81 (124.37)	90.89 (98.64)
Total personal cost (NZ$)	506.56 (664.58)	461.43 (574.32)	520.07 (2210.19)	396.52 (567.34)	373.79 (534.57)	370.27 (522.55)
GP cost to health funder (NZ$)	183.30 (384.96)	154.20 (313.15)	175.82 (315.18)	150.76 (285.15)	171.83 (335.04)	127.25 (231.47)
Inpatient costs (NZ$) to health funder	431.49 (1595.14)	551.24 (2238.69)	517.67 (2147.12)	484.90 (1769.15)	426.12 (1810.79)	435.60 (1782.25)
education department/outpatient department costs to health funder	160.54 (358.65)	159.08 (365.91)	99.62 (273.23)	106.37 (294.59)	121.97 (323.07)	114.24 (452.86)
Cost (NZ$) of time off work	415.76 (1881.58)	317.85 (917.73)	199.36 (505.60)	309.35 (1356.39)	200.33 (863.93)	197.11 (716.42)
Total provider cost and cost of loss of productivity	1191.09 (2994.18)	1182.37 (2780.15)	1036.95 (2567.90)	1091.26 (2801.01)	932.12 (2297.51)	856.81 (2114.89)
Total indirect costs (NZ$)	$1697.65 (3122.75)	$1643.80 (2898.17)	$1558.62 (3445.24)	$1490.78 (2866.56)	$1361.22 (2426.67)	$1274.49 (2205.88)

Figures reported are exclusive of goods and services tax.
*Mean (SD) costs per participant are presented for all cost components.

physical activity enhanced measures of the individual's physical fitness. If there were real and sustained gains in fitness, then the active group might show long-term savings in health costs.

R. J. Shephard, MD (Lond), PhD, DPE

References

1. Rose SB, Lawton BA, Elley CR, Dowell AC, Fenton AJ. The 'Women's Lifestyle Study,' 2-year randomized controlled trial of physical activity counselling in primary health care: rationale and study design. *BMC Public Health.* 2007;7:166.
2. Lawton BA, Rose SB, Elley CR, Dowell AC, Fenton A, Moyes SA. Exercise on prescription for women aged 40-74 recruited through primary care: two year randomised controlled trial. *BMJ.* 2008;337:a2509.
3. Stevens W, Hillsdon M, Thorogood M, McArdle D. Cost-effectiveness of a primary care based physical activity intervention in 45-74 year old men and women: a randomised controlled trial. *Br J Sports Med.* 1998;32:236-241.
4. Sevick MA, Napolitano MA, Papandonatos GD, Gordon AJ, Reiser LM, Marcus BH. Cost-effectiveness of alternative approaches for motivating activity in sedentary adults: results of Project STRIDE. *Prev Med.* 2007;45:54-61.
5. Dalziel K, Segal L, Elley CR. Cost utility analysis of physical activity counselling in general practice. *Aust N Z J Public Health.* 2006;30:57-63.

The Effects of Time and Intensity of Exercise on Novel and Established Markers of CVD in Adolescent Youth
Buchan DS, Ollis S, Young JD, et al (Univ of the West of Scotland, Hamilton, UK; et al)
Am J Hum Biol 23:517-526, 2011

Objectives.—This article examines the effects of brief, intense exercise in comparison with traditional endurance exercise on both novel and traditional markers of cardiovascular disease (CVD) in youth.

Methods.—Forty seven boys and ten girls (16.4 ± 0.7 years of age) were divided into a moderate (MOD), high intensity (HIT), or a control group. The MOD group (12 boys, 4 girls) and HIT group (15 boys, 2 girls) performed three weekly exercise sessions over 7 weeks. Each session consisted of either four to six repeats of maximal sprint running within a 20 m area with 20–30 s recovery (HIT) or 20 min continuous running within a 20 m area at ~70% maximal oxygen uptake (VO_2max).

Results.—Total exercise time commitment over the intervention was 420 min (MOD) and 63 min (HIT). Training volume was 85% lower for the HIT group. Total estimated energy expenditure was ~907.2 kcal (HIT) and ~4410 kcal (MOD). Significant improvements ($P \leq 0.05$) were found in systolic blood pressure, aerobic fitness, and body mass index (BMI) postintervention (HIT). In the MOD group, significant ($P \leq 0.05$) improvements were noted in aerobic fitness, percentage body fat (%BF), BMI, fibrinogen (Fg), plasminogen activator inhibitor-1, and insulin concentrations.

TABLE 3.—Physical and Physiological Variables (mean ± SD) Before (Pre) and After (Post) the Interventions

Variables Physical	Control n = 24		Moderate n = 16		High Intensity n = 17	
	PRE	POST	PRE	POST	PRE	POST
Stature (cm)	171.1 ± 8.7	172.5 ± 8.8[b]	172.7 ± 9.3	173.8 ± 9.3[b]	170.1 ± 7.8	172.6 ± 7.5[b]
Body Mass (kg)	66.11 ± 7.6	66.27 ± 8.0	66.60 ± 9.9	66.61 ± 9.8	63.38 ± 9.2	63.69 ± 9.3
BMI (kg/m^2)	22.70 ± 2.6	22.31 ± 2.5[c]	22.4 ± 3.3	22.10 ± 3.3[b]	21.61 ± 2.2	21.31 ± 2.1[c]
WHR	0.82 ± 0.0	0.84 ± 0.0[c]	0.78 ± 0.0 (15)[a]	0.78 ± 0.0 (15)[a]	0.86 ± 0.3	0.84 ± 0.1
Body Fat (%)	16.62 ± 6.8	16.62 ± 7.2	19.73 ± 8.6 (15)[a]	17.64 ± 6.5 (15)[ac]	18.65 ± 7.7	19.20 ± 5.8
SBP (mm Hg)	113 ± 10	109 ± 11	112 ± 11	108 ± 12	112 ± 10	106 ± 11[c]
DBP (mm Hg)	68 ± 8	64 ± 7[b]	66 ± 7	66 ± 4	67 ± 7	65 ± 6
Aerobic Fitness (shuttles)	81.33 ± 25.3	80.13 ± 24.712	73.56 ± 21.8	93.25 ± 23.2[b]	82.00 ± 25.8	88.78 ± 26.4[b]

[a]Where n ≠ denoted number, actual sample number is presented in brackets.
[b]Different from baseline, $P<0.01$.
[c]Different from baseline, $P<0.05$.

Conclusions.—These findings demonstrate that brief, intense exercise is a time efficient means for improving CVD risk factors in adolescents (Table 3).

▶ This article has already attracted quite a bit of attention in the national press, although at the time of reading, it is still only an electronic publication. The text addresses the superficially attractive idea that those who "do not have time for exercise" can gain equivalent benefit by training at a higher intensity of physical activity; the choices tested are intensities corresponding to 70% and 85% of the maximal oxygen intake. The importance of intensity relative to initial fitness as a determinant of an individual's cardiovascular training response has been recognized for many years.[1] However, it is less certain that other health benefits such as a reduction in body fat content are obtained to a similar extent from low- and higher-intensity training regimens. Although the authors claim a reduction in cardiovascular risk factors from both programs, their data (Table 3) indicate a much smaller total energy expenditure with the high-intensity program. And whereas the moderate-intensity group decreased their skinfold estimated body fat from 19.7% to 17.6% over the trial, the percentage of body fat actually increased in the high-intensity group. Surprisingly, the high-intensity group fared better than the moderate-intensity group in terms of increases in high-density lipoprotein cholesterol. The subjects of this study were teenagers, and although some members of this age group might be willing to engage in high-intensity activity, this is less certain and possibly less safe for older adults; indeed, some older sedentary individuals might baulk at sustaining exercise at 70% of their maximal oxygen intake. Rather than advocating high-intensity exercise as a remedy for "lack of time," it may be better to consider time-management tactics that will bring out the substantial amount of time that most patients could allocate to physical activity.

R. J. Shephard, MD (Lond), PhD, DPE

Reference

1. Shephard RJ. Intensity, duration and frequency of exercise as determinants of the response to a training regime. *Int Z Angew Physiol.* 1968;26:272-278.

Comparisons of leisure-time physical activity and cardiorespiratory fitness as predictors of all-cause mortality in men and women
Lee D-C, Sui X, Ortega FB, et al (Univ of South Carolina, Columbia; Karolinska Inst, Hugginge, Sweden; et al)
Br J Sports Med 45:504-510, 2011

Objective.—To examine the combined associations and relative contributions of leisure-time physical activity (PA) and cardiorespiratory fitness (CRF) with all-cause mortality.
Design.—Prospective cohort study.
Setting.—Aerobics centre longitudinal study.

Participants.—31 818 men and 10 555 women who received a medical examination during 1978–2002.

Assessment of Risk Factors.—Leisure-time PA assessed by self-reported questionnaire; CRF assessed by maximal treadmill test.

Main Outcome Measures.—All-cause mortality until 31 December 2003.

Results.—There were 1492 (469 per 10 000) and 230 (218 per 10 000) deaths in men and women, respectively. PA and CRF were positively correlated in men (r=0.49) and women (r=0.47) controlling for age (p<0.001 for both). PA was inversely associated with mortality in multivariable Cox regression analysis among men, but the association was eliminated after further adjustment for CRF. No significant association of PA with mortality was observed in women. CRF was inversely associated with mortality in men and women, and the associations remained significant after further adjustment for PA. In the PA and CRF combined analysis, compared with the reference group "not meeting the recommended PA (<500 metabolic equivalent-minute/week) and unfit", the relative risks (95% CIs) of mortality were 0.62 (0.54 to 0.72) and 0.61 (0.44 to 0.86) in men and women "not meeting the recommended PA and fit", 0.96 (0.61 to 1.53) and 0.93 (0.33 to 2.58) in men and women "meeting the recommended PA and unfit" and 0.60 (0.51 to 0.70) and 0.56 (0.37 to 0.85) in men and women "meeting the recommended PA and fit", respectively.

Conclusions.—CRF was more strongly associated with all-cause mortality than PA; therefore, improving CRF should be encouraged in unfit individuals to reduce risk of mortality and considered in the development of future PA guidelines.

▶ The study by Lee and colleagues probes whether leisure-time physical activity (PA) and cardiorespiratory fitness (CRF) have independent and combined effects on reducing all-cause mortality in women and men. The rationale for this investigation was that the current public health recommendations for physical activity present goals for time spent in physical activity (a behavior) rather than in terms of improving CRF (a physiological response). The data came from a large sample of approximately 32 000 healthy men and 10 500 women aged 20 to 82 years who completed physical activity questionnaires and treadmill tests one time and were then followed for 12 to 14 years. Cardiorespiratory fitness was defined as the total duration of a maximal treadmill test. Approximately 44% of the participants met the recommendation of 500 or more metabolic equivalent minutes/week of physical activity. The authors posed 4 questions: (1) Does the magnitude of the association with mortality risk differ between PA and CRF? (2) Do PA and CRF contribute to mortality risk independently of each other? (3) Does mortality risk differ between less active-fit and active-unfit? (4) Are the combined effects of PA and CRF with mortality stronger than either exposure by itself? Overall, the mortality risk reduction associated with CRF was larger than PA; in women, PA level was not associated with reduced risk of mortality. The independent contributions of PA and CRF were not clear, in part because of the small number of deaths in the fit women and men; however, in prediction models adjusted for PA or CRF, CRF remained associated with reduced mortality risk after adjustment for PA, but not vice versa. These models suggested an independent effect of CRF on mortality risk reduction. The mortality risk was lower in the less-active fit than the active-unfit. The combined effects of PA and CRF were somewhat larger than either factor alone but largely attributed to CRF. In total, it was suggested that the effect of PA on activity is mediated in large part by CRF. People who have a genetic predisposition to greater CRF may be protected from other physiological insults that contribute to mortality. The lack of association of PA with reduced mortality risk in women may be attributed to the physical activity questionnaire, which was developed for use in men and not validated for use in women. The authors proposed that future versions of the national physical activity recommendations place more emphasis on improving CRF, but this may be premature. A more rigorous approach to evaluating the relative contributions of PA and CRF to mortality risk would be to use activity monitors rather than self-reported activity and intensity levels and measured maximal oxygen consumption rather than estimation from time on treadmill.

C. M. Jankowski, PhD

Comparisons of leisure-time physical activity and cardiorespiratory fitness as predictors of all-cause mortality in men and women

Lee D-C, Sui X, Ortega FB, et al (Univ of South Carolina, Columbia; Karolinska Inst, Hugginge, Sweden; Seoul Natl Univ, South Korea; et al)
Br J Sports Med 45:504-510, 2011

Objective.—To examine the combined associations and relative contributions of leisure-time physical activity (PA) and cardiorespiratory fitness (CRF) with all-cause mortality.

Design.—Prospective cohort study.

Setting.—Aerobics centre longitudinal study.

Participants.—31 818 men and 10 555 women who received a medical examination during 1978–2002.

Assessment of Risk Factors.—Leisure-time PA assessed by self-reported questionnaire; CRF assessed by maximal treadmill test.

Main Outcome Measures.—All-cause mortality until 31 December 2003.

Results.—There were 1492 (469 per 10 000) and 230 (218 per 10 000) deaths in men and women, respectively. PA and CRF were positively correlated in men (r=0.49) and women (r=0.47) controlling for age (p<0.001 for both). PA was inversely associated with mortality in multivariable Cox regression analysis among men, but the association was eliminated after further adjustment for CRF. No significant association of PA with mortality was observed in women. CRF was inversely associated with mortality in men and women, and the associations remained significant after further adjustment for PA. In the PA and CRF combined analysis, compared with the reference group "not meeting the recommended PA (<500 metabolic equivalent-minute/week) and unfit", the relative risks (95% CIs) of mortality were 0.62 (0.54 to 0.72) and 0.61 (0.44 to 0.86) in men and women "not meeting the recommended PA and fit", 0.96 (0.61 to 1.53) and 0.93 (0.33 to 2.58) in men and women "meeting the recommended PA and unfit" and 0.60 (0.51 to 0.70) and 0.56 (0.37 to 0.85) in men and women "meeting the recommended PA and fit", respectively.

Conclusions.—CRF was more strongly associated with all-cause mortality than PA; therefore, improving CRF should be encouraged in unfit individuals to reduce risk of mortality and considered in the development of future PA guidelines (Table 4).

▶ Blair and his colleagues have previously compared the relative usefulness of physical activity and physical fitness in the prediction of adverse health outcomes, using the large database from the Cooper Clinic,[1] an upper socioeconomic stratum. Blair and associates have found that most health variables were more closely associated with an individual's initial physical fitness (as assessed by treadmill endurance time) than with physical activity (classified as inactive, sufficient, or recommended based on responses to a questionnaire), and they suggested that this might reflect in part errors inherent in the questionnaire assessment of physical activity.[2] It may also be that for health benefit, physical activity must reach an intensity sufficient to augment physical fitness.[3,4] A further factor is that the questionnaire they used did not assess a person's occupational activity, household chores, or possible active commuting. Their follow-up has now continued for up to 25 years, providing a substantial mortality experience in both men and women. In terms of overall mortality, their data continue to favor measures of physical fitness; in women, the reported physical activity category is unrelated to mortality, and in men, any association with physical activity category disappears after controlling for initial physical fitness, but the benefit of greater fitness persists after adjusting for reported physical activity (Table 4). Not

TABLE 4.—Relative Risk (95% CI)* of All-Cause Mortality by PA in CRF Stratified Analysis and by CRF in PA Stratified Analysis

	Men CRF[†]		Women CRF[†]	
	Unfit	Fit	Unfit	Fit
Recommended PA (MET-minutes/week)				
No (0–499)	1.00 (referent)	1.00 (referent)	1.00 (referent)	1.00 (referent)
Yes (≥500)	0.90 (0.56 to 1.45)	0.96 (0.85 to 1.09)	0.85 (0.29 to 2.44)	0.92 (0.65 to 1.29)

	Men Recommended PA (MET-minutes/week)		Women Recommended PA (MET-minutes/week)	
	No (0–499)	Yes (≥500)	No (0–499)	Yes (≥500)
CRF[†]				
Unfit	1.00 (referent)	1.00 (referent)	1.00 (referent)	1.00 (referent)
Fit	0.61 (0.53 to 0.71)	0.64 (0.39 to 1.04)	0.63 (0.45 to 0.89)	0.49 (0.16 to 1.46)

CRF, cardiorespiratory fitness; MET, metabolic equivalent; PA, physical activity.
*Adjusted for age, examination year, body mass index, smoking status, hypertension, diabetes, hypercholesterolemia and parental cardiovascular disease.
†Unfit was defined as the least fit 20% and fit was defined as the most fit 80% based on maximal treadmill test time.

only can physical fitness be measured with greater precision than physical activity, but the treadmill endurance time also reflects the influences of inheritance, obesity, and various pathologies that could shorten life span.

R. J. Shephard, MD (Lond), PhD, DPE

References

1. Blair SN, Cheng Y, Holder JS. Is physical activity or physical fitness more important in defining health benefits? *Med Sci Sports Exerc.* 2001;33:S379-S399.
2. Walsh MC, Hunter GR, Sirikul B, Gower BA. Comparison of self-reported with objectively assessed energy expenditure in black and white women before and after weight loss. *Am J Clin Nutr.* 2004;79:1013-1019.
3. McMurray RG, Ainsworth BE, Harrell JS, Griggs TR, Williams OD. Is physical activity or aerobic power more influential on reducing cardiovascular disease risk factors? *Med Sci Sports Exerc.* 1998;30:1521-1529.
4. Lakka TA, Venäläinen JM, Rauramaa R, Salonen R, Tuomilehto J, Salonen JT. Relation of leisure-time physical activity and cardiorespiratory fitness to the risk of acute myocardial infarction. *N Engl J Med.* 1994;330:1549-1554.

Minimum amount of physical activity for reduced mortality and extended life expectancy: a prospective cohort study
Wen CP, Wai JPM, Tsai MK, et al (Natl Health Res Insts, Zhunan, Taiwan; Natl Taiwan Sport Univ, Taoyuan; et al)
Lancet 378:1244-1253, 2011

Background.—The health benefits of leisure-time physical activity are well known, but whether less exercise than the recommended 150 min a week can have life expectancy benefits is unclear. We assessed the health benefits of a range of volumes of physical activity in a Taiwanese population.

Methods.—In this prospective cohort study, 416175 individuals (199265 men and 216910 women) participated in a standard medical screening programme in Taiwan between 1996 and 2008, with an average follow-up of 8·05 years (SD 4·21). On the basis of the amount of weekly exercise indicated in a self-administered questionnaire, participants were placed into one of five categories of exercise volumes: inactive, or low, medium, high, or very high activity. We calculated hazard ratios (HR) for mortality risks for every group compared with the inactive group, and calculated life expectancy for every group.

Findings.—Compared with individuals in the inactive group, those in the low-volume activity group, who exercised for an average of 92 min per week (95% CI 71—112) or 15 min a day (SD 1·8), had a 14% reduced risk of all-cause mortality (0·86, 0·81—0·91), and had a 3 year longer life expectancy. Every additional 15 min of daily exercise beyond the minimum amount of 15 min a day further reduced all-cause mortality by 4% (95% CI 2·5—7·0) and all-cancer mortality by 1% (0·3—4·5). These benefits were applicable to all age groups and both sexes, and to those with cardiovascular disease risks. Individuals who were inactive had a 17% (HR 1·17, 95% CI

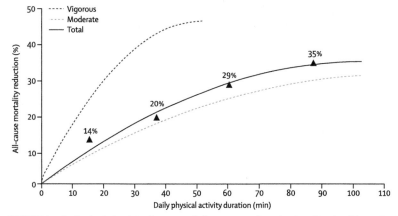

FIGURE 2.—Daily physical activity duration and all-cause mortality reduction. (Reprinted from Wen CP, Wai JPM, Tsai MK, et al. Minimum amount of physical activity for reduced mortality and extended life expectancy: a prospective cohort study. *Lancet.* 2011;378:1244-1253, Copyright 2011, with permission from Elsevier.)

1·10–1·24) increased risk of mortality compared with individuals in the low-volume group.

Interpretation.—15 min a day or 90 min a week of moderate-intensity exercise might be of benefit, even for individuals at risk of cardiovascular disease (Fig 2).

▶ In this large, prospective cohort, epidemiologic study, reductions in all-cause mortality as well as cancer, diabetes mellitus, and cardiovascular disease mortality, were reduced beginning at 15 min/d of physical activity. As shown in Fig 2, increasing activity duration and intensity were associated with even greater reductions in all-cause mortality. Compared with individuals in the inactive group, at age 30 years, life expectancy for individuals in the low-volume activity group was 2.6 years longer for men and 3.1 years longer for women. The 2008 Physical Activity Guidelines for Americans[1] concluded that 150 min/wk and more were needed for health and disease prevention. Picking an exact point on the physical activity continuum that reduces disease risk is a difficult academic task. A minimum physical activity threshold of 15 min/d is more acceptable for sedentary individuals and may result in a greater percentage of the population initiating and adhering to long-term lifestyle changes.

D. C. Nieman, DrPH

Reference

1. U.S. Department of Health and Human Services. *2008 Physical Activity Guidelines for Americans.* ODPHP; 2008. Publication No. U0036.

Depressive symptoms, physical inactivity and risk of cardiovascular mortality in older adults: the Cardiovascular Health Study
Win S, Parakh K, Eze-Nliam CM, et al (Johns Hopkins Univ School of Medicine, Baltimore, MD; et al)
Heart 97:500-505, 2011

Background.—Depressed older individuals have a higher mortality than older persons without depression. Depression is associated with physical inactivity, and low levels of physical activity have been shown in some cohorts to be a partial mediator of the relationship between depression and cardiovascular events and mortality.

Methods.—A cohort of 5888 individuals (mean 72.8 ± 5.6 years, 58% female, 16% African-American) from four US communities was followed for an average of 10.3 years. Self-reported depressive symptoms (10-item Center for Epidemiological Studies Depression Scale) were assessed annually and self-reported physical activity was assessed at baseline and at 3 and 7 years. To estimate how much of the increased risk of cardiovascular mortality associated with depressive symptoms was due to physical inactivity, Cox regression with time-varying covariates was used to determine the percentage change in the log HR of depressive symptoms for cardiovascular mortality after adding physical activity variables.

Results.—At baseline, 20% of participants scored above the cut-off for depressive symptoms. There were 2915 deaths (49.8%), of which 1176 (20.1%) were from cardiovascular causes. Depressive symptoms and physical inactivity each independently increased the risk of cardiovascular mortality and were strongly associated with each other (all p<0.001). Individuals with both depressive symptoms and physical inactivity had greater cardiovascular mortality than those with either individually (p<0.001, log rank test). Physical inactivity reduced the log HR of depressive symptoms for cardiovascular mortality by 26% after adjustment. This was similar for persons with (25%) and without (23%) established coronary heart disease.

Conclusions.—Physical inactivity accounted for a significant proportion of the risk of cardiovascular mortality due to depressive symptoms in older adults, regardless of coronary heart disease status (Fig 1).

▶ As summarized in Fig 1, high depression scores increased risk of cardiovascular mortality over a 10-year period by 67%, in concert with previous findings.[1] The major new finding of this study was that physical inactivity accounted for approximately 25% of the increased risk. These findings imply that depressed individuals can reduce their elevated risk of cardiovascular disease by becoming more physically active. In this study, individuals in the lowest physical activity group were more than 3 times as likely to have high depression scores as those in the most active group. The relationship between depression and physical inactivity is complex[2]: regular physical activity decreases the risk of depression,

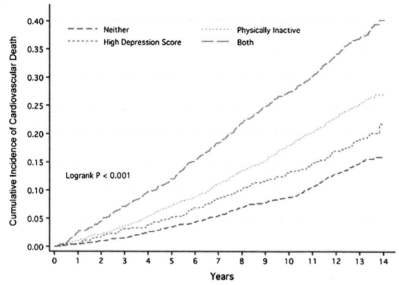

FIGURE 1.—Cumulative incidence of cardiovascular death according to depression score and physical activity status. Number of cardiovascular deaths 1176/5852 (20.1%). High depression score, Center for Epidemiological Studies Depression Score (CES-D) ≥8; physical inactivity, Physical Activity Score (PAS) ≤7. (Reprinted from Win S, Parakh K, Eze-Nliam CM, et al. Depressive symptoms, physical inactivity and risk of cardiovascular mortality in older adults: the Cardiovascular Health Study. *Heart.* 2011;97:500-505, Copyright 2011, with permission from the BMJ Publishing Group Ltd.)

whereas cessation of exercise increases the likelihood of depression. Depressed people tend to exercise less than those without depression.

D. C. Nieman, DrPH

References

1. Schulz R, Beach SR, Ives DG, et al. Association between depression and mortality in older adults: the Cardiovascular Health Study. *Arch Intern Med.* 2000;160: 1761-1768.
2. Wang JT, Hoffman B, Blumenthal JA. Management of depression in patients with coronary heart disease: association, mechanisms, and treatment implications for depressed cardiac patients. *Expert Opin Pharmacother.* 2011;12:85-98.

Impact of Body Mass Index, Physical Activity, and Other Clinical Factors on Cardiorespiratory Fitness (from the Cooper Center Longitudinal Study)
Lakoski SG, Barlow CE, Farrell SW, et al (Univ of Texas Southwestern Med School, Dallas; The Cooper Inst, Dallas, TX; et al)
Am J Cardiol 108:34-39, 2011

Cardiorespiratory fitness (CRF) is widely accepted as an important reversible cardiovascular risk factor. In the present study, we examined the non-modifiable and modifiable determinants of CRF within a large healthy

Caucasian population of men and women. The study included 20,239 patients presenting to Cooper Clinic (Dallas, Texas) for a comprehensive medical examination from 2000 through 2010. CRF was determined by maximal treadmill exercise testing. Physical activity categories were 0 metabolic equivalent tasks (METs)/min/week (no self-reported moderate or vigorous intensity physical activity), 1 to 449 METs/min/week (not meeting physical activity guideline), 450 to 749 METs/min/week (meeting guideline), and ≥750 METs/min/week (exceeding guideline). Linear regression modeling was used to determine the most robust clinical factors associated with achieved treadmill time. Age, gender, body mass index (BMI), and physical activity were the most important factors associated with CRF, explaining 56% of the variance ($R^2 = 0.56$). The addition of all other factors combined (current smoking, systolic blood pressure, blood glucose, high-density and low-density lipoprotein cholesterol, health status) were

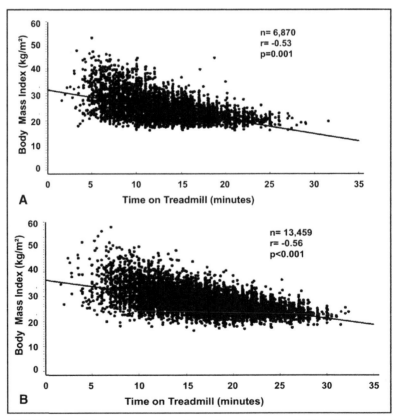

FIGURE 1.—Correlation between cardiorespiratory fitness (time on treadmill) and body mass index for Caucasian women (A) and men (B). (Reprinted from Lakoski SG, Barlow CE, Farrell SW, et al. Impact of body mass index, physical activity, and other clinical factors on cardiorespiratory fitness (from the Cooper center longitudinal study). *Am J Cardiol*. 2011;108:34-39, Copyright 2011, with permission from Elsevier.)

associated with CRF (p < 0.05) but additively only improved R^2 by 2%. There was a significant interaction between BMI and physical activity on CRF, such that normal-weight (BMI <25 kg/m^2) subjects achieved higher CRF for a given level of physical activity compared to obese subjects (BMI ≥30 kg/m^2). Percent body fat, not lean body mass, was the key factor driving this interaction. In conclusion, BMI was the most important clinical risk factor associated with CRF other than nonmodifiable risk factors age and gender. For a similar amount of physical activity, normal-weight subjects achieved a higher CRF level compared to obese subjects. These data suggest that obesity may offset the benefits of physical activity on achieved CRF, even in a healthy population of men and women (Fig 1).

▶ Age, gender, body mass index (BMI), and physical activity accounted for approximately 56% of the variance in cardiorespiratory fitness, and heritability probably accounted for the rest.[1] BMI was strongly related to cardiorespiratory fitness, such that women and men in the highest quintile had a mean BMI of 21.0 ± 2.1 and 25.3 ± 2.5 kg/m^2, respectively, whereas women and men in the lowest fitness quintile had a mean BMI of 27.5 ± 5.5 and 32.5 ± 5.7 kg/m^2, respectively. Thus, BMI was a key modifiable risk factor for fitness, and for each BMI unit increase, there was a decrease of 30 seconds on the treadmill (see Fig 1). Forty-two percent of subjects in the lowest fitness quintile reported not taking part in any form of organized physical activity compared with 6.9% of highly fit subjects.

D. C. Nieman, DrPH

Reference

1. Bouchard C, Daw EW, Rice T, et al. Familial resemblance for VO2max in the sedentary state: the HERITAGE family study. *Med Sci Sports Exerc.* 1998;30: 252-258.

Impact of an Active Video Game on Healthy Children's Physical Activity
Baranowski T, Abdelsamad D, Baranowski J, et al (Baylor College of Medicine, Houston, TX; et al)
Pediatrics 129:e636-e642, 2012

Objective.—This naturalistic study tests whether children receiving a new (to them) active video game spontaneously engage in more physical activity than those receiving an inactive video game, and whether the effect would be greater among children in unsafe neighborhoods, who might not be allowed to play outside.

Methods.—Participants were children 9 to 12 years of age, with a BMI >50th percentile, but <99th percentile; none of these children had a medical condition that would preclude physical activity or playing video games. A randomized clinical trial assigned children to receiving 2 active or 2 inactive video games, the peripherals necessary to run the games, and a Wii console. Physical activity was monitored by using accelerometers for 5 weeks over the course of a 13-week experiment. Neighborhood safety was assessed with a 12 item validated questionnaire.

Results.—There was no evidence that children receiving the active video games were more active in general, or at anytime, than children receiving the inactive video games. The outcomes were not moderated by parent perceived neighborhood safety, child BMI z score, or other demographic characteristics.

Conclusions.—These results provide no reason to believe that simply acquiring an active video game under naturalistic circumstances provides a public health benefit to children.

▶ This was a very timely and interesting article. The current generation of children and youth spend about 2 hours per day, on average, playing video games. So-called active video games, such as some of the sports games that are available on the Wii (eg, Dance Dance Revolution, EA Sports Active), have been advocated as an alternative to sedentary video games as a means of increasing physical activity levels. While the positive influence of such video games on energy expenditure has been studied and documented in tightly controlled laboratory settings, the impact they have on total physical activity outside the laboratory in a child's natural environment has not been studied.

The key finding of this study is that children who receive active video games do not increase their light or moderate-to-vigorous-intensity physical activity (MVPA) levels. In fact, in this study, the group of 41 children who received active video games as their intervention had an average MVPA of 27.4 min/d at baseline, and this MVPA level did not vary by more than 2 min/d throughout the 13-week intervention. Thus, based on these findings, there is no reason to believe that children who play active video games will have a better health profile than children who play more traditional sedentary video games. Sorry parents, sorry kids! Wii tennis, Wii snowboarding, Wii golf, and other such games are not a replacement for the real thing.

I. Janssen, PhD

Only lower limb controlled interactive computer gaming enables an effective increase in energy expenditure
Jordan M, Donne B, Fletcher D (Trinity College, Dublin, Ireland)
Eur J Appl Physiol 111:1465-1472, 2011

Limited research documents if new and existing interactive computer gaming "exergaming" increase energy expenditure and cardio-respiratory costs comparable to common exercise modalities. To address this, healthy male volunteers ($n = 15$) completed six by 12-min test elements: PlayStation2 (PS2$_{hand}$), Nintendo Wii boxing, walk at 5.6 km h^{-1}, cycle at 120 W, playing an adapted lower limb controlled PS2 (PS2$_{limb}$) and run at 9.6 km h^{-1}. In addition, they played PS2$_{limb}$ for 30 min and performed

TABLE 3.—Mean (SD) Percent of HR_{max} and VO_2peak During Sub-Maximal Exercise

	$PS2_{hand}$	Wii Boxing	Walk (5.6 km h^{-1})	Cycle (120 W)	$PS2_{limb}$	Run (9.6 km h^{-1})
%HR_{max}	36.7 (5.0)	65.5 (10.1)	52.7 (7.1)	71.8 (5.9)	71.5 (9.3)	85.4 (7.7)
%VO_2peak	8.5 (1.9)	41.0 (10.3)	33.8 (1.6)	52.1 (7.0)	55.9 (7.3)	73.6 (7.4)

an incremental treadmill test to exhaustion. Data were analysed using repeated measures ANOVA with post hoc Tukey tests, $P < 0.05$ inferred significance. $PS2_{limb}$ increased energy expenditure (EE) and post-exercise blood lactate (BLa) significantly higher ($P < 0.001$) than $PS2_{hand}$, Wii gaming or walking at 5.6 km h^{-1} (EE: 30.3 ± 4.9 vs. 4.7 ± 1.1, 22.0 ± 6.1 and 17.9 ± 1.9 kJ h^{-1} kg^{-1}; BLa: 2.4 ± 1.5 vs. 1.0 ± 0.3, 1.8 ± 0.8 and 0.9 ± 0.2 mmol L^{-1}), playing the $PS2_{limb}$ raised mean EE over six times greater than $PS2_{hand}$. Mean fat and carbohydrate oxidation rates during the 9- to 12-min period playing the $PS2_{limb}$ were five and ten times greater than $PS2_{hand}$ (0.25 ± 0.10 vs. 0.05 ± 0.10, 1.69 ± 0.52 vs. 0.15 ± 0.14 g min^{-1}, respectively). $PS2_{limb}$ met ACSM guidelines for cardiovascular fitness; however, current Wii technology failed. In conclusion, gaming interactive technology must be adapted or designed to include the lower limbs in order to provide a significant exercise stimulus (Table 3).

▶ There is growing recognition of an association between hours of computer use per week and ill health, and there has thus been interest in the development of computer games that require a significant physical response from the children using them (for example, dance mats and Nintendo Wii), but there has been little evaluation of the effectiveness of "exergaming" devices.[1] Although there is some increase of energy expenditure relative to entirely sedentary games,[2,3] it is far from clear whether this reaches the level needed to protect the health of children and adolescents.[4] The report of Jordan and associates examines the metabolic response to a PlayStation 2 device modified to require extensive use of the lower limbs. In contrast to other alternatives, this device brought the heart rate to 71.5% of its maximal value, with an oxygen consumption of some 7 METs, at 56% of the subjects' directly measured peak values (Table 3). These observations are encouraging, and suggest that computer games can be adapted to provide aerobic training and reduce body fat.

R. J. Shephard, MD (Lond), PhD, DPE

References

1. Daley AJ. Can exergaming contribute to improving physical activity levels and health outcomes in children? *Pediatrics.* 2009;124:763-771.
2. Graf DL, Pratt LV, Hester CN, Short KR. Playing active video games increases energy expenditure in children. *Pediatrics.* 2009;124:534-540.
3. Graves L, Stratton G, Ridgers ND, Cable NT. Energy expenditure in adolescents playing new generation computer games. *Br J Sports Med.* 2008;42:592-594.
4. Janssen I. Physical activity guidelines for children and youth. *Appl Physiol Nutr Metab.* 2007;32:S109-S121.

Sufficient Sleep, Physical Activity, and Sedentary Behaviors

Foti KE, Eaton DK, Lowry R, et al (Natl Ctr for Chronic Disease Prevention and Health Promotion, CDC, Atlanta, GA)

Am J Prev Med 41:596-602, 2011

Background.—Insufficient sleep among adolescents is common and has adverse health and behavior consequences. Understanding associations of physical activity and sedentary behaviors with sleep duration could shed light on ways to promote sufficient sleep.

Purpose.—The purpose of this study is to determine whether physical activity and sedentary behaviors are associated with sufficient sleep (8 or more hours of sleep on an average school night) among U.S. high school students.

Methods.—Data were from the 2009 national Youth Risk Behavior Survey and are representative of 9th–12th-grade students nationally ($n=14{,}782$). Associations of physical activity and sedentary behaviors with sufficient sleep were determined using logistic regression models controlling for confounders. Data were analyzed in October 2010.

Results.—Students who engaged in ≥60 minutes of physical activity daily during the 7 days before the survey had higher odds of sufficient sleep than those who did not engage in ≥60 minutes on any day. There was no association between the number of days students were vigorously active ≥20 minutes and sufficient sleep. Compared to their respective referent groups of 0 hours on an average school day, students who watched TV ≥4 hours/day had higher odds of sufficient sleep and students who played video or computer games or used a computer for something that was not school work ≥2 hours/day had lower odds of sufficient sleep.

Conclusions.—Daily physical activity for ≥60 minutes and limited computer use are associated with sufficient sleep among adolescents (Table 2).

▶ Lack of sleep is a common problem among teenagers, with one-third of US adolescents getting less than 5 hours of sleep per night.[1] The questionnaire-based analysis of Foti and associates appears to show a modest association (Table 2) between 60 minutes of vigorous physical activity 7 days of the week and an arbitrary assessment of adequate sleep (>8 hours per night) in a large sample of US students (n = 14 782) from grades 9 through 12. The large sample size allowed statistical adjustment of data for other risk factors linked to poor sleep patterns, and, for some reason not clearly explained by the authors, this removed much of the relationship between sleep and physical activity. Nevertheless, their analysis reinforces earlier small-scale studies suggesting that regular physical activity is related to both the volume and the quality of sleep in teenagers[2-7]; whether this is due to the activity itself or to a better-regulated lifestyle is less clear. Two important issues not addressed by the present study were the timing of physical activity (late-night physical activity could have an arousing effect) and possible lengthy travel for those involved in team sports.

R. J. Shephard, MD (Lond), PhD, DPE

TABLE 2.—Odds of Sufficient Sleep[a] by Physical Activity or Sedentary Behavior Category

	OR (95% CI)	AOR (95% CI)
Physical activity for ≥60 minutes (days during the past 7 days)		
0	ref	ref[b]
1	0.97 (0.78, 1.21)	0.92 (0.72, 1.17)
2	1.00 (0.87, 1.16)	0.95 (0.82, 1.10)
3	1.06 (0.88, 1.27)	0.93 (0.75, 1.14)
4	1.31 (1.09, 1.58)*	1.08 (0.85, 1.37)
5	1.26 (1.05, 1.51)*	0.99 (0.78, 1.25)
6	1.33 (1.10, 1.59)*	1.00 (0.81, 1.23)
7	1.67 (1.46, 1.91)*	1.24 (1.01, 1.51)*
Vigorous physical activity ≥20 minutes (days during the past 7 days)		
0	ref	ref[c]
1	0.95 (0.79, 1.14)	0.90 (0.72, 1.13)
2	0.85 (0.63, 1.15)	0.76 (0.53, 1.08)
3	1.00 (0.77, 1.29)	0.91 (0.68, 1.21)
4	1.07 (0.89, 1.29)	0.95 (0.78, 1.15)
5	1.25 (1.03, 1.53)*	1.05 (0.83, 1.33)
6	1.29 (1.04, 1.62)*	0.93 (0.71, 1.21)
7	1.61 (1.37, 1.89)*	1.10 (0.90, 1.34)
Watched TV (hours/day on an average school day)		
0	ref	ref[d]
<1	1.02 (0.90, 1.17)	0.92 (0.78, 1.09)
1	1.25 (1.00, 1.58)	1.16 (0.95, 1.41)
2	1.16 (0.97, 1.40)	1.12 (0.93, 1.34)
3	1.20 (0.99, 1.46)	1.22 (0.97, 1.53)
4	1.19 (0.95, 1.49)	1.25 (1.00, 1.55)*
≥5	1.15 (0.92, 1.44)	1.31 (1.00, 1.72)*
Used computers (hours/day on an average school day)		
0	ref	ref[e]
<1	1.00 (0.84, 1.20)	0.93 (0.74, 1.17)
1	1.06 (0.87, 1.30)	0.96 (0.77, 1.21)
2	0.85 (0.71, 1.02)	0.78 (0.64, 0.95)*
3	0.62 (0.50, 0.77)*	0.55 (0.42, 0.72)*
4	0.71 (0.58, 0.88)*	0.69 (0.56, 0.86)*
≥5	0.74 (0.63, 0.88)*	0.67 (0.54, 0.83)*

*$p<0.05$.

[a]Sufficient sleep is defined as ≥8 hours of sleep per night on an average school night.

[b]Controlling for: gender, race/ethnicity, grade, academic grades, being in a physical fight, feeling sad or hopeless, eating fruits and vegetables five or more times per day, drinking soda or pop at least one time per day, engaging in ≥20 minutes of vigorous physical activity per day on ≥3 days/week, using a computer ≥3 hours per day.

[c]Controlling for: gender, race/ethnicity, grade, academic grades, being in a physical fight, feeling sad or hopeless, current cigarette use, eating fruits and vegetables five or more times per day, drinking soda or pop at least one time per day, ≥60 minutes of physical activity per day on all 7 days/week, using a computer ≥3 hours per day.

[d]Controlling for: gender, race/ethnicity, grade, academic grades, being in a physical fight, current marijuana use, currently sexually active, drinking soda or pop at least one time per day, ≥60 minutes of physical activity per day on all 7 days/week, engaging in ≥20 minutes of vigorous physical activity per day on ≥3 days/week, using a computer ≥3 hours per day.

[e]Controlling for: gender, race/ethnicity, grade, academic grades, being in a physical fight, feeling sad or hopeless, drinking soda or pop at least one time per day, ≥60 minutes of physical activity per day on all 7 days/week, engaging in ≥20 minutes of vigorous physical activity per day on ≥3 days/week.

References

1. Eaton DK, McKnight-Eily LR, Lowry R, Perry GS, Presley-Cantrell L, Croft JB. Prevalence of insufficient, borderline, and optimal hours of sleep among high school students — United States, 2007. *J Adolesc Health*. 2010;46:399-401.

2. Chen MY, Wang EK, Jeng YJ. Adequate sleep among adolescents is positively associated with health status and health-related behaviors. *BMC Public Health*. 2006; 6:59.

3. Liu X, Uchiyama M, Okawa M, Kurita H. Prevalence and correlates of self-reported sleep problems among Chinese adolescents. *Sleep*. 2000;23:27-34.
4. Nelson MC, Gordon-Larsen P. Physical activity and sedentary behavior patterns are associated with selected adolescent health risk behaviors. *Pediatrics*. 2006; 117:1281-1290.
5. Dworak M, Wiater A, Alfer D, Stephan E, Hollmann W, Strüder HK. Increased slow wave sleep and reduced stage 2 sleep in children depending on exercise intensity. *Sleep Med*. 2008;9:266-272.
6. Brand S, Gerber M, Beck J, Hatzinger M, Pühse U, Holsboer-Trachsler E. High exercise levels are related to favorable sleep patterns and psychological functioning in adolescents: a comparison of athletes and controls. *J Adolesc Health*. 2010;46: 133-141.
7. Delisle TT, Werch CE, Wong AH, Bian H, Weiler R. Relationship between frequency and intensity of physical activity and health behaviors of adolescents. *J Sch Health*. 2010;80:134-140.

US Adolescent Nutrition, Exercise, and Screen Time Baseline Levels Prior to National Recommendations
Foltz JL, Cook SR, Szilagyi PG, et al (Univ of Rochester School of Medicine and Dentistry, NY)
Clin Pediatr (Phila) 50:424-433, 2011

Experts have recommended daily obesity prevention goals: ≥5 fruits/vegetables, <2 hours of screen time, >1 hour of physical activity, and no sugar-sweetened beverages (5-2-1-0). The authors analyzed National Health and Nutrition Examination Survey data for 1999-2002 to determine the proportion of US adolescents (12-19 years) who would have met each goal prior to dissemination of the 5-2-1-0 recommendations. Merely 0.4% would have met all goals; 41% would have met none. Only 9% consumed ≥5 fruits/vegetables, 27% reported <2 hours of screen time, 32% had >1 hour of physical activity, and 14% consumed no sugar-sweetened beverages per day. Demographic subgroups (eg, racial/ethnic minority and lower income) would have been even farther from meeting the goals. Clinicians are likely to encounter adolescents with nutrition, exercise, and screen time behaviors that are far from 5-2-1-0 goals, and can use these guidelines during clinical encounters to counsel adolescents regarding healthier lifestyles (Fig 2).

▶ Obesity rates among adolescents have risen strongly during the past several decades, with a current prevalence of 17%. The 5-2-1-0 guidelines investigated in this study are lofty: 5 or more servings per day of fruits and vegetables, less than 2 hours per day of screen time (television, computer, video games), at least 1 hour per day of physical activity (moderate or vigorous, including walking and sport play), and avoidance of all sugar-sweetened beverages. The majority of adolescents in the National Health and Nutrition Examination Survey database missed each 5-2-1-0 goal by a substantial amount (Fig 2). Nutritional behaviors were especially dismal, with close to half of all adolescents consuming 1 or less serving of fruits and vegetables daily and half consuming more than 3

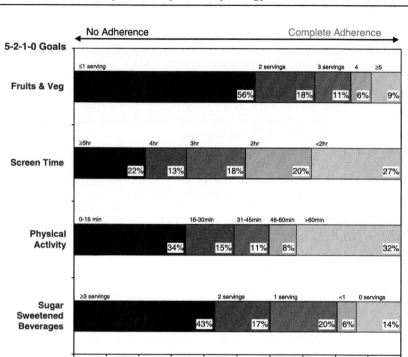

FIGURE 2.—Percentage of US adolescents who would have met each 5-2-1-0 goal in 1999-2002. Each bar represents one of the 5-2-1-0 goals; the degree of meeting the goal is listed above each bar segment. On the bottom is percentage of youth who adhered to or deviated from each goal; the corresponding numerical values are found imbedded in the bar segments. The right segment shows those who fully met the goal; left those who deviated most (eg, 56% ate ≤1 serving of fruits and vegetables, 9% ate ≥5). (Reprinted from Foltz JL, Cook SR, Szilagyi PG, et al. US adolescent nutrition, exercise, and screen time baseline levels prior to national recommendations. *Clin Pediatr (Phila)*. 2011;50:424-433, with permission from The Author(s)).

servings of sugar-sweetened beverages. Nearly one-fourth of adolescents had more than 5 hours of screen time daily (mean of 2.8 hours), and one-third reported only 0 to 15 minutes of daily physical activity. These are alarming data, and, unless schools and families band together with government officials to turn this around, obesity rates will continue to soar among US teenagers.

D. C. Nieman, DrPH

Sedentary Activity Associated With Metabolic Syndrome Independent of Physical Activity

Bankoski A, Harris TB, McClain JJ, et al (Natl Inst on Aging, Bethesda, MD; Natl Cancer Inst, Bethesda, MD; et al)
Diabetes Care 34:497-503, 2011

Objective.—This study examined the association between objectively measured sedentary activity and metabolic syndrome among older adults.

Research Design and Methods.—Data were from 1,367 men and women, aged ≥60 years who participated in the 2003–2006 National Health and Nutrition Examination Survey (NHANES). Sedentary time during waking hours was measured by an accelerometer (<100 counts per minute). A sedentary bout was defined as a period of time >5 min. A sedentary break was defined as an interruption in sedentary time (≥100 counts per minute). Metabolic syndrome was defined according to the Adult Treatment Panel (ATP) III criteria.

Results.—On average, people spent 9.5 h (65% of wear time) as sedentary. Compared with people without metabolic syndrome, people with metabolic syndrome spent a greater percentage of time as sedentary (67.3 vs. 62.2%), had longer average sedentary bouts (17.7 vs. 16.7 min), had lower intensity during sedentary time (14.8 vs. 15.8 average counts per minute), and had fewer sedentary breaks (82.3 vs. 86.7), adjusted for age and sex (all $P < 0.01$). A higher percentage of time sedentary and fewer sedentary breaks were associated with a significantly greater likelihood of metabolic syndrome after adjustment for age, sex, ethnicity, education, alcohol consumption, smoking, BMI, diabetes, heart disease, and physical activity. The association between intensity during sedentary time and metabolic syndrome was borderline significant.

Conclusions.—The proportion of sedentary time was strongly related to metabolic risk, independent of physical activity. Current results suggest older people may benefit from reducing total sedentary time and avoiding prolonged periods of sedentary time by increasing the number of breaks during sedentary time.

▶ Including exercise bouts within the daily schedule is not enough.[1] As supported by this study, reducing time spent in sedentary pursuits is also needed to lower the likelihood of the metabolic syndrome. This study used a large National Health and Nutrition Examination Survey database and showed that older people with metabolic syndrome spent more hours and a greater percentage of their time in sedentary pursuits without breaks. To reduce sedentary behavior, individuals can insert brief activity breaks to disrupt prolonged periods of sitting or by increasing movements while sitting.

D. C. Nieman, DrPH

Reference

1. Proper KI, Singh AS, van Mechelen W, Chinapaw MJ. Sedentary behaviors and health outcomes among adults: a systematic review of prospective studies. *Am J Prev Med.* 2011;40:174-182.

Physical activity levels, ownership of goods promoting sedentary behaviour and risk of myocardial infarction: results of the INTERHEART study

Held C, Iqbal R, Lear SA, et al (Uppsala Univ, Sweden; Aga Khan Univ, Pakistan; Simon Fraser Univ, Vancouver, British Columbia, Canada; et al)

Eur Heart J 2012 [Epub ahead of print]

Aims.—To evaluate the association between occupational and leisure-time physical activity (PA), ownership of goods promoting sedentary behaviour, and the risk of myocardial infarction (MI) in different socio-economic populations of the world. Studies in developed countries have found low PA as a risk factor for cardiovascular disease; however, the protective effect of occupational PA is less certain. Moreover, ownership of goods promoting sedentary behaviour may be associated with an increased risk.

Methods.—In INTERHEART, a case—control study of 10 043 cases of first MI and 14 217 controls who did not report previous angina or physical disability completed a questionnaire on work and leisure-time PA.

Results.—Subjects whose occupation involved either light [multivariable-adjusted odds ratio (OR) 0.78, confidence interval (CI) 0.71—0.86] or moderate (OR 0.89, CI 0.80—0.99) PA were at a lower risk of MI, whereas those who did heavy physical labour were not (OR 1.02, CI 0.88—1.19), compared with sedentary subjects. Mild exercise (OR 0.87, CI 0.81—0.93) as well as moderate or strenuous exercise (OR 0.76, CI 0.69—0.82) was protective. The effect of PA was observed across countries with low, middle, and high income. Subjects who owned both a car and a television (TV) (multivariable adjusted OR 1.27, CI 1.05—1.54) were at higher risk of MI compared with those who owned neither.

Conclusion.—Leisure-time PA and mild-to-moderate occupational PA, but not heavy physical labour, were associated with a reduced risk, while ownership of a car and TV was associated with an increased risk of MI across all economic regions (Table 8).

▶ Public health agencies have long fretted over the minimum amount of physical activity needed to reduce the risk of heart attacks and other manifestations of chronic ill health. Recommendations have changed periodically, with consequent adverse effects on credibility of their message. Currently, the consensus seems to recommend 30 minutes of moderate-intensity physical activity on most days of the week[1]; this verdict seems to have been reached by poring over the statistics of various epidemiologists, apparently with little recognition of the problem that the minimum dose yielding a statistically significant benefit depends upon the observer's accuracy in measuring patterns of physical activity, the nature and size of the sample examined, and the statistician's ability to allow for other confounding variables. I have long operated from a rather different philosophy. In my judgment, any physical activity is better than none, and as long as the intensity remains moderate, more is probably better than less; my personal daily dose is 60 to 90 minutes. The paper of Held and associates, based on data from 52 countries, certainly seems to strike at the heart of the

TABLE 8.—Association Between the Duration of Leisure-Time Physical Activity
and the Risk of MI

Duration of Leisure-Time Activity	OR Model[a]	OR Model[b]	OR Model[c]
No activity	1.00	1.00	1.00
>0–30 min/week	0.79 (0.60–1.06)	0.91 (0.67–1.24)	0.92 (0.67–1.28)
>30–60 min/week	0.60 (0.50–0.72)	0.69 (0.57–0.84)	0.72 (0.59–0.90)
>60–150 min/week	0.59 (0.51–0.68)	0.73 (0.63–0.85)	0.78 (0.67–0.91)
>150–210 min/week	0.61 (0.52–0.72)	0.75 (0.63–0.89)	0.75 (0.62–0.91)
>210 min/week	0.56 (0.51–0.62)	0.66 (0.60–0.73)	0.71 (0.63–0.79)

[a]Model adjusted for age, sex, and country level income.
[b]Model adjusted for age, sex, country level income, smoking status, alcohol, education, and WHR.
[c]Model adjusted for age, sex, country level income, smoking status, alcohol intake, education, household income, WHR, hypertension, diabetes, psychosocial factors, fruit intake, and vegetable intake.

current public health recommendation, with the suggestion of benefit from only 30 to 60 minutes of exercise per week (Table 8) and no added advantage from a greater weekly dosage of exercise. This assessment was based on a simple yes/no response to the question "Do you play sports or exercise during your leisure time?" Those giving a positive response were asked to indicate the number of minutes of physical activity per week and the number of months per year when they were active (with the results presented as minutes of activity per week, averaged over the year). Possibly, the simplicity of the question, uncertainty about what constituted sport or exercise, and the difficulty in eliciting consistent responses across many nations may have obscured the dose-response relationship that others have reported.[2] However, the data add weight to the view that there is some health benefit in even small amounts of exercise,[3] and this should certainly be a part of any more definitive public health recommendation.

R. J. Shephard, MD (Lond), PhD, DPE

References

1. Haskell WL, Lee IM, Pate RR, et al. Physical activity and public health: updated recommendation for adults from the American College of Sports Medicine and the American Heart Association. *Circulation.* 2007;116:1081-1093.
2. Lee IM, Sesso HD, Paffenbarger RS Jr. Physical activity and coronary heart disease risk in men: does the duration of exercise episodes predict risk? *Circulation.* 2000; 102:981-986.
3. Lovasi GS, Lemaitre RN, Siscovick DS, et al. Amount of leisure-time physical activity and risk of nonfatal myocardial infarction. *Ann Epidemiol.* 2007;17:410-416.

Body Mass Index and Physical Activity in Relation to the Incidence of Hip Fracture in Postmenopausal Women

Armstrong MEG, Valerie Beral for the Million Women Study Collaborators
(Univ of Oxford, UK; et al)
J Bone Miner Res 26:1330-1338, 2011

Hip fracture risk is known to increase with physical inactivity and decrease with obesity, but there is little information on their combined effects. We report on the separate and combined effects of body mass index (BMI) and physical activity on hospital admissions for hip fracture among postmenopausal women in a large prospective UK study. Baseline information on body size, physical activity, and other relevant factors was collected in 1996−2001, and participants were followed for incident hip fractures by record linkage to National Health Service (NHS) hospital admission data. Cox regression was used to calculate adjusted relative risks of hip fracture. Among 925,345 postmenopausal women followed for an average of 6.2 years, 2582 were admitted to hospital with an incident hip fracture. Hip fracture risk increased with decreasing BMI: Compared with obese women (BMI of 30+ kg/m^2), relative risks were 1.71 [95% confidence interval (CI) 1.47−1.97)] for BMI of 25.0 to 29.9 kg/m^2 and 2.55 (95% CI 2.22−2.94) for BMI of 20.0 to 24.9 kg/m^2. The increase in fracture risk per unit decrease in BMI was significantly greater among lean women than among overweight women ($p < .001$). For women in every category of BMI, physical inactivity was associated with an increased risk of hip fracture. There was no significant interaction between the relative effects of BMI and physical activity. For women who reported that they took any exercise versus no exercise, the adjusted relative risk of hip fracture was 0.68 (95% CI 0.62−0.75), with similar results for strenuous exercise. In this large cohort of postmenopausal women, BMI and physical activity had independent effects on hip fracture risk (Fig 4).

▶ In this 6.2-year study of almost a million postmenopausal women, hip fracture risk decreased with increasing body mass index (BMI) and was greater in

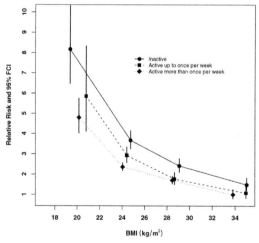

FIGURE 4.—Relative risk of hip fracture in postmenopausal women by frequency of any physical activity and BMI. Relative risks, adjusted for age, region, socioeconomic status, smoking, alcohol consumption, parity, use of HRT, height, heart disease/thrombosis, diabetes mellitus, thyroid disease, and rheumatoid arthritis/osteoarthritis. Relative risks are plotted against the mean measured BMI in each category. (Reprinted from Armstrong MEG, Valerie Beral for the Million Women Study Collaborators. Body mass index and physical activity in relation to the incidence of hip fracture in postmenopausal women. *J Bone Miner Res.* 2011;26:1330-1338, with permission from American Society for Bone and Mineral Research.)

inactive than active women (Fig 4). Women who reported participating in any or in strenuous exercise had a 30% reduction in fracture risk compared with women who exercised rarely or never. Physically active women had lower risks of hip fracture than inactive women at every level of BMI (Fig 4). Obesity protects against hip fractures[1] and is attributed to higher levels of bone mineral density from increased chronic strain on the bones, an increased production of estrogens from larger stores of adipose tissue, or a reduced impact from falls because of a greater cushioning by subcutaneous adipose tissue.

D. C. Nieman, DrPH

Reference

1. De Laet C, Kanis JA, Odén A, et al. Body mass index as a predictor of fracture risk: a meta-analysis. *Osteoporos Int.* 2005;16:1330-1338.

A new VO$_{2max}$ protocol allowing self-pacing in maximal incremental exercise
Mauger AR, Sculthorpe N (Univ of Bedfordshire, UK)
Br J Sports Med 46:59-63, 2012

Introduction.—The traditional maximal oxygen uptake (VO$_{2max}$) protocol has received criticism for being an unnatural form of exercise, lacking ecological validity and producing different VO$_{2max}$ responses depending on protocol duration and work rate increments.

Purpose.—The purpose of this investigation was to design and test a new VO$_{2max}$ protocol allowing subjects to self-pace their work rate while maintaining an incremental test structure.

Methods.—16 untrained subjects completed a self-paced VO$_{2max}$ protocol (SPV) and a traditional VO$_{2max}$ test in a counter-balanced, crossover design. The SPV used incremental 'clamps' of ratings of perceived exertion (RPE) over 5×2-min stages (10-min duration) while allowing subjects to vary their power output (PO) according to the required RPE.

Results.—Subjects achieved significantly higher ($p < 0.05$) VO$_{2max}$ values (40 ± 10 ml/kg/min vs 37 ± 8 ml/kg/min) and peak POs (273 ± 58 W vs 238 ± 55 W) in the SPV. Higher VO$_{2max}$ values were observed in the SPV even when a plateau (VO$_2$—time slope <0.05 l/min) occurred in the traditional test. No differences were found between any other measured physiological variable (minute ventilation, heart rate and respiratory exchange ratio).

Conclusions.—As SPV is a closed-loop test (10-min duration) that allows subjects to self-pace their work rate, it disregards the need for experimenters to estimate starting work rates, stage lengths and increments in order to bring about volitional exhaustion in 8—10 min. The observation that the SPV may also elicit higher VO$_{2max}$ values than a traditional test

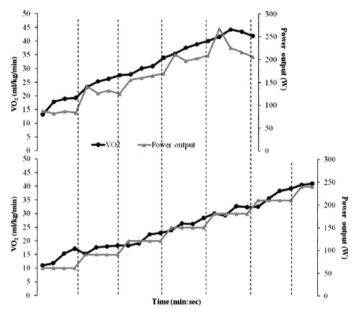

FIGURE 2.—VO_2 and power output data for the self-paced protocol and traditional protocol in a representative subject. A VO_2 plateau is observed in both occasions, yet a higher VO_{2max} is achieved in the self-paced test. A higher peak power output is also achieved in the self-paced test during the final stage (RPE 20). The plateau in both tests occurs in the presence of either a plateau or fall in power output, which in the SPV may be an anticipatory pacing response. (Reprinted from Mauger AR, Sculthorpe N. A new VO_{2max} protocol allowing self-pacing in maximal incremental exercise. *Br J Sports Med.* 2012;46:59-63, Copyright 2012, with permission from BMJ Publishing Group Ltd.)

warrants further research in this area and its consideration as standard measure to elicit VO_{2max} (Fig 2).

▶ It has been common practice in many types of exercise test, such as measurements of maximal muscle force or maximal oxygen intake, to encourage subjects by shouting at them and sometimes even bullying them. Mauger and Sculthorpe here make the intriguing suggestion that a greater effort can be achieved if the subject is allowed to reach his or her maximum effort without intervention from the observer, self-pacing increments of intensity using a series of five 2-minute gradations in the rating of perceived effort (RPE), 11, 13, 15, 17, and 20 on Borg's scale. Their justification for trying this approach was that previous observations had demonstrated that exercising at a fixed RPE offered less of a physiological challenge than exercising at a fixed power output.[1] They further reasoned that this would introduce a role for the brain, countering one criticism of the traditional maximal oxygen intake test previously advanced by Noakes.[2] The comparison of the traditional and the self-regulated test was made on a cycle ergometer, using a sample of 16 untrained 22-year-old subjects. The supposedly traditional test was around 13 minutes in duration, an adverse factor for achieving maximal effort,[3] and contrary to Instituting Best Practices/World Health Organization (IBP/WHO) recommendations.[4] It adopted a ramp protocol (30-W increments) beginning at an undesirably low intensity of effort (60 W). Moreover, the final heart rates (187/min for the self-paced test and 190/min for the traditional test) suggest that both tests may have achieved peak rather than true maximal values. Higher peak oxygen intakes were observed with the self-paced test; however, this seems partly because the self-paced test began substantially nearer to the subject's maximal value and reached peak effort more rapidly (Fig 2). Before dismissing the "brainless" traditional test of maximal aerobic power, it would be interesting to make a further comparison, using trained subjects and using as the basis of comparison the recommended IBP/WHO protocol, with subjects beginning a progressive test at 80% to 90% of their supposed maximal effort.

R. J. Shephard, MD (Lond), PhD, DPE

References

1. Lander PJ, Butterly RJ, Edwards AM. Self-paced exercise is less physically challenging than enforced constant pace exercise of the same intensity: influence of complex central metabolic control. *Br J Sports Med.* 2009;43:789-795.
2. Noakes TD. Testing for maximum oxygen consumption has produced a brainless model of human exercise performance. *Br J Sports Med.* 2008;42:551-555.
3. Yoon BK, Kravitz L, Robergs R. VO2max, protocol duration, and the VO2 plateau. *Med Sci Sports Exerc.* 2007;39:1186-1192.
4. Shephard RJ, Allen C, Benade AJ, et al. The maximum oxygen intake. An international reference standard of cardiorespiratory fitness. *Bull World Health Organ.* 1968;38:757-764.

Validity of the 6 min walk test in prediction of the anaerobic threshold before major non-cardiac surgery
Sinclair RCF, Batterham AM, Davies S, et al (The James Cook Univ Hosp, Middlesbrough, UK; Teesside Univ, Middlesbrough, UK)
Br J Anaesth 108:30-35, 2012

Background.—For perioperative risk stratification, a robust, practical test could be used where cardiopulmonary exercise testing (CPET) is unavailable. The aim of this study was to assess the utility of the 6 min walk test (6MWT) distance to discriminate between low and high anaerobic threshold (AT) in patients awaiting major non-cardiac surgery.

Methods.—In 110 participants, we obtained oxygen consumption at the AT from CPET and recorded the distance walked (in m) during a 6MWT. Receiver operating characteristic (ROC) curve analysis was used to derive two different cut-points for 6MWT distance in predicting an AT of <11 ml O_2 kg^{-1} min^{-1}; one using the highest sum of sensitivity and specificity (conventional method) and the other adopting a 2:1 weighting in favour of sensitivity. In addition, using a novel linear regression-based technique, we obtained lower and upper cut-points for 6MWT distance that are predictive of an AT that is likely to be ($P \geq 0.75$) <11 or >11 ml O_2 kg^{-1} min^{-1}.

Results.—The ROC curve analysis revealed an area under the curve of 0.85 (95 confidence interval, 0.77−0.91). The optimum cut-points were

<440 m (conventional method) and <502 m (sensitivity-weighted approach). The regression-based lower and upper 6MWT distance cut-points were <427 and >563 m, respectively.

Conclusions.—Patients walking >563 m in the 6MWT do not routinely require CPET; those walking <427 m should be referred for further evaluation. In situations of 'clinical uncertainty' (≥427 but ≤563 m), the number of clinical risk factors and magnitude of surgery should be incorporated into the decision-making process. The 6MWT is a useful clinical tool to screen and risk stratify patients in departments where CPET is unavailable (Fig 1).

▶ Health care in most countries is now reaching the point where it consumes an unsustainable proportion of the gross national product, and one factor contributing to this escalation in expenditures is an ever-increasing reliance of the physician on expensive laboratory tests. One such expense is the laboratory testing of cardiorespiratory performance before surgery; this is commonly regarded as an important component of risk stratification,[1-5] with anaerobic thresholds of 11 and 8 mL/[kg/min] serving to identify high- and very high-risk patients. One simpler alternative is to measure the distance the patient can walk at his or her chosen maximal pace in 6 minutes. The speed of walking bears a moderate relationship to a person's cardiorespiratory status, although it has been questioned whether its accuracy is sufficient to allow a useful evaluation of an individual's condition. The present data show a fair scatter between the anaerobic threshold and the 6-minute distance (Fig 1), with a standard error of estimation of 1.9 mL/[kg/min]. However, the 3-level evaluation proposed by Sinclair and colleagues seems a useful compromise: if the distance walked in 6 minutes is greater than 563 m, the anaerobic threshold is likely to be greater than 11 mL/[kg/min], and further laboratory evaluation is unnecessary; if it is less than 427 m, laboratory testing is advised, and between these 2 markers, the decision should be determined by the severity of the proposed surgery and the presence of other risk factors. One interesting aspect of this article is

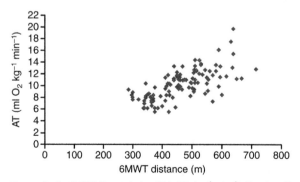

FIGURE 1.—Scatter plot for 6MWT distance (m) *vs* AT (ml O_2 kg^{-1} min^{-1}). (Reprinted from Sinclair RCF, Batterham AM, Davies S, et al. Validity of the 6 min walk test in prediction of the anaerobic threshold before major non-cardiac surgery. *Br J Anaesth*. 2012;108:30-35, by permission of The Board of Management and Trustees of the British Journal of Anaesthesia, Oxford University Press.)

the observation that subjective assessment[1,2] was not very helpful in risk stratification; only 1 of the 101 patients reported a peak capacity of less than the commonly accepted critical value of 4 metabolic equivalent scores (unable to climb a fight of stairs), but 58% had an anaerobic threshold of less than 11 mL/[kg/min] when tested in the laboratory. On this evidence, the 6-minute walk seems a better approach to screening than a simple questioning of the patient.

R. J. Shephard, MD (Lond), PhD, DPE

References

1. Fleisher LA, Beckman JA, Brown KA, et al. ACC/AHA 2007 guidelines on perioperative cardiovascular evaluation and care for noncardiac surgery: executive summary: a report of the American college of cardiology/American heart association task force on practice guidelines (writing committee to revise the 2002 guidelines on perioperative cardiovascular evaluation for noncardiac surgery): developed in collaboration with the American society of echocardiography, American society of nuclear cardiology, heart rhythm society, society of cardiovascular anesthesiologists, society for cardiovascular angiography and interventions, society for vascular medicine and biology, and society for vascular surgery. *Circulation.* 2007;116:1971-1996.
2. Poldermans D, Bax JJ, Boersma E, et al; European Society of Cardiology Guidelines. Guidelines for pre-operative cardiac risk assessment and perioperative cardiac management in non-cardiac surgery. *Eur Heart J.* 2009;30:2769-2812.
3. Snowden CP, Prentis JM, Anderson HL, et al. Submaximal cardiopulmonary exercise testing predicts complications and hospital length of stay in patients undergoing major elective surgery. *Ann Surg.* 2010;251:535-541.
4. Wilson RJ, Davies S, Yates D, Redman J, Stone M. Impaired functional capacity is associated with all-cause mortality after major elective intra-abdominal surgery. *Br J Anaesth.* 2010;105:297-303.
5. Older P, Smith R, Courtney P, Hone R. Preoperative evaluation of cardiac failure and ischemia in elderly patients by cardiopulmonary exercise testing. *Chest.* 1993; 104:701-704.

Left atrial volume index in highly trained athletes
D'Andrea A, Riegler L, Cocchia R, et al (Second Univ of Naples, Italy; et al)
Am Heart J 159:1155-1161, 2010

Background.—Increase of left atrial (LA) diameter in trained athletes has been regarded as another component of the "athlete's heart".

Aims.—To evaluate the possible impact of competitive training on LA volume and to define reference values of LA volume index in athletes.

Methods and Results.—Six hundred fifteen consecutive elite athletes (370 endurance- [ATE] vs 245 strength-trained athletes [ATS]; 385 men; 28.4 ± 10.2 years, range 18-40 years) underwent a comprehensive transthoracic echocardiography exam. LA maximal volume was measured at the point of mitral valve opening using the biplane area-length method, and corrected for body surface area. LA mild dilatation was defined as a LA volume index between 29 and 33 mL/m^2, while a moderate dilatation was identified by a LA volume index $\geq$34 mL/m^2. Left ventricular (LV) mass index and ejection fraction did not significantly differ between the 2 groups. Conversely, ATS showed increased body surface area, sum of wall thickness (septum + LV posterior wall), LV circumferential end-systolic stress (ESSc) and relative wall thickness, whereas LA volume index, LV stroke volume and LV end-diastolic volume were greater in ATE. The range of LA volume index was 26 to 36 mL/m^2 (mean 28.2 ± 9.2) in men and 22 to 33 mL/m^2 (mean 26.5 ± 7.2) in women ($P < .01$). LA volume index was mildly enlarged in 150 athletes (24.3%) and moderately enlarged only in 20, all males (3.2%). Mild mitral regurgitation was observed in 64 athletes (10.3%). LA volume index was significantly greater in ATE ($P < .01$). By multivariate analysis, the overall population type ($P < .01$) and duration ($P < .01$) of training and LV end-diastolic volume ($P < .001$) were the only independent predictors of LA volume index.

Conclusions.—In a large population of highly trained athletes, a mild enlargement of LA volume index was relatively common and may be regarded as a physiologic adaptation to exercise conditioning (Fig 2).

▶ This paper is from Naples, Italy, and although the 615 elite participants are consecutive referrals, the need to accumulate normative echocardiographic (ECG) data on both endurance and strength-training athletes no doubt reflects in part concerns raised by the side effects of mandatory ECG screening in that country. Current standards for the general population consider a left atrial volume of 29 to 33 mL/m^2 as mild dilatation, and a volume > 34 mL/m^2 as moderate dilatation.[1] There may be a problem in using a ratio to body surface area, because the body build of both endurance athletes and weight lifters differs from the population norms on which the body surface area formula is

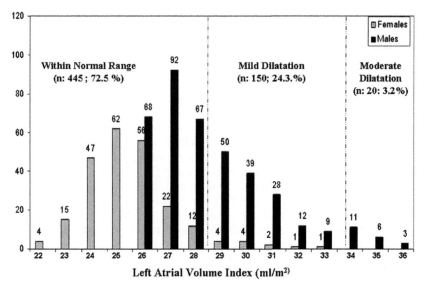

FIGURE 2.—Distribution of LA volume index in the overall population of 615 athletes. (Reprinted from D'Andrea A, Riegler L, Cocchia R, et al. Left atrial volume index in highly trained athletes. *Am Heart J*. 2010;159:1155-1161, Copyright 2010, with permission from Elsevier.)

based. With this qualification, most endurance and strength competitors have an atrial index well within normal limits (Fig 2). However, what would normally be regarded as mild enlargement was seen in 24% of the sample, and moderate enlargement in 3%, mainly in endurance competitors with an enlarged left ventricular end-diastolic volume who had been training for a long period. Such findings are probably physiological rather than pathological, reflecting a need for a high left atrial pressure to maintain ventricular filling,[2,3] and the authors of this report suggest setting the upper limits of normality at 33 mL/m^2 for female athletes, and 36 mL/m^2 for male athletes.

R. J. Shephard, MD (Lond), PhD, DPE

References

1. Lang RM, Bierig M, Devereux RB, et al; American Society of Echocardiography's Nomenclature and Standards Committee, Task Force on Chamber Quantification; American College of Cardiology Echocardiography Committee, American Heart Association, European Association of Echocardiography, European Society of Cardiology. Recommendations for chamber quantification. *Eur J Echocardiogr.* 2006;7:79-108.
2. Tsang TS, Barnes ME, Gersh BJ, Bailey KR, Seward JB. Left atrial volume as a morphophysiologic expression of left ventricular diastolic dysfunction and relation to cardiovascular risk burden. *Am J Cardiol.* 2002;90:1284-1289.
3. D'Andrea A, De Corato G, Scarafile R, et al. Left atrial myocardial function in either physiological or pathological left ventricular hypertrophy: a two-dimensional speckle strain study. *Br J Sports Med.* 2008;42:696-702.

The Effect of Nitric-Oxide-Related Supplements on Human Performance
Bescós R, Sureda A, Tur JA, et al (Univ of Barcelona, Spain; Univ of Balearic Islands, Spain)
Sports Med 42:99-117, 2012

Nitric oxide (NO) has led a revolution in physiology and pharmacology research during the last two decades. This labile molecule plays an important role in many functions in the body regulating vasodilatation, blood flow, mitochondrial respiration and platelet function. Currently, it is known that NO synthesis occurs via at least two physiological pathways: NO synthase (NOS) dependent and NOS independent. In the former, L-arginine is the main precursor. It is widely recognized that this amino acid is oxidized to NO by the action of the NOS enzymes. Additionally, L-citrulline has been indicated to be a secondary NO donor in the NOS-dependent pathway, since it can be converted to L-arginine. Nitrate and nitrite are the main substrates to produce NO via the NOS-independent pathway. These anions can be reduced *in vivo* to NO and other bioactive nitrogen oxides. Other molecules, such as the dietary supplement glycine propionyl-L-carnitine (GPLC), have also been suggested to increase levels of NO, although the physiological mechanisms remain to be elucidated.

The interest in all these molecules has increased in many fields of research. In relation with exercise physiology, it has been suggested that an increase in NO production may enhance oxygen and nutrient delivery to active muscles, thus improving tolerance to physical exercise and recovery mechanisms. Several studies using NO donors have assessed this hypothesis in a healthy, trained population. However, the conclusions from these studies showed several discrepancies. While some reported that dietary supplementation with NO donors induced benefits in exercise performance, others did not find any positive effect. In this regard, training status of the subjects seems to be an important factor linked to the ergogenic effect of NO supplementation. Studies involving untrained or moderately trained healthy subjects showed that NO donors could improve tolerance to aerobic and anaerobic exercise. However, when highly trained subjects were supplemented, no positive effect on performance was indicated. In addition, all this evidence is mainly based on a young male population. Further research in elderly and female subjects is needed to determine whether NO supplements can induce benefit in exercise capacity when the NO metabolism is impaired by age and/or estrogen status.

▶ Nitric oxide (NO) is a vascular dilator, and it thus has the potential to enhance the delivery of both oxygen and nutrients to active muscle, with a resulting enhancement of physical performance. Other beneficial effects may be linked to increased efficiency of the mitochondria[1] and of adenosine triphosphate turnover.[2] Potential sources of NO include arginine (and other compounds that can be metabolized to arginine) and the nitrates and nitrites present in many food products. Empirical studies (mostly performed in young men) seem to have found a beneficial effect on endurance performance in untrained or poorly trained subjects[3-5] but not in those who are already well trained (possibly because in the latter individuals, training has already brought about favorable changes in arterial architecture); this immediately reduces the likelihood that NO would be used as an ergogenic aid in an attempt to enhance the endurance performance of top athletes.

R. J. Shephard, MD (Lond), PhD, DPE

References

1. Larsen FJ, Schiffer TA, Borniquel S, et al. Dietary inorganic nitrate improves mitochondrial efficiency in humans. *Cell Metab.* 2011;13:149-159.
2. Bailey SJ, Fulford J, Vanhatalo A, et al. Dietary nitrate supplementation enhances muscle contractile efficiency during knee-extensor exercise in humans. *J Appl Physiol.* 2010;109:135-148.
3. Bailey SJ, Winyard PG, Vanhatalo A, et al. Acute L-arginine supplementation reduces the O2 cost of moderate-intensity exercise and enhances high-intensity exercise tolerance. *J Appl Physiol.* 2010;109:1394-1403.
4. Camic CL, Housh TJ, Zuniga JM, et al. Effects of arginine-based supplements on the physical working capacity at the fatigue threshold. *J Strength Cond Res.* 2010; 24:1306-1312.
5. Camic CL, Housh TJ, Mielke M, et al. The effects of 4 weeks of an arginine-based supplement on the gas exchange threshold and peak oxygen uptake. *Appl Physiol Nutr Metab.* 2010;35:286-293.

Modeling the Association between HR Variability and Illness in Elite Swimmers

Hellard P, Guimaraes F, Avalos M, et al (French Swimming Federation, Paris, France; INSERM U897, Bordeaux, France; et al)
Med Sci Sports Exerc 43:1063-1070, 2011

Purpose.—To determine whether HR variability (HRV), an indirect measure of autonomic control, is associated with upper respiratory tract and pulmonary infections, muscular affections, and all-type pathologies in elite swimmers.

Methods.—For this study, 7 elite international and 11 national swimmers were observed weekly for 2 yr. The indexes of cardiac autonomic regulation in supine and orthostatic position were assessed as explanatory variables by time domain (SD1, SD2) and spectral analyses (high frequency [HF] = 0.15−0.40 Hz, low frequency [LF] = 0.04−0.15 Hz, and HF/LF ratio) of HRV. Logistic mixed models described the relationship between the explanatory variables and the risk of upper respiratory tract and pulmonary infections, muscular affections, and all-type pathologies.

Results.—The risk of all-type pathologies was higher for national swimmers and in winter ($P < 0.01$). An increase in the parasympathetic indexes (HF, SD1) in the supine position assessed 1 wk earlier was linked to a higher risk of upper respiratory tract and pulmonary infections ($P < 0.05$) and to a higher risk of muscular affections (increase in HF, $P < 0.05$). Multivariate analyses showed (1) a higher all-type pathologies risk in winter and for an increase in the total power of HRV associated with a decline SD1 in supine position, (2) a higher all-type pathologies risk in winter associated with a decline in HF assessed 1 wk earlier in orthostatic position, and (3) a higher risk of muscular affections in winter associated with a decrease SD1 and an increase LF in orthostatic position.

Conclusions.—Swimmers' health maintenance requires particular attention when autonomic balance shows a sudden increase in parasympathetic indices in the supine position assessed 1 wk earlier evolving toward sympathetic predominance in supine and orthostatic positions.

▶ The search for measures that can demonstrate an excessive intensity of training in high-performance athletes has had little success. The surest indicators to date have seemed a deterioration in actual athletic performance and altered responses to simple psychological questionnaires.[1,2] Nevertheless, there is some evidence that periods of particularly heavy training can increase a competitor's vulnerability to upper respiratory infections,[3-5] and this in itself can have a disastrous impact on placing in races that are won by a small fraction of a second.[6] In the early stages of overtraining, sympathetic nerve activity seems to dominate, but if this ignored, the athlete may progress to the parasympathetic stage of overtraining.[7] Hellard et al speculated that there might be a causal relationship between such autonomic disturbances and vulnerability to infection, with the potential to use measures of heart rate variability in regulating the intensity of training. Parasympathetic dominance was assessed from Polar heart monitor recordings showing high-frequency heart rate variability and instantaneous variability (between successive beats), and infections were assessed from a weekly questionnaire. Unfortunately, the study did not distinguish between pathological and inflammatory forms of respiratory symptomatology, and no measures of either immune function or inflammatory markers were obtained. Parasympathetic dominance in the supine position was followed 1 week later by upper respiratory symptoms; however, heart rate variability in the supine position suggested a sympathetic dominance during the week when respiratory complaints were made. The lack of a consistent relationship between autonomic activity and upper respiratory infection reduces the practical value of such measurements in the prevention of illness and the regulation of training. It also argues against the existence of any simple causal relationship.

R. J. Shephard, MD (Lond), PhD, DPE

References

1. Verde T, Thomas S, Shephard RJ. Potential markers of heavy training in highly trained distance runners. *Br J Sports Med.* 1992;26:167-175.
2. Kuipers H. Training and overtraining: an introduction. *Med Sci Sports Exerc.* 1998;30:1137-1139.
3. Gleeson M, McDonald WA, Cripps AW, Pyne DB, Clancy RL, Fricker PA. The effect on immunity of long-term intensive training in elite swimmers. *Clin Exp Immunol.* 1995;102:210-216.
4. Gleeson M, McDonald WA, Pyne DB, et al. Salivary IgA levels and infection risk in elite swimmers. *Med Sci Sports Exerc.* 1999;31:67-73.
5. Mackinnon LT, Hooper SL. Mucosal (secretory) immune system responses to exercise of varying intensity and during overtraining. *Int J Sports Med.* 1994;15:S179-S183.
6. Pyne DB, Hopkins WG, Batterham AM, Gleeson M, Fricker PA. Characterising the individual performance responses to mild illness in international swimmers. *Br J Sports Med.* 2005;39:752-756.
7. Fry AC, Schilling BK, Weiss LW, Chiu LZ. beta2-Adrenergic receptor downregulation and performance decrements during high-intensity resistance exercise overtraining. *J Appl Physiol.* 2006;101:1664-1672.

Changes in salivary antimicrobial peptides, immunoglobulin A and cortisol after prolonged strenuous exercise
Usui T, Yoshikawa T, Orita K, et al (Osaka City Univ, Japan)
Eur J Appl Physiol 111:2005-2014, 2011

The aim of the present study was to examine whether amount of oral antimicrobial components, human β-defensin-2 (HBD-2), cathelicidin (LL-37), and immunoglobulin A (IgA), might be affected by prolonged strenuous exercise. Ten young male volunteers either exercised on recumbent ergometer at 75% $\dot{V}O_{2max}$ for 60 min (exercise session) or sat quietly (resting session). Saliva samples were obtained at 60-min intervals during sessions for measurements of saliva antimicrobial components (HBD-2, LL-37, and IgA), saliva cortisol and osmolality. Saliva flow rate was decreased and saliva osmolality was increased during the 60-min exercise. Saliva HBD-2 and LL-37 concentrations and secretion rates were

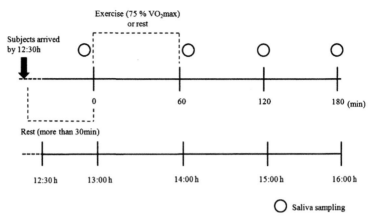

FIGURE 1.—Scheme of exercise and sampling protocol to investigate the change in saliva peptide levels caused by prolonged strenuous exercise in young adult males. Subjects were asked to visit to laboratory without having lunch by 12:30 p.m. After saliva sample was collected ($t = 0$), subjects were asked to wear a mask for continuous measurement of VO_2 during exercise. The subject either exercised on the recumbent ergometer at 75% $\dot{V}O_{2max}$ for 60 min (exercise session) or sat while allowed to read or write quietly (resting session). Immediately after the end of exercise, subjects took off the mask, followed by saliva collection ($t = 60$ min). Saliva samples were obtained at 60-min intervals after exercise ($t = 120, 180$ min). During resting session, saliva samples were collected at the same time points of exercise session ($t = 0, 60, 120, 180$ min). (Reprinted from Usui T, Yoshikawa T, Orita K, et al. Changes in salivary antimicrobial peptides, immunoglobulin A and cortisol after prolonged strenuous exercise. *Eur J Appl Physiol.* 2011;111:2005-2014, Copyright 2011, with kind permission of Springer Science+Business Media.)

increased during and after the exercise, whereas saliva IgA concentration and secretion rates were decreased after the exercise. Saliva cortisol was increased during and after the exercise. The areas under the curve of the time courses of saliva levels of HBD-2 and LL-37 were negatively correlated with those of cortisol levels in saliva. The present findings suggested that a single bout of prolonged strenuous exercise caused a transient increase in the oral HBD-2 and LL-37 levels (Fig 1).

▶ A novel class of antimicrobial peptides, defensins and cathelicidins, is currently attracting attention as a possible component in host defense of the oral mucosa.[1,2] The defensins are secreted by the epithelial cells lining the oral and respiratory tract. One of the cathelicidins (LL-37) is also secreted by macrophages and neutrophils.[3] Assuming that the antimicrobial role of these substances is confirmed, it becomes important to ascertain how their concentrations are affected by strenuous exercise or prolonged training. The study of Usui et al addresses the first of these issues, looking at the changes in salivary concentrations induced by 60 minutes of recumbent ergometer exercise at 75% of maximal aerobic power (Fig 1); although concentrations of immunoglobulin A in saliva collected by chewing decreased sharply after exercise, both the concentrations and the absolute secretions of a defensin (HBD-2) and LL-37 rose sharply during exercise and remained elevated for the following hour. These observations confirm a recent report from Davison et al.[4] Nevertheless, there remains a need to check the overall impact on the antibacterial activity of the saliva.

R. J. Shephard, MD (Lond), PhD, DPE

References

1. Doss M, White MR, Tecle T, Hartshorn KL. Human defensins and LL-37 in mucosal immunity. *J Leukoc Biol.* 2010;87:79-92.
2. Hancock RE, Diamond G. The role of cationic antimicrobial peptides in innate host defences. *Trends Microbiol.* 2000;8:402-410.
3. Nijnik A, Hancock RE. The roles of cathelicidin LL-37 in immune defences and novel clinical applications. *Curr Opin Hematol.* 2009;16:41-47.
4. Davison G, Allgrove J, Gleeson M. Salivary antimicrobial peptides (LL-37 and alpha-defensins HNP1-3), antimicrobial and IgA responses to prolonged exercise. *Eur J Appl Physiol.* 2009;106:277-284.

Nonalcoholic Beer Reduces Inflammation and Incidence of Respiratory Tract Illness

Scherr J, Nieman DC, Schuster T, et al (Technische Universitaet Muenchen, Munich, Germany; Appalachian State Univ and North Carolina Res Campus, Kannapolis; et al)
Med Sci Sports Exerc 44:18-26, 2012

Purpose.—Strenuous exercise significantly increases the incidence of upper respiratory tract illness (URTI) caused by transient immune dysfunction. Naturally occurring polyphenolic compounds present in food such as nonalcoholic beer (NAB) have strong antioxidant, antipathogenic, and anti-inflammatory properties. The objective of this study was to determine whether ingestion of NAB polyphenols for 3 wk before and 2 wk after a marathon would attenuate postrace inflammation and decrease URTI incidence.

Methods.—Healthy male runners ($N = 277$, age $= 42 \pm 9$ yr) were randomly assigned to $1-1.5 \, L \cdot d^{-1}$ of NAB or placebo (PL) beverage (double-blind design) for 3 wk before and 2 wk after the Munich Marathon. Blood samples were collected 4 and 1 wk before the race and immediately and 24 and 72 h after the race and analyzed for inflammation measures (interleukin-6 and total blood leukocyte counts). URTI rates, assessed by the Wisconsin Upper Respiratory Symptom Survey, were compared between groups during the 2-wk period after the race.

Results.—Change in interleukin-6 was significantly reduced in NAB compared with PL immediately after the race (median (interquartile range) $= 23.9$ $(15.9-38.7)$ vs 31.6 $(18.5-53.3)$ ng·L^{-1}, $P = 0.03$). Total blood leukocyte counts were also reduced in NAB versus PL by approximately 20% immediately and 24 h after the race ($P = 0.02$). Incidence of URTI was 3.25-fold lower (95% confidence interval $= 1.38$-7.66) ($P = 0.007$) in NAB compared with PL during the 2-wk postmarathon period.

Conclusions.—Consumption of $1-1.5 \, L \cdot d^{-1}$ of NAB for 3 wk before and 2 wk after marathon competition reduces postrace inflammation and URTI incidence.

▶ It seems a reasonable hypothesis that one of the factors increasing suscepti-bility to upper respiratory tract infections after very prolonged endurance exercise[1,2] is an increased production of reactive oxygen species. This being the case, treatment with antioxidants might be beneficial. Thus, Edith Peters demonstrated an apparent benefit from the administration of large doses of vitamin C a number of years ago,[3] although the administration of quercetin has been less beneficial.[4] Certain types of fruit and vegetables have also been commended because of the antioxidant properties of the phenols that they contain.[5] Red wine and beers have been held to provide a convenient source of phenols, although recently some questions of possible research fraud have been raised with regard to the apparent health-giving effects of red wine. The study of Scherr and associates, like many other studies of respiratory illness in athletes, has the limitation that diagnosis of infection was based on a respiratory symptom questionnaire, with a fair proportion of nonrespondents. Nevertheless, ingestion of 1.0 to 1.5 L/day of the nonalcoholic beer for 3 weeks before and 2 weeks after an international marathon event appears to have given an impressive reduction in the likelihood of both respiratory symptomatology and increased immune markers of inflammation in a substantial controlled trial. It is less clear whether it is necessary to give phenols as the complex brew of a nonalcoholic beer. The present study was funded by a brewer, and from my limited experience of nonalcoholic beers in Muslim countries, I am not sure whether I would want to drink 1.5 liters per day of such a beverage on a regular basis. There is thus a need to conduct a similar trial where the phenols are administered in tablet form.

R. J. Shephard, MD (Lond), PhD, DPE

References

1. Ekblom B, Ekblom O, Malm C. Infectious episodes before and after a marathon race. *Scand J Med Sci Sports*. 2006;16:287-293.
2. Murphy EA, Davis JM, Carmichael MD, Gangemi JD, Ghaffar A, Mayer EP. Exercise stress increases susceptibility to influenza infection. *Brain Behav Immun*. 2008;22:1152-1155.
3. Peters EM, Goetzsche JM, Grobbelaar B, Noakes TD. Vitamin C supplementation reduces the incidence of postrace symptoms of upper-respiratory-tract infection in ultramarathon runners. *Am J Clin Nutr*. 1993;57:170-174.
4. Nieman DC, Henson DA, Gross SJ, et al. Quercetin reduces illness but not immune perturbations after intensive exercise. *Med Sci Sports Exerc*. 2007;39:1561-1569.
5. Heinonen M. Antioxidant activity and antimicrobial effect of berry phenolics—a Finnish perspective. *Mol Nutr Food Res*. 2007;51:684-691.

Nonalcoholic Beer Reduces Inflammation and Incidence of Respiratory Tract Illness

Scherr J, Nieman DC, Schuster T, et al (Technische Universitaet Muenchen, Munich, Germany; Appalachian State Univ and North Carolina Res Campus, Kannapolis)

Med Sci Sports Exerc 44:18-26, 2012

Purpose.—Strenuous exercise significantly increases the incidence of upper respiratory tract illness (URTI) caused by transient immune dysfunction. Naturally occurring polyphenolic compounds present in food such as nonalcoholic beer (NAB) have strong antioxidant, antipathogenic, and anti-inflammatory properties. The objective of this study was to determine whether ingestion of NAB polyphenols for 3 wk before and 2 wk after a marathon would attenuate postrace inflammation and decrease URTI incidence.

Methods.—Healthy male runners ($N = 277$, age $= 42 \pm 9$ yr) were randomly assigned to $1-1.5$ L·d^{-1} of NAB or placebo (PL) beverage (double-blind design) for 3 wk before and 2 wk after the Munich Marathon. Blood samples were collected 4 and 1 wk before the race and immediately and 24 and 72 h after the race and analyzed for inflammation measures (interleukin-6 and total blood leukocyte counts). URTI rates, assessed by the Wisconsin Upper Respiratory Symptom Survey, were compared between groups during the 2-wk period after the race.

Results.—Change in interleukin-6 was significantly reduced in NAB compared with PL immediately after the race (median (interquartile range) $= 23.9$ ($15.9-38.7$) vs 31.6 ($18.5-53.3$) ng·L^{-1}, $P = 0.03$). Total blood leukocyte counts were also reduced in NAB versus PL by approximately 20% immediately and 24 h after the race ($P = 0.02$). Incidence of URTI was 3.25-fold lower (95% confidence interval $= 1.38-7.66$) ($P = 0.007$) in NAB compared with PL during the 2-wk postmarathon period.

Conclusions.—Consumption of $1-1.5$ L·d^{-1} of NAB for 3 wk before and 2 wk after marathon competition reduces postrace inflammation and URTI incidence (Fig 3).

▶ This study supports what many runners had long hoped was true—beer intake is beneficial, before and after running a marathon race. Marathoners drinking at least 2 pints per day of nonalcoholic beer for 3 weeks before and 2 weeks after racing the Munich Marathon experienced dramatically lowered rates of illness (Fig 3). The polyphenols in the beer also acted as an ibuprofen substitute in reducing marathon-induced inflammation. Polyphenols are plant chemicals and provide many of the colors in fruits, vegetables, nuts, seeds, and grains where they serve as defenders against microbes, radiation damage from the sun, and other insults. There is growing scientific support that polyphenols also provide multiple health and fitness benefits for athletes.[1-3] Polyphenol-rich plant extracts are being investigated as performance aids and countermeasures to exercise-induced inflammation, delayed-onset muscle soreness (DOMS), and oxidative stress. The dosing regimen is still under scientific scrutiny, but most studies support 1 to 3 weeks of supplementation with plant extracts or polyphenol-rich beverages before periods of heavy training or marathon competitions. Beer has more than 50 polyphenolic compounds from barley and hop and contains 366 to 875 mg polyphenols per liter, depending on the variety. Beer polyphenols are rapidly absorbed and increase antioxidant capacity to the same degree as wine. For 3 weeks before and 2 weeks after the Munich Marathon, athletes drank 1.0 to 1.5 L of nonalcoholic beer each day, either with polyphenols or without. New episodes of illness (primarily the common cold) were 3.25-fold lower in

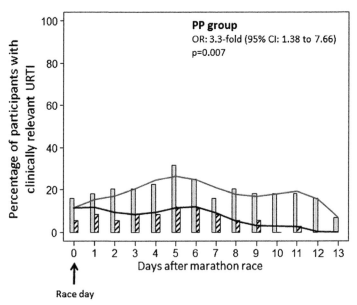

FIGURE 3.—Incidence of clinically relevant URTI after the marathon race in the intervention group (*black striped*) and control group (*gray*). (Reprinted from Scherr J, Nieman DC, Schuster T, et al. Nonalcoholic beer reduces inflammation and incidence of respiratory tract illness. *Med Sci Sports Exerc.* 2012;44:18-26, with permission from the American College of Sports Medicine.)

runners consuming beer with polyphenols than without during the 2-week period after the Munich Marathon, and postrace inflammation was 24% lower. These are impressive results and support the practice of ingesting polyphenolic-rich beverages and plant extracts before and after marathon competitions. Obviously, a high consumption of beer with alcohol tips the benefit-to-risk balance the wrong way. Beer with alcohol has a higher polyphenolic content than nonalcoholic beer, but health experts recommend an intake of no more than 2 cans of regular beer per day. The Munich marathoners consumed 3 to 4 cans of nonalcoholic beer per day, so runners can consider drinking 2 cans of regular beer and 1 or 2 cans of nonalcoholic beer each day during the weeks surrounding competitions or intense training.

D. C. Nieman, DrPH

References

1. Walsh NP, Gleeson M, Pyne DB, et al. Position statement. Part two: maintaining immune health. *Exerc Immunol Rev.* 2011;17:64-103.
2. Nieman DC, Stear SJ, Castell LM, Burke LM. A-Z of nutritional supplements: dietary supplements, sports nutrition foods and ergogenic aids for health and performance: part 15, flavonoids. *Br J Sports Med.* 2010;44:1202-1205.
3. Nieman DC. Immunonutrition support for athletes. *Nutr Rev.* 2008;66:310-320.

Mucosal Immune Responses to Treadmill Exercise in Elite Wheelchair Athletes

Leicht CA, Bishop NC, Goosey-Tolfrey VL (Loughborough Univ, UK)
Med Sci Sports Exerc 43:1414-1421, 2011

Purpose.—The study's purpose was to examine salivary secretory immunoglobulin A (sIgA) responses and α-amylase activity after constant load and intermittent exercise in elite wheelchair athletes.

Methods.—Twenty-three wheelchair athletes divided into three groups (eight tetraplegic (TETRA), seven paraplegic, and eight non–spinal cord–injured) performed two randomized and counterbalanced 60-min sessions on a treadmill. These consisted of constant load (60% peak oxygen uptake) and intermittent (80% and 40% peak oxygen uptake) exercise blocks. Timed unstimulated saliva samples were obtained before, mid, after, and 30 min after exercise and analyzed for sIgA and α-amylase. Furthermore, oxygen uptake, blood lactate concentration, and RPE were measured during both sessions.

Results.—SIgA secretion rate and α-amylase activity were increased during exercise in all groups ($P < 0.05$). However, the increase of sIgA secretion rate during exercise was greater in TETRA individuals (postexercise average data for both trials in comparison with preexercise data: TETRA = +60% ± 31%, paraplegic = +30% ± 35%, non–spinal cord–injured = +11% ± 25%; $P < 0.05$). Yet, groups were comparable with respect to blood lactate concentration and RPE for both exercise sessions.

Conclusions.—Despite the disruption of autonomic salivary gland innervation in TETRA athletes, their ability to increase sIgA secretion rate seems comparable to wheelchair athletes with intact autonomic salivary gland innervation. The similar responses between groups may stem from sympathetic reflex activity during exercise or a predominant contribution of parasympathetic activity, which are still intact systems in the TETRA population. The results of this study support the positive role of acute exercise on oral immune function in wheelchair athletes independent of disability type (Fig 2).

▶ It is now well recognized that periods of very intensive training can increase the risk of upper respiratory infections in athletes; this is probably related to a temporary suppression of mucosal immune function.[1,2] The issue is important for elite wheelchair athletes with quadriplegia. They are particularly vulnerable to upper respiratory tract infections because weakness of the chest and abdominal muscles limits their ability to cough up mucus,[3] and poor autonomic control may lead to abnormal patterns of bronchial secretion and airway hypersensitivity.[4] The study of Leicht et al was based on 60-minute bouts of exercise, either two 30-minute bouts at 60% of maximal oxygen intake or 20 alternating blocks of exercise at 40% and 80% of maximal oxygen intake. Both of these patterns of exercise would enhance rather than impair immune function in an able-bodied individual. During exercise, an immediate increase in immunoglobulin A (IgA)

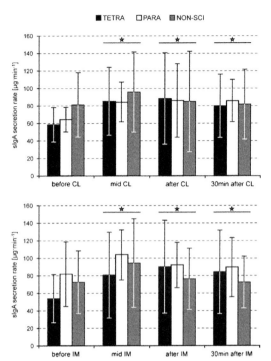

FIGURE 2.—Effect of a 60-min exercise trial on sIgA secretion rate. *Significantly different from before, at $P < 0.05$. (Reprinted from Leicht CA, Bishop NC, Goosey-Tolfrey VL. Mucosal immune responses to treadmill exercise in elite wheelchair athletes. *Med Sci Sports Exerc.* 2011;43:1414-1421, with permission from the American College of Sports Medicine.)

concentrations in unstimulated saliva samples was seen in individuals with paraplegia, much like that observed in wheelchair athletes without spinal cord injury, and the increase was even larger in those with tetraplegia (Fig 2). There was also the expected exercise-induced increase of salivary α-amylase, an enzyme that (by binding to oral bacteria) may facilitate the action of salivary IgA.[5] The main conclusion from this study is that despite the disruption of salivary secretion in people with tetraplegia, mucosal immune function remains unimpaired. There is one important qualification to this verdict: none of those who were tested demonstrated autonomic dysreflexia—a phenomenon that might well have an important impact on the distribution of immune cells.

R. J. Shephard, MD (Lond), PhD, DPE

References

1. Fahlman MM, Engels HJ. Mucosal IgA and URTI in American college football players: a year longitudinal study. *Med Sci Sports Exerc.* 2005;37:374-380.
2. Neville V, Gleeson M, Folland JP. Salivary IgA as a risk factor for upper respiratory infections in elite professional athletes. *Med Sci Sports Exerc.* 2008;40:1228-1236.

3. Haisma JA, van der Woude LH, Stam HJ, et al. Physical capacity in wheelchair-dependent persons with a spinal cord injury: a critical review of the literature. *Spinal Cord.* 2006;44:642-652.
4. Krassioukov A. Autonomic function following cervical spinal cord injury. *Respir Physiol Neurobiol.* 2009;169:157-164.
5. Scannapieco FA, Solomon L, Wadenya RO. Emergence in human dental plaque and host distribution of amylase-binding streptococci. *J Dent Res.* 1994;73:1627-1635.

5 Metabolism and Obesity, Nutrition and Doping

Nonprescribed physical activity energy expenditure is maintained with structured exercise and implicates a compensatory increase in energy intake

Turner JE, Markovitch D, Betts JA, et al (Univ of Bath, UK)

Am J Clin Nutr 92:1009-1016, 2010

Background.—Exercise interventions elicit only modest weight loss, which might reflect a compensatory reduction in nonprescribed physical activity energy expenditure (PAEE).

Objective.—The objective was to investigate whether there is a reduction in nonprescribed PAEE as a result of participation in a 6-mo structured exercise intervention in middle-aged men.

Design.—Sedentary male participants [age: 54 ± 5 y; body mass index (in kg/m^2): 28 ± 3] were randomly assigned to a 6-mo progressive exercise (EX) or control (CON) group. Energy expenditure during structured exercise (prescribed PAEE) and nonprescribed PAEE were determined with the use of synchronized accelerometry and heart rate before the intervention, during the intervention (2, 9, and 18 wk), and within a 2-wk period of detraining after the intervention.

Results.—Structured prescribed exercise increased total PAEE and had no detrimental effect on nonprescribed PAEE. Indeed, there was a trend for greater nonprescribed PAEE in the EX group ($P = 0.09$). Weight loss in the EX group ($-1.8 ± 2.2$ kg compared with $+0.2 ± 2.2$ kg in the CON group, $P < 0.02$) reflected only ≈40% of the 300−373 kcal/kg body mass potential energy deficit from prescribed exercise. Serum leptin concentration decreased by 24% in the EX group (compared with 3% in the CON group, $P < 0.03$), and we estimate that this was accompanied by a compensatory increase in energy intake of ≈100 kcal/d.

Conclusions.—The adoption of regular structured exercise in previously sedentary, middle-aged, and overweight men does not result in a negative compensatory reduction in nonprescribed physical activity. The less-than-predicted weight loss is likely to reflect a compensatory increase in

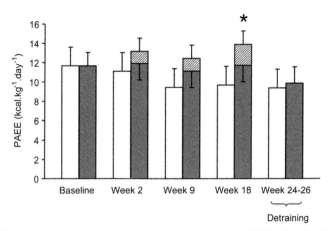

FIGURE 2.—Mean (95% CI) physical activity energy expenditure (PAEE) before (baseline), during (weeks 2—18), and after (weeks 24—26; detraining) the intervention in control (CON; open bars) and exercise (EX; closed bars) groups. Energy expended during the prescribed exercise intervention is shown for the EX group (prescribed PAEE; hatched bars). EX group, $n = 15$; CON group, $n = 14$. There was a significant time × group interaction effect for overall PAEE ($F = 2.9$, $P = 0.03$; 2-factor repeated-measures ANOVA). *Denotes that total PAEE in the EX group (prescribed and nonprescribed PAEE) is greater than in the CON group ($P = 0.004$, independent-samples t test). (Reprinted from Turner JE, Markovitch D, Betts JA, et al. Nonprescribed physical activity energy expenditure is maintained with structured exercise and implicates a compensatory increase in energy intake. *Am J Clin Nutr.* 2010;92:1009-1016, with permission from American Society for Nutrition.)

energy intake in response to a perceived state of relative energy insufficiency (Fig 2).

▶ Exercise training without diet intervention does not induce a meaningful loss in body mass.[1] Although surprising to some, explanations include compensatory decreases in pre-exercise and postexercise activity patterns (ie, resting reward behavior), eating more (ie, eating reward behavior), and failure to calculate net energy expenditure (ie, subtracting out resting metabolic rate and activities that would normally take place during exercise). As summarized in Fig 2, this study suggests that middle-aged men do not reduce nonprescribed physical activity energy expenditure. Other studies disagree, and the use of accelerometry and heart rate in this study does not provide a definitive answer. Further research with larger numbers of subjects is needed, but to enhance the beneficial effects of exercise training on weight loss, clinicians should urge individuals to aim for 60 minutes of exercise each day while avoiding the tendency to reward this good behavior with more rest and food.

D. C. Nieman, DrPH

Reference

1. Jakicic JM. The effect of physical activity on body weight. *Obesity (Silver Spring).* 2009;17:S34-S38.

Moderate to Vigorous Physical Activity and Sedentary Time and Cardiometabolic Risk Factors in Children and Adolescents

Ekelund U, for the International Children's Accelerometry Database (ICAD) Collaborators (Inst of Metabolic Science, Cambridge, UK; et al)

JAMA 307:704-712, 2012

Context.—Sparse data exist on the combined associations between physical activity and sedentary time with cardiometabolic risk factors in healthy children.

Objective.—To examine the independent and combined associations between objectively measured time in moderate- to vigorous-intensity physical activity (MVPA) and sedentary time with cardiometabolic risk factors.

Design, Setting, and Participants.—Pooled data from 14 studies between 1998 and 2009 comprising 20 871 children (aged 4-18 years) from the International Children's Accelerometry Database. Time spent in MVPA and sedentary time were measured using accelerometry after reanalyzing raw data. The independent associations between time in MVPA and sedentary time, with outcomes, were examined using metaanalysis. Participants were stratified by tertiles of MVPA and sedentary time.

Main Outcome Measures.—Waist circumference, systolic blood pressure, fasting triglycerides, high-density lipoprotein cholesterol, and insulin.

Results.—Times (mean [SD] min/d) accumulated by children in MVPA and being sedentary were 30 (21) and 354 (96), respectively. Time in MVPA was significantly associated with all cardiometabolic outcomes independent of sex, age, monitor wear time, time spent sedentary, and waist circumference (when not the outcome). Sedentary time was not associated with any outcome independent of time in MVPA. In the combined analyses, higher levels of MVPA were associated with better cardiometabolic risk factors across tertiles of sedentary time. The differences in outcomes between higher and lower MVPA were greater with lower sedentary time. Mean differences in waist circumference between the bottom and top tertiles of MVPA were 5.6 cm (95% CI, 4.8-6.4 cm) for high sedentary time and 3.6 cm (95% CI, 2.8-4.3 cm) for low sedentary time. Mean differences in systolic blood pressure for high and low sedentary time were 0.7 mm Hg (95% CI, −0.07 to 1.6) and 2.5 mm Hg (95% CI, 1.7-3.3), and for high-density lipoprotein cholesterol, differences were −2.6 mg/dL (95% CI, −1.4 to −3.9) and −4.5 mg/dL (95% CI, −3.3 to −5.6), respectively. Geometric mean differences for insulin and triglycerides showed similar variation. Those in the top tertile of MVPA accumulated more than 35 minutes per day in this intensity level compared with fewer than 18 minutes per day for those in the bottom tertile. In prospective analyses (N=6413 at 2.1 years' follow-up), MVPA and sedentary time were not associated with waist circumference at follow-up, but a higher waist circumference at baseline was associated with higher amounts of sedentary time at follow-up.

Conclusion.—Higher MVPA time by children and adolescents was associated with better cardiometabolic risk factors regardless of the amount of sedentary time.

▶ To my knowledge, this is by far the largest assembled cohort of children wherein physical activity and sedentary behavior were measured using an objective method. Thus, the International Children's Accelerometry Database provided Ekelund and colleagues with a unique opportunity to look at how moderate to vigorous physical activity (MVPA) and sedentary behavior relate to cardiometabolic risk factors such as obesity, blood pressure, and plasma lipids/lipoproteins (eg, high-density lipoprotein—cholesterol, triglycerides). Before discussing the findings, it is important to highlight that sedentary behavior is not the same as a lack of MVPA. In fact, the time children spend being sedentary, in a sitting or lying position during waking hours, is poorly correlated to how much time they spend in MVPA. There has been great interest in recent years among the physical activity research community in defining sedentary behavior and determining whether it has an independent effect on health.

The authors reported that the time children participated in MVPA was significantly and meaningfully associated with all the cardiometabolic outcomes examined in their study and that these relationships were independent of sex, age, and sedentary time. This was no surprise, as such relationships have been reported in dozens if not hundreds of previous studies. It was, however, reassuring to see such relationships replicated in such a large and diverse sample in which objective measures of physical activity were used. In contrast to MVPA, the time children spent in sedentary behavior was not an independent predictor of the cardiometabolic risk factors. This finding raises serious questions as to whether sedentary behavior per se is an important target for health promotion.

Although this is a very powerful study, the findings on sedentary behavior should be interpreted with caution. The accelerometers that were used to measure MVPA and sedentary behavior are more sensitive at measuring the former than the latter. While total sedentary time many not be important, specific sedentary behaviors such as television may have an independent effect on obesity and other cardiometabolic risk factors.[1]

I. Janssen, PhD

Reference

1. Carson V, Janssen I. Volume, patterns, and types of sedentary behavior and cardiometabolic health in children and adolescents: a cross-sectional study. *BMC Public Health.* 2011;11:274.

Relationship Between Active School Transport and Body Mass Index in Grades-4-to-6 Children

Larouche R, Lloyd M, Knight E, et al (Univ of Ottawa, Ontario, Canada)
Pediatr Exerc Sci 23:322-330, 2011

The current investigation assessed the impact of active school transportation (AST) on average daily step counts, body mass index (BMI) and waist circumference in 315 children in Grades 4—6 who participated to Cycle 2 of the Canadian Assessment of Physical Literacy (CAPL) pilot testing. T-tests revealed a significant association between AST and lower BMI values (18.7 ± 3.3 vs. 19.9 ± 3.8 kg/m^2). The active commuters accumulated an average of 662 more steps per day, and their waist circumference was lower by an average of 3.1 cm, but these differences were not statistically significant. ANCOVA analyses controlling for age and step counts, found trends toward lower BMI and waist circumference values among the active commuters. These results suggest that AST may be a valid strategy to prevent childhood obesity; further research is needed to determine more precisely the impact of AST on body composition, and the direction of the relationship.

▶ The proportion of children who use a form of active transportation to get to school, such as walking or bicycling, is at a historical low, and less than a third of children in North American now get to school in an active way.[1,2] This has economic and environmental impacts; traveling by bus to school is very expensive (about $1000 per child per year in my local school board) and the airborne diesel particles emitted from school buses are extremely toxic. The excessive reliance on motorized transport may also affect the total physical activity levels and health of our children.

This study of 315 children in grades 4 to 6 found that children who were active commuters accumulated 662 steps more than children who got to school by bus or car; this represented a 6% difference in activity levels between the 2 groups. The active commuters also had more favorable obesity measures; their BMI values were 1.2 kg/m^2 lower and their waist circumference values were 3 cm lower. Unfortunately, the biggest limitation of this study was the relatively small sample size; there were only 66 children who used active transportation as their sole means of getting to school, and this contributed to nonsignificant differences in the physical activity and obesity measures. Nonetheless, these are promising findings that speak to the importance of active transportation to school and the need for young people to incorporate less vigorous forms of physical activity into their daily routine. These findings also speak to the need for parents, teachers, and clinicians to encourage such forms of physical activity.

I. Janssen, PhD

References

1. Buliung RN, Mitra R, Faulkner G; Active school transportation in the Greater Toronto Area, Canada: an exploration of trends in space and time (1986—2006). *Prev Med.* 2009;48:507-512.

2. Ham SA, Martin S, Kohl HW 3rd; Changes in the percentage of students who walk or bike to school-United States, 1969 and 2001. *J Phys Act Health.* 2008; 5:205-215.

Metabolic flexibility and obesity in children and youth

Aucouturier J, Duché P, Timmons BW (McMaster Univ, Hamilton, Ontario, Canada; Blaise Pascal Univ, Clermont-Ferrand, France)
Obes Rev 12:e44-e53, 2011

The concept of metabolic flexibility describes the ability of skeletal muscle to switch between the oxidation of lipid as a fuel during fasting periods to the oxidation of carbohydrate during insulin stimulated period. Alterations in energy metabolism in adults with obesity, insulin resistance and/or type 2 diabetes induce a state of impaired metabolic flexibility, or metabolic inflexibility. Despite the increase in the prevalence of type 2 diabetes in obese children and youth, less is known about the factors involved in the development of metabolic inflexibility in the paediatric population. Metabolic flexibility is conditioned by nutrient partitioning in response to feeding, substrate mobilization and delivery to skeletal muscle during fasting or exercising condition, and skeletal muscle oxidative capacity. Our aim in this review was to identify among these factors those making obese children at risk of metabolic inflexibility. The development of ectopic rather than peripheral fat storage appears to be a factor strongly linked with a reduced metabolic flexibility. Tissue growth and maturation are determinants of impaired energy metabolism later in life but also as a promising way to reverse metabolic inflexibility given the plasticity of many tissues in youth. Finally, we have attempted to identify perspectives for future investigations of metabolic flexibility in obese children that will improve our understanding of the genesis of metabolic diseases associated with obesity.

▶ The increase in the prevalence of obesity in children and youth observed over the last few decades is alarming. As has been known for some time, obesity, and abdominal obesity in particular, is highly associated with resistance to the effects of insulin on peripheral glucose and free fatty acid usage, which often then leads to type II diabetes. Often termed *metabolic syndrome*, those children and youth so effected exhibit impaired metabolic function in glucose transport, insulin signaling, muscle oxidative capacity, and glycogen storage. The skeletal muscle in normal-weight children and youth is metabolically flexible so that there is an ability to switch from the oxidation of lipid as a fuel in the fasting state to the oxidation of carbohydrate (CHO) in hyperinsulinemic conditions. This is not the case in obese children and youth who exhibit metabolic inflexibility. In this review, Aucouturier and coauthors outline the problem very nicely by first pointing out that very little is known about the link between metabolic flexibility and the development of insulin resistance in children and youth. Associations are emphasized between physical activity levels and the determination of metabolic flexibility and the response to chronic high-fat or high-CHO diet. These issues are difficult to study in obese children and youth because of the ethical issues involved in invasive experimental procedures, such as muscle biopsies. However, a good case is made to use exercise as an experimental approach. For example, exercise is a wonderful model for studying metabolic flexibility to lipid and the ability to adapt fat utilization to availability. If this is impaired, then we see the accumulation of fat in ectopic fat deposits, thereby putting these children at higher risk of insulin resistance and cardiovascular disease. Finally, the authors suggest that interventions that include nutritional education and physical activity have the potential of reversing the metabolic dysfunction and enabling healthy growth and development.

V. Galea, PhD

Association between attention-deficit/hyperactivity disorder symptoms and obesity and hypertension in early adulthood: a population-based study
Fuemmeler BF, Østbye T, Yang C, et al (Duke Univ Med Ctr, Durham, NC; Duke Univ, Durham, NC)
Int J Obes 35:852-862, 2011

Objective.—To examine the associations between attention-deficit/hyperactivity disorder (ADHD) symptoms, obesity and hypertension in young adults in a large population-based cohort.

Design, Setting and Participants.—The study population consisted of 15 197 respondents from the National Longitudinal Study of Adolescent Health, a nationally representative sample of adolescents followed from 1995 to 2009 in the United States. Multinomial logistic and logistic models examined the odds of overweight, obesity and hypertension in adulthood in relation to retrospectively reported ADHD symptoms. Latent curve modeling was used to assess the association between symptoms and naturally occurring changes in body mass index (BMI) from adolescence to adulthood.

Results.—Linear association was identified between the number of inattentive (IN) and hyperactive/impulsive (HI) symptoms and waist circumference, BMI, diastolic blood pressure and systolic blood pressure (all P-values for trend <0.05). Controlling for demographic variables, physical activity, alcohol use, smoking and depressive symptoms, those with three or more HI or IN symptoms had the highest odds of obesity (HI 3+, odds ratio (OR) = 1.50, 95% confidence interval (CI) = 1.22–2.83; IN 3+, OR = 1.21, 95% CI = 1.02–1.44) compared with those with no HI or IN symptoms. HI symptoms at the 3+ level were significantly associated with a higher OR of hypertension (HI 3+, OR = 1.24, 95% CI = 1.01–1.51; HI continuous, OR = 1.04, 95% CI = 1.00–1.09), but associations were nonsignificant when models were adjusted for BMI. Latent growth modeling results indicated that compared with those reporting no HI or IN symptoms, those reporting 3 or more symptoms had higher initial levels of BMI during adolescence. Only HI symptoms were associated with change in BMI.

Conclusion.—Self-reported ADHD symptoms were associated with adult BMI and change in BMI from adolescence to adulthood, providing further evidence of a link between ADHD symptoms and obesity.

▶ The prevalence of attention-deficit/hyperactivity disorder (ADHD) has been shown to be higher than expected in obese children and adults. Although most of these studies were clinically based, the link between obesity and ADHD has been established in population-based studies. The study by Fuemmeler and colleagues is one such study where they set out to examine the associations between subthreshold retrospectively reported ADHD symptoms, obesity, and hypertension in young adults from a population-based cohort in the United States. This is the first population-based study to examine the role of inattentive (IN) and hyperactive/impulsive (HI) symptoms, alone and in combination, in the association between ADHD obesity and hypertension. Of interest to this readership are the compelling results from a final analysis sample of 11 666 participants. Specifically, those participants with 3 or more symptoms of HI or IN had the highest odds of obesity with odds ratios of 1.50 (95% confidence interval [CI] = 1.22-2.83) and 1.21 (95% CI = 1.02-1.44), respectively. Furthermore, those participants reporting 3 or more ADHD-related symptoms had higher initial values of body mass index (BMI) during adolescence and were more likely to show changes (increased) in BMI into adulthood if they reported 3 or more symptoms of HI. Evidence from studies specifically related to the comorbidity of ADHD with developmental coordination disorder then also becomes associated with decreased participation in physical activity, further promoting the likelihood of consequences of inactivity contributing to overweight, obesity, cardiovascular problems, and possibly Type II diabetes in later life. These children and adolescents are difficult to motivate to physical activity and therefore, it becomes important to address their specific needs when designing exercise programs if they are going to comply. Clearly, further research is required in this area.

V. Galea, PhD

Pericardial Fat Loss in Postmenopausal Women under Conditions of Equal Energy Deficit
Brinkley TE, Ding J, Carr JJ, et al (Wake Forest Univ School of Medicine, Winston-Salem, NC)
Med Sci Sports Exerc 43:808-814, 2011

Weight loss induced by caloric restriction (CR) or aerobic exercise can reduce pericardial fat, and these reductions may help improve cardiovascular health.

Purpose.—We examined whether combining CR with aerobic exercise enhances pericardial fat loss compared with a CR-only intervention designed to elicit equivalent reductions in body weight. We also examined the relationship between changes in pericardial fat and changes in maximal oxygen consumption ($\dot{V}O_{2max}$), a measure of cardiorespiratory fitness.

Methods.—Thirty-two abdominally obese postmenopausal women (mean age $= 58$ yr; 78% Caucasian) were randomly assigned to one of three interventions of equal energy deficit (~ 2800 kcal·wk^{-1}) for 20 wk: CR only ($n = 8$), CR + moderate-intensity exercise ($n = 15$), or CR + vigorous-intensity exercise ($n = 9$). The volume of pericardial fat around the coronary arteries was measured by computed tomography.

Results.—Women in the CR, CR + moderate-intensity, and CR + vigorous-intensity groups had similar baseline characteristics. The mean $\pm$ SD value for pericardial fat before weight loss was 79.07 ± 32.90 cm^3 (range $= 34.04 - 152.74$ cm^3), with no difference among groups ($P = 0.89$). All three interventions significantly reduced body weight (15%), waist circumference (10%), and abdominal visceral fat (28%) to a similar degree. There was also a 17% reduction in pericardial fat (-12.75 ± 6.29 cm^3, $P < 0.0001$), which did not differ among groups ($P = 0.84$). Changes in pericardial fat were inversely correlated with changes in $\dot{V}O_{2max}$ ($r = -0.37$, $P = 0.05$), but not after adjusting for intervention group and change in body weight.

Conclusions.—Weight loss interventions of equal energy deficit have similar effects on pericardial fat in postmenopausal women, regardless of whether the energy deficit is due to CR alone or CR plus aerobic exercise (Fig 1).

▶ Those involved in preventive medicine have long recognized that an abdominal fat accumulation has bad long-term implications for cardiovascular health. However, attention has shifted recently to the consequences of an accumulation of fat around the ventricles and the coronary vessels,[1-3] which is also associated with increased risk to cardiovascular health, possibly independent of effects due to any abdominal accumulation of fat. One study has further reported an inverse association between pericardial fat and cardiac output in obese individuals.[4] This article used computed tomography[5] to study pericardial fat accumulation in 32 women aged 50 to 70 years who were either overweight or obese. As I would have anticipated, a negative energy balance of 11.5 MJ/wk reduced the amount of this fat, whether it was brought about by dietary restriction alone or by a combination of dieting and exercise (Fig 1). The usual argument for adding exercise to a weight-reduction program is not that it increases the extent of fat loss but rather that it helps to conserve lean tissue; however, in this study, the 3 groups showed similar small decreases in lean tissue mass. The loss of 16% pericardial fat was similar to the change in overall body mass (15%), but it was substantially less than the reduction in abdominal visceral fat (28%). The authors attempted to prove that the reduction of pericardial fat had improved cardiovascular function by demonstrating a correlation ($r = -37$) between the loss of pericardial fat and an increase in maximal oxygen intake. However, the units chosen for the latter were mL/[kg.min], so that the observed association could equally reflect the decrease in body mass; as the authors admit, relationships to maximal

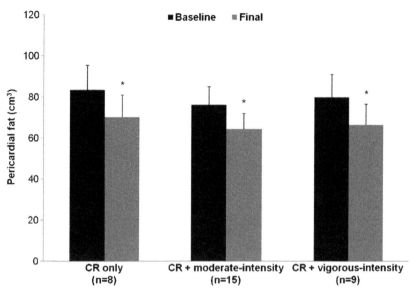

FIGURE 1.—Pericardial fat before and after weight loss by intervention group; *significantly different from baseline, $P < 0.05$. (Reprinted from Brinkley TE, Ding J, Carr JJ, et al. Pericardial fat loss in postmenopausal women under conditions of equal energy deficit. *Med Sci Sports Exerc.* 2011;43:808-814, with permission from the American College of Sports Medicine.)

oxygen intake became statistically insignificant when data were covaried for changes in overall body mass.

R. J. Shephard, MD (Lond), PhD, DPE

References

1. Ding J, Hsu FC, Harris TB, et al. The association of pericardial fat with incident coronary heart disease: the Multi-Ethnic Study of Atherosclerosis (MESA). *Am J Clin Nutr.* 2009;90:499-504.
2. Kim MK, Tanaka K, Kim MJ, et al. Epicardial fat tissue: relationship with cardio-respiratory fitness in men. *Med Sci Sports Exerc.* 2010;42:463-469.
3. Rosito GA, Massaro JM, Hoffmann U, et al. Pericardial fat, visceral abdominal fat, cardiovascular disease risk factors, and vascular calcification in a community-based sample: the Framingham Heart Study. *Circulation.* 2008;117:605-613.
4. Ruberg FL, Chen Z, Hua N, et al. The relationship of ectopic lipid accumulation to cardiac and vascular function in obesity and metabolic syndrome. *Obesity (Silver Spring).* 2010;18:1116-1121.
5. Ding J, Kritchevsky SB, Harris TB, et al. Multi-Ethnic Study of Atherosclerosis. The association of pericardial fat with calcified coronary plaque. *Obesity (Silver Spring).* 2008;16:1914-1919.

Is lost lean mass from intentional weight loss recovered during weight regain in postmenopausal women?

Beavers KM, Lyles MF, Davis CC, et al (Wake Forest Univ School of Medicine, Winston-Salem, NC; et al)
Am J Clin Nutr 94:767-774, 2011

Background.—Despite the well-known recidivism of obesity, surprisingly little is known about the composition of body weight during weight regain.

Objective.—The objective of this study was to determine whether the composition of body weight regained after intentional weight loss is similar to the composition of body weight lost.

Design.—The design was a follow-up to a randomized controlled trial of weight loss in which body composition was analyzed and compared in 78 postmenopausal women before the intervention, immediately after the intervention, and 6 and 12 mo after the intervention.

Results.—All body mass and composition variables were lower immediately after weight loss than at baseline (all $P < 0.05$). More fat than lean mass was lost with weight loss, which resulted in body-composition changes favoring a lower percentage of body fat and a higher lean-to-fat mass ratio ($P < 0.001$). Considerable interindividual variability in weight regain was noted (CV = 1.07). In women who regained ≥ 2 kg body weight, a decreasing trend in the lean-to-fat mass ratio was observed, which indicated greater fat mass accretion than lean mass accretion ($P < 0.001$). Specifically, for every 1 kg fat lost during the weight-loss intervention, 0.26 kg lean tissue was lost; for every 1 kg fat regained over the following year, only 0.12 kg lean tissue was regained.

Conclusions.—Although not all postmenopausal women who intentionally lose weight will regain it within 1 y, the data suggest that fat mass is regained to a greater degree than is lean mass in those who do experience some weight regain. The health ramifications of our findings remain to be seen (Fig 2).

▶ One of the most obvious negative effects of an intentional reduction in body mass is a substantial loss of lean tissue in addition to the unwanted abdominal fat. This problem can be alleviated to some extent by basing a fat-loss program on a combination of physical activity and a small negative energy balance rather than dieting alone; preservation of lean tissue is particularly likely if the regimen includes resistance exercise, but most studies show some loss of lean tissue. Given that only some 20% of patients are successful in maintaining their initial weight loss,[1] a related issue is whether the subsequent gain in body mass is simply fat or whether the lean tissue is also restored. In the study of Beavers and associates, 5 months of weight loss was based on a moderate energy deficit (about 1.68 MJ/d, 400 kcal/d), with 2 of 3 groups of patients supposedly undertaking moderate or vigorous aerobic exercise 3 times per week. One may wonder about the effectiveness of the prescribed exercise, because the loss of body mass and lean tissue did not differ between groups; losses averaged

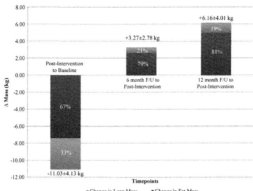

FIGURE 2.—Composition of weight lost during the 5-mo intervention and composition of weight regained over the 6- and 12-mo follow-up (F/U) period in women who regained ≥2 kg body mass. $n = 54$ at 5 mo after the intervention and at the 6-mo follow-up; $n = 44$ at the 12-mo follow-up. (Reprinted from Beavers KM, Lyles MF, Davis CC, et al. Is lost lean mass from intentional weight loss recovered during weight regain in postmenopausal women? *Am J Clin Nutr.* 2011;94:767-774, with permission from American Society for Nutrition.)

some 8 kg of fat and 3.7 kg of lean tissue. Over the subsequent 12 months, the only intervention was from a dietician, who provided 1 counseling session. However, the group members were said to be highly motivated. Nevertheless, about a third of the initial weight loss was regained (3.7 kg), more of this being fat than lean tissue (Fig 2). The typical patient history of frequent bouts of dieting and "weight cycling" may thus lead to a progressive sarcopenic obesity. It would be interesting to see how far this undesirable situation could be avoided through a combination of a high-protein diet and deliberate resistance training during the period that follows a bout of dieting.

R. J. Shephard, MD (Lond), PhD, DPE

Reference

1. McGuire MT, Wing RR, Hill JO. The prevalence of weight loss maintenance among American adults. *Int J Obes Relat Metab Disord.* 1999;23:1314-1319.

Overweight Adults May Have the Lowest Mortality—Do They Have the Best Health?

Zajacova A, Dowd JB, Burgard SA (Univ of Wyoming, Laramie; City Univ of New York; Univ of Michigan, Ann Arbor)
Am J Epidemiol 173:430-437, 2011

Numerous recent studies have found that overweight adults experience lower overall mortality than those who are underweight, normal-weight, or obese. These highly publicized findings imply that overweight may be the optimal weight category for overall health via its association with longevity—a conclusion with important public health implications. In this study, the authors examined the association between body mass index (BMI; (weight (kg)/height (m)^2)) and 3 markers of health risks using a nationally representative sample of US adults aged 20–80 years ($n = 9,255$) from the National Health and Nutrition Examination Survey (2005–2008). Generalized additive models, a type of semiparametric regression model, were used to examine the relations between BMI and biomarkers of inflammation, metabolic function, and cardiovascular function (C-reactive protein, hemoglobin A$_{1c}$, and high density lipoprotein cholesterol, respectively). The association between BMI and each biomarker was monotonic, with higher BMI being consistently associated with worse health risk profiles at all ages, in contrast to the U-shaped relation between BMI and mortality. Prior results

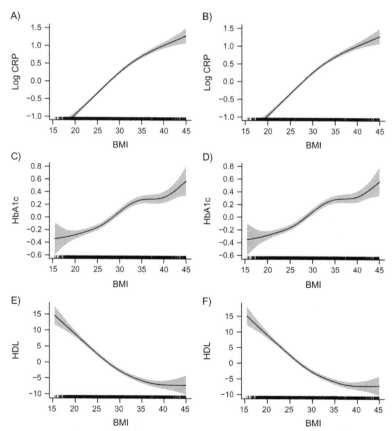

FIGURE 1.—Relations between body mass index (BMI; weight (kg)/height (m)^2) and selected biomarkers for men, National Health and Nutrition Examination Survey, 2005–2008. Results were adjusted for age only (left column) and for age plus smoking (right column). The first row (plots A and B) shows relations between BMI and C-reactive protein (CRP); the second row (plots C and D) shows relations between BMI and hemoglobin A$_{1c}$ (HbA1c); and the third row (plots E and F) show relations between BMI and high density lipoprotein cholesterol (HDL). The solid lines represent the estimated relation, and the shaded areas represent the 95% confidence interval. (Reprinted from Zajacova A, Dowd JB, Burgard SA. Overweight adults may have the lowest mortality—do they have the best health? *Am J Epidemiol.* 2011;173:430-437, with permission from Oxford University Press.)

suggesting that the overweight BMI category corresponds to the lowest risk of mortality may not be generalizable to indicators of health risk (Fig 1).

▶ The conventional wisdom on which most public health recommendations are based is that the optimal body mass index (BMI) of an adult lies in the range of 20 to 25 kg/m^2. The main foundation for this belief is a large study of North American Insurance data conducted by Dr Reuben Andres.[1] His data showed that the ratio of actual to expected mortality was lowest for those individuals with a "normal" body mass. He confirmed this trend for men in all age groups from 20 to 29 to 60 to 69 years and for most causes of death except suicide and pulmonary conditions, where optima were seen in the "overweight" range (25-30 kg/m^2). Limitations to his findings were sample selection (those choosing to purchase life insurance), an inability to distinguish between lean tissue and body fat, and reliance on reported values for the individual's height and body mass (the latter often being 2 kg or so less than the true body mass). Given that most of the North American population is now either overweight or obese (BMI > 30 kg/m^2), great popular interest was aroused by some more recent reports suggesting that mortality was no higher (and in some studies lower) for those who were overweight rather than of normal body mass.[2-7] Possibly, the relationship changes if observations continue into advanced age. A slightly greater body mass might be advantageous to survival into the oldest age categories, implying that the person concerned had a greater initial body mass (and thus a slower onset of sarcopenia and osteoporosis[8]) and/or a greater amount of body fat (which could boost androgen production in old age). In this article, Zajacova and associates emphasize that health experience during a person's lifespan is more important than simple longevity. There have been previous suggestions that those who are overweight have a poorer health experience than those with a normal body mass.[9,10] In this study, 3 biologic markers of health status offer good evidence that health status is poorer in those who are overweight than in those whose body mass falls in the normal range (Fig 1).

R. J. Shephard, MD (Lond), PhD, DPE

References

1. Andres R. Discussion: assessment of health status. In: Bouchard C, et al., eds. *Exercise, Fitness and Health*. Champaign, IL: Human Kinetics; 1990:133-136.
2. Troiano RP, Frongillo EA Jr, Sobal J, Levitsky DA. The relationship between body weight and mortality: a quantitative analysis of combined information from existing studies. *Int J Obes Relat Metab Disord*. 1996;20:63-75.
3. McGee DL, The Diverse Populations Collaboration. Body mass index and mortality. a meta-analysis based on person-level data from twenty-six observational studies. *Ann Epidemiol*. 2005;15:87-97.
4. Berraho M, Nejjari C, Raherison C, et al. Body mass index, disability, and 13-year mortality in older French adults. *J Aging Health*. 2010;22:68-83.
5. Janssen I. Morbidity and mortality risk associated with an overweight BMI in older men and women. *Obesity (Silver Spring)*. 2007;15:1827-1840.
6. Flegal KM, Graubard BI, Williamson DF, Gail MH. Cause-specific excess deaths associated with underweight, overweight, and obesity. *JAMA*. 2007;298:2028-2037.
7. Flicker L, McCaul KA, Hankey GJ, et al. Body mass index and survival in men and women aged 70 to 75. *J Am Geriatr Soc*. 2010;58:234-241.

8. Greenberg JA, Fontaine K, Allison DB. Putative biases in estimating mortality attributable to obesity in the US population. *Int J Obes (Lond)*. 2007;31: 1449-1455.

9. Must A, Spadano J, Coakley EH, Field AE, Colditz G, Dietz WH. The disease burden associated with overweight and obesity. *JAMA*. 1999;282:1523-1529.

10. Katz DA, McHorney CA, Atkinson RL. Impact of obesity on health-related quality of life in patients with chronic illness. *J Gen Intern Med*. 2000;15: 789-796.

Physical activity and gain in abdominal adiposity and body weight: prospective cohort study in 288,498 men and women
Ekelund U, Besson H, Luan J, et al (Inst of Metabolic Science, Cambridge, UK; et al)
Am J Clin Nutr 93:826-835, 2011

Background.—The protective effect of physical activity (PA) on abdominal adiposity is unclear.

Objective.—We examined whether PA independently predicted gains in body weight and abdominal adiposity.

Design.—In a prospective cohort study [the EPIC (European Prospective Investigation into Cancer and Nutrition)], we followed 84,511 men and 203,987 women for 5.1 y. PA was assessed by a validated questionnaire, and individuals were categorized into 4 groups (inactive, moderately inactive, moderately active, and active). Body weight and waist circumference were measured at baseline and self-reported at follow-up. We used multilevel mixed-effects linear regression models and stratified our analyses by sex with adjustments for age, smoking status, alcohol consumption, educational level, total energy intake, duration of follow-up, baseline body weight, change in body weight, and waist circumference (when applicable).

Results.—PA significantly predicted a lower waist circumference (in cm) in men ($\beta = -0.045$; 95% CI: -0.057, -0.034) and in women ($\beta = -0.035$; 95% CI: -0.056, -0.015) independent of baseline body weight, baseline waist circumference, and other confounding factors. The magnitude of associations was materially unchanged after adjustment for change in body weight. PA was not significantly associated with annual weight gain (in kg) in men ($\beta = -0.008$; 95% CI: -0.02, 0.003) and women ($\beta = -0.01$; 95% CI: -0.02, 0.0006). The odds of becoming obese were reduced by 7% ($P < 0.001$) and 10% ($P < 0.001$) for a one-category difference in baseline PA in men and women, respectively.

Conclusion.—Our results suggest that a higher level of PA reduces abdominal adiposity independent of baseline and changes in body weight and is thus a useful strategy for preventing chronic diseases and premature deaths (Table 3).

▶ Many nutritionists still maintain that physical activity has little role in the control of obesity. They point to the substantial distance that must be walked to metabolize a few grams of fat, ignoring the fact that the obesity has

TABLE 3.—Subgroup Analysis Stratified by Baseline BMI Status for the Prospective Associations Between Baseline Physical Activity and Annual Change in Waist Circumference in European Men and Women[1]

	β Coefficient (95% CI)	P for Linear Trend
Men		
Normal weight ($n = 12,439$)	−0.044 (−0.062, −0.026)	<0.001
Overweight ($n = 17,406$)	−0.047 (−0.062, −0.031)	<0.001
Obese ($n = 4298$)	−0.047 (−0.084, −0.009)	0.015
All ($n = 34,143$)	−0.045 (−0.057, −0.034)	<0.001
Women		
Normal weight ($n = 25,740$)	−0.034 (−0.062, −0.006)	0.018
Overweight ($n = 16,215$)	−0.040 (−0.061, −0.019)	0.0002
Obese ($n = 6106$)	−0.051 (−0.089, −0.013)	0.0079
All ($n = 48,061$)	−0.035 (−0.056, −0.015)	0.0008

[1]β Coefficients and 95% CIs (cm/y) are for comparisons of effects between one category and the adjacent category for overall physical activity (eg, from inactive to moderately inactive). Data were analyzed by mixed-effects linear regression. Average physical activity energy expenditures measured by the individually calibrated combined heart rate and movement sensing in an independent validation study ($n = 1941$) across categories of physical activity in men and women, respectively, were as follows: inactive (38.1 and 39.2 kJ · kg^{-1} · d^1), moderately inactive (47.5 and 39.9 kJ · kg^{-1} · d^{-1}), moderately active (48.5 and 44.7 kJ · kg^{-1} · d^{-1}), and active (56.8 and 49.3 kJ · kg^{-1} · d^{-1}).

developed over 10 to 20 years, rather than a few weeks. They also point to the limited benefit of physical activity as seen in controlled trials, again ignoring that most of these have been conducted for only 10 to 12 weeks, often evaluating success from changes in body mass (and ignoring the ability of a well-designed exercise program to convert fat into muscle tissue of similar weight). Against such nay-saying, I would point to the membership of the American College of Sports Medicine. Here is a group committed to physical activity, and there is scarcely a fat person among their 15 000 + members. It is hard to imagine that every member of this organization is inherently thinner than the rest of North American society; rather, we are looking at the effects of sustained physical activity. Previous population studies have found a weak relationship between habitual activity and body mass index.[1,2] The study of Ekelund and associates is based on a massive European trial that has followed 84 511 men and 203 987 women in 10 countries for an average of 5.1 years. It has for the first time related self-selected habitual physical activity (assessed by a validated questionnaire) to that most critical component of body fat—abdominal fat[3-5]—as seen in the waist circumference, after allowing for baseline values and a variety of potentially confounding variables. The nature and duration of activity were used to categorize participants into 4 activity groups. Over the 5 years, waist circumference increased by an average of 32 mm in men and 63 mm in women. However, irrespective of initial obesity, the gain in waist circumference was negatively associated with the reported level of physical activity (Table 3). This study supports the public health benefits of an increase in population activity; although absolute benefits of greater physical activity as imputed to the 5-year period were not large, this is probably due in part to difficulties in assessing physical activity from simple questionnaires.

R. J. Shephard, MD (Lond), PhD, DPE

References

1. Summerbell CD, Douthwaite W, Whittaker V, et al. The association between diet and physical activity and subsequent excess weight gain and obesity assessed at 5 years of age or older: a systematic review of the epidemiological evidence. *Int J Obes (Lond)*. 2009;33:S1-92.
2. Lee IM, Djoussé L, Sesso HD, Wang L, Buring JE. Physical activity and weight gain prevention. *JAMA*. 2010;303:1173-1179.
3. Wang Y, Rimm EB, Stampfer MJ, Willett WC, Hu FB. Comparison of abdominal adiposity and overall obesity in predicting risk of type 2 diabetes among men. *Am J Clin Nutr*. 2005;81:555-563.
4. Yusuf S, Hawken S, Ounpuu S, et al. Obesity and the risk of myocardial infarction in 27,000 participants from 52 countries: a case-control study. *Lancet*. 2005;366: 1640-1649.
5. Pischon T, Boeing H, Hoffmann K, et al. General and abdominal adiposity and risk of death in Europe. *N Engl J Med*. 2008;359:2105-2120.

Startup Circuit Training Program Reduces Metabolic Risk in Latino Adolescents
Davis JN, Gyllenhammer LE, Vanni AA, et al (Univ of Southern California, Los Angeles, CA)
Med Sci Sports Exerc 43:2195-2203, 2011

Purpose.—This study aimed to test the effects of a circuit training (CT; aerobic + strength training) program, with and without motivational interviewing (MI) behavioral therapy, on reducing adiposity and type 2 diabetes risk factors in Latina teenagers.

Methods.—Thirty-eight Latina adolescents (15.8 ± 1.1 yr) who are overweight/obese were randomly assigned to control (C; $n = 12$), CT ($n = 14$), or CT + MI ($n = 12$). The CT classes were held twice a week (60−90 min) for 16 wk. The CT + MI group also received individual or group MI sessions every other week. The following were measured before and after intervention: strength by one-repetition maximum; cardiorespiratory fitness ($\dot{V}O_{2max}$) by submaximal treadmill test; physical activity by accelerometry; dietary intake by records; height, weight, waist circumference; total body composition by dual-energy x-ray absorptiometry; visceral adipose tissue, subcutaneous adipose tissue, and hepatic fat fraction by magnetic resonance imaging; and glucose/insulin indices by fasting blood draw. Across-intervention group effects were tested using repeated-measures ANOVA with *post hoc* pairwise comparisons.

Results.—CT and CT + MI participants, compared with controls, significantly increased fitness (+16% and +15% vs −6%, $P = 0.03$) and leg press (+40% vs +20%, $P = 0.007$). Compared with controls, CT participants also decreased waist circumference (−3% vs +3%; $P < 0.001$), subcutaneous adipose tissue (−10% vs 8%, $P = 0.04$), visceral adipose tissue (−10% vs +6%, $P = 0.05$), fasting insulin (−24% vs +6%, $P = 0.03$), and insulin resistance (−21% vs −4%, $P = 0.05$).

Conclusions.—CT may be an effective starter program to reduce fat depots and improve insulin resistance in Latino youth who are overweight/obese, whereas the additional MI therapy showed no additive effect on these health outcomes.

▶ Most studies examining the health benefits of physical activity in children and youth have focused on aerobic-type exercises.[1] Fewer studies have examined resistance-type exercise, and the results from those studies suggest that resistance exercise does not provide the same benefits for most health outcomes (not bone density) as the same duration of aerobic exercise.[1] Fewer studies yet have examined circuit-type training, which if proved effective may be an attractive alternative for some youngsters.

This study tested the effectiveness of a 16-week circuit training (CT, aerobic + strength training) program on reducing adiposity and type 2 diabetes risk factors in Latina teenagers. CT classes were held twice a week, and each session lasted from 60 to 90 minutes. Given that current public health guidelines for physical activity in school-aged youth call for 60 or more minutes of activity on a daily basis, the dose of exercise prescribed in this program was quite modest. Compared with the control group, participants who received CT had significant improvement in cardiorespiratory fitness (approximately 20% difference), muscle strength (approximately 20% difference), visceral fat (approximately 16% difference), and insulin resistance (17% difference). Thus, the CT program was efficacious at improving cardiometabolic risk factors. What remains unclear is whether such programs are as beneficial as a similar volume of aerobic exercise alone and whether they are effective and not just efficacious, that is, this and other randomized controlled exercise trials of the pediatric population do not perform intent-to-treat analyses and they therefore test efficacy and not effectiveness. This is a major flaw. The samples in such studies also tend to be very small, and the results are not generalizable. These studies suffer from other important limitations (eg, do not report adverse events, do not include a priori power calculations) that would be unacceptable in many other disciplines (eg, pharmacological trials). This should not be interpreted as a criticism of this study per se. Rather, this should be interpreted as a rant by this reviewer and a call to others in the pediatric exercise science community to be aware of such methodological issues and to learn from this and design better exercise trials in the future.

I. Janssen, PhD

Reference

1. Janssen I, LeBlanc AG. Systematic review of the health benefits of physical activity and fitness in school-aged children and youth. *Int J Behav Nutr Phys Act.* 2010;7:40.

Separate and combined associations of body-mass index and abdominal adiposity with cardiovascular disease: collaborative analysis of 58 prospective studies
The Emerging Risk Factors Collaboration (Univ of Cambridge, UK; et al)
Lancet 377:1085-1095, 2011

Background.—Guidelines differ about the value of assessment of adiposity measures for cardiovascular disease risk prediction when information is available for other risk factors. We studied the separate and combined associations of body-mass index (BMI), waist circumference, and waist-to-hip ratio with risk of first-onset cardiovascular disease.

Methods.—We used individual records from 58 cohorts to calculate hazard ratios (HRs) per 1 SD higher baseline values (4·56 kg/m^2 higher BMI, 12·6 cm higher waist circumference, and 0·083 higher waist-to-hip ratio) and measures of risk discrimination and reclassification. Serial adiposity assessments were used to calculate regression dilution ratios.

Results.—Individual records were available for 221 934 people in 17 countries (14 297 incident cardiovascular disease outcomes; 1·87 million person-years at risk). Serial adiposity assessments were made in up to 63 821 people (mean interval 5·7 years [SD 3·9]). In people with BMI of 20 kg/m^2 or higher, HRs for cardiovascular disease were 1·23 (95% CI 1·17—1·29) with BMI, 1·27 (1·20—1·33) with waist circumference, and 1·25 (1·19—1·31) with waist-to-hip ratio, after adjustment for age, sex, and smoking status. After further adjustment for baseline systolic blood pressure, history of diabetes, and total and HDL cholesterol, corresponding HRs were 1·07 (1·03—1·11) with BMI, 1·10 (1·05—1·14) with waist circumference, and 1·12 (1·08—1·15) with waist-to-hip ratio. Addition of information on BMI, waist circumference, or waist-to-hip ratio to a cardiovascular disease risk prediction model containing conventional risk factors did not importantly improve risk discrimination (C-index changes of −0·0001, −0·0001, and 0·0008, respectively), nor classification of participants to categories of predicted 10-year risk (net reclassification improvement −0·19%, −0·05%, and −0·05%, respectively). Findings were similar when adiposity measures were considered in combination. Reproducibility was greater for BMI (regression dilution ratio 0·95, 95% CI 0·93—0·97) than for waist circumference (0·86, 0·83—0·89) or waist-to-hip ratio (0·63, 0·57—0·70).

Interpretation.—BMI, waist circumference, and waist-to-hip ratio, whether assessed singly or in combination, do not importantly improve cardiovascular disease risk prediction in people in developed countries when additional information is available for systolic blood pressure, history of diabetes, and lipids.

▶ This is a massive prospective trial, based on a synthesis of 58 trials and involving 221 934 people. After adjusting for age, sex, and smoking habits, the association of 10-year cardiovascular risk with either body mass index (BMI) or waist circumference is relatively weak, and after addition of information on systolic blood pressure, history of diabetes, total and high-density lipoprotein cholesterol, the risk attributable to either of these markers of adiposity was negligible (Table 2 in the original article). The inference is that laboratories with limited resources cannot substitute BMI for the measurement of cholesterol levels when assessing cardiovascular risk. Perhaps because of problems in measuring it accurately, waist circumference was no better than BMI. It would be interesting to test the effect of other simple measures of obesity, such as skinfold readings, to see whether they also add little to the prediction of cardiovascular risks.

R. J. Shephard, MD (Lond), PhD, DPE

The Effect of Time-of-Day and Ramadan Fasting on Anaerobic Performances
Chtourou H, Hammouda O, Chaouachi A, et al (Natl Ctr of Medicine and Science in Sports (CNMSS), Tunis, Tunisia)
Int J Sports Med 33:142-147, 2012

This study was designed to assess the effects of Ramadan-intermittent-fasting (RIF) and time-of-day on muscle power and fatigue during the Wingate test. In a randomized design, 10 football players completed a Wingate test at 07:00 and 17:00 h on 3 different occasions: one week before Ramadan (BR), the second week of Ramadan (SWR) and the fourth week of Ramadan (ER). There was an interval of 36-h between any 2 successive tests. During the Wingate test, peak power (PP), mean power (MP) and the fatigue index (FI) were recorded. While PP, MP and FI were greater in the evening than in the morning during BR ($p < 0.001$), these diurnal variations in muscle power disappeared during the month of Ramadan (i.e., SWR and ER) due to a significant decrease in PP and MP in the evening ($p < 0.001$). However, the diurnal variation in FI when measured at 17:00 h increased during this month ($p < 0.001$). In addition, ratings of perceived exertion and fatigue were higher in the evening during Ramadan in comparison with BR. These results suggest that Ramadan might modify the circadian rhythm of muscle power and fatigue during the Wingate test by decreasing power output and increasing muscle fatigue at the time of the acrophase (Fig 3).

▶ The 2012 Olympic competitions will occur during the month of Ramadan, and, with an increasing world population of Muslim athletes, the impact of Ramadan observance on their physical performance is attracting growing attention. The main adverse effect of this form of intermittent fasting (from sunrise to sunset) is probably because of the absence of fluid intake during daylight hours, although the need to eat the day's nutrient requirements during the hours of darkness sometimes causes loss of sleep, disturbances of mood state, and alterations in the type and amounts of food consumed.[1,2] Empirical reports on changes of performance during the month of Ramadan have been conflicting, and this may reflect the season of the year when Ramadan occurs, the type of event evaluated, and the time of day at which measurements were made. In most events, a loss of performance is most likely to be observed during the period

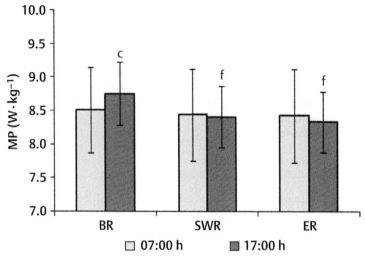

FIGURE 3.—MP (W·kg^{-1}) (mean ± SD) recorded during the Wingate test at 07:00 and 17:00 h during BR, SWR and ER. ^{c}: significant difference between 07:00 and 17:00 h (p < 0.001); ^{f}: significant difference in comparison with BR (p < 0.001). (Reprinted from Chtourou H, Hammouda O, Chaouachi A, et al. The effect of time-of-day and Ramadan fasting on anaerobic performances. *Int J Sports Med*. 2012;33:142-147, with permission from Thieme Medical Publishers, Inc.)

immediately before sunset,[3] and, indeed in Arab countries, it is common practice during Ramadan to rearrange schedules to avoid competing during the late afternoon or early evening. The present study demonstrates an impact of Ramadan observance on the performance of junior football players, with no control group. Observations were made during August, although presumably in Tunisia, where summer daylight hours are shorter than in London. There was little change in overall food intake over Ramadan, and the morning power output on the Wingate test was virtually unchanged. However, the evening performance was substantially worsened, with accompanying increased ratings of fatigue (but no other changes) on the profile of mood states and higher ratings of perceived exertion (Fig 3). The underlying mechanisms remain unclear, but a reduction of muscle carbohydrate reserves seems likely to have been one factor.[4,5] This could be explored by muscle biopsy, but, for the forthcoming Olympics, the recommendation for those athletes who wish to observe Ramadan may be to increase the carbohydrate content of their diet.

R. J. Shephard, MD (Lond), PhD, DPE

References

1. Chaouachi A, Leiper JB, Souissi N, Coutts AJ, Chamari K. Effects of Ramadan intermittent fasting on sports performance and training: a review. *Int J Sports Physiol Perform*. 2009;4:419-434.
2. Waterhouse J. Effects of Ramadan on physical performance: chronobiological considerations. *Br J Sports Med*. 2010;44:509-515.
3. Souissi N, Souissi H, Sahli S, et al. Effect of Ramadan on the diurnal variation in short-term high power output. *Chronobiol Int*. 2007;24:991-1007.

4. Ramadan J. Does fasting during Ramadan alter body composition, blood constituents and physical performance? *Med Princ Pract.* 2002;2:41-46.
5. el Ati J, Beji C, Danguir J. Increased fat oxidation during Ramadan fasting in healthy women: an adaptive mechanism for body-weight maintenance. *Am J Clin Nutr.* 1995;62:302-307.

Continuous glucose monitoring system during physical exercise in adolescents with type 1 diabetes
Adolfsson P, Nilsson S, Lindblad B (Univ of Gothenburg, Göteborg, Sweden; Chalmers Univ of Technology, Göteborg, Sweden)
Acta Paediatr 100:1603-1609, 2011

Aim.—Continuous glucose monitoring system (CGMS) provides detailed information on glucose fluctuations. The aim was to establish whether CGMS could be used during physical exercise and whether it detects more episodes of hypoglycaemia and hyperglycaemia than frequent blood glucose measurements.

Methods.—Adolescents with type 1 diabetes (12 girls and 47 boys) participated in three annual sports camps that lasted for 3—4 days and included different types of exercise: soccer, floorball + cross-country skiing and golf. During the study, blood glucose values, mean 8.7 ± 3.3 per day, were obtained with Hemocue in parallel with the CGMS.

Results.—Ninety-eight per cent of the participants used the sensor at all times during the camps. Eighty-seven per cent of the sensors gave adequate signals for 24 h and 66% for 48 h. Median durations of hypoglycaemia and hyperglycaemia were 1.7 h per day and 3.8 h per day, respectively. The CGMS identified significantly more episodes of hypoglycaemia (p < 0.005) and hyperglycaemia (p < 0.005) during the day and night than frequent blood glucose tests.

Conclusion.—We demonstrate that, even during days that included episodic strenuous physical exercise, CGMS could provide useful information on glucose fluctuations during day and night, albeit with significant failure rates (Table 2).

▶ A fear of inducing hypoglycemia is a strong negative motivational influence to sports participation in children with type 1 diabetes mellitus.[1,2] Moreover, a fear of hypoglycemia may contribute to high HbAc1 levels.[3] Repeated testing of blood sugar (> 4-5 times/day) is associated with lower HbAc1 levels,[4] but it is difficult to undertake such repeated testing during prolonged bouts of physical activity. Adolfsson and associates thus examined the practicality of using a continuous monitoring system (a device by Medtronic that samples subcutaneous glucose concentrations every 10 seconds). Results were compared with Hemocue estimates of glucose concentrations in capillary blood. The subjects included a substantial sample of adolescents attending a sports camp where they participated in various vigorous activities, including contact sports. Despite the vigor of these pursuits, 87% of sensors functioned well for 24 hours and

TABLE 2.—Number of Hyperglycaemic (>10 mmol/L) and Hypoglycaemic (<3.9 mmol/L) Events Per Individual and 24 h Detected by Blood Glucose (BG) and the Continuous Glucose Monitoring System (CGMS) During Three Sports Camps. Day = 08.00—24.00, Night = 24.00—08.00. Values are Given as Mean ± SD

Event	Camp	Day BG	Day CGMS	p	Night BG	Night CGMS	p
Hyperglycaemia (>10 mmol/L)	Soccer	2.4 ± 2.2	3.0 ± 2.0	ns	0.6 ± 0.6	0.9 ± 1.1	ns
	Floorball/Cross-country skiing	1.6 ± 1.4	3.3 ± 2.7	<0.005	0.2 ± 0.4	0.8 ± 0.9	<0.005
	Golf	1.8 ± 1.7	2.7 ± 1.9	<0.05	0.6 ± 0.8	0.8 ± 0.9	ns
	All camps aggregated	1.9 ± 1.8	3.0 ± 2.3	<0.005	0.5 ± 0.7	0.8 ± 0.9	<0.005
Hypoglycaemia (<3.9 mmol/L)	Soccer	1.3 ± 1.3	1.9 ± 1.8	<0.05	0.4 ± 0.6	0.8 ± 1.1	<0.05
	Floorball/Cross-country skiing	1.2 ± 1.1	2.5 ± 2.6	<0.005	0.1 ± 0.3	1.1 ± 1.6	<0.005
	Golf	1.5 ± 1.7	2.7 ± 2.2	<0.005	0.3 ± 0.5	0.9 ± 1.3	<0.005
	All camps aggregated	1.3 ± 1.4	2.4 ± 2.2	<0.005	0.2 ± 0.5	0.9 ± 1.4	<0.005

66% for 48 hours, with about a half of failures reflecting disconnection due to sweating and a loosening of tapes and the other half simply ceasing to function. The continuous monitor provided a better indication of both hyper- and hypo-glycemia than the spot checks of blood glucose for all of the sports examined (Table 2). The findings with the continuous monitor are sufficiently positive to negate warnings not to use this or similar equipment during exercise.[5-7] At the same time it must be acknowledged that subcutaneous data may not fully reflect rapidly changing blood glucose levels, particularly when subcutaneous blood flow is limited; there is probably a 10- to 20-minute lag between blood and subcutaneous readings.

R. J. Shephard, MD (Lond), PhD, DPE

References

1. Temple MY, Bar-Or O, Riddell MC. The reliability and repeatability of the blood glucose response to prolonged exercise in adolescent boys with IDDM. *Diabetes Care.* 1995;18:326-332.
2. Riddell MC, Perkins BA. Type 1 diabetes and vigorous exercise. Applications of exercise physiology to patient management. *Can J Diabetes.* 2006;30:63-71.
3. Nordfeldt S, Ludvigsson J. Fear and other disturbances of severe hypoglucaemia in children and adolescents with type 1 diabetes mellitus. *J Pediatr Endocrinol Metab.* 2005;18:83-91.
4. Haller MJ, Stalvey MS, Silverstein JH. Predictors of control of diabetes: monitoring may be the key. *J Pediatr.* 2004;144:660-661.
5. MiniMed CGMS. Continuous Glucose Monitoring System, Guidebook, GMP9190047—011C, 5/99. Medtronics, Northridge, CA.
6. Nunnold T, Colberg SR, Herriot MT, Somma CT. Use of noninvasive GlucoWatch Biographer during exercise of varying intensity. *Diabetes Technol Ther.* 2004;6:454-462.
7. Fayolle C, Brun JF, Bringer J, Mercier J, Renard E. Accuracy of continuous subcutaneous glucose monitoring with the GlucoDay in type 1 diabetic patients treated by subcutaneous insulin infusion during exercise of low versus high intensity. *Diabetes Metab.* 2006;32:313-320.

Physical Activity Advice Only or Structured Exercise Training and Association With HbA₁c Levels in Type 2 Diabetes: A Systematic Review and Meta-analysis

Umpierre D, Ribeiro PAB, Kramer CK, et al (Hosp de Clínicas de Porto Alegre, Brazil; et al)

JAMA 305:1790-1799, 2011

Context.—Regular exercise improves glucose control in diabetes, but the association of different exercise training interventions on glucose control is unclear.

Objective.—To conduct a systematic review and meta-analysis of randomized controlled clinical trials (RCTs) assessing associations of structured exercise training regimens (aerobic, resistance, or both) and physical activity advice with or without dietary cointervention on change in hemoglobin A_{1c} (HbA$_{1c}$) in type 2 diabetes patients.

Data Sources.—MEDLINE, Cochrane-CENTRAL, EMBASE, Clinical Trials.gov, LILACS, and SPORTDiscus databases were searched from January 1980 through February 2011.

Study Selection.—RCTs of at least 12 weeks' duration that evaluated the ability of structured exercise training or physical activity advice to lower HbA$_{1c}$ levels as compared with a control group in patients with type 2 diabetes.

Data Extraction.—Two independent reviewers extracted data and assessed quality of the included studies.

Data Synthesis.—Of 4191 articles retrieved, 47 RCTs (8538 patients) were included. Pooled mean differences in HbA$_{1c}$ levels between intervention and control groups were calculated using a random-effects model. Overall, structured exercise training (23 studies) was associated with a decline in HbA$_{1c}$ level (-0.67%; 95% confidence interval [CI], -0.84% to -0.49%; I^2, 91.3%) compared with control participants. In addition, structured aerobic exercise (-0.73%; 95% CI, -1.06% to -0.40%; I^2, 92.8%), structured resistance training (-0.57%; 95% CI, -1.14% to -0.01%; I^2, 92.5%), and both combined (-0.51%; 95% CI, -0.79% to -0.23%; I^2, 67.5%) were each associated with declines in HbA$_{1c}$ levels compared with control participants. Structured exercise durations of more than 150 minutes per week were associated with HbA$_{1c}$ reductions of 0.89%, while structured exercise durations of 150 minutes or less per week were associated with HbA$_{1c}$ reductions of 0.36%. Overall, interventions of physical activity advice (24 studies) were associated with lower HbA$_{1c}$ levels (-0.43%; 95% CI, -0.59% to -0.28%; I^2, 62.9%) compared with control participants. Combined physical activity advice and dietary advice was associated with decreased HbA$_{1c}$ (-0.58%; 95% CI, -0.74% to -0.43%; I^2, 57.5%) as compared with control participants. Physical activity advice alone was not associated with HbA$_{1c}$ changes.

Conclusions.—Structured exercise training that consists of aerobic exercise, resistance training, or both combined is associated with HbA$_{1c}$ reduction in patients with type 2 diabetes. Structured exercise training of more than 150 minutes per week is associated with greater HbA$_{1c}$ declines than that of 150 minutes or less per week. Physical activity advice is associated with lower HbA$_{1c}$, but only when combined with dietary advice.

▶ With the current emphasis on "evidence-based" practice, many accepted facets of treatment are being exposed to the scrutiny of exhaustive meta-analyses. Umpierre and colleagues have conducted such an analysis to examine the effectiveness of various forms of exercise[1,2] in the treatment of type 2 diabetes mellitus, using reductions in the patient's hemoglobin A1c as the marker of successful therapy. The standard lifestyle advice is at present similar to that offered to the general population: take at least 150 minutes of moderate aerobic exercise per week, supplementing this by resistance exercise on 3 days per week. Two large recent trials have reached conflicting conclusions concerning such a recommendation. One study found benefit from either aerobic or resistance activity, but the best results were seen with a combination of the 2 modalities.[3] The second report found benefit only when a combination of the 2 types of exercise was adopted.[4] Less is known about the value of medical advice to exercise more, and one of the important objectives of Umpierre and colleagues was to compare such advice with structured physical activity undertaken in a formal exercise class. The meta-analysis seems to have been conducted carefully, and a large number of patients (8538) were finally accepted. The benefit seen with structured physical activity was similar across all 3 types of classes (aerobic, resistance, or both types of exercise [Fig 1 in the original article]), with the new finding of greater benefit if classes provided more than 150 minutes of exercise per week. The mean response, a decrease in hemoglobin A1c of 0.67%, compared favorably with the benefits obtained from addition of noninsulin antidiabetic drugs to maximal metformin therapy.[5] In contrast, medical advice to become more active had only minor benefit unless it was accompanied by dieting, a finding reiterated in a recent randomized control trial from Italy.[6] There are 2 comments on the apparent need for structured activities. First, many of the formal classes were of only 12 weeks' duration, and it is less clear how effective they would have remained over a longer term. Second, classes probably included dietary advice, and this may have accounted for a fair part of the benefit that was observed.

R. J. Shephard, MD (Lond), PhD, DPE

References

1. American Diabetes Association. Standards of medical care in diabetes—2011. *Diabetes Care.* 2011;34:S11-S61.
2. Colberg SR, Sigal RJ, Fernhall B, et al. American College of Sports Medicine, American Diabetes Association. Exercise and type 2 diabetes: the American College of Sports Medicine and the American Diabetes Association: joint position statement. *Diabetes Care.* 2010;33:e147-e167.
3. Sigal RJ, Kenny GP, Boulé NG, et al. Effects of aerobic training, resistance training, or both on glycemic control in type 2 diabetes: a randomized trial. *Ann Intern Med.* 2007;147:357-369.
4. Church TS, Blair SN, Cocreham S, et al. Effects of aerobic and resistance training on hemoglobin A1c levels in patients with type 2 diabetes: a randomized controlled trial. *JAMA.* 2010;304:2253-2262.

5. Phung OJ, Scholle JM, Talwar M, Coleman CI. Effect of noninsulin antidiabetic drugs added to metformin therapy on glycemic control, weight gain, and hypoglycemia in type 2 diabetes. *JAMA*. 2010;303:1410-1418.
6. Balducci S, Zanuso S, Nicolucci A, et al. Italian Diabetes Exercise Study (IDES) Investigators. Effect of an intensive exercise intervention strategy on modifiable cardiovascular risk factors in subjects with type 2 diabetes mellitus: a randomized controlled trial: the Italian Diabetes and Exercise Study (IDES). *Arch Intern Med.* 2010;170:1794-1803.

Physical Activity Advice Only or Structured Exercise Training and Association With HbA$_{1c}$ Levels in Type 2 Diabetes: A Systematic Review and Meta-analysis

Umpierre D, Ribeiro PAB, Kramer CK, et al (Hospital de Clínicas de Porto Alegre, Brazil; et al)
JAMA 305:1790-1799, 2011

Context.—Regular exercise improves glucose control in diabetes, but the association of different exercise training interventions on glucose control is unclear.

Objective.—To conduct a systematic review and meta-analysis of randomized controlled clinical trials (RCTs) assessing associations of structured exercise training regimens (aerobic, resistance, or both) and physical activity advice with or without dietary cointervention on change in hemoglobin A$_{1c}$ (HbA$_{1c}$) in type 2 diabetes patients.

Data Sources.—MEDLINE, Cochrane-CENTRAL, EMBASE, Clinical Trials.gov, LILACS, and SPORTDiscus databases were searched from January 1980 through February 2011.

Study Selection.—RCTs of at least 12 weeks' duration that evaluated the ability of structured exercise training or physical activity advice to lower HbA$_{1c}$ levels as compared with a control group in patients with type 2 diabetes.

Data Extraction.—Two independent reviewers extracted data and assessed quality of the included studies.

Data Synthesis.—Of 4191 articles retrieved, 47 RCTs (8538 patients) were included. Pooled mean differences in HbA$_{1c}$ levels between intervention and control groups were calculated using a random-effects model. Overall, structured exercise training (23 studies) was associated with a decline in HbA$_{1c}$ level (−0.67%; 95% confidence interval [CI], −0.84% to −0.49%; I^2, 91.3%) compared with control participants. In addition, structured aerobic exercise (−0.73%; 95% CI, −1.06% to −0.40%; I^2, 92.8%), structured resistance training (−0.57%; 95% CI, −1.14% to −0.01%; I^2, 92.5%), and both combined (−0.51%; 95% CI, −0.79% to −0.23%; I^2, 67.5%) were each associated with declines in HbA$_{1C}$ levels compared with control participants. Structured exercise durations of more than 150 minutes per week were associated with HbA1c reductions of 0.89%, while structured exercise durations of 150 minutes or less per week were associated with HbA$_{1C}$ reductions of 0.36%. Overall, interventions of physical activity advice (24 studies) were associated with lower HbA_{1c} levels (-0.43%; 95% CI, -0.59% to -0.28%; I^2, 62.9%) compared with control participants. Combined physical activity advice and dietary advice was associated with decreased HbA_{1c} (-0.58%; 95% CI, -0.74% to -0.43%; I^2, 57.5%) as compared with control participants. Physical activity advice alone was not associated with HbA_{1c} changes.

Conclusions.—Structured exercise training that consists of aerobic exercise, resistance training, or both combined is associated with HbA_{1c} reduction in patients with type 2 diabetes. Structured exercise training of more than 150 minutes per week is associated with greater HbA_{1c} declines than that of 150 minutes or less per week. Physical activity advice is associated with lower HbA_{1c}, but only when combined with dietary advice.

▶ This is the first systematic review to assess the association between physical activity advice interventions and glycemic control. A key point of this review is that physical activity advice is only associated with hemoglobin A1c (HbA1c) reduction when accompanied by a dietary co-intervention. This highlights the need for a combined recommendation of these lifestyle interventions. Previous meta-analyses found that structured exercise training, including aerobic and resistance exercises, reduces HbA1c levels by approximately 0.6%.[1,2]

D. C. Nieman, DrPH

References

1. Snowling NJ, Hopkins WG. Effects of different modes of exercise training on glucose control and risk factors for complications in type 2 diabetic patients: a meta-analysis. *Diabetes Care.* 2006;29:2518-2527.
2. Thomas DE, Elliott EJ, Naughton GA. Exercise for type 2 diabetes mellitus. *Cochrane Database Syst Rev.* 2006;(3):CD002968.

Acute Calcium Ingestion Attenuates Exercise-Induced Disruption of Calcium Homeostasis

Barry DW, Hansen KC, van Pelt RE, et al (Univ of Colorado, Aurora)
Med Sci Sports Exerc 43:617-623, 2011

Purpose.—Exercise is associated with a decrease in bone mineral density under certain conditions. One potential mechanism is increased bone resorption due to an exercise-induced increase in parathyroid hormone (PTH), possibly triggered by dermal calcium loss. The purpose of this investigation was to determine whether calcium supplementation either before or during exercise attenuates exercise-induced increases in PTH and C-terminal telopeptide of Type I collagen (CTX; a marker of bone resorption).

Methods.—Male endurance athletes ($n = 20$) completed three 35-km cycling time trials under differing calcium supplementation conditions: 1) 1000 mg of calcium 20 min before exercise and placebo during, 2) placebo before and 250 mg of calcium every 15 min during exercise (1000 mg total), or 3) placebo before and during exercise. Calcium was delivered in a 1000-mg·L^{-1} solution. Supplementation was double-blinded, and trials were performed in random order. PTH, CTX, bone-specific alkaline phosphatase (BAP; a marker of bone formation), and ionized calcium (iCa) were measured before and immediately after exercise.

Results.—CTX increased and iCa decreased similarly in response to exercise under all test conditions. When compared with placebo, calcium supplementation before exercise attenuated the increase in PTH (mean ± SE: 55.8 ± 15.0 vs 74.0 ± 14.2 pg·mL^{-1}, $P = 0.04$); there was a similar trend (58.0 ± 17.4, $P = 0.07$) for calcium supplementation during exercise. There were no effects of calcium on changes in CTX, BAP, and iCa.

Conclusions.—Calcium supplementation before exercise attenuated the disruption of PTH. Further research is needed to determine the effects of repeated increases in PTH and CTX on bone (i.e., exercise training) and

TABLE 2.—Serum Concentrations of PTH, CTX, BAP, iCa, and Hct Before and After Exercise

Variable	Placebo	Condition Ca Before	Ca During
PTH (pg·mL^{-1})			
Before	51.44 ± 4.58	44.13 ± 4.27	54.80 ± 5.57
After	125.47 ± 16.14	99.89 ± 16.61	112.81 ± 20.06
After$_{adj}$	121.54 ± 16.01	96.19 ± 16.47	108.01 ± 20.04
Change	74.03 ± 14.22*	55.77 ± 15.03*†	58.01 ± 17.43*‡
Change$_{adj}$	70.10 ± 14.18*	52.06 ± 15.01*†	53.21 ± 17.48*‡
CTX (ng·mL^{-1})			
Before	0.59 ± 0.05	0.68 ± 0.05	0.60 ± 0.05
After	0.82 ± 0.09	0.85 ± 0.07	0.88 ± 0.07
After$_{adj}$	0.77 ± 0.08	0.79 ± 0.07	0.82 ± 0.07
Change	0.24 ± 0.06*	0.17 ± 0.05*	0.28 ± 0.06*
Change$_{adj}$	0.19 ± 0.06*	0.11 ± 0.05*	0.23 ± 0.06*
BAP (U·L^{-1})			
Before	23.60 ± 1.40	21.98 ± 1.53	22.35 ± 1.42
After	24.95 ± 1.71	23.23 ± 1.51	24.04 ± 1.51
After$_{adj}$	24.95 ± 1.71	21.62 ± 1.49	21.96 ± 1.40
Change	1.35 ± 0.90	1.25 ± 0.79	1.69 ± 0.82**
Change$_{adj}$	−0.40 ± 0.93	−0.36 ± 0.72	−0.38 ± 0.86
iCa (mmol·L^{-1})			
Before	1.20 ± 0.01	1.24 ± 0.01	1.21 ± 0.01
After	1.14 ± 0.01	1.17 ± 0.01	1.16 ± 0.01
After$_{adj}$	1.05 ± 0.01	1.08 ± 0.01	1.05 ± 0.01
Change	−0.06 ± 0.01*	−0.06 ± 0.01*	−0.06 ± 0.01*
Change$_{adj}$	−0.16 ± 0.02*	−0.16 ± 0.01*	−0.17 ± 0.02*
Hct (%)			
Before	44.80 ± 0.53	44.85 ± 0.63	44.65 ± 0.63
After	46.80 ± 0.51	46.90 ± 0.54	47.05 ± 0.58
Change	2.00 ± 0.36*	2.05 ± 0.59*	2.40 ± 0.24*

Values are means ± SE.
Before versus ± s after exercise, * $P < 0.01$, **$P = 0.05$.
Change different from placebo, †$P \le 0.04$, ‡$P = 0.07$.
Adj, adjusted for hemoconcentration; Hct, hematocrit.

whether calcium supplementation can diminish any exercise-induced demineralization (Table 2).

▶ Although moderate physical activity has a beneficial effect on bone density,[1] excessive training can cause loss of bone calcium (particularly if there is a negative protein balance and the sport is weight supported, as in distance cycling[2,3]). One hypothesis is that the calcium loss in sweat triggers a chain of events to defend blood calcium levels. These events include an increased secretion of the bone-resorbing parathyroid hormone (PTH), with a resulting increase in plasma levels of the osteoclastic marker C terminal telopeptide of type I collagen (CTX).[4] The study of Guillemant et al[4] found decreases in both PTH and CTX when a calcium-rich beverage was consumed beginning 1 hour before exercising. The present double-blind placebo-controlled trial examined the effects of calcium supplementation over 35-km time trials performed on a laboratory cycle ergometer (duration of about 1 hour, a time previously shown to disrupt calcium homeostasis). In 2 of the 3 time ergometer trials, a sports beverage was supplemented with calcium (1000 mg/L). The calcium supplement reduced PTH levels, particularly if it was administered before exercising (Table 2), but there were no changes in CTX. The latter finding is contrary to previous observations[4] and suggests that in these experiments, bone resorption was not reduced by acute calcium supplementation. It may be that with a single bout of exercise, the dermal calcium loss was insufficient to demonstrate benefit. Further trials in which calcium supplements are provided regularly over several months of training are necessary.

R. J. Shephard, MD (Lond), PhD, DPE

References

1. Suominen H. Bone mineral density and long term exercise. An overview of cross-sectional athlete studies. *Sports Med.* 1993;16:316-330.
2. Rector RS, Rogers R, Ruebel M, Hinton PS. Participation in road cycling vs running is associated with lower bone mineral density in men. *Metabolism.* 2008;57:226-232.
3. Nichols JF, Palmer JE, Levy SS. Low bone mineral density in highly trained male master cyclists. *Osteoporos Int.* 2003;14:644-649.
4. Guillemant J, Accarie C, Peres G, Guillemant S. Acute effects of an oral calcium load on markers of bone metabolism during endurance cycling exercise in male athletes. *Calcif Tissue Int.* 2004;74:407-414.

Effect of Mouth-Rinsing Carbohydrate Solutions on Endurance Performance
Rollo I, Williams C (Loughborough Univ, UK)
Sports Med 41:449-461, 2011

Ingesting carbohydrate-electrolyte solutions during exercise has been reported to benefit self-paced time-trial performance. The mechanism responsible for this ergogenic effect is unclear. For example, during short duration (≤1 hour), intense (>70% maximal oxygen consumption) exercise, euglycaemia is rarely challenged and adequate muscle glycogen

TABLE 1.—Summary Table of Studies Completed Investigating the Influence of Mouth Rinsing Carbohydrate (CHO) Solutions on Endurance Performance

Study (y)	No. of Subjects and Sex	$\dot{V}O_{2max}$ (mL/kg/min) [mean ± SD]	Mode	Time Trial [mean ± SD]	Fasting Duration	Beverage	CHO (%)	No. of Mouth Rinses (Duration [sec])	HR (beats/min) [Mean ± SD]	RPE [Mean ± SD]	Result [Mean ± SD]	% Diff.
Carter et al[19] (2004)	7 M, 2 F	63.2 ± 2.7	Cycle	914 ± 40 kJ	4 h	Maltodextrin	6.4	8 (5)	172 ± 1	16 ± 1	59.57 ± 1.50 min[a]	2.9
						Water	0	8 (5)	171 ± 1	16 ± 1	61.37 ± 1.56 min	
Pottier et al[21] (2010)	12 M	61.7 ± 3.1	Cycle	975 ± 85 kJ	3 h	Sucrose (5.4 g/glucose (0.46 g)	6	8 (5)	161 ± 12	15.4 ± 1.4	61.7 ± 5.1 min[a]	3.7[b]
						Placebo	0		157 ± 12	15.5 ± 1.7	64.1 ± 6.5 min	
Beelen et al[22] (2009)	14 M	NR	Cycle	1053 ± 48 kJ	2 h	Maltodextrin	6.4	8 (5)	169 ± 2	16.4 ± 0.3	68.14 ± 1.14 min	NA
						Water	0		168 ± 2	16.7 ± 0.3	67.52 ± 1.00 min	
Chambers et al[25] (2009)	8 M	60.8 ± 4.1	Cycle	914 ± 29 kJ	Overnight	Glucose	6.4	8 (10)	180 ± 3	16 ± 1.8	60.4 ± 3.7 min[a]	2.0 ± 1.5
						Placebo	0		177 ± 4	16 ± 1.6	61.6 ± 3.8 min	
	6 M, 2 F	57.8 ± 3.2	Cycle	837 ± 68 kJ	Overnight	Maltodextrin	6.4	8 (10)	181 ± 10	15 ± 1.8	62.6 ± 4.7 min[a]	3.1 ± 1.7
						Placebo	0		180 ± 10 (peak HR)	15 ± 1.5	64.6 ± 4.9 min	
Whitham and McKinney[26] (2007)	7 M	57.8 ± 2.7	Run	45 min	4 h	Maltodextrin	6	10 (5)	NR	NR	9333 ± 988 km	NA
						Placebo	0		~160 ± 20	NR	9309 ± 993 km	
Rollo et al[36] (2010)	10 M	63.9 ± 4.3	Run	1 h	13–15 h	Glucose/maltodextrin	6.4	4 (5)	163 ± 13	14 ± 1	14298 ± 685 km[a]	1.5[b]
						Placebo	0		163 ± 12	14 ± 1	14086 ± 732 km	

F = female; **HR** = heart rate; **M** = male; **NA** = not applicable; **NR** = not reported; **RPE** = ratings of perceived exertion; $\dot{V}O_{2max}$ = maximal oxygen consumption; % **Diff.** = percentage performance differences.

Editor's Note: Please refer to original journal article for full references.

[a] Indicates reported significant difference between CHO and placebo trials.

[b] % **Diff.** indicates performances differences beyond day-to-day variation in testing method.

remains at the cessation of exercise. The absence of a clear metabolic explanation has led authors to speculate that ingesting carbohydrate solutions during exercise may have a 'non-metabolic' or 'central effect' on endurance performance. This hypothesis has been explored by studies investigating the performance responses of subjects when carbohydrate solutions are mouth rinsed during exercise. The solution is expectorated before ingestion, thus removing the provision of carbohydrate to the peripheral circulation. Studies using this method have reported that simply having carbohydrate in the mouth is associated with improvements in endurance performance. However, the performance response appears to be dependent upon the pre-exercise nutritional status of the subject. Furthermore, the ability to identify a central effect of a carbohydrate mouth rinse maybe affected by the protocol used to assess its impact on performance. Studies using functional MRI and transcranial stimulation have provided evidence that carbohydrate in the mouth stimulates reward centres in the brain and increases corticomotor excitability, respectively. However, further research is needed to determine whether the central effects of mouth-rinsing carbohydrates, which have been seen at rest and during fatiguing exercise, are responsible for improved endurance performance (Table 1).

▶ This short review examines the influence of mouth rinsing (using a variety of simple carbohydrates: glucose, sucrose, and maltodextrin) on physical performance. Three of 6 authors report either a shorter time to complete a fixed amount of work on a cycle ergometer, or a greater distance covered in a 45- or 60-minute run (I presume the reviewers intended to express the distance covered in meters rather than km!) (Table 1); the remaining 3 investigators report unchanged rather than decreased performance. One factor contributing to interstudy differences in response is probably the duration of fasting prior to a trial.[1,2] The durations of physical activity (45-60 minutes) are too short to postulate development of a major drop in blood glucose levels, and some other explanation of benefit is required. The tongue contains receptors that identify sweet stimuli,[3] and magnetic resonance imaging studies suggest that this information activates reward centers in the brain, as well as increases excitability of the motor cortex. Runners who develop gastrointestinal complaints when ingesting typical sports drinks might consider using carbohydrate mouth washes as an alternative method of enhancing their performance,[4] although reports do not yet suggest that this approach is effective in reducing gastrointestinal complaints.[5,6] Mouth rinsing could also find possible application as a calorie-free means of stimulating the intensity of physical activity in those who are attempting to lose weight.

R. J. Shephard, MD (Lond), PhD, DPE

References

1. Beelen M, Berghuis J, Bonaparte B, Ballak SB, Jeukendrup AE, van Loon LJ. Carbohydrate mouth rinsing in the fed state: lack of enhancement of time-trial performance. *Int J Sports Nutr Exerc Metab.* 2009;19:400-409.

2. Chambers ES, Bridge MW, Jones DA. Carbohydrate sensing in the human mouth: effects on exercise performance and brain activity. *J Physiol.* 2009;578:1779-1794.
3. Berthoud HR. Neural systems controlling food intake and energy balance in the modern world. *Curr Opin Clin Nutr Metab Care.* 2003;6:615-620.
4. Brouns F, Beckers E. Is the gut an athletic organ? Digestion, absorption and exercise. *Sports Med.* 1993;15:242-257.
5. Rollo I, Williams C. Influence of ingesting a carbohydrate-electrolyte solution before and during a 1-hr running performance test. *Int J Sport Nutr Exerc Metab.* 2009;19:645-658.
6. Rollo I, Cole M, Miller R, Williams C. Influence of mouth rinsing a carbohydrate solution on 1-h running performance. *Med Sci Sports Exerc.* 2010;42:798-804.

Effect of a 2-h hyperglycemic–hyperinsulinemic glucose clamp to promote glucose storage on endurance exercise performance

Maclaren DPM, Mohebbi H, Nirmalan M, et al (Liverpool John Moores Univ, UK; Wythenshawe Hosp, Manchester, UK)
Eur J Appl Physiol 111:2105-2114, 2011

Carbohydrate stores within muscle are considered essential as a fuel for prolonged endurance exercise, and regimes for enhancing such stores have proved successful in aiding performance. This study explored the effects of a hyperglycaemic–hyperinsulinemic clamp performed 18 h previously on subsequent prolonged endurance performance in cycling. Seven male subjects, accustomed to prolonged endurance cycling, performed 90 min of cycling at $\sim 65\%$ VO_{2max} followed by a 16-km time trial 18 h after a 2-h hyperglycemic–hyperinsulinemic clamp (HCC). Hyperglycemia (10 mM) with insulin infused at 300 mU/m^2/min over a 2-h period resulted in a total glucose uptake of 275 g (assessed by the area under the curve) of which glucose storage accounted for about 73% (i.e. 198 g). Patterns of substrate oxidation during 90-min exercise at 65% VO_{2max} were not altered by HCC. Blood glucose and plasma insulin concentrations were higher during exercise after HCC compared with control ($p < 0.05$) while plasma NEFA was similar. Exercise performance was improved by 49 s and power output was 10–11% higher during the time trial ($p < 0.05$) after HCC. These data suggest that carbohydrate loading 18 h previously by means of a 2-h HCC improves cycling performance by 3.3% without any change in pattern of substrate oxidation.

▶ It is becoming progressively more difficult to draw a clear line between a legitimate exploitation of normal human physiology and procedures that must be banned, such as doping. A new frontier in this controversy is the laboratory boosting of muscle glycogen levels through use of a glucose clamp. The process of glycogen loading by exercising to exhaustion and then ingesting a high-carbohydrate diet for several days has long been an accepted practice among endurance athletes,[1-5] although success in exploiting this technique demands considerable commitment from both the competitor and his or her advisers. Maclaren and associates have thus proposed using a clinical type of glucose clamp procedure, with a 2-hour laboratory intravenous infusion of glucose and insulin. This yielded a surprisingly large 3.3% gain in performance over a 16-km time trial on the following day. Not all athletes will want to undergo a glucose clamp procedure of this type before they engage in a major competition, but the reported benefit is sufficiently large that it needs to be considered by those regulating doping. The glucose clamp boosted muscle reserves of glycogen by 200 g, and although the authors found no significant increase in the metabolism of glucose under these conditions, this seems mainly a reflection of an inadequate sample size (n = 7); the average rate of carbohydrate oxidation during their time trial was 39.6 versus 33.7 mg/kg/min without the glucose clamp.

R. J. Shephard, MD (Lond), PhD, DPE

References

1. Bergström J, Hermansen L, Hultman E, Saltin B. Diet, muscle glycogen and physical performance. *Acta Physiol Scand.* 1967;71:140-150.
2. Bosch AN, Dennis SC, Noakes TD. Influence of carbohydrate loading on fuel substrate turnover and oxidation during prolonged exercise. *J Appl Physiol.* 1993;74:1921-1927.
3. Lamb DR, Snyder AC, Baur TS. Muscle glycogen loading with a liquid carbohydrate supplement. *Int J Sports Nutr.* 1991;1:52-60.
4. Widrick JJ, Costill DL, Fink WJ, Hickey MS, McConell GK, Tanaka H. Carbohydrate feedings and exercise performance: effect of initial muscle glycogen concentration. *J Appl Physiol.* 1993;74:2998-3005.
5. DeFronzo RA, Tobin JD, Andres R. Glucose clamp technique: a method for quantifying insulin secretion and resistance. *Am J Physiol.* 1979;237:E214-E223.

Urine Concentrations of Repetitive Doses of Inhaled Salbutamol

Elers J, Pedersen L, Henninge J, et al (Bispebjerg Hosp, København NV, Denmark; Bispebjerg Hosp, Copenhagen NV, Denmark; Aker Univ Hosp, Oslo, Norway)
Int J Sports Med 32:574-579, 2011

We examined blood and urine concentrations of repetitive doses of inhaled salbutamol in relation to the existing cut-off value used in routine doping control. We compared the concentrations in asthmatics with regular use of beta2-agonists prior to study and healthy controls with no previous use of beta2-agonists. We enrolled 10 asthmatics and 10 controls in an open-label study in which subjects inhaled repetitive doses of 400 microgram salbutamol every second hour (total 1 600 microgram), which is the permitted daily dose by the World Anti-Doping Agency (WADA). Blood samples were collected at baseline, 30 min, 1, 2, 3, 4, and 6 h after the first inhalations. Urine samples were collected at baseline, 0−4 h, 4−8 h, and 8−12 h after the first inhalations. Median urine concentrations peaked in the period 4−8 h after the first inhalations in the asthmatics and between 8−12 h in controls and the median ranged from 268 to 611 ng×mL^{-1}. No samples exceeded the WADA threshold value of 1000 ng×mL^{-1} when corrected for the urine specific gravity. When not corrected one sample exceeded the cut-off value with urine concentration of 1082 ng×mL^{-1}.

In conclusion we found no differences in blood and urine concentrations between asthmatic and healthy subjects. We found high variability in urine concentrations between subjects in both groups. The variability between subjects was still present after the samples were corrected for urine specific gravity (Fig 1).

▶ Since 2010, the World Anti-Doping Association has allowed competitors to inhale therapeutic doses of salbutamol or salmeterol (up to 1.6 mg daily) without first obtaining a formal therapeutic exemption. Monitoring to prevent athletes taking more than the therapeutic dose is based mainly on a monitoring of urinary concentrations of beta-2 agonists, with a maximum allowable concentration of 1000 ng/mL of urine. If this value is exceeded, then the athlete must attend a laboratory and demonstrate that his or her urine can attain a value > 1000 ng/mL during normal therapeutic use of the drug. The aim of previous studies was to compare the urinary response to a single inhalation of salbutamol with that which was seen following oral ingestion of salbutamol.[1-3] Elers and colleagues here evaluate a more likely scenario, in which an asthmatic athlete may use an inhaler several times during the day, reaching the permitted maximum of 1.6 mg; the drug was inhaled as a dry powder, and deposition might have been greater if a pressurized metered dose inhaler had been used. When data were corrected for specific gravity, none of the urinary salbutamol samples exceeded the permitted limit (Fig 1). In 1 subject, a crude maximum value of 1082 ng/mL was observed, but this was reduced to an acceptable value of 746 ng/mL after correcting for a concentrated urine specimen. There has been 1 other case report where values for glucoronized plus sulfonated salbutamol apparently exceeded the legal limit; the competitor was a Swiss track and field athlete who had taken repeated (but permitted) inhalations of salbutamol.[4] An important limitation of

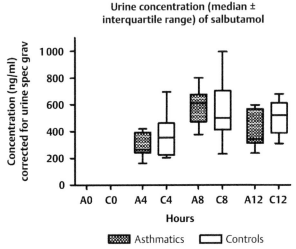

FIGURE 1.—Salbutamol concentrations in urine. (Reprinted from Elers J, Pedersen L, Henninge J, et al. Urine concentrations of repetitive doses of inhaled salbutamol. *Int J Sports Med.* 2011;32:574-579, with permission from Georg Thieme Verlag KG Stuttgart, New York.)

the present study is that subjects were not exercising; this could affect both drug metabolism and urinary concentrations, and data still need to be collected on a substantial group of both men and women under the likely scenario of competition.

R. J. Shephard, MD (Lond), PhD, DPE

References

1. Pichon A, Venisse N, Krupka E, Pérault-Pochat MC, Denjean A. Urinary and blood concentrations of beta2-agonists in trained subjects: comparison between routes of use. *Int J Sports Med.* 2006;27:187-192.
2. Sporer BC, Sheel AW, McKenzie DC. Dose response of inhaled salbutamol on exercise performance and urine concentrations. *Med Sci Sports Exerc.* 2008;40:149-157.
3. Sporer BC, Sheel AW, Taunton J, Rupert JL, McKenzie DC. Inhaled salbutamol and doping control: effects of dose on urine concentrations. *Clin J Sport Med.* 2008;18:282-285.
4. Schweizer C, Saugy M, Kamber M. Doping test reveals high concentrations of salbutamol in a Swiss track and field athlete. *Clin J Sport Med.* 2004;14:312-315.

Current markers of the Athlete Blood Passport do not flag microdose EPO doping

Ashenden M, Gough CE, Garnham A, et al (SIAB Res Consortium, Queensland, Australia; Australian Inst of Sport, Belconnen, Australia; Deakin Univ, Burwood, Victoria, Australia; et al)
Eur J Appl Physiol 111:2307-2314, 2011

The Athlete Blood Passport is the most recent tool adopted by anti-doping authorities to detect athletes using performance-enhancing drugs such as recombinant human erythropoietin (rhEPO). This strategy relies on detecting abnormal variations in haematological variables caused by doping, against a background of biological and analytical variability. Ten subjects were given twice weekly intravenous injections of rhEPO for up to 12 weeks. Full blood counts were measured using a Sysmex XE-2100 automated haematology analyser, and total haemoglobin mass via a carbon monoxide rebreathing test. The sensitivity of the passport to flag abnormal deviations in blood values was evaluated using dedicated Athlete Blood Passport software. Our treatment regimen elicited a 10% increase in total haemoglobin mass equivalent to approximately two bags of reinfused blood. The passport software did not flag any subjects as being suspicious of doping whilst they were receiving rhEPO. We conclude that it is possible for athletes to use rhEPO without eliciting abnormal changes in the blood variables currently monitored by the Athlete Blood Passport.

▶ It has not been very long since the athletic passport was deemed a conclusive response to problems of blood doping. However, as with other issues of doping control, dishonest athletes quickly find a way to circumvent any new rules that are imposed. The introduction of a relatively effective blood-testing procedure quickly caused a dip in the average hemoglobin level of International Ski Federation contestants from an average of 162 g/L in 1997 to 148 g/L in 1999, but values have subsequently crept back up to suspiciously high levels, with a parallel drop in reticulocyte counts.[1] Data for long-distance cyclists show a similar disturbing biphasic trend over the same period.[2] Ashenden and colleagues have suggested that one way athletes currently avoid detection of blood doping is to make repeated injections of very small doses of recombinant human erthyropoietin (rhEPO).[3] In the present study, volunteers were given 20 to 30 IU/kg of rhEPO intravenously twice weekly, leading to a 10% increase in total hemoglobin mass (the equivalent of 2 pints of reinfused blood, and a dose that is known to be effective in increasing maximal oxygen intake). However, none of the hematological data, including the algorithm based on hemoglobin level and reticulocyte count,[4] fell outside the permitted limits during the period when the injections were being administered. Plainly, those regulating endurance sport need to rethink the question of athlete passports.

R. J. Shephard, MD (Lond), PhD, DPE

References

1. Morkeberg J, Saltin B, Belhage B, Damsgaard R. Blood profiles in elite cross-country skiers: a 6-year follow-up. *Scand J Med Sci Sports.* 2009;19:198-205.
2. Zorzoli M. Blood monitoring in anti-doping setting. In: Schanzer WHG, Gotzmann A, eds. *Recent advances in doping analysis.* Koln, Germany: Sport und Buch Strauss; 2005:255-264.
3. Ashenden M, Varlet-Marie E, Lasne F, Audran M. The effects of microdose recombinant human erythropoietin regimens in athletes. *Haematologica.* 2006; 91:1143-1144.
4. Gore CJ, Parisotto R, Ashenden MJ, et al. Second-generation blood tests to detect erythropoietin abuse by athletes. *Haematologica.* 2003;88:333-344.

Growth Hormone Abuse and Biological Passport: Is Mannan-Binding Lectin a Complementary Candidate?
Such-Sanmartín G, Bosch J, Segura J, et al (IMIM-Hosp del Mar, Barcelona, Spain)
Clin J Sport Med 21:441-443, 2011

Objective.—In the detection of human growth hormone (GH) abuse, the approach based on altered GH-related biomarkers is also being considered with respect to its application within the context of a biological passport. As a potential biomarker, mannan-binding lectin (MBL), which is reported to respond to recombinant GH (rGH) administration, is evaluated here.

Design.—Randomized and single blind and approved by the Ethical Committee (Comité Ético de Investigación Clínica—Instituto Municipal de Asistencia Sanitaria).

Participants.—One group of 12 male subjects (24.2 ± 2.2 years; 76.1 ± 6.1 kg) was studied.

Interventions.—Mannan-binding lectin concentration was measured in 12 healthy individuals after subcutaneous daily doses of 6 IU of rGH administration. Mannan-binding lectin serum concentration increased after rGH administration. Mannan-binding lectin concentration increases were observed 48 hours after the first administration and remained elevated for several days after the final dose.

Main Outcome Measures.—Mannan-binding lectin concentration increase and elapsed time to recover initial MBL values after the last rGH administration.

Results.—Absolute values displayed high interindividual variability, and 1 individual did not show any MBL increase (potential MBL deficiency). Mannan-binding lectin protein showed a clear concentration increase after continued rGH administration, despite the high heterogeneity found between individuals.

Conclusions.—The use of MBL as a complementary GH-related biomarker could be of interest, taking advantage of the high increases (up to 700%) and the relatively slow recovery time (Fig).

▶ The direct detection of human growth hormone (HGH) and its variants following the abuse of such preparations is possible for only 24 to 36 hours.[1] The use of biomarkers of HGH has a longer time window, but there are then

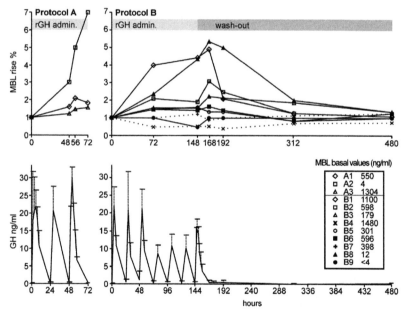

FIGURE.—Evolution of MBL (top) and rGH (bottom) serum concentrations in individuals receiving rGH in protocol A (3 days) (top left) and protocol B (7 days) (top right). Mannan-binding lectin values are expressed in percentages as compared with each basal concentration. Mannan-binding lectin basal concentrations are included (bottom right). Recombinant GH values are expressed in absolute concentrations. Subjects B4 and B7 did not receive rGH. (Reprinted from Such-Sanmartín G, Bosch J, Segura J, et al. Growth hormone abuse and biological passport: is mannan-binding lectin a complementary candidate? *Clin J Sport Med.* 2011;21:441-443, with permission from Lippincott Williams & Wilkins.)

problems from sex and ethnic differences in basal values.[2] One way around this latter problem might be the creation of an individualized "biological passport," analogous to that currently used to monitor athletes for blood doping.[3,4] A possible candidate marker to enter on such a passport would be mannan-binding lectin (MBL); this substance is thought to increase after administration of recombinant growth hormone (rGH),[5,6] although basal serum levels of MBL vary widely from 500 to 5000 ng/mL between different individual competitors. The study of Such-Sanmartin and colleagues tests the consistency in rise of MBL following the administration of rGH and the time needed to regain basal values. Their subjects were 12 young male recreational athletes who were given the rGH (6 IU subcutaneously) daily for either 3 or 7 days. Every subject except 1 showed an increase of MBL within 48 hours of beginning rGH administration, and in 9 of 12 subjects a significant elevation of MBL persisted for at least 48 hours following treatment, although there was much interindividual variation in both the initial MBL response and its persistence (Fig). The findings seem sufficiently promising to merit further testing of this marker on a larger sample that includes female athletes.

R. J. Shephard, MD (Lond), PhD, DPE

References

1. Barroso O, Schamasch P, Rabin O. Detection of GH abuse in sport: past, present and future. *Growth Horm IGF Res.* 2009;19:369-374.
2. Sönksen P. The International Olympic Committee (IOC) and GH-2000. *Growth Horm IGF Res.* 2009;19:341-345.
3. Wozny M. The biological passport and doping in athletics. *Lancet.* 2010;376:79.
4. Sottas PE, Saugy M, Saudan C. Endogenous steroid profiling in the athlete biological passport. *Endocrinol Metab Clin North Am.* 2010;39:59-73.
5. Hansen TK, Thiel S, Dall R, et al. GH strongly affects serum concentrations of mannan-binding lectin: evidence for a new IGF-I independent immunomodulatory effect of GH. *J Clin Endocrinol Metab.* 2001;86:5383-5388.
6. Gravholt CH, Leth-Larsen R, Lauridsen AL, et al. The effects of GH and hormone replacement therapy on serum concentrations of mannan-binding lectin, surfactant protein D and vitamin D binding protein in Turner syndrome. *Eur J Endocrinol.* 2004;150:355-362.

Proteomic Profiling of K-11706 Responsive Proteins
Horie M, Kawashima Y, Naka A, et al (Univ of Tsukuba, Japan; Kitasato Univ, Sagamihara, Japan; et al)
Int J Sports Med 32:559-564, 2011

Erythropoietin promotes the production of red blood cells. Recombinant human erythropoietin is illicitly used to improve performance in endurance sports. Expression of the *Erythropoietin* gene is negatively controlled by the transcription factor GATA-binding protein (GATA). Specific GATA inhibitors have recently been developed as novel drugs for the management of anemia. These drugs could, therefore, be illicitly used like recombinant human erythropoietin to improve performance in sports. To examine alterations in levels of plasma protein after administration of GATA inhibitors, proteomic analyses were conducted on mouse plasma samples treated with the potent GATA inhibitor K-11706. The analysis based on gel electrophoresis identified 41 protein spots differentially expressed when compared with normal plasma. Each spot was identified with liquid chromatography coupled to tandem mass spectrometry and 2 of them, fetuin-B and prothrombin, were verified by Western blotting. The results showed that the expression of fetuin-B in mice plasma was increased by K-11706, but not by recombinant human erythropoietin or hypoxia. These results suggest the potential of proteomic-based approaches as tools to identify biomarkers for the illegal use of novel drugs (e.g., GATA inhibitors). Also, fetuin-B could be a sensitive marker for the detection of abuse of GATA inhibitors (Fig 1).

▶ There seems no end to the ways that laboratories can find to enhance human performance, with corresponding new challenges for antidoping laboratories. Expression of the erythropoietin gene (and thus circulating hemoglobin levels) is positively controlled by a hypoxia-inducible factor but is downregulated by the transcription factor GATA-binding protein (which blocks the corresponding site on the erythropoietin gene promoter[1]). Thus, the administration of GATA inhibitors such as K-11706 can increase erythropoietin levels, reticulocyte counts, and hemoglobin concentrations.[2-4] The study by Horie et al suggests that the effect of K-11706 is roughly equivalent to that of 20 days' living at a simulated altitude of 3500 m for 20 h/d but is much less than that which could be obtained from use of recombinant erythropoietin (Fig 1). Experiments were conducted on mice rather than humans, but they do demonstrate the potential to detect the use of GATA inhibitors by using electrophoresis and

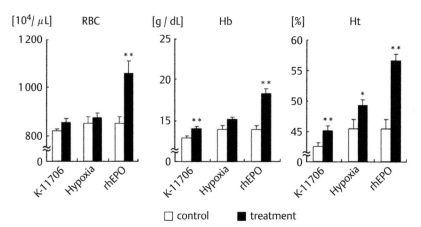

□ control   ■ treatment

FIGURE 1.—The effect of each treatment on hematological parameters. Data represent red blood cell (RBC) numbers, hemoglobin (Hb) concentration, and hematocrit (Ht) value in each treatment group (K-11706 control n = 13, K-11706 treated n = 13, Hypoxia control n = 11, Hypoxia n = 16, rhEPO control n = 10, rhEPO treated n = 6). Error bars represent SE. * p < 0.05 and ** p < 0.01 vs. each control. (Reprinted from Horie M, Kawashima Y, Naka A, et al. Proteomic profiling of K-11706 responsive proteins. *Int J Sports Med.* 2011;32:559-564, with permission from Georg Thieme Verlag KG Stuttgart.)

Western blotting to look at changes in plasma protein levels, particularly increases in fetuin-B levels. Unfortunately, the analysis is relatively complex and, presumably, correspondingly costly to complete.

R. J. Shephard, MD (Lond), PhD, DPE

References

1. Imagawa S, Suzuki N, Ohmine K, et al. GATA suppresses erythropoietin gene expression through GATA site in mouse erythropoietin gene promoter. *Int J Hematol.* 2002;75:376-381.
2. Imagawa S, Nakano Y, Obara N, et al. A GATA-specific inhibitor (K-7174) rescues anemia induced by IL-1β, TNF-α, or L-NMMA. *FASEB J.* 2003;17:1742-1744.
3. Nakano Y, Imagawa S, Matsumoto K, et al. Oral administration of K-11706 inhibits GATA binding activity, enhances hypoxia-inducible factor 1 binding activity, and restores indicators in an in vivo mouse model of anemia of chronic disease. *Blood.* 2004;104:4300-4307.
4. Umetani M, Nakao H, Doi T, et al. A novel cell adhesion inhibitor, K-7174, reduces the endothelial VCAM-1 induction by inflammatory cytokines, acting through the regulation of GATA. *Biochem Biophys Res Commun.* 2000;272:370-374.

6 Cardiorespiratory Disorders

Markers of Chronic Inflammation with Short-Term Changes in Physical Activity

Lund AJS, Hurst TL, Tyrrell RM, et al (Univ of Bath, UK; Unilever Discover, Colworth Park, Sharnbrook, Bedfordshire, UK)
Med Sci Sports Exerc 43:578-583, 2011

Purpose.—Regular exercise is inversely related to markers of chronic inflammation, but we do not know to what extent these changes are the product of recent exercise behavior. The aim of the present investigation was to examine the stability of markers of chronic inflammation in the face of short-term positive and negative changes in physical activity in middle-aged men.

Methods.—Two studies were conducted using a randomized counterbalanced design. In the first study (Study 1), eight highly active men (age = 56 ± 5 yr, body mass index (BMI) = 23.3 ± 3.2 kg m^{-2}, $\dot{V}O_{2max}$ = 50.7 ± 7.0 mL kg^{-1} min^{-1}) undertook two trials; withdrawal of exercise for 1 wk versus control (normal exercise behavior). In the second study (Study 2), 10 sedentary men (age = 57 ± 2 yr, BMI = 27.9 ± 3.6 kg m^{-2}, $\dot{V}O_{2max}$ = 30.4 ± 4.6 mL kg^{-1} min^{-1}) undertook 30 min of daily walking at 60% $\dot{V}O_{2max}$ for 1 wk versus control (normal sedentary behavior).

Results.—The withdrawal of exercise for 1 wk in highly active men (Study 1) and the imposition of 1 wk of daily exercise in sedentary men (Study 2) did not elicit any substantial changes in the inflammatory proteins C-reactive protein (CRP), IL-6, and TNF-α and circulating leukocyte concentration. The differences in inflammatory proteins between active (Study 1) and sedentary (Study 2) men were marked; for example, baseline CRP was 0.85 ± 0.79 and 3.02 ± 2.30 mg L^{-1}, respectively.

Conclusions.—The inflammatory markers CRP, IL-6, and TNF-α are stable and not affected by large short-term positive or negative alterations in exercise behavior. This stability strengthens the use of these markers in clinical and research settings because differences and changes are not simply the product of recent exercise behavior (Fig 1).

▶ The authors of this article suggest that no one has previously carried out controlled experiments to test how far the classical clinical markers of chronic inflammation and risk of cardiovascular disease (C-reactive protein [CRP],

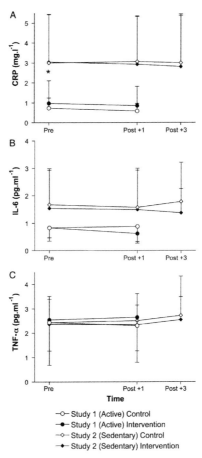

FIGURE 1.—CRP (A), IL-6 (B), and TNF-α (C) concentrations for Study 1 and Study 2 before intervention (Pre), at 1 d after intervention (Post + 1), and at 3 d after intervention (Study 2 only) and control trials. Values are mean ± SD. $n = 8$ for (A) and (C) and $n = 7$ for (B) for the active group (Study 1). $n = 10$ for the sedentary group (Study 2). *Significant difference between sedentary and active groups based on the average of both trials at baseline. (Reprinted from Lund AJS, Hurst TL, Tyrrell RM, et al. Markers of chronic inflammation with short-term changes in physical activity. *Med Sci Sports Exerc*. 2011;43:578-583, with permission from the American College of Sports Medicine.)

interleukin-6 [IL-6], and tumor necrosis factor alpha)[1-3] are affected by short-term changes in an individual's level of physical activity rather than the individual's habitual behavior. Two parallel experiments were performed: the withdrawal of all exercise for 7 days in a group of previously very active middle-aged men (maximal oxygen intake 51 mL/[kg.min] normally undertaking 6 hours of exercise per day) and an increase of physical activity (introduction of a daily 30-minute walk at 60% of their maximal oxygen intake) in very sedentary men (maximal oxygen intake 30 mL/[kg.min]) of a similar age. As a consequence of their habitual activity, the active men had much lower initial levels of IL-6 and CRP than the sedentary group, but in neither group were levels affected by the short-term changes in activity patterns tested in this study (Fig 1). It would be interesting to repeat these experiments with activities that involved eccentric exercise, but currently it seems that the inflammatory markers can be used as an index of long-term risks, irrespective of any recent physical activity a patient may have undertaken.

R. J. Shephard, MD (Lond), PhD, DPE

References

1. Libby P. Inflammation in atherosclerosis. *Nature.* 2002;420:868-874.
2. Petersen AM, Pedersen BK. The anti-inflammatory effect of exercise. *J Appl Physiol.* 2005;98:1154-1162.
3. Ridker PM. Clinical application of C-reactive protein for cardiovascular disease detection and prevention. *Circulation.* 2003;107:363-369.

Exercise Training Versus Propranolol in the Treatment of the Postural Orthostatic Tachycardia Syndrome
Fu Q, VanGundy TB, Shibata S, et al (Texas Health Presbyterian Hosp Dallas; et al)
Hypertension 58:167-175, 2011

We have found recently that exercise training is effective in the treatment of the postural orthostatic tachycardia syndrome (POTS). Whether this nondrug treatment is superior to "standard" drug therapies, such as β-blockade, is unknown. We tested the hypothesis that exercise training but not β-blockade treatment improves symptoms, hemodynamics, and renal-adrenal responses in POTS patients. Nineteen patients (18 women and 1 man) completed a double-blind drug trial (propranolol or placebo) for 4 weeks, followed by 3 months of exercise training. Fifteen age-matched healthy individuals (14 women and 1 man) served as controls. A 2-hour standing test was performed before and after drug treatment and training. Hemodynamics, catecholamines, plasma renin activity, and aldosterone were measured supine and during 2-hour standing. We found that both propranolol and training significantly lowered standing heart rate. Standing cardiac output was lowered after propranolol treatment ($P=0.01$) but was minimally changed after training. The aldosterone:renin ratio during 2-hour standing remained unchanged after propranolol treatment (4.1 ± 1.7 [SD] before versus 3.9 ± 2.0 after; $P=0.46$) but modestly increased after training (5.2 ± 2.9 versus 6.5 ± 3.0; $P=0.05$). Plasma catecholamines were not affected by propranolol or training. Patient quality of life, assessed using the 36-item Short-Form Health Survey, was improved after training (physical functioning score 33 ± 10 before versus 50 ± 9 after; social functioning score 37 ± 9 versus 48 ± 6; both $P<0.01$) but not after propranolol treatment (34 ± 10 versus 36 ± 11, $P=0.63$; 39 ± 7 versus 39 ± 5, $P=0.73$). These results suggest that, for patients with POTS, exercise training is superior to propranolol at restoring upright hemodynamics,

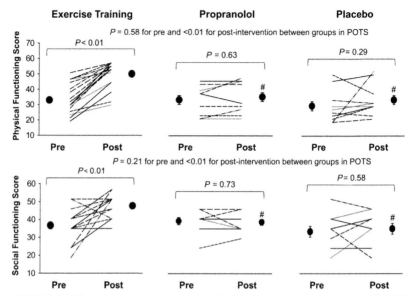

FIGURE 6.—Effects of exercise training, propranolol, and placebo treatment on patient quality of life assessed by the 36-item Short-Form Health Survey. Values are expressed as individuals and mean ± SE. (Reprinted from Fu Q, VanGundy TB, Shibata S, et al. Exercise training versus propranolol in the treatment of the postural orthostatic tachycardia syndrome. *Hypertension*. 2011;58:167-175, with permission from American Heart Association.)

normalizing renal-adrenal responsiveness, and improving quality of life (Fig 6).

▶ Physicians are sometimes tempted to treat apparently abnormal numbers rather than the pathology that underlies a patient's symptoms. Thus, individuals with postural orthostatic tachycardia syndrome are often prescribed β-blockers, such as propranolol, to bring their heart rates within what is perceived as a normal range.[1,2] However, the condition probably reflects an inadequate cardiac stroke volume secondary to poor peripheral venous tone and/or a decrease of blood volume rather than a dysfunction of baroreflexes. Such issues are associated with inadequate habitual physical activity and/or life in a zero-gravity environment, and, thus, cardiologists have recently developed an interest in a progressive aerobic training regimen as a means of treating the disorder.[3-5] In the present report, Fu and associates compared the traditional propranolol treatment (80 mg of long-acting propranolol) and progressive aerobic training (beginning with semirecumbent activity but progressing over 2-3 months to 5-6 hours of vigorous aerobic and resistance exercise per week) against placebo capsules in a small group of patients who met the "inclusion without exclusion" criteria for the syndrome. Both forms of active treatment restored a more normal heart rate; but training was only effective in restoring a normal blood volume and the aldosterone:renin ratio in response to 2 hours of standing and above all in reducing symptoms and enhancing the patient's quality of life as assessed by the 36-item Short-Form questionnaire (Fig 6). The exercise program brought many other health advantages, in contrast to the side effects commonly encountered during drug treatment. Many of the symptoms associated with the postural orthostatic tachycardia syndrome seem related to a progressive physical inactivity, self-imposed by the patient in response to the syndrome, and this underlines a growing perception by physicians that other chronic and poorly understood syndromes, such as chronic fatigue syndrome and fibromyalgia,[1] may be ameliorated by a progressive increase in habitual physical activity.

R. J. Shephard, MD (Lond), PhD, DPE

References

1. Joyner MJ. Exercise training in postural orthostatic tachycardia syndrome: blocking the urge to block β-receptors? *Hypertension.* 2011;58:136-137.
2. Raj SR, Black BK, Biaggioni I, et al. Propranolol decreases tachycardia and improves symptoms in the postural tachycardia syndrome: less is more. *Circulation.* 2009; 120:725-734.
3. Joyner MJ, Masuki S. POTS versus deconditioning: the same or different? *Clin Auton Res.* 2008;18:300-307.
4. Fu Q, VanGundy TB, Galbreath MM, et al. Cardiac origins of the postural orthostatic tachycardia syndrome. *J Am Coll Cardiol.* 2010;55:2858-2868.
5. Winker R, Barth A, Bidmon D, et al. Endurance exercise training in orthostatic intolerance: a randomized, controlled trial. *Hypertension.* 2005;45:391-398.

Cardiorespiratory Fitness and Classification of Risk of Cardiovascular Disease Mortality

Gupta S, Rohatgi A, Ayers CR, et al (Univ of Texas Southwestern Med Ctr, Dallas; et al)
Circulation 123:1377-1383, 2011

Background.—Cardiorespiratory fitness (fitness) is associated with cardiovascular disease (CVD) mortality. However, the extent to which fitness improves risk classification when added to traditional risk factors is unclear.

Methods and Results.—Fitness was measured by the Balke protocol in 66 371 subjects without prior CVD enrolled in the Cooper Center Longitudinal Study between 1970 and 2006; follow-up was extended through 2006. Cox proportional hazards models were used to estimate the risk of CVD mortality with a traditional risk factor model (age, sex, systolic blood pressure, diabetes mellitus, total cholesterol, and smoking) with and without the addition of fitness. The net reclassification improvement and integrated discrimination improvement were calculated at 10 and 25 years. Ten-year risk estimates for CVD mortality were categorized as <1%, 1% to <5%, and ≥5%, and 25-year risk estimates were categorized as <8%, 8% to 30%, and ≥30%. During a median follow-up period of 16 years, there were 1621 CVD deaths. The addition of fitness to the traditional risk factor model resulted in reclassification of 10.7% of the men, with significant net reclassification improvement at both 10 years (net reclassification improvement=0.121) and 25 years (net reclassification improvement=0.041) (P<0.001 for both). The integrated discrimination improvement was 0.010 at 10 years (P<0.001), and the relative integrated discrimination improvement was 29%. Similar findings were observed for women at 25 years.

Conclusions.—A single measurement of fitness significantly improves classification of both short-term (10-year) and long-term (25-year) risk for CVD mortality when added to traditional risk factors (Table 2).

▶ The identification of an individual patient's cardiac risk is difficult, because currently the general population is at low risk, and as Bayes' theorem indicates,[1] attempts to determined an individual's risk are hampered by high false-positive and false-negative rates. There have been previous reports suggesting that a low level of cardio respiratory fitness has some adverse effect upon an individual's cardiac prognosis, even after taking into account traditional Framingham cardiac risk factors[2-5]; one contributing factor may be that a fit heart retains more functional myocardium than the heart of a sedentary person after a heart attack. The inclusion of simple fitness testing might thus improve the sensitivity and specificity of cardiac prognoses. The article by Gupta and associates makes a long-lasting prospective study of prognostic utility (average duration 17 and 12 years, in men and women, respectively) in a large group of patients who were attending the Cooper Clinic in Dallas, Texas. Fitness was classified by treadmill times, using the Balke protocol, and given their initial age of 44 years, both sexes were relatively fit (respective estimates of maximal oxygen intake 40 and 33 mL/[kg.min]). Most participants also had fairly low Framingham

TABLE 2.—Reclassification of 10-Year Risk of CVD Mortality in Men Using Models With and Without Quintiles of Fitness (n=43 041)

Model Without Fitness	0% to <1%	1% to <5%	≥5%	Overall	Model With Fitness Reclassified as Higher Risk	Reclassified as Lower Risk	Net Correctly Reclassified
Participants with CVD death					49	19	0.113*
0% to <1%	60	27	0	87			
1% to <5%	13	81	22	116			
≥5%	0	6	56	62			
Overall	73	114	78	265			
Participants without CVD death					1622	1882	0.008*
0% to <1%	25 650	1298	0	26 948			
1% to <5%	1636	3719	324	5679			
≥5%	0	246	428	674			
Overall	27 286	5263	752	33 301			
Net reclassification improvement							0.121*
Net reclassification improvement (1% to <5% risk only)							0.309*

CVD indicates cardiovascular disease.
*P<0.001.

risk scores. Thus, despite the large sample size and long follow-up period, there were relatively few cardiac deaths. Nevertheless, in this sample, the inclusion of information on fitness significantly improved the classification of risk relative to use of traditional risk factors on their own (Table 2). The added information was more pertinent at 10 years than at 25 years, perhaps because activity patterns changed with time. It would be helpful to confirm this finding on another sample of lower socioeconomic status and with a higher initial level of risk factors. It is also important to note that there are now a variety of other risk markers, such as high-density lipoprotein cholesterol and immune markers of chronic inflammation, that were not included in this analysis.

R. J. Shephard, MD (Lond), PhD, DPE

References

1. Bayes T, Price R. An Essay towards solving a Problem in the Doctrine of Chance. *Philos Trans R Soc Lond.* 1763;53:370-418.
2. Ekelund LG, Haskell WL, Johnson JL, et al. Physical fitness as a predictor of cardiovascular mortality in asymptomatic North American men. The Lipid Research Clinics Mortality Follow-up Study. *N Engl J Med.* 1988;319:1379-1384.
3. De Backer G, Ambrosioni E, Borch-Johnsen K, et al. European guidelines on cardiovascular disease prevention in clinical practice. Third Joint Task Force of European and other Societies on Cardiovascular Disease Prevention in Clinical Practice. *Atherosclerosis.* 2004;173:381-391.
4. Lloyd-Jones DM, Dyer AR, Wang R, Daviglus ML, Greenland P. Risk factor burden in middle age and lifetime risks for cardiovascular and non-cardiovascular death (Chicago Heart Association Detection Project in Industry). *Am J Cardiol.* 2007; 99:535-540.
5. Lloyd-Jones DM, Leip EP, Larson MG, et al. Prediction of lifetime risk for cardiovascular disease by risk factor burden at 50 years of age. *Circulation.* 2006;113: 791-798.

Impact of Cardiac Rehabilitation on Mortality and Cardiovascular Events After Percutaneous Coronary Intervention in the Community
Goel K, Lennon RJ, Tilbury RT, et al (Mayo Clinic, Rochester, MN)
Circulation 123:2344-2352, 2011

Background.—Although numerous studies have reported that cardiac rehabilitation (CR) is associated with reduced mortality after myocardial infarction, less is known about its association with mortality after percutaneous coronary intervention.

Methods and Results.—We performed a retrospective analysis of data from a prospectively collected registry of 2395 consecutive patients who underwent percutaneous coronary intervention in Olmsted County, Minnesota, from 1994 to 2008. The association of CR with all-cause mortality, cardiac mortality, myocardial infarction, or revascularization was assessed with 3 statistical techniques: propensity score—matched analysis (n=1438), propensity score stratification (n=2351), and regression adjustment with propensity score in a 3-month landmark analysis (n=2009). During a median follow-up of 6.3 years, 503 deaths (199 cardiac), 394 myocardial infarctions, and 755 revascularization procedures occurred in the study subjects. Participation in CR, noted in 40% (964 of 2395) of the cohort, was associated with a significant decrease in all-cause mortality by all 3 statistical techniques (hazard ratio, 0.53 to 0.55; $P<0.001$). A trend toward decreased cardiac mortality was also observed in CR participants; however, no effect was observed for subsequent myocardial infarction or revascularization. The association between CR participation and reduced mortality rates was similar for men and women, for older and younger patients, and for patients undergoing elective or nonelective percutaneous coronary intervention.

Conclusions.—We found that CR participation after percutaneous coronary intervention was associated with a significant reduction in mortality rates. These findings add support to published clinical practice guidelines, performance measures, and insurance coverage policies that recommend CR for patients after percutaneous coronary intervention (Table 2).

▶ Meta-analyses of various randomized controlled trials have shown that involvement in a program of formal rehabilitation following myocardial infarction reduces the risk of a subsequent cardiac fatality by 20% to 30%,[1,2] and it

TABLE 2.—Factors Associated With Cardiac Rehabilitation Participation After Percutaneous Coronary Intervention

Variables	Estimate	OR	95% CI	P
Age, y*				<0.001
65 (vs 55)	0.0896	1.09	0.90−1.33	
75 (vs 55)	−0.2956	0.74	0.60−0.92	
85 (vs 55)	−1.3560	0.26	0.19−0.36	
History of acute MI*	0.6274	1.87	1.13−3.09	0.014
History of MI (>7 d)	−0.4189	0.66	0.49−0.88	0.006
Current smoker	−0.3840	0.68	0.52−0.89	0.005
Diabetes mellitus	−0.2606	0.77	0.61−0.98	0.032
Prior PCI	−0.6147	0.54	0.32−0.92	0.024
Prior CABG	−0.3893	0.68	0.43−1.06	0.090
COPD	−0.3088	0.73	0.53−1.02	0.062
PCI date*				<0.001
January 1, 2000 (vs January 1, 1994)	0.2945	1.34	1.06−1.71	
January 1, 2005 (vs January 1, 1994)	−0.0548	0.95	0.75−1.19	
January 1, 2008 (vs January 1, 1994)	0.7564	2.13	1.50−3.02	
Minor branches (any lesion)	0.2470	1.28	1.06−1.55	0.012
Drug-eluting stents	−0.3670	0.69	0.49−0.98	0.041
Glycoprotein IIa/IIIb therapy	0.3782	1.46	1.14−1.87	0.003
In-hospital MI/CABG/PCI	0.5558	1.74	1.18−2.58	0.006
Calcium channel blockers	−0.3107	0.73	0.55−0.98	0.039
Lipid-lowering drugs	0.3496	1.42	1.13−1.78	0.003
Cardiac glycoside	−0.4934	0.61	0.38−0.98	0.043

OR indicates odds ratio; CI, confidence interval; MI, myocardial infarction; PCI, percutaneous coronary intervention; CABG, coronary artery bypass graft; and COPD, chronic obstructive pulmonary disease. Acute MI is defined as a history of MI within 24 hours of the procedure The following variables had a significant univariate association with cardiac rehabilitation participation ($\alpha<0.15$) but were not associated with it after adjustment in the multiple logistic regression model: definite/probable angina on presentation; New York Heart Association class; heart failure; family history of CAD; peripheral vascular disease, cerebrovascular accident, moderate/severe renal disease, and cancer; predominant symptom of chest pain or positive exercise test; presence of thrombus; PCI in the right coronary artery, PCI in a severe bend, or Thrombolysis in Myocardial Infarction grade 3 flow after the procedure; vein graft intervention; and use of aspirin, β-blockers, diuretics, oral nitrates, anticoagulants, and antihypertensives at discharge.

*Age and procedure date were modeled as 3-*df* splines. See Figure 2 for more details. The hazard ratios here represent the fit of those splines at specific points within the variable range with other variables set to the sample mean.

is thus logical to anticipate that a similar benefit might be seen in patients undergoing percutaneous coronary vascular interventions for coronary vascular disease. Some of the benefit from a prolonged course of cardiac rehabilitation is physiological,[3,4] but the study of Goel et al also looks at other factors, such as group support and counseling on preventive tactics[5,6]; their minimum criterion of "participation" was attendance at 1 or more sessions of rehabilitation; the average number of sessions attended was 13, but this is a far cry from the 6 to 12 months of daily exercise that we have examined in Toronto, or even the 13 weeks of thrice weekly sessions adopted in many U.S. centers. Although overall mortality was lower in the rehabilitation group, there was no difference in the incidence of recurrent myocardial infarctions or revascularization rates. Importantly, Goel et al are reporting an association rather than a randomized clinical trial, and as with the 45% to 47% lower rates of all-cause mortality that they have observed, very high apparent rates of benefit were seen in many early nonrandomized trials of rehabilitation following myocardial infarction. The main reason for such spurious benefits is that many of the factors influencing prognosis also affect participation in a rehabilitation program (Table 2), including age, smoking habits, and a history of diabetes mellitus. There remains a need for a randomized controlled trial to provide categoric proof of benefit from rehabilitation following percutaneous interventions.

R. J. Shephard, MD (Lond), PhD, DPE

References

1. Suaya JA, Stason WB, Ades PA, Normand SL, Shepard DS. Cardiac rehabilitation and survival in older coronary patients. *J Am Coll Cardiol.* 2009;54:25-33.
2. O'Connor GT, Buring JE, Yusuf S, et al. An overview of randomized trials of rehabilitation with exercise after myocardial infarction. *Circulation.* 1989;80:234-244.
3. Lavie CJ, Thomas RJ, Squires RW, Allison TG, Milani RV. Exercise training and cardiac rehabilitation in primary and secondary prevention of coronary heart disease. *Mayo Clin Proc.* 2009;84:373-383.
4. Marchionni N, Fattirolli F, Fumagalli S, et al. Improved exercise tolerance and quality of life with cardiac rehabilitation of older patients after myocardial infarction: results of a randomized, controlled trial. *Circulation.* 2003;107:2201-2206.
5. Lavie CJ, Milani RV. Adverse psychological and coronary risk profiles in young patients with coronary artery disease and benefits of formal cardiac rehabilitation. *Arch Intern Med.* 2006;166:1878-1883.
6. Shah ND, Dunlay SM, Ting HH, et al. Long-term medication adherence after myocardial infarction: experience of a community. *Am J Med.* 2009;122: 961.e7-961.e13.

Physical Activity and Cardiovascular Mortality Risk: Possible Protective Mechanisms?
Hamer M, Ingle L, Carroll S, et al (Univ College London, UK; Leeds Metropolitan Univ, UK; Univ of Hull, UK)
Med Sci Sports Exerc 44:84-88, 2012

Introduction.—The biological mechanisms through which increased physical activity or structured exercise training lowers the risk of recurrent cardiac events are incompletely understood. We examined the extent to which modification of primary risk markers explains the association between physical activity and cardiovascular death in participants with diagnosed cardiovascular disease (CVD).

Methods and Results.—In a prospective study of 1429 participants with physician-diagnosed CVD living in England and Scotland (age = 66.5 ± 11.1 yr (mean ± SD), 54.2% men), we measured physical activity and several risk markers (body mass index, total-to-HDL cholesterol ratio, diagnosed diabetes, systolic blood pressure, resting heart rate, C-reactive protein) at baseline. The main outcome was CVD death. There were a total of 446 all-cause deaths during an average of 7.0 ± 3.1 yr of follow-up, of which 213 were attributed to cardiovascular causes. Participation in moderate to vigorous physical activity at least three sessions per week was associated with lower risk of CVD death (hazard ratio = 0.61, 95% confidence interval = 0.38–0.98). Physically active participants demonstrated significantly lower levels of body mass index, diabetes, and inflammatory risk (C-reactive protein). Metabolic (body mass index, total-to-HDL cholesterol ratio, and physician-diagnosed diabetes) and inflammatory risk factors explained an estimated 12.8% and 15.4%, respectively, of the association between physical activity and CVD death.

Conclusions.—Physical activity may reduce the risk of secondary CVD events, in part, by improving metabolic and inflammatory risk markers.

▶ It is now generally agreed that a progressive exercise training regimen improves prognosis in patients with coronary vascular disease, both reducing the risk of critical incidents and increasing survival prospects.[1] However, the mechanism(s) of benefit are less clearly established. Hamer and associates here report a 7-year follow-up of 1429 patients with physician-diagnosed cardiovascular disease (unfortunately, their sample included some cases of stroke, which complicates the analysis). Physical activity was assessed by an interview that assessed the patient's participation in moderate physical activity (sessions > 30 min of activity > 3 metabolic syndrome in the previous 4 weeks). Those patients who were physically active had a substantially lower risk of mortality over the 7 years (0.61), with metabolic and inflammatory risk factors apparently accounting for only a small part of their advantage. No data were obtained on endothelial function, which may also have contributed to the advantage of the exercisers.[2] But because the subjects were not randomly assigned to exercise and control groups, it is likely that those who exercised were also more likely to abstain from smoking and to adopt other manifestations of a prudent lifestyle; furthermore, those who were less prone to exercise probably had more severe initial disease. Certainly, the apparent benefit of exercise seen in this series was larger than what has been observed in randomized, controlled trials (20% to 30%),[3] emphasizing the problems that can arise when drawing conclusions from observational studies.

R. J. Shephard, MD (Lond), PhD, DPE

References

1. Clark AM, Hartling L, Vandermeer B, McAlister FA. Meta-analysis: secondary prevention programs for patients with coronary artery disease. *Ann Intern Med.* 2005;143:659-672.
2. Wisløff U, Støylen A, Loennechen JP, et al. Superior cardiovascular effect of aerobic interval training versus moderate continuous training in heart failure patients: a randomized study. *Circulation.* 2007;115:3086-3094.
3. Taylor RS, Unal B, Critchley JA, Capewell S. Mortality reductions in patients receiving exercise-based cardiac rehabilitation: how much can be attributed to cardiovascular risk factor improvements? *Eur J Cardiovasc Prev Rehabil.* 2006; 13:369-374.

Physical inactivity and idiopathic pulmonary embolism in women: prospective study

Kabrhel C, Varraso R, Goldhaber SZ, et al (Massachusetts General Hosp, Boston; CESP Centre for Res in Epidemiology and Population Health, Villejuif, France; Harvard Med School, Boston, MA; et al)
BMJ 342:d3867, 2011

Objectives.—To determine the association between physical inactivity (that is, a sedentary lifestyle) and incident idiopathic pulmonary embolism.

Design.—Prospective cohort study.

Setting.—Nurses' Health Study.

Participants.—69 950 female nurses who completed biennial questionnaires from 1990 to 2008.

Main Outcome Measures.—The primary outcome was idiopathic pulmonary embolism confirmed in medical records. Multivariable Cox proportional hazards models controlled for age, body mass index (BMI), energy intake, smoking, pack years, race, spouse's educational attainment, parity, menopause, non-aspirin non-steroidal anti-inflammatory drugs, warfarin, multivitamin supplements, hypertension, coronary heart disease, rheumatological disease, and dietary patterns. The primary exposure was physical inactivity, measured in hours of sitting each day. The secondary exposure was physical activity, measured in metabolic equivalents a day.

Results.—Over the 18 year study period, there were 268 cases of incident idiopathic pulmonary embolism. There was an association between time of sitting and risk of idiopathic pulmonary embolism (41/104 720 v 16/14 565 cases in most inactive v least inactive in combined data; P<0.001 for trend). The risk of pulmonary embolism was more than twofold in women who spent the most time sitting compared with those who spent the least time sitting (multivariable hazard ratio 2.34, 95% confidence interval 1.30 to 4.20). There was no association between physical activity and pulmonary embolism (P=0.53 for trend).

TABLE 2.—Association Between Physical Inactivity and Incident Idiopathic Pulmonary Embolism, Nurses' Health Study (n=69 950), with Hazard Ratios (HR) for Trend

| | Amount of Time Sitting* (Score 2=Lowest, 6=Highest), Combined Data From 1988 and 1990 | | | | | HR (95% CI) for Trend, P Value |
	2	3	4	5	6	
No of cases/person years	41/104 720	53/175 518	104/209 002	54/88 228	16/14 565	—
Age adjusted HR (95% CI)	1.00	0.79 (0.52 to 1.19)	1.31 (0.90 to 1.88)	1.62 (1.08 to 2.44)	2.73 (1.53 to 4.88)	1.29 (1.15 to 1.45), <0.001
Multivariable HR (95% CI)†	1.00	0.79 (0.52 to 1.19)	1.29 (0.90 to 1.85)	1.61 (1.07 to 2.42)	2.68 (1.50 to 4.79)	1.29 (1.15 to 1.45), <0.001
Multivariable HR (95% CI)‡	1.00	0.79 (0.53 to 1.19)	1.29 (0.89 to 1.85)	1.51 (1.01 to 2.28)	2.34 (1.30 to 4.20)	1.25 (1.12 to 1.40), <0.001

*Amount of time sitting available from 1988 questionnaire, and amount of time sitting at home available from 1990 questionnaire.
†Adjusted for age, coronary heart disease, hypertension, menopausal status, multivitamin use, use of non-aspirin non-steroidal anti-inflammatory drugs, parity, race, rheumatological disease, spouse's highest educational attainment, smoking status and pack years of smoking, and warfarin use.
‡Additionally adjusted for BMI, total energy intake, physical activity, and dietary pattern.

Conclusions.—Physical inactivity is associated with incident pulmonary embolism in women. Interventions that decrease time sitting could lower the risk of pulmonary embolism (Table 2).

▶ There is increasing recognition of the risk of incurring a venous thrombosis and a resulting pulmonary embolism after a period of prolonged immobility, as when wedged into an economy-class seat on a long air trip. However, previous reports on the influence of habitual physical activity have been less consistent. Although some authors have found a 30% to 50% decrease in the risks of pulmonary embolism in active individuals,[1-3] other studies, possibly weighted by the acute effects of exercise,[4,5] have seen an increased incidence of pulmonary embolism following strenuous exertion. The report of Kabrhel et al is based on a massive 18-year follow-up of US nurses (mainly white women, age > 55 years). Study participants were asked to rate the total amount of time they spent sitting per week (at work, at home, and driving) both in 1988 and in 1990; on each occasion, their score was rated from 1 to 3, and addition of the 2 scores yielded a composite rating that ranged from 2 to 6. After appropriate adjustment for other risk factors, the hazard ratio for an idiopathic pulmonary embolus (an incident unrelated to trauma, surgery, or malignancy) more than doubled as the self-reported sedentarity score increased over the range 2 to 6 (Table 2). It would be nice to be reassured that cardiovascular disease was not the cause of the inactivity, and that the levels of sedentarity as reported in 1988 and 1990 continued through to the end of the study. It also remains to be determined whether the apparent increase of risk is related directly to venous stasis or whether other concomitants of inactivity, such as changes in platelets and fibrinogen levels, are implicated. Finally, the crucial experiment will be to test whether reducing a person's amount of daily sitting reduces the risk of venous embolism, particularly in individuals who undertake a fair amount of physical activity at other times during the day.

R. J. Shephard, MD (Lond), PhD, DPE

References

1. van Stralen KJ, Le Cessie S, Rosendaal FR, Doggen CJ. Regular sports activities decrease the risk of venous thrombosis. *J Thromb Haemost.* 2007;5:2186-2192.
2. van Stralen KJ, Rosendaal FR, Doggen CJ. Minor injuries as a risk factor for venous thrombosis. *Arch Intern Med.* 2008;168:21-26.
3. Cushman M, Kuller LH, Prentice R, et al. Estrogen plus progestin and risk of venous thrombosis. *JAMA.* 2004;292:1573-1580.
4. van Stralen KJ, Blom JW, Doggen CJ, Rosendaal FR. Strenuous sport activities involving the upper extremities increase the risk of venous thrombosis of the arm. *J Thromb Haemost.* 2005;3:2110-2111.
5. van Stralen KJ, Doggen CJ, Lumley T, et al. The relationship between exercise and risk of venous thrombosis in elderly people. *J Am Geriatr Soc.* 2008;56:517-522.

Cardiac Arrest during Long-Distance Running Races

Kim JH, for the Race Associated Cardiac Arrest Event Registry (RACER) Study Group (Massachusetts General Hosp and Harv Med School, Boston; et al)
N Engl J Med 366:130-140, 2012

Background.—Approximately 2 million people participate in long-distance running races in the United States annually. Reports of race-related cardiac arrests have generated concern about the safety of this activity.

Methods.—We assessed the incidence and outcomes of cardiac arrest associated with marathon and half-marathon races in the United States from January 1, 2000, to May 31, 2010. We determined the clinical characteristics of the arrests by interviewing survivors and the next of kin of nonsurvivors, reviewing medical records, and analyzing postmortem data.

Results.—Of 10.9 million runners, 59 (mean [$\pm$SD] age, 42 ± 13 years; 51 men) had cardiac arrest (incidence rate, 0.54 per 100,000 participants; 95% confidence interval [CI], 0.41 to 0.70). Cardiovascular disease accounted for the majority of cardiac arrests. The incidence rate was significantly higher during marathons (1.01 per 100,000; 95% CI, 0.72 to 1.38) than during half-marathons (0.27; 95% CI, 0.17 to 0.43) and among men (0.90 per 100,000; 95% CI, 0.67 to 1.18) than among women (0.16; 95% CI, 0.07 to 0.31). Male marathon runners, the highest-risk group, had an increased incidence of cardiac arrest during the latter half of the study decade (2000–2004, 0.71 per 100,000 [95% CI, 0.31 to 1.40]; 2005–2010, 2.03 per 100,000 [95% CI, 1.33 to 2.98]; P = 0.01). Of the 59 cases of cardiac arrest, 42 (71%) were fatal (incidence, 0.39 per 100,000; 95% CI, 0.28 to 0.52). Among the 31 cases with complete clinical data, initiation of bystander-administered cardiopulmonary resuscitation and an underlying diagnosis other than hypertrophic cardiomyopathy were the strongest predictors of survival.

Conclusions.—Marathons and half-marathons are associated with a low overall risk of cardiac arrest and sudden death. Cardiac arrest, most commonly attributable to hypertrophic cardiomyopathy or atherosclerotic coronary disease, occurs primarily among male marathon participants; the incidence rate in this group increased during the past decade.

▶ Medical opinion about participation in marathon events has varied widely. At one end of the spectrum, the Toronto Rehabilitation Centre has entered many postcoronary patients in marathon events around the world; they have been thoroughly trained and have participated under close medical supervision, apparently without ill effect.[1] However, the Bassler hypothesis that distance running of this type ensures immunity against fatal coronary atherosclerosis[2] is now categorically disproved.[3] Some physicians also cite the fate of Pheidippides, the original Greek marathon man, who burst into the Athenian assembly crying *Nenikékamen* ("We have won") before collapsing and dying in the chamber. Some historians now argue that Pheidippides had done rather more than a standard marathon race: he had probably completed a rugged, mountainous 2-way run of 480 km to Sparta over the previous 3 days, and then marched with the Athenian army to the plain of Marathon, fighting the Persians in full armor, before he even began the 42-km side trip to Athens to convey the news of victory. Moreover, he packed an extraordinary 4 days of physical activity into the heat of the Mediterranean summer; afternoon temperatures on his final run from Marathon to Athens would likely have led to cancellation of a marathon run, with dry-bulb temperatures of around 32°C, rising to 38°C as the runner approached Athens.[4] The article by Baggish and associates now provides a definitive answer on the risk under modern conditions, with an analysis of findings in US marathon and half-marathon events from nearly 11 million runners who participated in the race-associated cardiac arrest event registry. Their answer: there is some immediate increase in the risk of cardiac arrest (generally fatal) during the race and within 1 hour of finishing, although the danger is quite low (0.5 per 100 000 participants) even when compared with that accepted in collegiate athletics. Deaths from cardiac arrest were more frequent in younger participants, suggesting to the authors that in this age group, hypertrophic cardiomyopathy was responsible for the incident; unfortunately, it was possible to obtain detailed clinical data for only a half of the incidents. It is also unfortunate that data were not obtained on the race experience of those who succumbed.

R. J. Shephard, MD (Lond), PhD, DPE

References

1. Shephard RJ, Kavanagh T, Tuck J, et al. Marathon jogging in post-myocardial infarction patients. *J Cardiopulm Rehabil.* 1983;3:321-329.
2. Bassler TJ. Marathon running and immunity to atherosclerosis. *Ann N Y Acad Sci.* 1977;301:579-592.
3. Noakes T, Opie L, Beck W, McKechnie J, Benchimol A, Desser K. Coronary heart disease in marathon runners. *Ann N Y Acad Sci.* 1977;301:593-619.
4. Shephard RJ. The developing understanding of human health and fitness. 3. The Classical Era. Health Fitness. *J Can.* 2012; In press.

Snow shovel-related injuries and medical emergencies treated in US EDs, 1990 to 2006
Watson DS, Shields BJ, Smith GA (The Res Inst at Nationwide Children's Hosp, Columbus, OH)
Am J Emerg Med 29:11-17, 2011

Background.—Injuries and medical emergencies associated with snow shovel use are common in the United States.

Methods.—This is a retrospective analysis of data from the National Electronic Injury Surveillance System. This study analyzes the epidemiologic features of snow shovel—related injuries and medical emergencies treated in US emergency departments (EDs) from 1990 to 2006.

Results.—An estimated 195 100 individuals (95% confidence interval, 140 400-249 800) were treated in US EDs for snow shovel—related incidents during the 17-year study period, averaging 11 500 individuals annually (SD, 5300). The average annual rate of snow shovel–related injuries and medical emergencies was 4.15 per 100 000 population. Approximately two thirds (67.5%) of these incidents occurred among males. Children younger than 18 years comprised 15.3% of the cases, whereas older adults (55 years and older) accounted for 21.8%. The most common diagnosis was soft tissue injury (54.7%). Injuries to the lower back accounted for 34.3% of the cases. The most common mechanism of injury/nature of medical emergency was acute musculoskeletal exertion (53.9%) followed by slips and falls (20.0%) and being struck by a snow shovel (15.0%). Cardiac-related ED visits accounted for 6.7% of the cases, including all of the 1647 deaths in the study. Patients required hospitalization in 5.8% of the cases. Most snow shovel–related incidents (95.6%) occurred in and around the home.

Conclusions.—This is the first study to comprehensively examine snow shovel–related injuries and medical emergencies in the United States using a nationally representative sample. There are an estimated 11 500 snow

TABLE 1.—Characteristics of Snow Shovel–Related Injuries and Medical Emergencies Treated in US EDs, 1990 to 2006

Description	Actual Cases (n)	Weighted Estimate (%)	95% CI
Age (y)			
<18	746	29 872 (15.3)	22 468-37 276
18-54	2981	122 699 (62.9)	86 310-159 088
≥55	1005	42 499 (21.8)	29 726-55 272
Not documented	1	NA	NA
Sex			
Male	3168	131 559 (67.5)	94 497-168 622
Female	1564	63 475 (32.5)	45 374-81 576
Not documented	1	NA	NA
Diagnosis			
Soft tissue injury	2521	106 484 (54.7)	74 399-138 569
Fracture	329	12 866 (6.6)	9321-16 411
Laceration	742	31 040 (16.0)	23 760-38 320
Other	1128	44 158 (22.7)	28 418-59 896
Not documented	13	NA	NA
Body part injured			
Head	724	28 573 (14.7)	21 397-35 750
Trunk	2630	109 684 (56.5)	74 404-144 964
Arm/hand	736	30 915 (15.9)	22 727-39 104
Leg/foot	497	20 290 (10.5)	15 044-25 536
Other	120	4595 (2.4)	2882-6308
Not documented	26	1044	NA
Disposition			
Treated/released/against medical advice	4417	182 146 (93.4)	130 539-233 754
Hospitalized	272	11 248 (5.8)	7467-15 029
Fatality	41	1647 (0.8)	827-2466
Not documented	3	NA	NA
Location			
Home/farm	2847	120 368 (95.6)	86 244-154 491
Street/public property/sports-recreational facility	129	5575 (4.4)	3261-7889
Not documented	1757	69 158	NA

NA indicates not applicable.

shovel—related injuries and medical emergencies treated annually in US EDs (Table 1).

▶ Snow-shoveling has long been regarded as a rather dangerous pastime for the middle-aged, coronary-prone businessman, although the information has mostly been anecdotal, and the precise elevation of risk has remained unclear.[1-3] It has been known for a long time that vigorous physical activity increases the immediate risk of a cardiac catastrophe by a factor of at least 5 relative to most sedentary pursuits.[4] Watson and associates' article presents some definitive statistics for the United States over a 17-year period. The first point to underline is that the risks to muscles, tendons, and bones are greater than the risk to the heart (Table 1). Nevertheless, the present study estimated that about 100 cardiac deaths per year were attributable to snow-shoveling. We still do not know the proportion of men who engage in such activities, but a reasonable guess might be 30 000 000 men needing to engage in vigorous shoveling 4 days during a winter, or about 330 000 person-years of exposure. This would in turn indicate a risk of 1 in 3300, not very different from the typical risk in a sedentary middle-aged man. Factors that may contribute to an adverse outcome include very cold weather,[5] wet or frozen snow, and attempts to clear a driveway against the clock. Current statistics should not discourage older adults from finding useful winter exercise by clearing snow at a reasonable pace, however.

R. J. Shephard, MD (Lond), PhD, DPE

References

1. Auliciems A, Frost D. Temperature and cardiovascular deaths in Montreal. *Int J Biometeorol.* 1989;33:151-156.
2. Burgess AM Jr. Snow-shoveling deaths. A report of eight cases in January 1964, during a single storm. *R I Med J.* 1965;48:131-133.
3. Franklin BA, Bonzheim K, Gordon S, Timmis GC. Snow shoveling: a trigger for acute myocardial infarction and sudden coronary death. *Am J Cardiol.* 1996;77:855-858.
4. Shephard RJ. Sudden death—a significant hazard of exercise? *Br J Sports Med.* 1974;8:101-110.
5. Jason LA. Modifying snow shoveling behaviors in an urban area. *Am J Public Health.* 1981;71:861.

Incidental Physical Activity Is Positively Associated with Cardiorespiratory Fitness

Ross R, McGuire KA (Queen's Univ, Kingston, Ontario, Canada)
Med Sci Sports Exerc 43:2189-2194, 2011

Purpose.—The primary aim was to determine whether incidental physical activity (IPA), expressed either as duration or intensity, was associated with cardiorespiratory fitness (CRF).

Methods.—Participants were inactive abdominally obese men ($n = 43$, waist circumference ≥ 102 cm) and women ($n = 92$, waist circumference

≥88 cm) recruited from Kingston, Canada. IPA (>100 counts per minute) was determined by accelerometry during 7 d and categorized into duration (min·d^{-1}) and intensity (counts per minute). In secondary analyses, IPA was further categorized as light physical activity (LPA, 100–1951 counts per minute) and sporadic moderate physical activity (MPA, ≥1952 counts per minute accumulated in bouts <10 consecutive minutes). CRF was assessed using a maximal treadmill exercise test.

Results.—Participants accumulated 308.2 ± 98.8 (mean ± SD) min of IPA per day of which 19.2 ± 13.5 min was spent in sporadic MPA. Mean CRF was 26.8 ± 4.7 mL·kg^{-1} body weight·min^{-1}. IPA duration was positively associated with CRF in the univariate model ($r^2 = 0.03$, $P < 0.05$) and after control for gender and body mass index ($r^2 = 0.53$, $P < 0.01$). Likewise, IPA intensity was positively associated with CRF in univariate ($r^2 = 0.18$, $P < 0.001$) and multivariate analyses ($r^2 = 0.56$, $P < 0.01$). After further control for each other, IPA duration was not associated with CRF ($P = 0.05$), whereas IPA intensity remained a significant predictor ($r^2 = 0.57$, $P < 0.001$). In secondary analyses, LPA was not associated with CRF ($P > 0.05$). Sporadic MPA was associated with CRF ($r^2 = 0.20$, $P < 0.001$) and remained a positive correlate after control for gender, body mass index, and the other physical activity variables ($r^2 = 0.60$, $P < 0.001$).

Conclusions.—In this study, both duration and intensity of IPA were positively associated with CRF among inactive abdominally obese adults. Sporadic MPA, but not LPA, was an independent predictor of CRF (Fig 1).

▶ The traditional view, based on both laboratory study[1] and self-reports of physical activity,[2] has been that light physical activity is not associated with cardiorespiratory fitness. However, some recent authors have suggested that

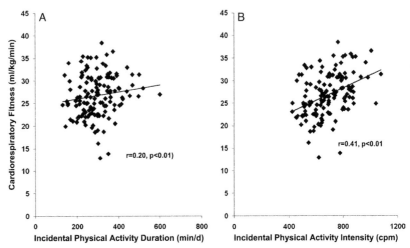

FIGURE 1.—Associations between IPA duration (A) and intensity (B) with CRF. (Reprinted from Ross R, McGuire KA. Incidental physical activity is positively associated with cardiorespiratory fitness. *Med Sci Sports Exerc.* 2011;43:2189-2194, with permission from the American College of Sports Medicine.)

incidental, nonpurposeful daily activity, not captured by questionnaires, may also have importance for health.[3] Ross and McGuire sought objective evidence on this issue; they used an Actigraph accelerometer to monitor incidental activity over at least 4 days and correlated these data with maximal oxygen intake (mL/[kg.min]) as measured on a treadmill. Activity was regarded as incidental if it occurred in bouts that were shorter than 10 minutes in duration. A modest cross-sectional correlation between such incidental activity and cardiorespiratory fitness was apparently observed (Fig 1). However, further evaluation of their data showed that much of the relationship was attributable to short bouts of moderate rather than light intensity physical activity, as defined for the Actigraph by Freedson and associates.[4] Moreover, the subjects studied by Ross and McGuire were quite obese (average body mass index, 33 kg/m^2), and the relationship that was observed could reflect a small cumulative effect of incidental activity on obesity rather than cardiorespiratory fitness. The question originally raised by Hardman[5] as to whether short bouts of physical activity benefit cardiovascular health remains important, but to establish the basic hypothesis concerning the value of such incidental activity, it would be necessary to recalculate correlations using absolute rather than relative maximal oxygen intake values.

R. J. Shephard, MD (Lond), PhD, DPE

References

1. Shephard RJ. Intensity, duration and frequency of exercise as determinants of the response to a training regimen. *Int Z Angew Physiol.* 1968;26:272-278.
2. Leon AS, Jacobs DR Jr, DeBacker G, Taylor HL. Relationship of physical characteristics and life habits to treadmill exercise capacity. *Am J Epidemiol.* 1981;113:653-660.
3. Tremblay MS, Colley RC, Saunders TJ, Healy GN, Owen N. Physiological and health implications of a sedentary lifestyle. *Appl Physiol Nutr Metab.* 2010;35:725-740.
4. Freedson PS, Melanson E, Sirard J. Calibration of the Computer Science and Applications, Inc. accelerometer. *Med Sci Sports Exerc.* 1998;30:777-781.
5. Hardman AE. Accumulation of physical activity for health gains: what is the evidence? *Br J Sports Med.* 1999;33:87-92.

Gender differences in the prognostic value of exercise treadmill test characteristics
Daugherty SL, Magid DJ, Kikla JR, et al (Univ of Colorado Denver, Aurora; Longmont United Hosp, CO; et al)
Am Heart J 161:908-914, 2011

Background.—Although exercise treadmill testing (ETT) is less sensitive and specific for diagnosis of coronary disease in women, little is known about gender differences in the prognostic importance of ETT variables.

Methods.—We studied 9,569 consecutive patients (46.8% women) referred for ETT between July 2001 and June 2004 in a community-based system. We assessed the association between ETT variables (exercise capacity, symptoms, ST-segment deviations, heart rate recovery, and chronotropic response) and time to all-cause death and myocardial infarction (MI), adjusting for patient and stress test characteristics. Models were stratified by gender to determine the relationship between ETT variables and outcomes.

Results.—In the entire population, exercise capacity and heart rate recovery were significantly associated with all-cause death, whereas exercise capacity, chest pain, and ST-segment deviations were significantly associated with subsequent MI. The relationship between ETT variables and outcomes were similar between men and women, except for abnormal exercise capacity, which had a significantly stronger association with death in men (men: hazard ratio [HR] 2.89 and 95% CI 1.89-4.44, women: HR 0.99 and 95% CI 0.52-1.93, and interaction $P = .01$), and chronotropic incompetence, which had a significantly stronger relationship with MI in women (men: HR 1.29 and 95% CI 0.74-2.20, women: HR 2.79 and 95% CI 0.94-8.27, and interaction $P = .04$).

Conclusions.—Although many traditional ETT variables had similar prognostic value in both men and women, exercise capacity was more prognostically important in men, and chronotropic incompetence was more important in women. Future studies should confirm these findings in additional populations (Table 1).

▶ Early investigators used exercise stress tests to assess a patient's prognosis primarily in terms of depression of the ST segment of the electrocardiogram. In male patients, the risk of premature death was increased at least 2-fold in those showing a horizontal or downsloping ST depression > 2 mm (0.2 mV) during vigorous exercise. However, for a variety of reasons, exercise-induced ST depression was a less reliable indicator of prognosis in women.[1,2] More recently, cardiologists have directed attention to other components of the exercise response that can also affect prognosis, including exercise capacity,[3] heart rate recovery curves,[4] and chronotropic incompetence.[5] The Duke treadmill score, for instance, is a composite figure, based on ST segment changes, treadmill time, and exercise-induced angina.[6] The question arises as to how far these additional variables overcome the sex bias inherent in prognoses predicted on ST segmental changes alone. The treadmill endurance time (and measurements of peak oxygen intake expressed in the traditional units of mL/[kg.min]) reflects both peak cardiac performance and the individual's body mass. In those who have already sustained a heart attack, cardiac performance is probably the dominant variable, and our data show that peak oxygen intake gives a good indication of prognosis in women as well as in men.[7] The article by Daugherty and associates compares the prognostic potential of various treadmill test measurements in a large community sample of older individuals (n = 9569; average age, 55 years) referred for exercise testing mainly because of chest pain or dyspnea on exertion; all-cause mortality (142 cases) and the onset of myocardial infarction (130 cases) were assessed over a follow-up period averaging 3.2 years. In such a group, exercise time is probably influenced more strongly by obesity than by cardiac function, and perhaps for this reason the treadmill endurance provided a much better indication of the risk of all-cause

TABLE 1.—Baseline Characteristics of the Study Population Referred for an ETT

Characteristic	Total, n = 9569	Men, n = 5094	Women, n = 4475	P
Age (y)	56 (48, 65)	55 (47, 65)	57 (49, 66)	<.01
Current smoking	1348 (14.1)	729 (14.3)	619 (13.8)	.52
Clinical history				
Diabetes mellitus	1341 (14.1)	781 (15.3)	560 (12.5)	<.01
Hypertension	4664 (48.7)	2463 (48.4)	2201 (49.2)	.43
Hyperlipidemia	6083 (63.6)	3279 (64.4)	2804 (62.7)	.09
Coronary artery disease	1305 (13.7)	972 (19.1)	333 (7.4)	<.01
Chronic obstructive pulmonary disease	463 (4.8)	234 (4.6)	229 (5.1)	.23
Peripheral vascular disease	175 (1.8)	122 (2.4)	53 (1.2)	<.01
Cerebral vascular disease	237 (2.5)	115 (2.3)	122 (2.7)	.14
Obstructive sleep apnea	417 (4.4)	273 (5.4)	144 (3.2)	<.01
Cancer	468 (4.9)	238 (4.7)	230 (5.1)	.29
Depression	1485 (15.5)	561 (11.0)	924 (20.6)	<.01
Family history of coronary disease	3498 (36.6)	1738 (34.1)	1760 (39.3)	<.01
Reason for ETT referral				
Atypical chest pain	4489 (47.0)	2386 (46.8)	2103 (47.9)	.49
Chest pain	1679 (17.6)	835 (16.4)	844 (18.9)	<.01
Dyspnea on exertion	862 (9.0)	453 (8.9)	409 (9.1)	.68
Other or missing	2541 (26.5)	1288 (25.3)	1253 (28.0)	<.01
Exercise treadmill variables				
Chest pain	868 (9.1)	385 (7.6)	483 (10.8)	<.01
Exercise capacity <85%*	2330 (24.4)	1084 (21.3)	1246 (27.8)	<.01
Ischemic ST-segment change	1905 (19.9)	1008 (19.8)	897 (20.0)	.77
HRR ≤12 beat/min†	2947 (30.8)	1486 (29.2)	1461 (32.6)	<.01
Chronotropic incompetence <0.8	2288 (23.9)	1173 (23.0)	1115 (24.9)	.03
Maximal heart rate	155 (142, 168)	155 (142, 169)	155 (142, 166)	<.01
Maximal systolic BP	168 (152, 182)	170 (160, 188)	164 (150, 180)	<.01
Maximal diastolic BP	80 (76, 90)	82 (78, 90)	80 (76, 90)	<.01
Ectopy in recovery‡	194 (2.0)	124 (2.4)	69 (1.5)	<.01
Medications				
Aspirin	2541 (26.6)	1531 (30.1)	1010 (22.6)	<.01
β-Blockers	2287 (24.0)	1258 (24.7)	1029 (23.0)	.05
Diuretics	1819 (19.1)	780 (15.3)	1039 (23.2)	<.01
Calcium-channel blockers	658 (6.9)	335 (6.7)	323 (7.2)	.22
ACE and/or ARB	1777 (18.6)	1091 (21.4)	686 (15.3)	<.01
Statins	2234 (23.4)	1424 (27.9)	810 (18.1)	<.01

Continuous variables are shown as median (25th, 75th percentiles). Categorical variables are shown as exact count (%). ACE indicates angiotensin-converting enzyme; ARB, angiotensin receptor blocker.
Editor's Note: Please refer to original journal article for full references.
*Proportion of age and gender predicted METs.[12,16]
†A cutoff value of ≤12 beat/min for HRR was considered abnormal.[6]
‡Presence of ≥6 premature ventricular beats per minute in recovery.[5]

mortality in men than in women (Table 1). In contrast, chronotropic incompetence appeared to provide a stronger measure of the risk of myocardial infarction in women than in men, after adjustment of the data for "competing causes of death"; however, perhaps because the total number of events was small in the women, the relationship with chronotropic incompetence only bordered on statistical significance. The authors of this report recommend continuing the use of composite treadmill scores but urge the development of new and sex-specific methods of combining data.

R. J. Shephard, MD (Lond), PhD, DPE

References

1. Kwok Y, Kim C, Grady D, Segal M, Redberg R. Meta-analysis of exercise testing to detect coronary artery disease in women. *Am J Cardiol.* 1999;83:660-666.
2. Gibbons RJ, Balady GJ, Bricker JT, et al. ACC/AHA 2002 guideline update for exercise testing: summary article: a report of the American College of Cardiology/American Heart Association Task Force on Practice Guidelines (Committee to Update the 1997 Exercise Testing Guidelines). *Circulation.* 2002;106:1883-1892.
3. Peterson PN, Magid DJ, Ross C, et al. Association of exercise capacity on treadmill with future cardiac events in patients referred for exercise testing. *Arch Intern Med.* 2008;168:174-179.
4. Vivekananthan DP, Blackstone EH, Pothier CE, Lauer MS. Heart rate recovery after exercise is a predictor of mortality, independent of the angiographic severity of coronary disease. *J Am Coll Cardiol.* 2003;42:831-838.
5. Dresing TJ, Blackstone EH, Pashkow FJ, Snader CE, Marwick TH, Lauer MS. Usefulness of impaired chronotropic response to exercise as a predictor of mortality, independent of the severity of coronary artery disease. *Am J Cardiol.* 2000;86:602-609.
6. Nishime EO, Cole CR, Blackstone EH, Pashkow FJ, Lauer MS. Heart rate recovery and treadmill exercise score as predictors of mortality in patients referred for exercise ECG. *JAMA.* 2000;284:1392-1398.
7. Kavanagh T, Mertens DJ, Hamm LF, et al. Peak oxygen intake and cardiac mortality in women referred for cardiac rehabilitation. *J Am Coll Cardiol.* 2003;42:2139-2143.

Effect of Air Travel on Exercise-Induced Coagulatory and Fibrinolytic Activation in Marathon Runners

Parker B, Augeri A, Capizzi J, et al (Hartford Hosp, CT)
Clin J Sport Med 21:126-130, 2011

Objective.—Air travel and exercise change hemostatic parameters. This study investigated the effect of air travel on exercise-induced coagulation and fibrinolysis in endurance athletes.

Design.—A prospective longitudinal study.

Setting.—The 114th Boston Marathon (April 19, 2010).

Participants.—Forty-one adults were divided into travel (T: 23 participants, living >4-hour plane flight from Boston) and nontravel (C: 18 participants, living <2-hour car trip from Boston) groups.

Independent Variables.—Age, anthropometrics, vital signs, training mileage, and finishing time were collected.

Main Outcome Measures.—Subjects provided venous blood samples the day before (PRE), immediately after (FINISH), and the day following the marathon after returning home (POST). Blood was analyzed for thrombin–antithrombin complex (TAT), tissue plasminogen activator (t-PA), hematocrit (Hct), and the presence of Factor V Leiden R506Q mutation.

Results.—Thrombin–antithrombin complex increased more in T subjects in PRE to FINISH samples (5.0 ± 4.0 to 12.9 ± 15.6 µg/L) than in C subjects (4.0 ± 1.2 to 6.1 ± 1.2 µg/L; P = 0.02 for comparison). The t-PA increased in both the T (5.4 ± 2.3 to 25.1 ± 12.2 ng/mL) and C (5.6 ± 2.0 to 27.7 ± 11.3 ng/mL) groups in PRE to FINISH samples, and this response did not differ between groups (P = 0.23 for comparison). Both

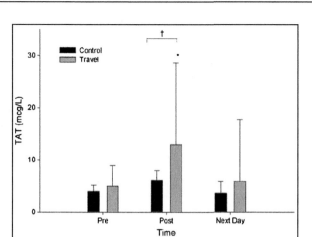

FIGURE 2.—Group means (±SD) of thrombin-antithrombin complex (TAT) before (Pre), immediately after (Post), and the day after the marathon (Next Day). *Significant effect change relative to the baseline (Pre) value at P P < 0.05. (Reprinted from Parker B, Augeri A, Capizzi J, et al. Effect of air travel on exercise-induced coagulatory and fibrinolytic activation in marathon runners. *Clin J Sport Med.* 2011;21:126-130.)

groups exhibited similar t-PA and TAT values at POST that were not different than PRE (all P > 0.35). Age was related to the FINISH TAT values in T (r2 = 0.19; P = 0.04) but not in C (r2 = 0.03; P = 0.53) subjects.

Conclusions.—Results suggest that the combination of air travel and marathon running induces an acute hypercoaguable state; this hemostatic imbalance is exaggerated with increasing age (Fig 2).

▶ Strenuous exercise, such as a marathon run, is well recognized as causing an activation of both coagulatory[1-3] and fibrinolytic[4,5] systems, although it is less clear whether changes in the 2 opposing systems alter the risk of blood clot formation. However, long plane or car journeys can increase the risks of deep vein thrombosis and pulmonary embolism,[6,7] and several anecdotal reports suggest that this can be a problem for athletes who are traveling to distant competitions. The current data suggest a significant interaction between the thrombin-antithrombin complex and travel (a plane journey averaging 5.6 hours, completed 53 hours prior to the event) that was not countered by increased fibrolytic activity and could increase the risk of a deep vein thrombosis (Fig 2); further, this risk remained elevated for the next day. One possible weakness in the argument is that those who traveled were substantially older (42 vs 32 years) than those who did not. Particular care seems necessary if there are other factors predisposing to clotting, such as age or use of oral contraceptives.

R. J. Shephard, MD (Lond), PhD, DPE

References

1. Cerneca E, Simeone R, Bruno G, Gombacci A. Coagulation parameters in senior athletes practicing endurance sporting activity. *J Sports Med Phys Fitness.* 2005; 45:576-579.

2. Prisco D, Paniccia R, Bandinelli B, et al. Evaluation of clotting and fibrinolytic activation after protracted physical exercise. *Thromb Res.* 1998;89:73-78.
3. Siegel AJ, Stec JJ, Lipinska I, et al. Effect of marathon running on inflammatory and hemostatic markers. *Am J Cardiol.* 2001;88:918-920.
4. Sumann G, Fries D, Griesmacher A, et al. Blood coagulation activation and fibrinolysis during a downhill marathon run. *Blood Coagul Fibrinolysis.* 2007;18: 435-440.
5. Röcker L, Taenzer M, Drygas WK, Lill H, Heyduck B, Altenkirch HU. Effect of prolonged physical exercise on the fibrinolytic system. *Eur J Appl Physiol Occup Physiol.* 1990;60:478-481.
6. Lehman S. *Blood Clots and the Endurance Athlete.* 2009. http://pressurepositive. wordpress.com/2009/03/30/blood-clots-and-the-endurance-athlete/2009. Accessed April 4, 2011.
7. Schreijer AJ, Cannegieter SC, Meijers JC, Middeldorp S, Büller HR, Rosendaal FR. Activation of coagulation system during air travel: a crossover study. *Lancet.* 2006; 367:832-838.

Lower prevalence of silent brain infarcts in the physically active: The Northern Manhattan Study

Willey JZ, Moon YP, Paik MC, et al (Columbia Univ, NY; et al)
Neurology 76:2112-2118, 2011

Objective.—To examine the independent association between physical activity and subclinical cerebrovascular disease as measured by silent brain infarcts (SBI) and white matter hyperintensity volume (WMHV).

Methods.—The Northern Manhattan Study (NOMAS) is a population-based prospective cohort examining risk factors for incident vascular disease, and a subsample underwent brain MRI. Our primary outcomes were SBI and WMHV. Baseline measures of leisure-time physical activity were collected in person. Physical activity was categorized by quartiles of the metabolic equivalent (MET) score. We used logistic regression models to examine the associations between physical activity and SBI, and linear regression to examine the association with WMHV.

Results.—There were 1,238 clinically stroke-free participants (mean age 70 ± 9 years) of whom 60% were women, 65% were Hispanic, and 43% reported no physical activity. A total of 197 (16%) participants had SBI. In fully adjusted models, compared to those who did not engage in physical activity, those in the upper quartile of MET scores were almost half as likely to have SBI (adjusted odds ratio 0.6, 95% confidence interval 0.4−0.9). Physical activity was not associated with WMHV.

Conclusions.—Increased levels of physical activity were associated with a lower risk of SBI but not WMHV. Engaging in moderate to heavy physical activities may be an important component of prevention strategies aimed at reducing subclinical brain infarcts (Table 3).

▶ Subclinical cerebrovascular disease (SCVD), or silent strokes, and associated white matter hyperintensity (WMH) on MRI are significant developments in the elderly, often being harbingers of impaired mobility and falls,[1,2] cognitive dysfunction,[3,4] and overt strokes.[5] The report of Willey and colleagues examined

TABLE 3.—Association Between Measures of Physical Activity and Subclinical Brain
Infarctions

	Univariate Analysis, OR (95% CI)	Model 1,[a] OR (95% CI)	Model 2,[b] OR (95% CI)
MET score >14 (upper quartile)[c]	0.8 (0.5−1.2)	0.6 (0.4−1.0)	0.6 (0.4−0.9)
MET score 3−14 (third quartile)[c]	1.0 (0.7−1.5)	0.9 (0.6−1.4)	1.0 (0.7−1.4)
Total intensity of physical activity (moderate to heavy vs none)	0.8 (0.5−1.2)	0.6 (0.4−1.0)	0.6 (0.4−0.9)
Total intensity of physical activity (light vs none)	1.0 (0.7−1.4)	0.8 (0.6−1.2)	0.8 (0.6−1.2)
Any physical activity vs none	0.9 (0.7−1.3)	0.7 (0.5−1.0)	0.8 (0.5−1.1)

Abbreviations: CI = confidence interval; MET = metabolic equivalent; OR = odds ratio.
[a]Model 1: adjusted for age, race-ethnicity, sex, insurance (Medicaid/none vs others), and completing high school education.
[b]Model 2: further adjusted for low-density lipoprotein cholesterol, high-density lipoprotein cholesterol, current tobacco use, moderate alcohol use, systolic blood pressure, diastolic blood pressure, glomerular filtration rate, and diabetes.
[c]Reference: lowest 2 quartiles of the MET score.

associations between a person's reported habitual activity (a questionnaire reported on physical activity undertaken during the previous 2 weeks and was used to classify subjects by quartiles of activity, expressed in metabolic equivalent [MET] levels of intensity), subclinical brain infarcts (SBI) as seen on MRI (diagnosed with a cavitation of at least 3 mm diameter), and WMH (obtained from semiautomated pixel intensity measurements on cerebrospinal fluid and white and grey matter). The subjects were a substantial multiethnic, urban, and community-based sample of elderly individuals who had no history of clinical strokes, although about 1 in 6 had SBIs. After adjusting for sociodemographic influences and traditional stroke risk factors, a lower incidence of SBI was seen among exercisers, but this was confined to the most active quartile, who reported moderate to heavy intensity activity (Table 3). There was no association between WMH and habitual physical activity, possibly because WMH can arise from a variety of pathologies other than SBI. Although a cross-sectional study of this type cannot establish a causal relationship between inactivity and SCVD, it does strengthen the case of those who continue to promote vigorous rather than light physical activity for elderly individuals.

R. J. Shephard, MD (Lond), PhD, DPE

References

1. Whitman GT, Tang Y, Lin A, Baloh RW. A prospective study of cerebral white matter abnormalities in older people with gait dysfunction. *Neurology.* 2001;57:990-994.
2. Longstreth WT Jr, Arnold AM, Beauchamp NJ Jr, et al. Incidence, manifestations, and predictors of worsening white matter on serial cranial magnetic resonance imaging in the elderly: the Cardiovascular Health Study. *Stroke.* 2005;36:56-61.
3. Wright CB, Festa JR, Paik MC, et al. White matter hyperintensities and subclinical infarction: associations with psychomotor speed and cognitive flexibility. *Stroke.* 2008;39:800-805.
4. Debette S, Beiser A, DeCarli C, et al. Association of MRI markers of vascular brain injury with incident stroke, mild cognitive impairment, dementia, and mortality: the Framingham Offspring Study. *Stroke.* 2010;41:600-606.

5. Debette S, Markus HS. The clinical importance of white matter hyperintensities on brain magnetic resonance imaging: systematic review and meta-analysis. *BMJ.* 2010;341:c3666.

Analysis of ST/HR hysteresis improves long-term prognostic value of exercise ECG test

Kronander H, Hammar N, Fischer-Colbrie W, et al (Royal Inst of Technology, Stockholm, Sweden; Karolinska Institutet, Stockholm, Sweden; Mälar Hosp, Eskilstuna, Sweden)
Int J Cardiol 148:64-69, 2011

Background.—ST/HR hysteresis is one of the better diagnostic exercise ECG variables for coronary artery disease. This study evaluates the long-term prognostic value of ST/HR hysteresis in predicting acute myocardial infarction (AMI) and all-cause mortality in men and women.

Methods.—The study population consisted of 8317 patients who had undergone routine exercise test on bicycle ergometer at one Swedish centre. Information on AMI and all-cause mortality was obtained from national Swedish registers covering a mean follow-up period of 9.5 years.

Results.—The adjusted hazard ratio for AMI at a diagnostic cut point of ≤ −20 µV for ST/HR hysteresis was 1.88 (95% CI, 1.62−2.17) in men and 2.31 (95% CI, 1.83−2.91) in women. For all-cause death the adjusted hazard ratio was 1.72 (95% CI, 1.52−1.96) in men and 1.90 (95% CI, 1.57−2.29) in women. The corresponding hazard ratios for ST-segment depression with horizontal or down-sloping ST-segment, ST-segment depression, ST/HR index, and ST/HR slope were lower. For comparison, the adjusted hazard ratio for AMI using maximal workload in percent of predicted was 2.02 (95% CI, 1.77−2.32) in men and 2.14 (95% CI, 1.71−2.67) in women. Area under the ROC curves for prediction of AMI was significantly larger using ST/HR hysteresis than using any of three other evaluated ECG indicators.

Conclusions.—ST/HR hysteresis appears to improve the prognostic ability of an exercise ECG test for AMI and all-cause mortality in a long-term perspective compared to conventional ST-segment and ST/HR indicators in both genders and clearly more markedly in women (Table 2).

▶ A horizontal or downward-sloping ST segment or the ST/heart rate (HR) relationship during a graded exercise test have long been the standard criteria of myocardial ischemia,[1-4] but the data of Kronander et al (Table 2) suggest that the presence of ST hysteresis during the recovery phase is substantially more informative. The information is solidly based—an average follow-up of 9.5 years, with almost no losses from the survey. ST/HR hysteresis is a somewhat complicated calculation and presumes the availability of a specialized computer program for analysis of the electrocardiogram records; unfortunately, this is not yet widely available, although these data may encourage its wider dissemination. The hysteresis is estimated as the difference in ST depression

TABLE 2.—Relative Risk of All-Cause Mortality and AMI Respectively in Relation to Exercise Test Variables

	All-Cause Death Relative Risk (95% CI)	P-Value	AMI Relative Risk (95% CI)	P-Value
Men (n=4834)				
Crude				
ST dep HD ≥1 mm	2.60 (2.29–2.95)	<0.001	2.62 (2.28–3.02)	<0.001
ST dep ≥1 mm	2.03 (1.80–2.29)	<0.001	2.30 (2.01–2.62)	<0.001
ST/HR index ≥1.60 µV (bpm)$^{-1}$	2.31 (2.05–2.61)	<0.001	2.41 (2.11–2.75)	<0.001
ST/HR slope ≥2.40 µV (bpm)$^{-1}$	2.20 (1.95–2.48)	<0.001	2.56 (2.23–2.93)	<0.001
ST/HR hysteresis ≤−20 µV	3.08 (2.72–3.49)	<0.001	3.27 (2.85–3.75)	<0.001
Maximal workload <85% of predicted	1.83 (1.62–2.06)	<0.001	1.84 (1.62–2.10)	<0.001
HR recovery ≤18 (bpm)	3.66 (3.24–4.14)	<0.001	3.00 (2.61–3.45)	<0.001
Adjusted	*		†	
ST dep HD ≥1 mm	1.51 (1.32–1.72)	<0.001	1.56 (1.35–1.80)	<0.001
ST dep ≥1 mm	1.20 (1.06–1.36)	0.003	1.46 (1.28–1.68)	<0.001
ST/HR index ≥1.60 µV (bpm)$^{-1}$	1.29 (1.14–1.46)	<0.001	1.41 (1.23–1.62)	<0.001
ST/HR slope ≥2.40 µV (bpm)$^{-1}$	1.22 (1.08–1.38)	0.002	1.49 (1.29–1.71)	<0.001
ST/HR hysteresis ≤−20 µV	1.72 (1.52–1.96)	<0.001	1.88 (1.62–2.17)	<0.001
Maximal workload <85% of predicted	2.19 (1.94–2.48)	<0.001	2.02 (1.77–2.32)	<0.001
HR recovery ≤18 (bpm)	1.82 (1.59–2.07)	<0.001	1.59 (1.37–1.84)	<0.001
Women (n=3483)				
Crude				
ST dep HD ≥1 mm	2.17 (1.73–2.73)	<0.001	2.33 (1.79–3.05)	<0.001
ST dep ≥1 mm	1.24 (1.02–1.50)	0.028	1.44 (1.15–1.80)	0.001
ST/HR index ≥1.60 µV (bpm)$^{-1}$	1.84 (1.54–2.21)	<0.001	2.47 (1.99–3.06)	<0.001
ST/HR slope ≥2.40 µV (bpm)$^{-1}$	1.40 (1.16–1.68)	<0.001	2.20 (1.78–2.73)	<0.001
ST/HR hysteresis ≤−20 µV	3.13 (2.61–3.74)	<0.001	4.08 (3.28–5.07)	<0.001
Maximal workload <85% of predicted	2.14 (1.79–2.56)	<0.001	2.26 (1.82–2.80)	<0.001
HR recovery ≤18 (bpm)	4.11 (3.43–4.92)	<0.001	3.33 (2.68–4.14)	<0.001
Adjusted	*		‡	
ST dep HD ≥1 mm	1.53 (1.21–1.93)	<0.001	1.50 (1.14–1.97)	0.004
ST dep ≥1 mm	1.11 (0.92–1.35)	0.285	1.25 (1.00–1.57)	0.051
ST/HR index ≥1.60 µV (bpm)$^{-1}$	1.30 (1.08–1.56)	0.005	1.71 (1.37–2.13)	<0.001
ST/HR slope ≥2.40 µV (bpm)$^{-1}$	1.03 (0.85–1.24)	0.795	1.51 (1.21–1.88)	<0.001
ST/HR hysteresis ≤−20 µV	1.90 (1.57–2.29)	<0.001	2.31 (1.83–2.91)	<0.001
Maximal workload <85% of predicted	2.43 (2.02–2.91)	<0.001	2.14 (1.71–2.67)	<0.001
HR recovery ≤18 (bpm)	2.32 (1.92–2.82)	<0.001	1.74 (1.38–2.21)	<0.001

AMI − acute myocardial infarction, HR − heart rate.
*Adjusted for age and diabetes mellitus.
†Adjusted for age and cardiovascular medication.
‡Adjusted for age, diabetes mellitus, and cardiovascular medication.

between the exercise and the recovery phases, integrated over the HR from the minimum HR during the first 3 min of recovery to the maximal HR reached during exercise, and then by the HR difference over the integration interval to normalize data relative to the recovery HR decrement.[5] The limitations of the study are that so far the value of hysteresis has been demonstrated only for cycle ergometer tests, and no information was available on dyslipidemia, hypertension, and smoking habits. Nevertheless, the findings are sufficiently impressive as to warrant further study.

R. J. Shephard, MD (Lond), PhD, DPE

References

1. Detrano R, Salcedo E, Passalacqua M, Friis R. Exercise electrocardiographic variables: a critical appraisal. *J Am Coll Cardiol.* 1986;8:836-847.
2. Kligfield P, Ameisen O, Okin PM. Relation of the exercise ST/HR slope to simple heart rate adjustment of ST segment depression. *J Electrocardiol.* 1987;20: 135-140.
3. Elamin MS, Mary DA, Smith DR, Linden RJ. Prediction of severity of coronary artery disease using slope of submaximal ST segment/heart rate relationship. *Cardiovasc Res.* 1980;14:681-691.
4. Kligfield P, Ameisen O, Okin PM. Heart rate adjustment of ST segment depression for improved detection of coronary artery disease. *Circulation.* 1989;79:245-255.
5. Lehtinen R, Sievänen H, Viik J, Turjanmaa V, Niemelä K, Malmivuo J. Accurate detection of coronary artery disease by integrated analysis of the ST-segment depression/heart rate patterns during the exercise and recovery phases of the exercise electrocardiography test. *Am J Cardiol.* 1996;78:1002-1006.

Coronary Computed Tomography Angiography After Stress Testing: Results From a Multicenter, Statewide Registry, ACIC (Advanced Cardiovascular Imaging Consortium)
Chinnaiyan KM, Raff GL, Goraya T, et al (William Beaumont Hosp, Royal Oak, MI; Michigan Heart, Ann Arbor; et al)
J Am Coll Cardiol 59:688-695, 2012

Objectives.—This study was conducted to evaluate the correlation between stress test results and coronary computed tomography angiography (CCTA) findings and comparative diagnostic performance of the 2 modalities in patients undergoing invasive coronary angiography (ICA).

Background.—Recent data suggest that only a third of patients undergoing ICA have obstructive coronary artery disease (CAD); accurate pre-ICA risk stratification is needed.

Methods.—At 47 centers participating in the ACIC (Advanced Cardiovascular Imaging Consortium) in Michigan, patients without known CAD who were undergoing CCTA within 3 months of a stress test were studied. Demographics, risk factors, symptoms, and stress test results were correlated with obstructive CAD (>50% stenosis) on CCTA and ICA.

Results.—Among 6,198 patients (age 56 ± 12 years, 48% men), >50% stenosis was seen in 1,158 (18.7%) on CCTA. Independent predictors included male sex (odds ratio [OR]: 2.37, 95% confidence interval [CI]: 1.83 to 3.06), current smoking (OR: 2.23, 95% CI: 1.57 to 3.17), older age (OR per 10-year increment: 2.14, 95% CI: 1.89 to 2.41), hypertension (OR: 1.8, 95% CI: 1.37 to 2.34), and typical angina (OR: 1.48, 95% CI: 1.03 to 2.12). Stress test results were not predictive. Among patients undergoing ICA (n = 621), there was a strong correlation of ICA with CCTA findings (OR: 9.09, 95% CI: 5.57 to 14.8, p < 0.001), but not stress results (OR: 0.79, 95% CI: 0.56 to 1.11, p = 0.17).

Conclusions.—Stress test findings did not predict obstructive CAD on CCTA, observed in <20% of patients in this large study group. The strong

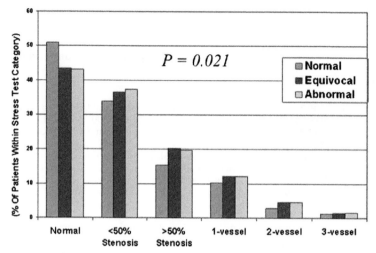

FIGURE 2.—Relationship Between Stress Test Results and CCTA. Distribution and severity of coronary artery disease as detected by coronary computed tomography angiography (CCTA) is shown by stress test result groups: normal (**green bars**), equivocal (**blue bars**), and abnormal (**gray bars**). For interpretation of the references to color in this figure legend, the reader is referred to web version of this article. (Reprinted from Chinnaiyan KM, Raff GL, Goraya T, et al. Coronary computed tomography angiography after stress testing: results from a multicenter, statewide registry, ACIC (Advanced Cardiovascular Imaging Consortium). *J Am Coll Cardiol*. 2012;59:688-695, Copyright 2012, with permission from American College of Cardiology.)

association of CCTA with ICA suggests that it may serve as an effective "gatekeeper" to invasive testing in patients needing adjudication of stress test results. (Advanced Cardiovascular Imaging Consortium: A Collaborative Quality Improvement Project [ACIC]; NCT00640068) (Fig 2).

▶ Health systems in many parts of the world are facing growing financial strain from the overuse of laboratory tests. One area of particular concern is testing for possible coronary artery occlusion; a growing number of patients are undergoing not only treadmill stress testing but also costly cardiac imaging.[1,2] The article by Chinnaiyan et al reports on the stress test and coronary computed tomographic angiography (CCTA) findings for a large sample of middle-aged adults who were initially free of known coronary disease. The clinical record (sex, age, smoking habits, blood pressure, and symptoms of angina) contributed significantly to the prediction of greater than 50% narrowing as seen on CCTA, and, as in previous trials,[3,4] there was a good correlation between the findings from CCTA and intracoronary angiography (ICA). CCTA added substantially to the information gleaned from clinical reports. However, the stress test data (obtained within the previous 3 months) were unrelated to the findings at either CCTA or ICA (Fig 2), and stress testing added little to clinical diagnosis alone. This finding at first glance seems a little at variance with some earlier reports, and it may reflect in part the use of a 50% rather than a 70% criterion of coronary obstruction on an ostensibly healthy population. The conclusion of the present authors is that CCTA should be used as a "gatekeeper" for ICA,[5,6] but a further important lesson to be drawn is that important information can be garnered by a careful clinical examination, without the expense of laboratory testing; this is important to remember, given that CCTA is not exactly a cheap procedure.

R. J. Shephard, MD (Lond), PhD, DPE

References

1. Bonow RO. Sixth Annual Mario S. Verani, MD Memorial Lecture: cardiovascular imaging—added value or added cost? *J Nucl Cardiol.* 2008;15:170-177.
2. Gibbons RJ. Finding value in imaging: what is appropriate? *J Nucl Cardiol.* 2008; 15:178-185.
3. Mowatt G, Cook JA, Hillis GS, et al. 64-Slice computed tomography angiography in the diagnosis and assessment of coronary artery disease: systematic review and meta-analysis. *Heart.* 2008;94:1386-1393.
4. Meijboom WB, Meijs MF, Schuijf JD, et al. Diagnostic accuracy of 64-slice computed tomography coronary angiography: a prospective, multicenter, multivendor study. *J Am Coll Cardiol.* 2008;52:2135-2144.
5. Lesser JR, Flygenring B, Knickelbine T, et al. Clinical utility of coronary CT angiography: coronary stenosis detection and prognosis in ambulatory patients. *Catheter Cardiovasc Interv.* 2007;69:64-72.
6. Cole JH, Chunn VM, Morrow JA, Buckley RS, Phillips GM. Cost implications of initial computed tomography angiography as opposed to catheterization in patients with mildly abnormal or equivocal myocardial perfusion scans. *J Cardiovasc Comput Tomogr.* 2007;1:21-26.

Hydrotherapy added to endurance training versus endurance training alone in elderly patients with chronic heart failure: A randomized pilot study
Caminiti G, Volterrani M, Marazzi G, et al (IRCCS San Raffaele Roma, Italy)
Int J Cardiol 148:199-203, 2011

Purpose.—To assess if Hydrotherapy (HT) added to endurance training (ET) is more effective than ET alone in order to improve exercise tolerance of elderly male patients with chronic heart failure (CHF).

Methods.—Twenty-one male CHF patients, age 68 ± 7 (mean ± DS) years; ejection fraction 32 ± 9. NYHA II-III were enrolled. Eleven pts were randomized to combined training (CT) group performing HT+ ET and 10 patients to ET group (ET only). At baseline and after 24 weeks all patients underwent: 6-minute walking test (6 MWT), assessment of quadriceps maximal voluntary contraction (MVC) and peak torque (PT), blood pressure and heart rate (HR), echocardiography and non-invasive hemodynamic evaluation. HT was performed 3 times/week in upright position at up to the xyphoid process at a temperature of 31°C. ET was performed 3 times/week.

Results.—Exercise was well tolerated. No patients had adverse events. Distance at 6 MWT improved in both groups (CT group: 150 ± 32 m; ET group: 105 ± 28 m) with significant intergroup differences (p 0.001). On land diastolic BP and HR significantly decreased in the CT group while remained unchanged in the ET group (−11 mm Hg ± 2, p 0.04;

e — 12 bpm, p 0.03; respectively). CO and SV had a relative despite no significant increase in CT group. TPR on land significantly decreased in CT group (-23 ± 3 mm Hg/l/m; p 0.01) while remained unchanged in ET group. Patients of CT group had no significant higher increase of both MVC and PT than ET group.

Conclusions.—CT training, significantly improves exercise tolerance and hemodynamic profile of patients with CHF.

▶ Chronic heart failure is a leading cause of hospitalization, disability, and mortality in the elderly. Rehabilitation programs have been shown to be beneficial. Determining what type of rehabilitation program is best suited for patients with heart failure is important. This small, randomized trial illustrates that the addition of a hydrotherapy program to endurance training in men with heart failure increases exercise tolerance as measured by the 6-minute walk distance. Compared with the group that received endurance training only, there was a decrease in rest heart rate, total peripheral resistance, and diastolic blood pressure and increase in cardiac output after 24 weeks among the group that received both hydrotherapy and endurance training. One limitation of the study (admitted by the authors) is that there may have been an elevated level of training in the group that received both interventions. According to the described methodology, the group that received both interventions received 30 minutes of hydrotherapy on one day and 30 minutes of endurance training on the next day, whereas those who received endurance training received only 2 sessions of 30 minutes on the same day (one of calisthenics and one of either cycling or walking). Fatigue may have been a factor for this latter group, reducing their level of training. Despite this, the authors have shown that both groups improved with respect to exercise tolerance and that there was no adverse effect to water immersion for men with heart failure. The challenge will be for health systems to provide these types of services for patients with heart failure.

D. E. Feldman, PT, PhD

Long-Term Effects of Changes in Cardiorespiratory Fitness and Body Mass Index on All-Cause and Cardiovascular Disease Mortality in Men: The Aerobics Center Longitudinal Study

Lee D-C, Sui X, Artero EG, et al (Univ of South Carolina, Columbia; et al)
Circulation 124:2483-2490, 2011

Background.—The combined associations of changes in cardiorespiratory fitness and body mass index (BMI) with mortality remain controversial and uncertain.

Methods and Results.—We examined the independent and combined associations of changes in fitness and BMI with all-cause and cardiovascular disease (CVD) mortality in 14 345 men (mean age 44 years) with at least 2 medical examinations. Fitness, in metabolic equivalents (METs),

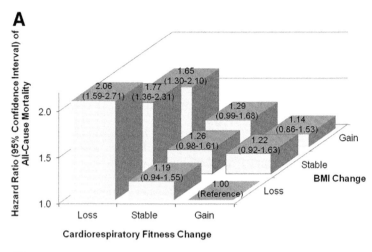

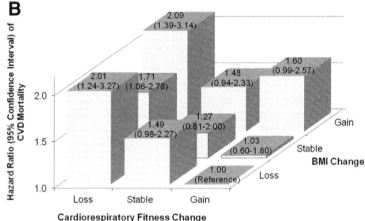

FIGURE 2.—Hazard ratios (95% confidence intervals) of all-cause (**A**) and cardiovascular disease (CVD) (**B**) mortality by combinations of changes in fitness and BMI in 14 345 men. All data were adjusted for age, examination year, parental CVD, BMI, and maximal METs at baseline, the combination patterns of each lifestyle factor (smoking status, alcohol intake, and physical activity) and each medical condition (abnormal ECG, hypertension, diabetes, and hypercholesterolemia) at the baseline and last examinations, and the number of clinic visits between the baseline and last examinations. The number of men (number of all-cause deaths) in the fitness loss, stable, and gain groups were 717 (82), 1240 (91), and 2824 (208) in the BMI loss group; 1732 (101), 2129 (113), and 921 (63) in the stable BMI group; and 2333 (115), 1412 (79), and 1037 (62) in the BMI gain group, respectively. The number of men (number of CVD deaths) in the fitness loss, stable, and gain groups were 658 (23), 1184 (35), and 2686 (70) in the BMI loss group; 1660 (29), 2050 (34), and 874 (16) in the stable BMI group; and 2259 (41), 1361 (28), and 999 (24) in the BMI gain group, respectively. (Reprinted from Lee D-C, Sui X, Artero EG, et al. Long-term effects of changes in cardiorespiratory fitness and body mass index on all-cause and cardiovascular disease mortality in men the Aerobics Center Longitudinal Study. *Circulation.* 2011;124:2483-2490, with permission from American Heart Association, Inc.)

was estimated from a maximal treadmill test. BMI was calculated using measured weight and height. Changes in fitness and BMI between the baseline and last examinations over 6.3 years were classified into loss, stable, or gain groups. During 11.4 years of follow-up after the last examination, 914 all-cause and 300 CVD deaths occurred. The hazard ratios (95% confidence intervals) of all-cause and CVD mortality were 0.70 (0.59–0.83) and 0.73 (0.54–0.98) for stable fitness, and 0.61 (0.51–0.73) and 0.58 (0.42–0.80) for fitness gain, respectively, compared with fitness loss in multivariable analyses including BMI change. Every 1-MET improvement was associated with 15% and 19% lower risk of all-cause and CVD mortality, respectively. BMI change was not associated with all-cause or CVD mortality after adjusting for possible confounders and fitness change. In the combined analyses, men who lost fitness had higher all-cause and CVD mortality risks regardless of BMI change.

Conclusions.—Maintaining or improving fitness is associated with a lower risk of all-cause and CVD mortality in men. Preventing age-associated fitness loss is important for longevity regardless of BMI change (Fig 2).

▶ These data are novel and support a strategy of preventing fitness loss with age to reduce mortality risk, regardless of whether body mass index (BMI) changes (see Fig 2). The authors also speculate that maintaining or improving fitness may also attenuate some potentially negative effects of weight gain on mortality. Much attention has been given to weight management and the influence of BMI on mortality and cardiovascular disease,[1] but the data support more of a focus on building and maintaining aerobic fitness over the long term. Thus increased attention needs to be placed on strategies to maintain or improve aerobic fitness.

D. C. Nieman, DrPH

Reference

1. Berrington de Gonzalez A, Hartge P, Cerhan JR, et al. Body-mass index and mortality among 1.46 million white adults. *N Engl J Med.* 2010;363:2211-2219.

Systematic review of exercise training or percutaneous transluminal angioplasty for intermittent claudication
Frans FA, Bipat S, Reekers JA, et al (Academic Med Centre, Amsterdam, The Netherlands)
Br J Surg 99:16-28, 2012

Background.—The aim was to summarize the results of all randomized clinical trials (RCTs) comparing percutaneous transluminal angioplasty (PTA) with (supervised) exercise therapy ((S)ET) in patients with intermittent claudication (IC) to obtain the best estimates of their relative effectiveness.

Methods.—A systematic review was performed of relevant RCTs identified from the MEDLINE, Embase and Cochrane Library databases. Eligible RCTs compared PTA with (S)ET, included patients with IC due to suspected or known aortoiliac and/or femoropopliteal artery disease, and compared their effectiveness in terms of functional outcome and/or quality of life (QoL).

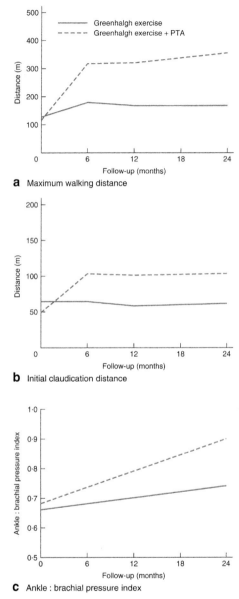

a Maximum walking distance

b Initial claudication distance

c Ankle : brachial pressure index

FIGURE 2.—Results for **a** maximum walking distance, **b** initial claudication distance and **c** ankle : brachial pressure index in patients with aortoiliac artery disease. PTA, percutaneous transluminal angioplasty. (Reprinted from Frans FA, Bipat S, Reekers JA, et al. Systematic review of exercise training or percutaneous transluminal angioplasty for intermittent claudication. *Br J Surg.* 2012;99:16-28, Copyright 2012, British Journal of Surgery Society Ltd. Reproduced with permission. Permission is granted by John Wiley & Sons Ltd on behalf of the BJSS Ltd.)

Results.—Eleven of 258 articles identified (reporting data on eight randomized clinical trials) met the inclusion criteria. One trial included patients with isolated aortoiliac artery obstruction, three trials studied those with femoropopliteal artery obstruction and five included those with combined lesions. Two trials compared PTA with advice on ET, four PTA with SET, two PTA plus SET with SET and two PTA plus SET with PTA. Although the endpoints in most trials comprised walking distances and QoL, pooling of data was impossible owing to heterogeneity. Generally, the effectiveness of PTA and (S)ET was equivalent, although PTA plus (S)ET improved walking distance and some domains of QoL scales compared with (S)ET or PTA alone.

Conclusion.—As IC is a common healthcare problem, defining the optimal treatment strategy is important. A combination of PTA and exercise (SET or ET advice) may be superior to exercise or PTA alone, but this needs to be confirmed (Fig 2).

▶ An increase in the distance that can be walked without the onset of calf pain makes a major contribution to the quality of life in patients with intermittent claudication.[1,2] Although various types of surgery, particularly percutaneous transluminal angioplasty (PTA), have long been the mainstay of treatment, there is growing recognition that exercise programs can also be beneficial for this class of patients,[3,4] particularly if activities are carefully supervised.[5,6] Involvement in an exercise program has the potential advantage of making a change in the patient's lifestyle, with a possibility of inducing benefit that may be more long lasting than that obtained with surgery. It is thus of interest to compare the relative benefits of the 2 treatment options. One immediate point, as in so many Cochrane-type meta-analyses, is that the number of acceptable trials relative to the number of published reports (11 of 258) is extremely low. This underlines the need for a much tighter control of the quality of articles by journal editors. Problems in many studies have included poor randomization and inadequate blinding of subjects and observers to what is a symptomatic problem. Data for a total of 702 patients were finally accepted for the Cochrane Review. Even among this highly selected group of studies, several articles gave few or no details about the complications arising from surgery, and others were vague about the extent of compliance with the exercise program. At 6 and 24 months, benefit in terms of walking distance seemed rather similar for surgery and exercise (Fig 2), but further investigation is needed to confirm this. Most of the existing trials have been small and underpowered, with a heterogeneity of patients and a lack of consistent surgical or exercise interventions precluding clear conclusions. The ultimate answer will probably prove to be a combination of the 2 treatments, but the long-term benefit and the optimal intensity, duration, and frequency of exercise remain to be specified.

R. J. Shephard, MD (Lond), PhD, DPE

References

1. Meru AV, Mittra S, Thyagarajan B, Chugh A. Intermittent claudication: an overview. *Atherosclerosis.* 2006;187:221-237.

2. Breek JC, Hamming JF, De Vries J, Aquarius AE, van Berge Henegouwen DP. Quality of life in patients with intermittent claudication using the World Health Organisation (WHO) questionnaire. *Eur J Vasc Endovasc Surg.* 2001;21:118-122.

3. Bosch JL, Hunink MG. Meta-analysis of the results of percutaneous transluminal angioplasty and stent placement for aortoiliac occlusive disease. *Radiology.* 1997; 204:87-96.

4. Gardner AW, Poehlman ET. Exercise rehabilitation programs for the treatment of claudication pain. A meta-analysis. *JAMA.* 1995;274:975-980.

5. Bendermacher BL, Willigendael EM, Teijink JA, Prins MH. Supervised exercise therapy versus non-supervised exercise therapy for intermittent claudication. *Cochrane Database Syst Rev.* 2006;(2):CD005263.

6. Wind J, Koelemay MJ. Exercise therapy and the additional effect of supervision on exercise therapy in patients with intermittent claudication. Systematic review of randomised controlled trials. *Eur J Vasc Endovasc Surg.* 2007;34:1-9.

Interval training for patients with coronary artery disease: a systematic review

Cornish AK, Broadbent S, Cheema BS (Massey Univ, Wellington, New Zealand; Victoria Univ, Melbourne, Australia; Univ of Western Sydney, Campbelltown, New South Wales, Australia)
Eur J Appl Physiol 111:579-589, 2011

Interval training (IT) may induce physiological adaptations superior to those achieved with conventional moderate-intensity continuous training (MCT) in patients with coronary artery disease (CAD). Our objectives were (1) to systematically review studies which have prescribed IT in CAD, (2) to summarize the findings of this research including the safety and physiological benefits of IT, and (3) to identify areas for further investigation. A systematic review of the literature using computerized databases was performed. The search yielded two controlled trials and five randomized controlled trials (RCTs) enrolling 213 participants. IT prescribed in isolation or in combination with resistance training was shown to induce significant and clinically important physiological adaptations in cardiac patients. IT was also shown to improve cardiorespiratory fitness (e.g. VO_{2max}, VO_{2AT}), endothelial function, left ventricle morphology and function (e.g. ejection fraction) to a significantly greater extent when compared with conventional MCT. No adverse cardiac or other life-threatening events occurred secondary to exercise participation in these studies. However, these findings must be interpreted with caution, as methodological limitations were present in all trials reviewed. In conclusion, robustly designed RCTs with thorough and standardized reporting are required to determine the risk and benefits of IT in the broader cardiac patient population. Further research is required to determine optimal IT protocols for the use in cardiac rehabilitation programmes, potentially contributing to novel exercise prescription guidelines for this patient population.

▶ The idea of using interval training for postcoronary rehabilitation goes back many years.[1] We saw it as a potential method of improving the physical condition of patients with angina who had severe pain when attempting to undertake continuous exercise at an intensity likely to improve their cardiorespiratory fitness. The efficacy of continuous training was underlined by a meta-analysis of 32 randomized, controlled trials involving 8440 patients.[2] Nevertheless, athletes can often reach a higher maximal oxygen intake through interval training, and because maximal oxygen intake is an important indicator of prognosis in coronary heart disease,[3] several authors have suggested that interval training might be the best approach to rehabilitation of the average postcoronary patient.[4-6] Cornish and associates here draw together details of the findings from 7 trials of interval training involving 213 participants. Gains are demonstrated in terms of maximal oxygen intake, endothelial function, and left ventricular ejection. However, further evidence, including direct comparisons of gains with continuous training and assessments of safety on a larger population, are needed before an overall change in policy can be recommended. Weaknesses of some of the existing studies include failure to use the "intention to treat" methodology, inadequate reporting of comorbidities, and lack of blinding among those assessing outcomes.

R. J. Shephard, MD (Lond), PhD, DPE

References

1. Kavanagh T, Shephard RJ. Conditioning of postcoronary patients: comparison of continuous and interval training. *Arch Phys Med Rehabil.* 1975;56:72-76.
2. Jolliffe JA, Rees K, Taylor RS, Thompson D, Oldridge N, Ebrahim S. Exercise-based rehabilitation for coronary heart disease. *Cochrane Database Syst Rev.* 2001;(1):CD001800.
3. Kavanagh T, Mertens DJ, Hamm LF, et al. Prediction of long-term prognosis in 12 169 men referred for cardiac rehabilitation. *Circulation.* 2002;106:666-671.
4. Rognmo Ø, Hetland E, Helgerud J, Hoff J, Slørdahl SA. High intensity aerobic interval exercise is superior to moderate intensity exercise for increasing aerobic capacity in patients with coronary artery disease. *Eur J Cardiovasc Prev Rehabil.* 2004;11:216-222.
5. Warburton DE, Mckenzie DC, Haykowsky MJ, et al. Effectiveness of high-intensity interval training for the rehabilitation of patients with coronary artery disease. *Am J Cardiol.* 2005;95:1080-1084.
6. Wisløff U, Støylen A, Loennechen JP, et al. Superior cardiovascular effect of aerobic interval training versus moderate continuous training in heart failure patients: a randomized study. *Circulation.* 2007;115:3086-3094.

Effects of Physical Activity on Teen Smoking Cessation

Horn K, Dino G, Branstetter SA, et al (West Virginia Univ, Morgantown; Pennsylvania State Univ)
Pediatrics 128:e801-e811, 2011

Objective.—To understand the influence of physical activity on teen smoking-cessation outcomes.

Methods.—Teens ($N = 233$; 14–19 years of age) from West Virginia high schools who smoked >1 cigarette in the previous 30 days were included. High schools with >300 students were selected randomly and assigned to brief intervention (BI), Not on Tobacco (N-O-T) (a proven teen cessation program), or N-O-T plus a physical activity module (N-O-T+FIT). Quit rates were determined 3 and 6 months after baseline by using self-classified and 7-day point prevalence quit rates, and carbon monoxide validation was obtained at the 3-month follow-up evaluation.

Results.—Trends for observed and imputed self-classified and 7-day point prevalence rates indicated that teens in the N-O-T+FIT group had significantly higher cessation rates compared with those in the N-O-T and BI groups. Effect sizes were large. Overall, girls quit more successfully with N-O-T compared with BI (relative risk [RR]: >∞) 3 months after baseline, and boys responded better to N-O-T+FIT than to BI (RR: 2−3) or to N-O-T (RR: 1−2). Youths in the N-O-T+FIT group, compared with those in the N-O-T group, had greater likelihood of cessation (RR: 1.48) at 6 months. The control group included an unusually large proportion of participants in the precontemplation stage at enrollment, but there were no significant differences in outcomes between BI and N-O-T ($z = 0.94$; $P = .17$) or N-O-T + FIT ($z = 1.12$; $P = .13$) participants in the precontemplation stage.

Conclusions.—Adding physical activity to N-O-T may enhance cessation success, particularly among boys.

▶ I reviewed this article because I was fascinated with its title. We typically think of physical activity as being an isolated behavior. However, a lack of physical activity often clusters with other important lifestyle risk factors such as smoking, diet, and substance use (eg, alcohol, drug use).[1] This particular experimental study examined whether smoking cessation among teenagers is mediated or affected by physical activity participation. Mediating mechanisms of physical activity could include such things as reducing withdrawal symptoms and cigarette cravings. The most striking finding was that teens who were provided with a physical activity program in addition to a proven smoking cessation program (Not on Tobacco [N-O-T] + FIT) were about 50% more likely to have quit smoking at 6 months compared with teens who were only provided with the N-O-T smoking cessation program. Interestingly, the effects of physical activity on smoking cessation were driven almost entirely by the responses seen in boys (100% difference between N-O-T vs N-O-T + FIT), as only a subtle effect of physical activity was observed within girls (13% difference between N-O-T vs N-O-T + FIT). These findings speak to a broad and expansive role that physical activity has in health promotion and disease prevention within teenagers. These findings also suggest that physical activity plays an important role in interventions that are focused on improving other lifestyle behaviors.

I. Janssen, PhD

Reference

1. Héroux M, Janssen I, Lee DC, Sui X, Hebert JR, Blair SN. Clustering of unhealthy behaviors in the aerobics center longitudinal study. *Prev Sci.* 2012;13:183-195.

Effect of Warm-Up Exercise on Exercise-Induced Bronchoconstriction

Stickland MK, Rowe BH, Spooner CH, et al (Univ of Alberta, Edmonton, Canada)
Med Sci Sports Exerc 44:383-391, 2012

Purpose.—Exercise-induced bronchoconstriction (EIB) occurs when vigorous exercise induces bronchoconstriction. Preexercise warm-up routines are frequently used to elicit a refractory period and thus reduce or prevent EIB. This study aimed to conduct a systematic review to evaluate the effectiveness of preexercise routines to attenuate EIB.

Methods.—A comprehensive literature search was performed, with steps taken to avoid publication and selection bias. Preexercise warm-up routines were classified into four groups: interval high intensity, continuous low intensity, continuous high intensity, and variable intensity (i.e., a combination of low intensity up to very high intensity). The EIB response was measured by the percent fall in the forced expiratory volume in 1 s (FEV_1) after exercise, and the mean differences (MDs) and 95% confidence intervals (CI) are reported.

Results.—Seven randomized studies met the inclusion criteria. The pooled results showed that high intensity (MD = −10.6%, 95% CI = −14.7% to −6.5%) and variable intensity (MD = −10.9%, 95% CI = −14.37% to −7.5%) exercise warm-up attenuated the fall in FEV_1. However, continuous low-intensity warm-up (MD = −12.6%, 95% CI = −26.7% to 1.5%) and continuous high-intensity warm-up (MD = −9.8%, 95% CI = −26.0% to 6.4%) failed to result in a statistically significant reduction in bronchoconstriction.

Conclusions.—The most consistent and effective attenuation of EIB was observed with high-intensity interval and variable intensity preexercise warm-ups. These findings indicate that an appropriate warm-up strategy that includes at least some high-intensity exercise may be a short-term nonpharmacological strategy to reducing EIB (Fig 2).

▶ It is usually a good idea to exploit a normal physiological mechanism rather than to use drugs to address minor medical problems. Is this the case for exercise-induced bronchoconstriction (EIB)? About half of the athletes who experience EIB have a refractory period of 1 to 4 hours following a warm-up; during this time, symptoms from a further bout of exercise are lessened if not abolished.[1] The underlying mechanisms are poorly understood, but one plausible hypothesis is that the initial exercise bout causes a degranulation of mast cells.[2] The systematic review of Stickland concluded that only 7 of 1634 warm-up studies initially identified met their selection criteria; this gave them a limited pool of 128 subjects. The most effective approach to preventing EIB seemed to be either a series of short high-intensity interval sprints or variable-intensity sprints; both these attenuated subsequent EIB by around 10% to 11% (Fig 2), a clinically useful response. In contrast, continuous exercise, whether high or low intensity, was of no benefit. One potential objection to reliance on warm-up is that, unlike an inhaled bronchodilator, the warm-up

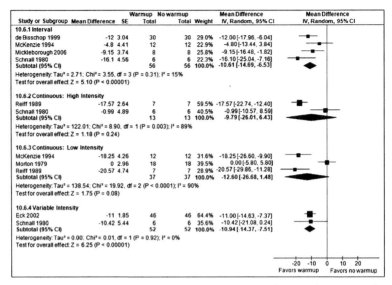

FIGURE 2.—Warm-up versus no warm-up in preexercise treatment of EIB: maximum percent decrease in FEV_1 or peak expiratory flow. (Reprinted from Stickland MK, Rowe BH, Spooner CH, et al. Effect of warm-up exercise on exercise-induced bronchoconstriction. *Med Sci Sports Exerc.* 2012;44:383-391, with permission from the American College of Sports Medicine.)

probably does not act directly on the airways. Further, the conclusion of clinically significant benefit reached by Stickland and associates is based on a very small number of subjects; this finding could easily be negated if only a few studies were not published because no benefit was seen. Finally, because the refractory period is seen in only half of the patients, the remainder will certainly require those patterns of medication accepted by antidoping authorities.

R. J. Shephard, MD (Lond), PhD, DPE

References

1. Randolph C. Exercise-induced asthma: update on pathophysiology, clinical diagnosis, and treatment. *Curr Probl Pediatr.* 1997;27:53-77.
2. Anderson SD, Holzer K. Exercise-induced asthma: is it the right diagnosis in elite athletes? *J Allergy Clin Immunol.* 2000;106:419-428.

Misdiagnosis of exercise-induced bronchoconstriction in professional soccer players

Ansley L, Kippelen P, Dickinson J, et al (Univ of Northumbria, Newcastle, UK; Brunel Univ, Uxbridge, UK; Liverpool John Moore's Univ, UK)
Allergy 67:390-395, 2012

Background.—Physicians typically rely heavily on self-reported symptoms to make a diagnosis of exercise-induced bronchoconstriction (EIB).

However, in elite sport, respiratory symptoms have poor diagnostic value. In 2009, following a change in international sports regulations, all elite athletes suspected of asthma and/or EIB were required to undergo pulmonary function testing (PFT) to permit the use of inhaled β_2-agonists. The aim of this study was to examine the diagnostic accuracy of physician diagnosis of asthma/EIB in English professional soccer players.

Methods.—Sixty-five players with a physician diagnosis of asthma/EIB were referred for pulmonary function assessment. Medication usage and respiratory symptoms were recorded by questionnaire. A bronchial provocation test with dry air was conducted in 42 players and a mannitol challenge in 18 players. Five players with abnormal resting spirometry performed a bronchodilator test.

Results.—Of the 65 players assessed, 57 (88%) indicated regular use of asthma medication. Respiratory symptoms during exercise were reported by 57 (88%) players. Only 33 (51%) of the players tested had a positive bronchodilator or bronchial provocation test. Neither symptoms nor the use of inhaled corticosteroids were predictive of pulmonary function tests' outcome.

Conclusion.—A high proportion of English professional soccer players medicated for asthma/EIB (a third with reliever therapy only) do not present reversible airway obstruction or airway hyperresponsiveness to indirect stimuli. This underlines the importance of objective PFT to support a symptoms-based diagnosis of asthma/EIB in athletes.

▶ The proportion of athletes who are treated for exercise-induced bronchospasm (EIB) is much higher than in the general population.[1] There are several reasons this might be anticipated: breathing occurs through the mouth rather than the nose (allowing cold, dry air to penetrate directly into the bronchi), respiratory minute volume is greatly increased, and (for some sports) exercise must be performed outdoors under very cold conditions and in the presence of mold and other allergens.[2,3] Nevertheless, perhaps in part because baseline spirometry has a limited predictive value,[4] much of the diagnosis of EIB in athletes is symptomatic, and some competitors may imagine symptoms or exaggerate their problems with the mistaken impression that bronchodilator treatment may give them a competitive edge. The article by Ansley and colleagues comparing the frequency of symptomatic and objective diagnoses is thus welcome, and it points to the need to extend current international rules requiring objective evidence of spasm when authorizing competitors to use bronchodilators.[5,6] There has been little previous study of bronchospasm in soccer.[7] The subjects of the present study were a sample of 65 professional soccer players, and a dramatic 57 of 65 (88%) of this group were taking anti-asthmatic medication on a regular basis. All 57 of bronchodilator users reported symptoms when they were exercising, but only 33 of 57 of them had a positive response to an objective test for EIB (an increase of forced expiratory volume [FEV]$_{1.0}$ >12% following administration of a bronchodilator, or a fall of $FEV_{1.0}$ with a provocative inhalation of mannitol or voluntary hyperventilation). Ansley et al found no relationship between the number of symptoms reported and the likelihood of finding a positive objective test response. This article provides an important warning of the current overuse of a medication that can adversely affect performance (by causing tremor and tachycardia) and can occasionally lead to fatal complications.

R. J. Shephard, MD (Lond), PhD, DPE

References

1. Dickinson JW, Whyte GP, McConnell AK, Harries MG. Impact of changes in the IOC-MC asthma criteria: a British perspective. *Thorax.* 2005;60:629-632.
2. Anderson SD, Kippelen P. Exercise-induced bronchoconstriction: pathogenesis. *Curr Allergy Asthma Rep.* 2005;5:116-122.
3. Bangsbo J, Mohr M, Krustrup P. Physical and metabolic demands of training and match-play in the elite football player. *J Sports Sci.* 2006;24:665-674.
4. Bonini M, Lapucci G, Petrelli G, et al. Predictive value of allergy and pulmonary function tests for the diagnosis of asthma in elite athletes. *Allergy.* 2007;62:1166-1170.
5. Anderson SD, Fitch K, Perry CP, et al. Responses to bronchial challenge submitted for approval to use inhaled beta2-agonists before an event at the 2002 Winter Olympics. *J Allergy Clin Immunol.* 2003;111:45-50.
6. World Anti-Doping Agency. International Standard for Therapeutic Use Exemptions. http://www.wada-ama.org/. Accessed March 11, 2012.
7. Dickinson J, McConnell A, Whyte G. Diagnosis of exercise-induced bronchoconstriction: eucapnic voluntary hyperpnoea challenges identify previously undiagnosed elite athletes with exercise-induced bronchoconstriction. *Br J Sports Med.* 2011;45:1126-1131.

The Effect of Exercise Training on Obstructive Sleep Apnea and Sleep Quality: A Randomized Controlled Trial
Kline CE, Crowley EP, Ewing GB, et al (Univ of Pittsburgh School of Medicine, PA; Univ of South Carolina, Columbia; et al)
Sleep 34:1631-1640, 2011

Study Objectives.—To evaluate the efficacy of a 12-week exercise training program for reducing obstructive sleep apnea (OSA) severity and improving sleep quality, and to explore possible mechanisms by which exercise may reduce OSA severity.

Design.—Randomized controlled trial.

Setting.—Clinical exercise physiology center, sleep laboratory.

Participants.—Forty-three sedentary and overweight/obese adults aged 18-55 years with at least moderate-severity untreated OSA (screening apnea-hypopnea index [AHI] $\geq$ 15).

Interventions.—Participants randomized to exercise training (n = 27) met 4 times/week for 12 weeks and performed 150 min/week of moderate-intensity aerobic activity, followed by resistance training twice/week. Participants randomized to a stretching control (n = 16) met twice weekly for 12 weeks to perform low-intensity exercises designed to increase whole-body flexibility.

Measurements and Results.—OSA severity was assessed with one night of laboratory polysomnography (PSG) before and following the 12-week intervention. Measures of sleep quality included PSG, actigraphy (7-10 days), and the Pittsburgh Sleep Quality Index. Compared with stretching, exercise resulted in a significant AHI reduction (exercise: 32.2 ± 5.6 to 24.6 ± 4.4, stretching: 24.4 ± 5.6 to 28.9 ± 6.4; P < 0.01) as well as significant changes in oxygen desaturation index (ODI; P = 0.03) and stage N3 sleep (P = 0.03). Reductions in AHI and ODI were achieved without a significant decrease in body weight. Improvements in actigraphic sleep and subjective sleep quality were also noted following exercise compared with stretching.

Conclusions.—Exercise training had moderate treatment efficacy for the reduction of AHI in sedentary overweight/obese adults, which suggests that exercise may be beneficial for the management of OSA beyond simply facilitating weight loss.

Trial Registration.—Clinicaltrials.gov identification number NCT0095 6423.

▶ The association between obesity and sleep disorders has been recognized at least since the time of Charles Dickens. Obstructive apnea is a substantial problem in general practice, with a population prevalence of up to 15%.[1] Moreover, there are various associated disorders such as cognitive impairment, cardiovascular disease, diabetes, and premature mortality, perhaps related as much to obesity as a lack of sleep. Traditional treatment options are limited. It is difficult to sustain compliance with positive pressure therapy, and there are often side effects from upper airway surgery. Given the association between the apnea and obesity, it seems logical to assess the value of exercise therapy, and there have been several previous small and generally uncontrolled trials suggesting benefit from such an approach.[2-6] The study of Kline et al offers a small-scale 12-week randomized controlled trial of moderate exercise (progressing to 150 min of aerobic activity per week at 60% of heart rate reserve, spread over 4 sessions, plus a substantial range of resistance exercises on 2 days per week) for patients with moderate sleep-related obstructive apnea. Control patients were given stretching exercises, so that they also anticipated some beneficial response. On average, the benefit to the experimental group was statistically quite convincing, but only about a quarter of the exercise group achieved what would be regarded as a clinical success. This success rate is lower than what has been claimed for alternative (but more invasive) therapies, although unlike positive airway pressure, the benefit persisted for at least a day after ceasing exercise. It remains unclear why exercise should have been beneficial, because there was no decrease in body mass or body fat, and no significant gains in respiratory muscle strength or peak expiratory flow rate. Although compliance with the exercise program was said to be good, another weakness in the report is failure to indicate objective changes in maximal oxygen intake in response to the training program. Nevertheless, if even 1 in 4 patients can be helped by an exercise program that will bring other health benefits, it is worth considering.

R. J. Shephard, MD (Lond), PhD, DPE

References

1. Young T, Shahar E, Nieto FJ, et al. Predictors of sleep-disordered breathing in community-dwelling adults: the Sleep Heart Health Study. *Arch Intern Med.* 2002;162:893-900.
2. Peppard PE, Young T. Exercise and sleep-disordered breathing: an association independent of body habitus. *Sleep.* 2004;27:480-484.
3. Quan SF, O'Connor GT, Quan JS, et al. Association of physical activity with sleep-disordered breathing. *Sleep Breath.* 2007;11:149-157.
4. Giebelhaus V, Strohl KP, Lormes W, et al. Physical exercise as an adjunct therapy in sleep apnea—an open trial. *Sleep Breath.* 2000;4:173-176.
5. Norman JF, Von Essen SG, Fuchs RH, et al. Exercise training effect on obstructive sleep apnea syndrome. *Sleep Res Online.* 2000;3:121-129.
6. Sengul YS, Ozalevli S, Oztura I, et al. The effect of exercise on obstructive sleep apnea: a randomized and controlled trial. *Sleep Breath.* 2011;15:49-56.

Intrahospital Weight and Aerobic Training in Children with Cystic Fibrosis: A Randomized Controlled Trial

Sosa ES, Groeneveld IF, Gonzalez-Saiz L, et al (European Univ of Madrid, Spain; Univ of Amsterdam, The Netherlands; et al)
Med Sci Sports Exerc 44:2-11, 2012

Purpose.—The purpose of our study was to assess the effects of an 8-wk intrahospital combined circuit weight and aerobic training program performed by children with cystic fibrosis (of low—moderate severity and stable clinical condition) on the following outcomes: cardiorespiratory fitness ($\dot{V}O_{2peak}$) and muscle strength (five-repetition maximum (5RM) bench press, 5RM leg press, and 5RM seated row) (primary outcomes) and pulmonary function (forced vital capacity, forced expiratory volume in 1 s), weight, body composition, functional mobility (Timed Up and Down Stairs and 3-m Timed Up and Go tests), and quality of life (secondary outcomes). We also determined the effects of a detraining period (4 wk) on the aforementioned outcomes.

Methods.—We performed a randomized controlled trial design. Eleven participants in each group (controls: 7 boys, age $= 11 \pm 3$ yr, body mass index $= 17.2 \pm 0.8$ kg·m^{-2} (mean $\pm$ SEM); intervention: 6 boys, age $= 10 \pm 2$ yr, body mass index $= 18.4 \pm 1.0$ kg·m^{-2}) started the study.

Results.—Adherence to training averaged 95.1% $\pm$ 7.4%. We observed a significant group $\times$ time interaction effect ($P = 0.036$) for $\dot{V}O_{2peak}$. In the intervention group, $\dot{V}O_{2peak}$ significantly increased with training by 3.9 mL·kg^{-1}·min^{-1} (95% confidence interval $= 1.8-6.1$ mL·kg^{-1}·min^{-1}, $P = 0.002$), whereas it decreased during the detraining period (-3.4 mL·kg^{-1}·min^{-1}, 95% confidence interval $= -5.7$ to -1.7 mL·kg^{-1}·min^{-1}, $P = 0.001$). In contrast, no significant changes were observed during the study period within the control group. Although significant improvements were also observed after training for all 5RM strength tests ($P < 0.001$ for the interaction effect), the training improvements were not significantly decreased after the detraining period in the intervention group (all $P > 0.1$

for after training vs detraining). We found no significant training benefits in any of the secondary outcomes.

Conclusions.—A short-term combined circuit weight and aerobic training program performed in a hospital setting induces significant benefits in the cardiorespiratory fitness and muscle strength of children with cystic fibrosis.

▶ On January 5, 2011 my wife and I received the scare of our life. Our family physician informed us that our 3-week-old daughter had screened positive for cystic fibrosis (CF) on her newborn screening test. Over the next 2 weeks, as we waited for the sweat chloride diagnostic test, which to our great relief ended up being negative, I learned as much as I could about CF. Among my research I discovered that about a handful of studies had examined the health and fitness effects of exercise training in patients with CF. The findings of these studies were quite encouraging, as recently reviewed.[1,2] In their study, Sosa and colleagues describe how they built off the existing literature by bringing their combined aerobic and resistance exercise intervention directly into the hospital setting by creating a specialized, intrahospital pediatric exercise gym. CF patients came to this gym 3 times a week for 8 weeks. The most meaningful impact of the exercise program was on cardiorespiratory fitness—$\dot{V}O_{2peak}$ improved by 4 mL/kg/min. This improvement was lost within 4 weeks during the detraining phase of the study, which speaks to the importance for CF patients to maintain a constantly active lifestyle. Muscle strength also improved in response to training by about 25%, which is quite substantive for such a short intervention.

I can only speculate as to what accounts for the excellent adherence rate (95%) to the 24 exercise sessions that were prescribed for this intervention. Perhaps it speaks to the desire that patients with CF have to improve their health, perhaps it speaks to the dedication and motivation of their parents, perhaps it speaks to the exercise facility and design of the exercise program itself, or perhaps it speaks to the exercise training staff at the hospital. Regardless, I was encouraged by the impact that this brief 8-week training program had on the cardiorespiratory and muscular fitness of these children.

I. Janssen, PhD

References

1. Bradley JM, Moran FM, Elborn JS. Evidence for physical therapies (airway clearance and physical training) in cystic fibrosis: an overview of five Cochrane systematic reviews. *Respir Med.* 2006;100:191-201.
2. van Doorn N. Exercise programs for children with cystic fibrosis: a systematic review of randomized controlled trials. *Disabil Rehabil.* 2010;32:41-49.

Physical Activity Is the Strongest Predictor of All-Cause Mortality in Patients With COPD: A Prospective Cohort Study

Waschki B, Kirsten A, Holz O, et al (Pulmonary Res Inst at Hosp Grosshansdorf, Germany; Hosp Grosshansdorf Ctr for Pneumology and Thoracic Surgery, Germany; et al)
Chest 140:331-342, 2011

Background.—Systemic effects of COPD are incompletely reflected by established prognostic assessments. We determined the prognostic value of objectively measured physical activity in comparison with established predictors of mortality and evaluated the prognostic value of noninvasive assessments of cardiovascular status, biomarkers of systemic inflammation, and adipokines.

Methods.—In a prospective cohort study of 170 outpatients with stable COPD (mean FEV_1, 56% predicted), we assessed lung function by spirometry and body plethysmography; physical activity level (PAL) by a multisensory armband; exercise capacity by 6-min walk distance test; cardiovascular status by echocardiography, vascular Doppler sonography (ankle-brachial index [ABI]), and N-terminal pro-B-type natriuretic peptide level; nutritional and muscular status by BMI and fat-free mass index; biomarkers by levels of high-sensitivity C-reactive protein, IL-6, fibrinogen, adiponectin, and leptin; and health status, dyspnea, and depressive symptoms by questionnaire. Established prognostic indices were calculated. The median follow-up was 48 months (range, 10-53 months).

Results.—All-cause mortality was 15.4%. After adjustments, each 0.14 increase in PAL was associated with a lower risk of death (hazard ratio [HR], 0.46; 95% CI, 0.33-0.64; $P < .001$). Compared with established predictors, PAL showed the best discriminative properties for 4-year survival (C statistic, 0.81) and was associated with the highest relative risk of death per standardized decrease. Novel predictors of mortality were adiponectin level (HR, 1.34; 95% CI, 1.06-1.71; $P = .017$), leptin level (HR, 0.81; 95% CI, 0.65-0.99; $P = .042$), right ventricular function (Tei-index) (HR, 1.26; 95% CI, 1.04-1.54; $P = .020$), and ABI <1.00 (HR, 3.87; 95% CI, 1.44-10.40; $P = .007$). A stepwise Cox regression revealed that the best model of independent predictors was PAL, adiponectin level, and ABI. The composite of these factors further improved the discriminative properties (C statistic, 0.85).

Conclusions.—We found that objectively measured physical activity is the strongest predictor of all-cause mortality in patients with COPD. In addition, adiponectin level and vascular status provide independent prognostic information in our cohort (Table 1).

▶ I began my career as a respiratory physiologist, and I still remember the time that I and many of my peers devoted to perfecting measures of lung dynamics and pulmonary gas mixing to assess the status of patients with chronic pulmonary disorders. The information that we obtained was useful in terms of predicting both performance and prognosis. However, from the viewpoint of the

TABLE 1.—Patient Characteristics by Survival Status

Characteristic	Survivors	Nonsurvivors	P Value
Description			
Patients	143 (84.6)	26 (15.4)	
Age, y	63.6 (6.6)	66.1 (6.4)	.083
Men	107 (74.8)	20 (76.9)	.82
Current smokers	62 (43.4)	9 (34.6)	.41
Pack-y smoked	52 (26)	52 (20)	.98
Lung function			
FEV$_1$, % predicted	58.8 (21.1)	41.4 (21.9)	< .001
IC/TLC	34.5 (9.6)	25.2 (11.0)	< .001
Physical activity			
Physical activity level	1.55 (0.27)	1.27 (0.18)	< .001
Steps per day	6424 (3679)	3006 (2081)	< .001
Exercise capacity			
6-min walk distance, m	450 (107)	317 (144)	< .001
Nutritional status			
BMI, kg/m^2	26.7 (5.1)	23.5 (4.3)	.004
Muscular status			
Fat-free mass index, kg/m^2	18.9 (2.6)	17.6 (2.4)	.023
Muscle depletion[a]	13 (9.5)	7 (26.9)	.013
Cardiovascular status			
LVEF ≤50%	4 (3)	1 (4)	.79
E-wave/A-wave	0.93 (0.21)	0.88 (0.20)	.32
Tei index	0.41 (0.11)	0.47 (0.15)	.033
NT-proBNP, pg/mL	64 (38-106)	98 (49-209)	.038
ABI	1.02 (0.92-1.11)	0.93 (0.79-1.01)	.012
ABI <1.00	66 (46)	21 (81)	.001
Adipokines			
Adiponectin, ng/mL	5649 (3,998-8,689)	9042 (3,402-19,453)	.039
Leptin, ng/mL	7348 (3,325-14,898)	5548 (1,902-10,555)	.057
Systemic inflammation			
hs-CRP, mg/L	2.8 (1.2-6.3)	2.9 (1.1-5.6)	.96
IL-6, pg/mL	2.8 (1.7-4.9)	3.0 (1.5-6.2)	.68
Fibrinogen, mg/dL	431 (96)	462 (105)	.13
Questionnaires			
MMRC grade	2 (1-3)	3 (2-4)	.002
SGRQ (total score)	43 (20)	54 (20)	.014
SGRQ (activity score)	56 (24)	70 (19)	.004
Beck Depression Inventory	7 (3-13)	7 (3-12)	.74
Mortality scores			
BODE index	2 (0-3)	4 (2-7)	< .001
Updated BODE index	1 (0-3)	6 (2-10)	< .001
ADO index	3 (2-4)	5 (4-6)	< .001

Variables that were normally distributed are presented as mean (SD) and were tested by two-tailed t test or, in case of heteroscedasticity (steps per day), by Mann-Whitney U test. Skewed variables are presented as median (interquartile range) and were tested log-transformed. Categorized variables are presented as median (interquartile range) and were tested by Mann-Whitney U test. Dichotomous variables are presented as No. (%) and were tested by χ^2 test. Data were missing for fat-free mass index and muscle depletion (n = 5), LVEF (n = 3), E-wave/A-wave (n = 8), Tei index (n = 24), and leptin level (n = 7). ABI = ankle-brachial index; ADO = age, dyspnea, and airflow obstruction; BODE = BMI, airflow obstruction, dyspnea, and exercise capacity; hs-CRP = high-sensitivity C-reactive protein; IC/TLC = inspiratory to total lung capacity ratio; LVEF = left ventricular ejection fraction; MMRC = modified Medical Research Council; NT-proBNP = N-terminal pro-B-type natriuretic peptide; SGRQ = St George Respiratory Questionnaire.
[a]Muscle depletion was defined as fat-free mass index <17.05 kg/m^2 in men and <14.62 kg/m^2 in women.

patient, the key question is the individual's ability to move about and undertake the activities of daily living. Thus, it makes greater intuitive sense to base assessment on a measure that integrates other, nonpulmonary aspects of physical function, including possible abnormalities in cardiac output, pulmonary arterial pressures, muscle strength, skeletal metabolism, and mood state.[1-3] As in other clinical conditions, laboratories should look at the peak oxygen transport, walking speed, or level of habitual physical activity. Waschki and associates followed 170 patients with chronic obstructive pulmonary disease (COPD) for a period of 4 years, looking at their overall survival. Physical activity level was determined by dividing the total daily energy expenditure by the sleeping energy expenditure; those with a ratio of 1.70 or higher were defined as being active.[4] Among a wide variety of possible methods to determine survival, this assessment of physical activity level, the daily step count, and the 6-minute walking distance each provided highly significant predictions, although standard lung volumes and 2 composite indices[5,6] also offered valuable indications of prognosis (Table 1). The present study confirms a previous report that found an association between a low level of physical activity (as reported by questionnaire) and a poor survival over 12 years.[7] Waschki and associates estimated that in their sample of COPD patients, the risk of death over the 4-year interval doubled for every 800 to 1000 kJ decrease in daily energy expenditure. Predictions were further enhanced by adding data on adiponectin and ankle-brachial index to a composite score. The observations need confirming with a larger, randomly selected sample and/or a longer follow-up to increase the number of deaths available for analysis.

R. J. Shephard, MD (Lond), PhD, DPE

References

1. Vestbo J, Prescott E, Almdal T, et al. Body mass, fat-free body mass, and prognosis in patients with chronic obstructive pulmonary disease from a random population sample: findings from the Copenhagen City Heart Study. *Am J Respir Crit Care Med*. 2006;173:79-83.
2. Dahl M, Vestbo J, Lange P, Bojesen SE, Tybjaerg-Hansen A, Nordestgaard BG. C-reactive protein as a predictor of prognosis in chronic obstructive pulmonary disease. *Am J Respir Crit Care Med*. 2007;175:250-255.
3. Fan VS, Ramsey SD, Giardino ND, et al. Sex, depression, and risk of hospitalization and mortality in chronic obstructive pulmonary disease. *Arch Intern Med*. 2007;167:2345-2353.
4. Watz H, Waschki B, Meyer T, Magnussen H. Physical activity in patients with COPD. *Eur Respir J*. 2009;33:262-272.
5. Celli BR, Cote CG, Marin JM, et al. The body-mass index, airflow obstruction, dyspnea, and exercise capacity index in chronic obstructive pulmonary disease. *N Engl J Med*. 2004;350:1005-1012.
6. Puhan MA, Garcia-Aymerich J, Frey M, et al. Expansion of the prognostic assessment of patients with chronic obstructive pulmonary disease: the updated BODE index and the ADO index. *Lancet*. 2009;374:704-711.
7. Garcia-Aymerich J, Lange P, Benet M, Schnohr P, Antó JM. Regular physical activity reduces hospital admission and mortality in chronic obstructive pulmonary disease: a population based cohort study. *Thorax*. 2006;61:772-778.

Aerobic exercise attenuates pulmonary injury induced by exposure to cigarette smoke

Toledo AC, Magalhaes RM, Hizume DC, et al (Univ of Sao Paulo, Brazil)
Eur Respir J 39:254-264, 2012

It has recently been suggested that regular exercise reduces lung function decline and risk of chronic obstructive pulmonary disease (COPD) among active smokers; however, the mechanisms involved in this effect remain poorly understood.

The present study evaluated the effects of regular exercise training in an experimental mouse model of chronic cigarette smoke exposure.

Male C57BL/6 mice were divided into four groups (control, exercise, smoke and smoke+exercise). For 24 weeks, we measured respiratory mechanics, mean linear intercept, inflammatory cells and reactive oxygen species (ROS) in bronchoalveolar lavage (BAL) fluid, collagen deposition in alveolar walls, and the expression of antioxidant enzymes, matrix metalloproteinase 9, tissue inhibitor of metalloproteinase (TIMP)1, interleukin (IL)-10 and 8-isoprostane in alveolar walls.

Exercise attenuated the decrease in pulmonary elastance (p<0.01) and the increase in mean linear intercept (p=0.003) induced by cigarette smoke exposure. Exercise substantially inhibited the increase in ROS in BAL fluid and 8-isoprostane expression in lung tissue induced by cigarette smoke. In addition, exercise significantly inhibited the decreases in IL-10, TIMP1 and CuZn superoxide dismutase induced by exposure to cigarette smoke. Exercise also increased the number of cells expressing glutathione peroxidase.

Our results suggest that regular aerobic physical training of moderate intensity attenuates the development of pulmonary disease induced by cigarette smoke exposure (Fig 2).

▶ There have been various studies of human subjects suggesting that regular physical activity can diminish the adverse pulmonary consequences of smoking, but it has been difficult to evaluate such reports, because both the social

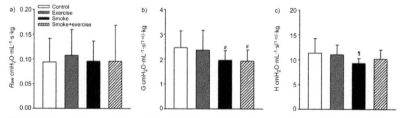

FIGURE 2.—a) Airway resistance (*Raw*), b) tissue damping (tissue resistance; G) and c) pulmonary elastance (H) obtained in the four experimental groups, after 24 weeks of the experimental protocol. Data are presented as means and SD. The values were normalised to body weight. #: p<0.01 compared with the two groups that were not exposed to smoke; ¶: p<0.01 compared with the other three groups. (Reprinted from Toledo AC, Magalhaes RM, Hizume DC, et al. Aerobic exercise attenuates pulmonary injury induced by exposure to cigarette smoke. *Eur Respir J.* 2012;39:254-264, with permission from ERS.)

circumstances and patterns of smoking usually differ between active and inactive individuals.[1] It is certainly clear that not everyone who smokes develops chronic obstructive pulmonary disease. Interindividual differences in susceptibility have been attributed to both genetic differences in bronchial enzymes and socioenvironmental influences, possibly including the altitude of residence.[2] The animal study of Toledo and associates allows control of many extraneous variables such as the type and amount of exercise, the extent of exposure to cigarette smoke, and genetic and environmental factors. With control of all these extraneous influences, a program of moderate but sustained regular exercise (60 min/d at 50% of maximal effort, 5 d/wk for 24 weeks) considerably attenuated the loss of pulmonary elastance seen at postmortem in the mice exposed to cigarette smoke (Fig 2). Exercise is known to increase a person's resistance to oxidative stress[3] and to diminish the risk of developing diseases associated with oxidative stress.[4] Given the high concentration of free radicals found in cigarette smoke[5] and the fact that lung levels of 8-isoprostane, a marker of oxidant stress, were lower in exercised animals, the authors of this report make the very reasonable suggestion that a reduction of oxidant levels may be the main basis of the protection that exercise offers against cigarette smoke. A further possibility is that exercise may be increasing the activity of anti-inflammatory mediators such as IL-10.[6]

R. J. Shephard, MD (Lond), PhD, DPE

References

1. Garcia-Aymerich J, Lange P, Benet M, Schnohr P, Antó JM. Regular physical activity modifies smoking-related lung function decline and reduces risk of chronic obstructive pulmonary disease: a population-based cohort study. *Am J Respir Crit Care Med.* 2007;175:458-463.
2. Menezes AM, Perez-Padilla R, Jardim JR, et al. Chronic obstructive pulmonary disease in five Latin American cities (the PLATINO study): a prevalence study. *Lancet.* 2005;366:1875-1881.
3. Radák Z, Naito H, Kaneko T, et al. Exercise training decreases DNA damage and increases DNA repair and resistance against oxidative stress of proteins in aged rat skeletal muscle. *Pflugers Arch.* 2002;445:273-278.
4. Radak Z, Chung HY, Goto S. Systemic adaptation to oxidative challenge induced by regular exercise. *Free Radic Biol Med.* 2008;44:153-159.
5. Church DF, Pryor WA. Free-radical chemistry of cigarette smoke and its toxicological implications. *Environ Health Perspect.* 1985;64:111-126.
6. Petersen AM, Pedersen BK. The anti-inflammatory effect of exercise. *J Appl Physiol.* 2005;98:1154-1162.

7 Other Medical Conditions

Influences of purposeful activity versus rote exercise on improving pain and hand function in pediatric burn
Omar MTA, Hegazy FA, Mokashi SP (Cairo Univ, Egypt; King Saud Univ, Saudi Arabia)
Burns 38:261-268, 2012

Purpose.—To explore the influences of purposeful activities versus rote exercises on pain, range of motion and hand function in children with hand burn.

Methods.—Thirty patients with superficial and deep partial and full-thickness burns, including hand and wrist with less than 25% total body surface area (TBSA), were included in this study. The patients were randomly allocated to one of the two groups; purposeful activity group (PA-group, $n = 15$) and rote exercises group (Rex-group, $n = 15$). Outcomes measured were pain severities using the self-report faces scale and analogue scale (VAS), total active motion (TAM) using standard dorsal hand goniometer, and hand function using Jebsen-Taylor hand function test (JTHFT). Measurements were recorded 72 h post-burn, after 1, 2, and 3 weeks, at the time of discharge and at 3 months follow up.

Results.—In PA-group, results regarding to pain modulation ($p < 0.05$), TAM ($p < 0.01$), and JTHFT ($p < 0.01$) were statistically significant in comparison to Rex-group.

Conclusion.—This study supports the belief that the purposeful activity based on playing, and games can reduce pain, improve hand movement and functions better than rote exercise. As well as its reusability and versatility, suggesting another option in the rehabilitation of children with hand burn (Fig 1).

▶ Regular physical activity is usually more likely to be sustained if it is purposeful rather than performed simply as a rote medical requirement. For instance, a patient is more likely to complete a daily walk on a cold, wet, and windy day if it includes a visit to a neighborhood coffee shop and the post office or local supermarket, rather than a simple walk down a wet street behind an umbrella. This generalization seems even more relevant if the required activity has the potential to be painful, as when exercising following severe burns.[1-3] In children, play offers a purposeful activity, and it has previously been shown that such

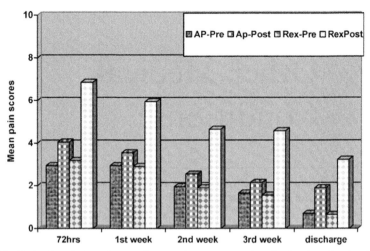

FIGURE 1.—Cumulative pain scores between the groups at each evaluation time. (Reprinted from Omar MTA, Hegazy FA, Mokashi SP. Influences of purposeful activity versus rote exercise on improving pain and hand function in pediatric burn. *Burns*. 2012;38:261-268, Copyright 2012, with permission from International Society for Burn Injuries.)

activity offers an effective nonpharmacological approach to pain relief.[4] The study by Omar and associates was conducted in children aged 8 to 14 years, and, given this wide age spread, each of the patients in the experimental group was allowed to choose a game or hobby or to play with a toy that he or she enjoyed, provided that it could be used within the treatment facility. In some cases, the activity was carried out in sterile water, and this may have helped to reduce pain. Responses were compared with the usual daily free and assisted range-of-motion exercises. Subjective reports of pain were much lower for the play group (Fig 1), and the final recovery of motion was also better than for the controls who received rote treatment. The only notes of caution are that a skilled occupational therapist is required to adapt the game, toy, or hobby to the child's specific needs, and the patient may become overinvolved in the game to the point of causing excessive movement, pain, and subsequent reluctance to exercise.

R. J. Shephard, MD (Lond), PhD, DPE

References

1. Umraw N, Chan Y, Gomez M, Cartotto RC, Fish JS. Effective hand function assessment after burn injuries. *J Burn Care Rehabil*. 2004;25:134-139.
2. van-Zuijlen PP, Kreis RW, Vloemans AF, Groenevelt F, Mackie DP. The prognostic factors regarding long-term functional outcome of full-thickness hand burns. *Burns*. 1999;25:709-714.
3. Ehde DM, Patterson DR, Fordyce WE. The quota system in burn rehabilitation. *J Burn Care Rehabil*. 1998;19:436-440.
4. McGrath PA. *Pain in children: nature, assessment, and treatment*. New York: Guilford; 1990.

Beneficial Effect of Creatine Supplementation in Knee Osteoarthritis
Neves M Jr, Gualano B, Roschel H, et al (Univ of São Paulo, Brazil)
Med Sci Sports Exerc 43:1538-1543, 2011

Introduction.—The aim of this study was to investigate the efficacy of creatine (CR) supplementation combined with strengthening exercises in knee osteoarthritis (OA).

Methods.—A randomized, double-blind, placebo-controlled trial was performed. Postmenopausal women with knee OA were allocated to receive either CR (20 g·d^{-1} for 1 wk and 5 g·d^{-1} thereafter) or placebo (PL) and were enrolled in a lower limb resistance training program. They were assessed at baseline (PRE) and after 12 wk (POST). The primary outcome was the physical function as measured by the timed-stands test. Secondary outcomes included lean mass, quality of life, pain, stiffness, and muscle strength.

Results.—Physical function was significantly improved only in the CR group ($P = 0.006$). In addition, a significant between-group difference was observed (CR: PRE $= 15.7 \pm 1.4$, POST $= 18.1 \pm 1.8$; PL: PRE $= 15.0 \pm 1.8$, POST $= 15.2 \pm 1.2$; $P = 0.004$). The CR group also presented improvements in physical function and stiffness subscales as evaluated by the Western Ontario and McMaster Universities Osteoarthritis Index ($P = 0.005$ and $P = 0.024$, respectively), whereas the PL group did not show any significant changes in these parameters ($P > 0.05$). In addition, only the CR group presented a significant improvement in lower limb lean mass ($P = 0.04$) as well as in quality of life ($P = 0.01$). Both CR and PL groups demonstrated significant reductions in pain ($P < 0.05$). Similarly, a main effect for time revealed an increase in leg-press one-repetition maximum ($P = 0.005$) with no significant differences between groups ($P = 0.81$).

Conclusions.—CR supplementation improves physical function, lower limb lean mass, and quality of life in postmenopausal women with knee OA undergoing strengthening exercises (Fig 2).

▶ This is an interesting empirical study of a small group of relatively elderly women with moderate rather than severe osteoarthritis. My first explanation of the beneficial effect of creatine was that many of the population in São Paulo had low incomes and therefore were not getting sufficient protein in their diet. However, given the booming Brazilian economy, my impressions of São Paulo are undoubtedly dated, and an assessment of the subjects' normal food intake (using a photo album of real foods and a Brazilian dietary analysis computer program) suggested a daily protein intake of 77 g (probably about 1 g/kg) and enough to meet normal dietary requirements. Creatine supplements are known to facilitate the response to resistance training in young athletes, and this may be the mechanism of benefit in elderly women. Certainly, those receiving creatine showed an increase in lower limb lean mass and a speeding of timed stands over their 12 weeks of training, whereas the controls did not (Fig 2). The development of stronger muscles might in turn control movement at the damaged joints and

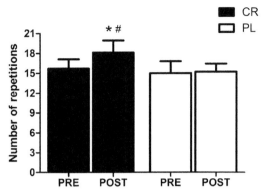

FIGURE 2.—Effects of CR supplementation combined with resistance training on physical function (as assessed by the timed-stands test) in patients with knee OA. *Time effect (PRE vs POST), $P = 0.006$. #Interaction effect (CR vs PL), $P = 0.004$. (Reprinted from Neves M Jr, Gualano B, Roschel H, et al. Beneficial effect of creatine supplementation in knee osteoarthritis. *Med Sci Sports Exerc.* 2011;43:1538-1543, with permission from the American College of Sports Medicine.)

thus permit healing. In support of this explanation, another study that provided creatine supplements without muscle training did not observe any speeding of recovery in response to the dietary supplement.[1] One potential mechanism of benefit is that the creatine boosts the phosphocreatine energy system, allowing resistance training to proceed more effectively.[2] Creatine kinase and phosphocreatine may also be important to cartilage metabolism,[3-5] allowing creatine supplements to contribute more directly to the healing process, although such healing would probably take longer than the 12 weeks studied here. The benefit from creatine seems appreciable, and it merits both confirmation and a further exploration of the mechanisms.

R. J. Shephard, MD (Lond), PhD, DPE

References

1. Roy BD, de Beer J, Harvey D, Tarnopolsky MA. Creatine monohydrate supplementation does not improve functional recovery after total knee arthroplasty. *Arch Phys Med Rehabil.* 2005;86:1293-1298.
2. Terjung RL, Clarkson P, Eichner ER, et al. American College of Sports Medicine roundtable: the physiological and health effects of oral creatine supplementation. *Med Sci Sports Exerc.* 2000;32:706-717.
3. Gerber I, ap Gwynn I, Alini M, Wallimann T. Stimulatory effects of creatine on metabolic activity, differentiation and mineralization of primary osteoblast-like cells in monolayer and micromass cell cultures. *Eur Cell Mater.* 2005;10:8-22.
4. Katoh R, Iyoda K, Oohira A, Kato K, Nogami H. Zonal and age-related difference in the amounts of creatine kinase subunits in cartilage. *Clin Orthop Relat Res.* 1991:283-287.
5. Wallimann T, Hemmer W. Creatine kinase in non-muscle tissues and cells. *Mol Cell Biochem.* 1994:133-134.

What Is the Effect of Physical Activity on the Knee Joint? A Systematic Review

Urquhart DM, Tobing JFL, Hanna FS, et al (Monash Univ, Melbourne, Victoria, Australia)
Med Sci Sports Exerc 43:432-442, 2011

Purpose.—Although several studies have examined the relationship between physical activity and knee osteoarthritis, the effect of physical activity on knee joint health is unclear. The aim of this systematic review was to examine the relationships between physical activity and individual joint structures at the knee.

Methods.—Computer-aided searches were conducted up until November 2008, and the reference lists of key articles were examined. The methodological quality of selected studies was assessed based on established criteria, and a best-evidence synthesis was used to summarize the results.

Results.—We found that the relationships between physical activity and individual joint structures at the knee differ. There was strong evidence for a positive association between physical activity and tibiofemoral osteophytes. However, we also found strong evidence for the absence of a relationship between physical activity and joint space narrowing, a surrogate method of assessing cartilage. Moreover, there was limited evidence from magnetic resonance imaging studies for a positive relationship between physical activity and cartilage volume and strong evidence for an inverse relationship between physical activity and cartilage defects.

Conclusions.—This systematic review found that knee structures are affected differently by physical activity. Although physical activity is associated with an increase in radiographic osteophytes, there was no related increase in joint space narrowing, rather emerging evidence of an associated increase in cartilage volume and decrease in cartilage defects on magnetic resonance imaging. Given that optimizing cartilage health is important in preventing osteoarthritis, these findings indicate that physical activity is beneficial, rather than detrimental, to joint health.

▶ It remains unclear whether physical activity is associated with greater incidence of osteoarthritis (OA) or progression of OA or is protective of OA. Disparate opinions and conclusions are the result of methodologic differences, such as the subjects included (previously injured, professional, amateur, recreational) and orthopedic evaluations of OA. The authors of this systematic review took a unique approach to the association of physical activity and knee health by considering multiple structural components of the knee that are used to evaluate OA. They synthesized the results of 28 studies that (1) were investigations of the association between physical activity and the development or progression of knee OA and (2) reported radiographic or MRI evidence of knee OA or healthy knees. They included longitudinal, cross-sectional, and case-controlled studies. The age range of subjects was 45 to 79 years. They found the associations of physical activity and knee OA to differ depending on the joint structure evaluated. Physical activity was positively associated with knee joint osteophytes but not joint space narrowing. There was strong evidence that greater physical activity was associated with fewer cartilage defects, whereas a positive relationship was found between cartilage volume and physical activity. The authors suggest that osteophytes in the knee joint could be the result of mechanical adaptation to force and are not indicative of knee OA in the absence of joint space narrowing or cartilage damage. The message that physical activity is detrimental to knees, that it causes or worsens knee OA, is not supported by this review.

C. M. Jankowski, PhD

Exercise Capacity in Pediatric Patients with Inflammatory Bowel Disease
Ploeger HE, Takken T, Wilk B, et al (Univ of Groningen, The Netherlands; Univ Med Ctr Utrecht, The Netherlands; McMaster Univ, Hamilton, Ontario, Canada)
J Pediatr 158:814-819, 2011

Objective.—To examine exercise capacity in youth with Crohn's disease (CD) and ulcerative colitis (UC).

Study Design.—Eleven males and eight females with CD and six males and four females with UC participated. Patients performed standard exercise tests to assess peak power (PP) and mean power (MP) and peak aerobic mechanical power (W_{peak}) and peak oxygen uptake (VO_{2peak}). Fitness variables were compared with reference data and also correlated with relevant clinical outcomes.

Results.—Pediatric patients with inflammatory bowel disease had lower PP ($\sim 90\%$ of predicted), MP ($\sim 88\%$ of predicted), W_{peak} ($\sim 91\%$ of predicted), and VO_{2peak} ($\sim 75\%$ of predicted) compared with reference values. When patients with CD or UC were compared separately to reference values, W_{peak} was significantly lower only in the CD group. No statistically significant correlations were found between any exercise variables and disease duration ($r = 0.01$ to 0.14, $P = .47$ to $.95$) or disease activity ($r = -0.19$ to -0.31, $P = .11$ to $.38$), measured by pediatric CD activity index or pediatric ulcerative colitis activity index. After controlling for chronological age, recent hemoglobin levels were significantly correlated with PP ($r = 0.45$, $P = .049$), MP ($r = 0.63$, $P = .003$), VO_{2peak} ($r = 0.62$, $P = .004$), and W_{peak} ($r = 0.70$, $P = .001$).

Conclusions.—Pediatric patients with inflammatory bowel disease exhibit impaired aerobic and anaerobic exercise capacity compared with reference values (Table 2).

▶ Previous authors have demonstrated a sedentary lifestyle[1] and a low level of cardiorespiratory fitness[2,3] in adults with chronic bowel disease. Ploeger and associates note a similar trend in cycle ergometer tests of maximal anaerobic and aerobic power in a relatively small sample of teenagers with either Crohn disease or ulcerative colitis (Table 2). Among the possible causes they suggest are low hemoglobin levels,[4] cachexia associated with increased circulating levels of tumor necrosis factor-α[5] and pro-inflammatory cytokines, and therapeutic

TABLE 2.—Anaerobic and Aerobic Exercise Measurements

	n	CD Mean ± SD	n	UC Mean ± SD	n	Total Mean ± SD
Anaerobic power test						
PP (Watts·kg^{-1})	19	8.9 ± 1.4*	10	8.1 ± 1.2*	29	8.6 ± 1.3[†]
MP (Watts·kg^{-1})[‡]	19	6.6 ± 1.2*	10	6.2 ± 1.0*	29	6.5 ± 1.1*
Fatigue index (%)	19	46.2 ± 10.0	10	43.6 ± 10.5	29	45.3 ± 10.0
Aerobic power test						
W$_{peak}$ (Watts·kg^{-1})	18	2.9 ± 0.7*	10	3.1 ± 0.6	28	3.0 ± 0.7*
VO$_{2peak}$ (L·min^{-1})	17	1.9 ± 0.6[†]	10	1.8 ± 0.5*	27	1.8 ± 0.6[†]
VO$_{2peak}$ (mL·kg^{-1}·min^{-1})	17	34.9 ± 6.5[†]	10	37.8 ± 7.7*	27	36.0 ± 7.0[†]

*$P < .05$ compared with reference values.
[†]$P < .001$ compared with reference values.
[‡]Level of significance based on CD, n = 11; UC, n = 7.

administration of corticosteroids,[6] although in this study, physical performance was no better in those who were not receiving corticosteroids. One issue that is not discussed is the possible exacerbation of bowel instability by exercise; this might well discourage these patients from prolonged and vigorous physical activity. It seems desirable to encourage children with chronic bowel inflammation to undertake more physical activity to augment both maximal aerobic power and muscle strength, although further study of effects on the course of the underlying disease process is also warranted.

R. J. Shephard, MD (Lond), PhD, DPE

References

1. Narula N, Fedorak RN. Exercise and inflammatory bowel disease. *Can J Gastroenterol.* 2008;22:497-504.
2. Brevinge H, Berglund B, Bosaeus I, Tölli J, Nordgren S, Lundholm K. Exercise capacity in patients undergoing proctocolectomy and small bowel resection for Crohn's disease. *Br J Surg.* 1995;82:1040-1045.
3. Wiroth JB, Filippi J, Schneider SM, et al. Muscle performance in patients with Crohn's disease in clinical remission. *Inflamm Bowel Dis.* 2005;11:296-303.
4. Christodoulou DK, Tsianos EV. Anemia in inflammatory bowel disease — the role of recombinant human erythropoietin. *Eur J Intern Med.* 2000;11:222-227.
5. Roubenoff R. Exercise and inflammatory disease. *Arthritis Rheum.* 2003;49:263-266.
6. Schakman O, Gilson H, Kalista S, Thissen JP. Mechanisms of muscle atrophy induced by glucocorticoids. *Horm Res.* 2009;72:36-41.

Body Mass, Training, Menses, and Bone in Adolescent Runners: A 3-yr Follow-up

Barrack MT, Van Loan MD, Rauh MJ, et al (Univ of California Davis; Rocky Mountain Univ of Health Professions, Provo, UT; et al)
Med Sci Sports Exerc 43:959-966, 2011

Endurance runners with low bone mass during adolescence may risk attaining a low peak bone mineral density (BMD) in adulthood. Alternatively, they may mature late and undergo delayed bone mineral accumulation.

Purpose.—The purpose of this study was to evaluate 40 adolescent runners (aged 15.9 ± 0.2 yr) at two time points, approximately 3 yr apart, to assess bone mass status and identify variables associated with bone mass change.

Methods.—Follow-up measures included a questionnaire to assess menstrual status, training, and sports participation history, height and weight, and a dual-energy x-ray absorptiometry scan to assess total body, total hip, and lumbar spine BMD, bone mineral content (BMC), BMD z-score, and body composition. We used −1 and −2 BMD z-score cutoffs to categorize runners with low bone mass.

Results.—Eighty-seven percent of girls with low BMD at baseline had low BMD at the follow-up. Girls with low compared with normal baseline BMD had lower follow-up adjusted total body (2220.4 ± 65.8 vs 2793.1 ± 68.2 g, $P < 0.001$), total hip (27.0 ± 1 vs 33.9 ± 1.0 g, $P < 0.05$), and lumbar spine (47.8 ± 2.0 vs 66.3 ± 2.2 g, $P < 0.001$) BMC values. Variables related to 3-yr training volume, menstrual function, age, developmental stage, and change in body mass explained 29%−54% of the variability in BMC change.

Conclusions.—The majority of adolescent runners with low BMD at baseline had low BMD after a 3-yr follow-up. Our observations suggest that "catch-up" accrual may be difficult and, thus, emphasize the importance of gaining adequate bone mineral during the early adolescent years.

▶ Osteoporosis can develop at older ages because of accelerated bone loss during adulthood or because of inadequate bone accumulation during childhood. It is well known that bone mass is lower in adolescent female athletes who have a low body weight and a history of menstrual irregularities. This study addressed, for the first time, whether low bone mass among adolescent female athletes, in this case competitive long-distance runners, is irreversible. In other words, is it possible for adolescent girls with a low bone mass to catch up to their peers in subsequent years and have a healthy bone mass at entry into adulthood? Unfortunately, the findings of this study suggest that such catch-up is highly unlikely. In fact, almost 9 in 10 girls with a low bone mass at age 15 still had a low bone mass at age 18. The small proportion of girls who were able to catch up tended to be younger at baseline, have younger gynecologic ages, and reported lower running mileage. These findings stress the importance of optimizing bone mineral accrual during the early to mid-adolescent years.

I. Janssen, PhD

Sclerostin and Its Association with Physical Activity, Age, Gender, Body Composition, and Bone Mineral Content in Healthy Adults
Amrein K, Amrein S, Drexler C, et al (Med Univ of Graz, Austria; et al)
J Clin Endocrinol Metab 97:148-154, 2012

Context.—Sclerostin is produced by osteocytes and inhibits bone formation through the Wnt/β-catenin-signaling pathway. Only limited data are available on circulating sclerostin levels in healthy subjects.

Objective.—We aimed to evaluate the correlation between sclerostin and physical activity, anthropometric, and biochemical variables.

Design, Setting, and Participants.—We conducted a cross-sectional observational study in 161 healthy adult men and premenopausal women aged 19 to 64 yr (mean age, 44 ± 10).

Intervention(s).—There were no interventions.

Main Outcome Measure(s).—Serum sclerostin levels were associated with body composition, bone mineral density, physical activity, and various biochemical parameters.

Results.—A positive correlation between age and sclerostin in both men (r = 0.37; $P < 0.001$) and premenopausal women (r = 0.66; $P < 0.001$) was found. Men had significantly higher sclerostin levels than women (49.8 ± 17.6 vs. 37.2 ± 15.2 pmol/liter; $P < 0.001$). However, after adjustment for age, bone mineral content (BMC), physical activity, body mass index (BMI), and renal function, sclerostin levels did not differ ($P = 0.543$). Partial correlation analysis adjusted for age, gender, and kidney function revealed a significant positive correlation between sclerostin levels and BMC, bone mineral density, BMI, and android/gynoid fat and a significant negative correlation with serum osteocalcin and calcium. The most physically active quartile had significantly lower sclerostin levels compared to the least active quartile in a univariate analysis.

Conclusions.—In healthy adults, sclerostin serum levels correlate positively with age, BMI, and BMC and negatively with osteocalcin and calcium. Further studies in larger populations are needed to confirm our findings and to better understand their clinical implications.

▶ An important function of osteocytes is to transduce mechanical strain signals to stimulate bone turnover. Sclerostin is a glycoprotein, produced by osteocytes, that inhibits osteoblast differentiation and bone formation. In animal models, there is a dose-dependent decrease in osteocyte sclerostin expression with mechanical loading and an increase in SOST expression with unloading; these responses favor bone formation. Sclerostin, and in particular sclerostin inhibition, is a target for novel therapies to preserve bone mass. The relation of sclerostin with physical activity in humans in not well defined. In this cross-sectional study by Amrein et al, circulating sclerostin was positively correlated with age and negatively correlated with self-reported physical activity in healthy men and premenopausal women. Men had higher circulating sclerostin than women, but this gender difference did not remain after adjustment for age, bone mineral content, body mass index, and physical activity. The research horizon is likely to include longitudinal studies of a dose response between exercise and sclerostin and the relations of sclerostin to bone mineral density and fracture risk.

C. M. Jankowski, PhD

Physical Activity and Change in Mammographic Density: The Study of Women's Health Across the Nation

Conroy SM, Butler LM, Harvey D, et al (Cancer Res Ctr of Hawai'i, Honolulu; Univ of California at Davis; et al)
Am J Epidemiol 171:960-968, 2010

One potential mechanism by which physical activity may protect against breast cancer is by decreasing mammographic density. Percent mammographic density, the proportion of dense breast tissue area to total breast area, declines with age and is a strong risk factor for breast cancer. The authors hypothesized that women who were more physically active would have a greater decline in percent mammographic density with age, compared with less physically active women. The authors tested this hypothesis using longitudinal data (1996−2004) from 722 participants in the Study of Women's Health Across the Nation (SWAN), a multiethnic cohort of women who were pre- and early perimenopausal at baseline, with multivariable, repeated-measures linear regression analyses. During an average of 5.6 years, the mean annual decline in percent mammographic density was 1.1% (standard deviation $= 0.1$). A 1-unit increase in total physical activity score was associated with a weaker annual decline in percent mammographic density by 0.09% (standard error $= 0.03$; $P = 0.01$). Physical activity was inversely associated with the change in non-dense breast area ($P < 0.01$) and not associated with the change in dense breast area ($P = 0.17$). Study results do not support the hypothesis that physical activity reduces breast cancer through a mechanism that includes reduced mammographic density (Table 3).

▶ It has been suggested that the percentage of dense mammary tissue relative to total breast tissue area is a measure of cumulative exposure to hormones and growth factors, and thus the potential for accumulation of genetic damage.[1]

TABLE 3.—Unadjusted and Adjusted Longitudinal Analyses for Change in Percent Mammographic Density[a] by Physical Activity Indices, Study of Women's Health Across the Nation, 1996−2004

Physical Activity Index[b]	β	Model 1[c] 95% Confidence Interval	β	Model 2[d] 95% Confidence Interval	β	Model 3[e] 95% Confidence Interval
Total activity	0.037	−0.027, 0.102	0.066	0.003, 0.130	0.087	0.024, 0.150
Sports/exercise	0.022	−0.083, 0.128	0.064	−0.040, 0.168	0.115	0.011, 0.219
Daily routine	0.045	−0.100, 0.190	0.128	−0.016, 0.272	0.149	0.009, 0.289
Household/caregiving	0.104	−0.036, 0.245	0.099	−0.038, 0.237	0.085	−0.051, 0.221

[a]Values are maximum likelihood estimates of coefficients for modification to annual change in percent density and 95% confidence intervals from mixed-effects regression models.
[b]One unit change in index measured on a 1−15 scale for total activity and a 1−5 scale for individual domains.
[c]Model 1 represents univariate models for each activity index.
[d]Model 2 represents individual models for each activity index adjusted for body mass index.
[e]Model 3 represents single models for each activity index adjusted for age, body mass index, menopausal status, race/ethnicity, study site, parity, past use of hormones (contraceptive and postmenopausal hormones), smoking, change in body mass index, and change in menopausal status.

Given the ability of regular physical activity to reduce the risk of breast cancer independently of changes in body mass,[2-4] Conroy and associates thought it interesting to examine how far a change in mammary density contributed to this trend through a modulation of endogenous reproductive hormones.[5] Mammographic density declines with age, this being particularly obvious at menopause.[6,7] The study was thus conducted on 722 U.S. perimenopausal women, including those using hormone replacement therapy. Physical activity was assessed using the Kaiser questionnaire 4 times over a period averaging 5.6 years. Statistical analysis that included a substantial number of covariates showed a 1.1% decrease in mammographic density per year. However, contrary to the initial hypothesis, activity actually seemed to slow the decline in breast density (Table 3). One limitation of the analysis is that the study included few women who were either very active or very sedentary. However, it may also be that much of the protection associated with physical activity comes via some other mechanisms. The excess risk associated with a large body mass index is also unrelated to breast density.

R. J. Shephard, MD (Lond), PhD, DPE

References

1. Martin LJ, Boyd NF. Mammographic density. Potential mechanisms of breast cancer risk associated with mammographic density: hypotheses based on epidemiological evidence. *Breast Cancer Res.* 2008;10:201 [electronic article].
2. IARC Working Group. *IARC handbooks of cancer prevention.* In: *Weight Control and Physical Activity.* Vol 6. Lyon, France: International Agency for Research on Cancer; 2002.
3. Maruti SS, Willett WC, Feskanich D, Rosner B, Colditz GA. A prospective study of age-specific physical activity and premenopausal breast cancer. *J Natl Cancer Inst.* 2008;100:728-737.
4. Friedenreich CM, Cust AE. Physical activity and breast cancer risk: impact of timing, type and dose of activity and population subgroup effects. *Br J Sports Med.* 2008;42:636-647.
5. Pike MC, Spicer DV, Dahmoush L, Press MF. Estrogens, progestogens, normal breast cell proliferation, and breast cancer risk. *Epidemiol Rev.* 1993;15:17-35.
6. Boyd N, Martin L, Stone J, Little L, Minkin S, Yaffe M. A longitudinal study of the effects of menopause on mammographic features. *Cancer Epidemiol Biomarkers Prev.* 2002;11:1048-1053.
7. Kelemen LE, Pankratz VS, Sellers TA, et al. Age-specific trends in mammographic density: the Minnesota Breast Cancer Family Study. *Am J Epidemiol.* 2008;167: 1027-1036.

Does Physical Activity Reduce the Risk of Prostate Cancer? A Systematic Review and Meta-analysis

Liu Y, Hu F, Li D, et al (Harbin Med Univ, Heilongjiang, People's Republic of China; et al)
Eur Urol 60:1029-1044, 2011

Context.—Numerous observational epidemiologic studies have evaluated the association between physical activity and prostate cancer (PCa); however, the existing results are inconsistent.

Objective.—To determine the association between physical activity and risk of PCa.

Evidence Acquisition.—A systematic search was performed using the Medline, Embase, and Web of Science databases through 15 May 2011 to identify all English-language articles that examined the effect of physical activity on the risk of PCa. This meta-analysis was conducted according to the guidelines for the meta-analysis of observational studies in epidemiology.

Evidence Synthesis.—This meta-analysis consisted of 88 294 cases from 19 eligible cohort studies and 24 eligible case-control studies. When data from both types of studies were combined, total physical activity (TPA) was significantly associated with a decreased risk of PCa (pooled relative risk [RR]: 0.90; 95% confidence interval [CI], 0.84−0.95). The pooled RR for occupational physical activity (OPA) and recreational physical activity (RPA) were 0.81 (95% CI, 0.73−0.91) and 0.95 (95% CI, 0.89−1.00), respectively. Notably, for TPA, we observed a significant PCa risk reduction for individuals between 20 and 45 yr of age (RR: 0.93; 95% CI, 0.89−0.97) and between 45 and 65 yr of age (RR: 0.91; 95% CI, 0.86−0.97) who performed activities but not for individuals <20 yr of age or >65 yr of age.

Conclusions.—There appears to be an inverse association between physical activity and PCa risk, albeit a small one. Given that increasing physical activity has numerous other health benefits, men should be encouraged to increase their physical activity in both occupational and recreational time to improve their overall health and potentially decrease their risk of PCa (Fig 2).

▶ Prostate cancer is the sixth most common cause of cancer death,[1,2] yet the possible benefits of an increase in physical activity to this point have remained

Subgroups (Number of studies)		Pooled RR (95% CI)	P	I^2 (%)
TPA				
Cohort studies (24)		0.94 (0.91-0.98)	0.002	4.06
Case-control studies (34)		0.86 (0.75-0.97)	0.02	69.82
Subtotal (58)		0.90 (0.84-0.95)	0.001	61.65
OPA				
Cohort studies (9)		0.91 (0.87-0.95)	<0.001	0.00
Case-control studies (18)		0.73 (0.62-0.87)	<0.001	66.42
Subtotal (27)		0.81 (0.73-0.91)	<0.001	68.19
RPA				
Cohort studies (19)		0.95 (0.90-1.00)	0.04	15.15
Case-control studies (15)		0.98 (0.85-1.14)	0.81	62.27
Subtotal (34)		0.95 (0.89-1.00)	0.07	43.43

0.5   1   2

FIGURE 2.—The pooled relative risk estimates for total, occupational, and recreational physical activity by study design. RR = relative risk; CI = confidence interval; TPA = total physical activity; OPA = occupational physical activity; RPA = recreational physical activity. (Reprinted from Liu Y, Hu F, Li D, et al. Does physical activity reduce the risk of prostate cancer? A systematic review and meta-analysis. *Eur Urol.* 2011;60:1029-1044, Copyright 2011, with permission from the European Association of Urology.)

unclear. Positive effects from a modulation of androgens, insulin, and insulin-like growth factors seem plausible,[3-6] and indeed androgen suppressants are now often administered to those with advanced prostate cancer following radiation treatment. A reduced likelihood of obesity and an enhancement of immune function are other possible ways in which regular physical activity could reduce risk. The present article is the first formal meta-analysis of this issue, with careful control for the quality of studies, the validity of the assessment of physical activity history, the length of follow-up, and possible confounding factors. A substantial volume of data from both cohort and case-control studies has been examined (in all, 88 294 cases). There is a small but statistically significant benefit from both occupational and recreational physical activity, although somewhat surprisingly, the occupational effect seems stronger than that due to recreational activity (Fig 2), and the magnitude of benefit is smaller (although still statistically significant) in the better-quality studies. One possible confounding factor tending to mask the benefit of exercise is that men who choose to engage in recreational physical activity may also undergo more regular checks for prostate cancer, so that the percentage of undetected cancers is lower in those who are physically active. The study also leaves unanswered the issue of dose-response relationships; if the mechanism of benefit is hormonal, then a response is only likely to be seen in those who are taking quite vigorous activity.

R. J. Shephard, MD (Lond), PhD, DPE

References

1. Baade PD, Youlden DR, Krnjacki LJ. International epidemiology of prostate cancer: geographical distribution and secular trends. *Mol Nutr Food Res.* 2009; 53:171-184.
2. Jemal A, Bray F, Center MM, Ferlay J, Ward E, Forman D. Global cancer statistics. *CA Cancer J Clin.* 2011;61:69-90.
3. Hsing AW, Chua S Jr, Gao YT, et al. Prostate cancer risk and serum levels of insulin and leptin: a population-based study. *J Natl Cancer Inst.* 2001;93:783-789.
4. Lehrer S, Diamond EJ, Stagger S, Stone NN, Stock RG. Increased serum insulin associated with increased risk of prostate cancer recurrence. *Prostate.* 2002;50:1-3.
5. Chan JM, Stampfer MJ, Giovannucci E, et al. Plasma insulin-like growth factor-I and prostate cancer risk: a prospective study. *Science.* 1998;279:563-566.
6. Hackney AC, Sinning WE, Bruot BC. Reproductive hormonal profiles of endurance-trained and untrained males. *Med Sci Sports Exerc.* 1988;20:60-65.

Acute Versus Chronic Exposure to Androgen Suppression for Prostate Cancer: Impact on the Exercise Response
Galvão DA, Taaffe DR, Spry N, et al (Edith Cowan Univ, Joondalup, Western Australia, Australia; Univ of Newcastle, Ourimbah, New South Wales, Australia; Univ of Western Australia, Nedlands, Australia)
J Urol 186:1291-1297, 2011

Purpose.—Exercise has been proposed as an effective countermeasure for androgen suppression therapy induced side effects. Since the magnitude of fat gain and muscle loss is most pronounced during the early phases of androgen suppression therapy, the exercise response may differ by the duration of androgen suppression therapy. We investigated whether the exercise response varied by the prior duration of exposure to androgen suppression therapy, that is acute—less than 6 months vs later—6 months or greater.

Materials and Methods.—A total of 50 men 55 to 84 years old undergoing androgen suppression therapy for nonbone metastatic prostate cancer completed a progressive resistance and cardiovascular exercise program for 12 weeks, including 16 with acute and 34 with chronic androgen suppression therapy exposure. We assessed fat and lean mass by dual energy x-ray absorptiometry as well as muscle strength, functional performance, quality of life and blood biomarkers.

Results.—Patients on acute androgen suppression showed an increase in total body fat compared to those on chronic androgen suppression (0.9 kg, p = 0.018). Each group experienced increased appendicular skeletal muscle (about 0.5 kg, p <0.01). Triglycerides decreased in the chronic group and increased in the acute group (p = 0.027). Change in triglycerides were associated with the change in total body fat (r = 0.411, p = 0.004). There were no differences between the groups in prostate specific antigen, testosterone, glucose, insulin, total cholesterol, low and high density lipoprotein, cholesterol, C-reactive protein, homocysteine or quality of life. The 2 groups showed similar improvement in muscle strength and function, and cardiovascular fitness.

Conclusions.—Apart from differences in body fat and triglycerides the beneficial effects of exercise are similar in patients on acute or chronic androgen suppression therapy.

▶ Androgen deprivation therapy has substantially improved prognosis following radiation therapy for intermediate- or high-risk prostate cancer, particularly if prostate-specific antigen levels show an early relapse. At the same time, such treatment carries side effects of sarcopenia, obesity, hyperglycemia, insulin resistance, diabetes, and an increase in morbidity and deaths from cardiovascular disease.[1-4] The current survival of prostate cancer patients into old age makes it important to counter all of these side effects. The temptation is to prescribe a wide range of medications such as antithrombotics, antihypertensives, and lipid-lowering drugs.[1] However, a much simpler and more appropriate remedy may be to encourage an adequate amount of physical activity. Galvão and associates here report on the benefits observed following a 12-week program of combined aerobic and resistance exercise; the control group received usual care for 12 weeks until the study had been completed. The aerobic component of the experimental program comprised cycling or jogging for 15 to 20 minutes twice per week at 65% to 80% of the maximal heart rate and a very thorough 40-minute resistance component that involved the main muscle groups twice per week. Benefits were seen both during acute (< 6 months) and in chronic cases (> 6 months) of antiandrogen therapy. Muscle strength and endurance and cardiorespiratory fitness and function were all enhanced at the end of the 12 weeks of training, although in the acute cases, body fat was increased despite participation in the exercise program. The volume of prescribed aerobic activity was less than the commonly recommended 30 minutes at least 5 days per week, and this probably needs to be increased, with some regulation of food intake, if continuing fat accumulation is to be avoided. Further, only about half of the 97 patients completed the program, and until methods of increasing the participation rate are found, pharmaceutical remedies will probably still be required for some cases.

R. J. Shephard, MD (Lond), PhD, DPE

References

1. Levine GN, D'Amico AV, Berger P, et al. Androgen-deprivation therapy in prostate cancer and cardiovascular risk: a science advisory from the American Heart Association, American Cancer Society, and American Urological Association: endorsed by the American Society for Radiation Oncology. *Circulation*. 2010;121:833-840.
2. Keating NL, O'Malley AJ, Smith MR. Diabetes and cardiovascular disease during androgen deprivation therapy for prostate cancer. *J Clin Oncol*. 2006;24:4448-4456.
3. D'Amico AV, Denham JW, Crook J, et al. Influence of androgen suppression therapy for prostate cancer on the frequency and timing of fatal myocardial infarctions. *J Clin Oncol*. 2007;25:2420-2425.
4. Van Hemelrijck M, Garmo H, Holmberg L, et al. Absolute and relative risk of cardiovascular disease in men with prostate cancer: results from the Population-Based PCBaSe Sweden. *J Clin Oncol*. 2010;28:3448-3456.

Evaluation of a Nordic Walking Program on Shoulder Joint Mobility and Isometric Force in Breast Cancer Patients
Rösner M (Clinic Bavaria Kreischa, Germany)
Dtsch Z Sportmed 62:120-124, 2011

Problem.—Functional restrictions of the shoulder joint are treatment-related consequences of breast cancer patients. Reduced strength and restriction of shoulder movements are consequences of muscular atrophy and joint contraction. This strength and mobility decline negatively influences the general health state and leads to psychological problems.

Methods.—In a randomized study 50 women after operation, radiation, and/or chemotherapy were included in the study. The treatment group (n=26) carried out nordic walking three times per week for 60 minutes a day lasting a total of four weeks. The control group (n=24) did not carry out any nordic walking. Otherwise both groups received the same treatment and therapies. The following parameters were tested: maximum isometric strength in arm and shoulder, shoulder movement and the state of health evaluated with the questionnaire SF 12.

Results.—The test group reached strength gains of 70.6 % for shoulder adduction (control group 14.3 %) and 53.3 % (control group 20%) for abduction. Strength gains of 35% (control group 6%) were recorded for elbow flexion and 53.8 % (control group 16.6 %) for elbow extension. Shoulder mobility improved 14.4 % in adduction (control group 9.9 %) and 23.6 % in abduction (control group 1%), also in ante version with

10.7 % (control group 5%) and in retro version with 15.1 % (control group 6%). The increases of strength and shoulder mobility had a positive effect on general health in the test group, whereas no effects were observed in the control group.

Discussion.—Nordic walking was used in this study as a supplementary treatment to the overall therapy concept. The comparison with the control group shows that the test group made considerably better progress in both physical and emotional health. Nordic walking can therefore be regarded as a beneficial supplementary therapy for breast cancer patients.

▶ The loss of arm function following surgery for breast cancer imposes significant physical and emotional problems for many women. This German-language paper offers a simple but effective controlled study demonstrating the effectiveness of Nordic walking as a simple means of restoring arm function. The gains of muscle strength in those following the required regimen are very impressive relative to a well-matched group of usual treatment controls. The amount of activity demanded of the successful patients (60 minutes per session, 3 times per week) may nevertheless be somewhat demanding for some patients.

R. J. Shephard, MD (Lond), PhD, DPE

Physical Activity after Diagnosis and Risk of Prostate Cancer Progression: Data from the Cancer of the Prostate Strategic Urologic Research Endeavor
Richman EL, Kenfield SA, Stampfer MJ, et al (Brigham and Women's Hosp and Harvard Med School, Boston, MA; et al)
Cancer Res 71:3889-3895, 2011

Vigorous activity after diagnosis was recently reported to be inversely associated with prostate cancer—specific mortality. However, men with metastatic disease may decrease their activity due to their disease; thus, a causal interpretation is uncertain. We therefore prospectively examined vigorous activity and brisk walking after diagnosis in relation to risk of prostate cancer progression, an outcome less susceptible to reverse causation, among 1,455 men diagnosed with clinically localized prostate cancer. Cox proportional hazards regression was used to examine vigorous activity, nonvigorous activity, walking duration, and walking pace after diagnosis and risk of prostate cancer progression. We observed 117 events (45 biochemical recurrences, 66 secondary treatments, 3 bone metastases, 3 prostate cancer deaths) during 2,750 person-years. Walking accounted for nearly half of all activity. Men who walked briskly for 3 h/wk or more had a 57% lower rate of progression than men who walked at an easy pace for less than 3 h/wk (HR = 0.43; 95% CI: 0.21–0.91; $P = 0.03$). Walking pace was associated with decreased risk of progression independent of duration (HR brisk vs. easy pace = 0.52; 95% CI: 0.29–0.91; $P_{trend} = 0.01$). Few men engaged in vigorous activity, but there was a suggestive inverse association (HR ≥3 h/wk vs. none = 0.63;

95% CI: 0.32—1.23; $P_{trend} = 0.17$). Walking duration and total nonvigorous activity were not associated with risk of progression independent of pace or vigorous activity, respectively. Brisk walking after diagnosis may inhibit or delay prostate cancer progression among men diagnosed with clinically localized prostate cancer.

▶ With most forms of cancer, treatment is initiated on a priority basis. However, prostate cancer is often an exception to this rule, and particularly in older patients, one option may be a period of observation to decide whether definitive treatment is needed, or whether the patient is likely to die before the tumor has a significant impact on overall health. This immediately raises the question as to how the prognosis is likely to be influenced by the amount of physical activity performed during this period of watchful waiting. The study reported by Richman and colleagues was based on 1445 men aged about 65 years, with localized prostate cancer. Previous observations by the same investigators had already suggested that vigorous physical activity in those with nonmetastatic cancer was associated with a 61% lower prostate-specific mortality.[1] However, critics of this earlier study argued that more severe disease could have limited the individual's physical activity rather than the reverse. The present study was initiated to address this criticism. The response as seen in a prospective trial of those beginning with minimal disease was similar to that reported earlier: over a follow-up averaging 22 months, the prognosis was 57% better in those taking 3 hours a week of brisk walking (Fig 1 in the original article). Benefit was assessed in terms of disease progression (biochemical progression, the need for secondary treatment, or [rarely] metastases or death). The observed benefit seems logical, because physical activity leads to reductions in insulin-like growth factor and inflammatory cytokines, with a potential to reduce proliferation and encourage apoptosis of cancer cells.[2-5] However, one limitation of the current findings is that there were fewer smokers among the more active patients; also, relatively few of the sample fell into the active category, limiting the statistical power of the comparison.

R. J. Shephard, MD (Lond), PhD, DPE

References

1. Kenfield SA, Stampfer MJ, Giovannucci E, et al. Physical activity and survival after prostate cancer diagnosis in the health professionals follow-up study. *J Clin Oncol.* 2011;29:726-732.
2. Haverkamp J, Charbonneau B, Ratliff TL. Prostate inflammation and its potential impact on prostate cancer: a current review. *J Cell Biochem.* 2008;103:1344-1353.
3. Frasca F, Pandini G, Sciacca L, et al. The role of insulin receptors and IGF-I in cancer and other diseases. *Arch Physiol Biochem.* 2008;114:23-37.
4. Barb D, Williams CJ, Neuwirth AK, Mantzoros CS. Adiponectin in relation to malignancies: a review of existing basic research and clinical evidence. *Am J Clin Nutr.* 2007;86:s858-s866.
5. Barnard RJ, Ngo TH, Leung PS, Aronson WJ, Golding LA. A low-fat diet and/or strenuous exercise alters the IGF axis in vivo and reduces prostate tumor cell growth in vitro. *Prostate.* 2003;56:201-206.

Physical activity, energy restriction, and the risk of pancreatic cancer: a prospective study in the Netherlands
Heinen MM, Verhage BAJ, Goldbohm RA, et al (Maastricht Univ Med Centre+, Netherlands; TNO Quality of Life, Leiden, Netherlands; et al)
Am J Clin Nutr 94:1314-1323, 2011

Background.—Because of their influence on insulin concentrations, we hypothesized that both physical activity and energy restriction may reduce the risk of pancreatic cancer.

Objective.—We examined the associations between physical activity, proxies for energy restriction, and pancreatic cancer risk.

Design.—The Netherlands Cohort Study consisted of 120,852 individuals who completed a baseline questionnaire in 1986. After 13.3 y of follow-up, 408 cases were available for analysis. Self-reported information on physical activity was collected. Three indicators were used as proxies for energy restriction: father's employment status during the Economic Depression (1932–1940) and place of residence during the World War II years (1940–1944) and the Hunger winter (1944–1945).

Results.—For past sports activities, we observed a significantly decreased risk of pancreatic cancer (HR: 0.80; 95% CI: 0.64, 0.99). Proxies for energy restriction were not related to pancreatic cancer risk. When the results for energy restriction were stratified by height, a significant multiplicative interaction was observed for the Economic Depression period ($P = 0.002$). Shorter individuals (height less than the sex-specific median adult height) with an unemployed father during the Economic Depression period had a significantly lower cancer risk (HR: 0.31; 95% CI: 0.14, 0.66) than did taller individuals with an employed father. No significant interactions were observed for exposure to energy restriction during the World War II years and the Hunger winter.

Conclusions.—Our results suggest a modestly decreased risk of pancreatic cancer associated with past sports activity. With respect to proxies for energy restriction, our findings suggest that shorter individuals exposed to energy restriction during adolescence may have a reduced risk, whereas taller individuals may not (Table 2).

▶ Carcinoma of the pancreas is the fourth leading cause of death in the United States[1] and has a 5-year survival rate < 6%.[2] It is also very hard to diagnose, so any method of prevention is doubly important. The study of Heinen et al is based on a very large sample of the Dutch population who were followed up over a 13-year period; this yielded more than 400 cases of microscopically verified pancreatic cancer. They obtained data on both occupational and nonoccupational physical activity for their sample. The occupational activity had no apparent influence on prognosis (Table 2), but there was a suggestion of protection against pancreatic carcinoma with > 90 minutes per day of leisure time physical activity, and this became statistically significant on distinguishing those who had engaged in sports (arbitrarily defined as activities that demanded energy expenditures > 2.5 metabolic equivalents). Benefit was most apparent in those

TABLE 2.—Age-Adjusted and Multivariable-Adjusted HRs (and 95% CIs) for Pancreatic Cancer According to Physical Activity (Both Nonoccupational and Occupational): NLCS, 1986—1999[1]

Exposure Variable	Person-Years[2]	Cases[2]	All Pancreatic Cancer Cases HR (95% CI)[3]	HR (95% CI)[4]
Nonoccupational physical activity				
At baseline[5]				
<30 min/d[6]	9420	67	1.00	1.00
30 to <60 min/d	15,582	119	1.07 (0.78, 1.46)	1.09 (0.79, 1.50)
60 to <90 min/d	10,620	89	1.20 (0.86, 1.68)	1.22 (0.88, 1.71)
≥90 min/d	13,493	87	0.88 (0.63, 1.22)	0.87 (0.62, 1.22)
P-trend			0.30	0.24
History of sports participation[5]				
Never[6]	24,671	198	1.00	1.00
Ever	24,965	165	0.81 (0.65, 1.01)	0.80 (0.64, 0.99)
Frequency of past sports participation				
<2 h/wk	3605	30	1.11 (0.74, 1.67)	1.18 (0.78, 1.79)
2 to <4 h/wk	7651	42	0.69 (0.48, 0.97)	0.67 (0.47, 0.96)
≥4 h/wk	12,564	84	0.79 (0.61, 1.04)	0.76 (0.57, 1.00)
P-trend			0.10	0.05
Duration of past sports participation				
<15 y	14,267	81	0.71 (0.54, 0.93)	0.69 (0.53, 0.91)
15 to <30 y	5281	37	0.85 (0.59, 1.23)	0.85 (0.58, 1.23)
≥30 y	3712	35	1.11 (0.76, 1.63)	1.08 (0.73, 1.58)
P-trend			0.81	0.91
Occupational physical activity[7]				
Longest held job				
Sitting time				
>6 h/d[6]	5409	39	1.00	1.00
2—6 h/d	9616	66	0.93 (0.61, 1.40)	0.92 (0.61, 1.40)
<2 h/d	5718	57	1.36 (0.88, 2.08)	1.25 (0.81, 1.93)
P-trend			0.15	0.28
Energy expenditure				
<8 kJ/min[6]	12,466	96	1.00	1.00
8—12 kJ/min	5296	44	1.06 (0.73, 1.55)	0.96 (0.66, 1.41)
>12 kJ/min	2981	22	0.93 (0.57, 1.52)	0.85 (0.52, 1.39)
P-trend			0.91	0.54
Last job				
Sitting time				
>6 h/d[6]	5738	46	1.00	1.00
2—6 h/d	10,132	70	0.85 (0.58, 1.26)	0.84 (0.57, 1.25)
<2 h/d	5647	53	1.16 (0.76, 1.75)	1.05 (0.69, 1.60)
P-trend			0.49	0.79
Energy expenditure				
<8 kJ/min[6]	13,383	103	1.00	1.00
8—12 kJ/min	5080	41	1.04 (0.71, 1.53)	0.95 (0.64, 1.39)
>12 kJ/min	3053	25	1.05 (0.66, 1.67)	0.96 (0.60, 1.55)
P-trend			0.79	0.82

[1]HRs and 95% CIs were calculated by using Cox proportional hazards models. NLCS, Netherlands Cohort Study.
[2]Number of cases and person-years do not add up to the total number because of missing values for covariables.
[3]Adjusted for age (y).
[4]Adjusted for age (y), smoking (current smoking: yes or no; number of cigarettes smoked per day; number of years of smoking), BMI (in kg/m2), energy intake (kcal/d), and intake of vegetables (g/d).
[5]Additionally adjusted for sex.
[6]Reference category.
[7]Women were excluded from analyses because most women of this generation had not held a job or had worked for only a short period of time, mostly in the distant past.

devoting > 2 hours per week to sports. These findings supplement the meta-analysis of Bao and Michaud,[3] who found a 25% reduction of risk with a history of heavy occupational activity. In most cases, sports participation began before the age of 20 years, and this early start may be important in terms of cancer prevention, although given the weakness of people's long-term memory, it is a difficult question to evaluate. Childhood nutrition was gauged as in some other Dutch studies from proxy information: the father's employment history during the Great Depression and the area of residence during the "hungry winter" of the Nazi occupation. There was little evidence that the supply of nutrients during youth affected risk unless the subcategory of shorter individuals was considered (the post-hoc examination of such subgroups is anathema to most statisticians). One possible mechanism of benefit could be the influence of physical activity upon the insulin-like growth factors axis.[4]

R. J. Shephard, MD (Lond), PhD, DPE

References

1. Jemal A, Siegel R, Ward E, et al. Cancer statistics, 2008. *CA Cancer J Clin.* 2008; 58:71-96.
2. Karim-Kos HE, de Vries E, Soerjomataram I, et al. Recent trends of cancer in Europe: a combined approach of incidence, survival and mortality for 17 cancer sites since the 1990s. *Eur J Cancer.* 2008;44:1345-1389.
3. Bao Y, Michaud DS. Physical activity and pancreatic cancer risk: a systematic review. *Cancer Epidemiol Biomarkers Prev.* 2008;17:2671-2682.
4. Kaaks R, Lukanova A. Energy balance and cancer: the role of insulin and insulin-like growth factor-I. *Proc Nutr Soc.* 2001;60:91-106.

Physical activity and risk of colon adenoma: a meta-analysis
Wolin KY, Yan Y, Colditz GA (Washington Univ School of Medicine in St Louis and Alvin J Siteman Cancer Ctr, MO)
Br J Cancer 104:882-885, 2011

Background.—Little evidence is available on the relation of physical activity with colon adenomas, a colon cancer precursor.

Methods.—We conducted a systematic literature review and meta-analysis of published studies (in English) through April 2010, examining physical activity or exercise and risk or prevalence of colon adenoma or polyp. Random effects models were used to estimate relative risks (RRs) and corresponding confidence intervals (CIs). A total of 20 studies were identified that examined the association and provided RRs and corresponding 95% CIs.

Results.—A significant inverse association between physical activity and colon adenomas was found with an overall RR of 0.84 (CI: 0.77−0.92). The association was similar in men (RR=0.81, CI: 0.67−0.98) and women (RR=0.87, CI: 0.74−1.02). The association appeared slightly stronger in large/advanced polyps (RR=0.70, CI: 0.56−0.88).

Conclusion.—This study confirms previous reports of a significant inverse association of physical activity and colon adenoma, and suggests that physical activity can have an important role in colon cancer prevention.

▶ The strong inverse relationship between physical activity and colon cancer risk is well established, more so than for any other type of cancer. Adenomas are often cut out of the colon before colon cancer develops. This comprehensive meta-analysis supports a significant 16% risk reduction when comparing the most with the least physically active. Risk reductions were similar for men and women and held when limited to studies designated as the best approach. The association was stronger when analyses were limited to advanced or large polyps, with a risk reduction of 35%. Potential mechanisms include exercise-induced influences on immune function, lowered inflammation, and improved insulin sensitivity.[1]

D. C. Nieman, DrPH

Reference

1. Wolin KY, Patel AV, Campbell PT, et al. Change in physical activity and colon cancer incidence and mortality. *Cancer Epidemiol Biomarkers Prev.* 2010;19: 3000-3004.

Does Physical Activity Reduce the Risk of Prostate Cancer? A Systematic Review and Meta-Analysis
Liu Y, Hu F, Li D, et al (Harbin Med Univ, Heilongjiang, People's Republic of China)
Eur Urol 60:1029-1044, 2011

Context.—Numerous observational epidemiologic studies have evaluated the association between physical activity and prostate cancer (PCa); however, the existing results are inconsistent.

Objective.—To determine the association between physical activity and risk of PCa.

Evidence Acquisition.—A systematic search was performed using the Medline, Embase, and Web of Science databases through 15 May 2011 to identify all English-language articles that examined the effect of physical activity on the risk of PCa. This meta-analysis was conducted according to the guidelines for the meta-analysis of observational studies in epidemiology.

Evidence Synthesis.—This meta-analysis consisted of 88 294 cases from 19 eligible cohort studies and 24 eligible case-control studies. When data from both types of studies were combined, total physical activity (TPA) was significantly associated with a decreased risk of PCa (pooled relative risk [RR]: 0.90; 95% confidence interval [CI], 0.84–0.95). The pooled RR for occupational physical activity (OPA) and recreational physical activity (RPA) were 0.81 (95% CI, 0.73–0.91) and 0.95 (95% CI, 0.89–1.00), respectively. Notably, for TPA, we observed a significant

Subgroups (Number of studies)		Pooled RR (95% CI)	*P*	I^2 (%)
TPA				
Cohort studies (24)		0.94 (0.91-0.98)	0.002	4.06
Case-control studies (34)		0.86 (0.75-0.97)	0.02	69.82
Subtotal (58)		0.90 (0.84-0.95)	0.001	61.65
OPA				
Cohort studies (9)		0.91 (0.87-0.95)	<0.001	0.00
Case-control studies (18)		0.73 (0.62-0.87)	<0.001	66.42
Subtotal (27)		0.81 (0.73-0.91)	<0.001	68.19
RPA				
Cohort studies (19)		0.95 (0.90-1.00)	0.04	15.15
Case-control studies (15)		0.98 (0.85-1.14)	0.81	62.27
Subtotal (34)		0.95 (0.89-1.00)	0.07	43.43

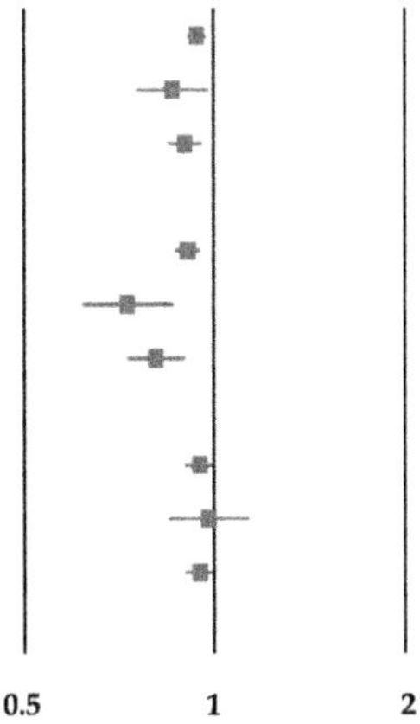

0.5   1   2

FIGURE 2.—The pooled relative risk estimates for total, occupational, and recreational physical activity by study design. RR = relative risk; CI = confidence interval; TPA = total physical activity; OPA = occupational physical activity; RPA = recreational physical activity. (Reprinted from European Urology. Liu Y, Hu F, Li D, et al. Does physical activity reduce the risk of prostate cancer? A systematic review and meta-analysis. *Eur Urol.* 2011;60:1029-1044, Copyright 2011, with permission from the European Association of Urology.)

PCa risk reduction for individuals between 20 and 45 yr of age (RR: 0.93; 95% CI, 0.89−0.97) and between 45 and 65 yr of age (RR: 0.91; 95% CI, 0.86−0.97) who performed activities but not for individuals <20 yr of age or >65 yr of age.

Conclusions.—There appears to be an inverse association between physical activity and PCa risk, albeit a small one. Given that increasing physical activity has numerous other health benefits, men should be encouraged to increase their physical activity in both occupational and recreational time to improve their overall health and potentially decrease their risk of PCa (Fig 2).

▶ This comprehensive meta-analysis found a 19% risk reduction for prostate cancer for higher levels of occupational physical activity and a 5% reduction for recreational physical activity (Fig 2). Physical activity may reduce the risk of prostate cancer through alteration in levels of androgens, insulin, insulin-like growth factors, and testosterone.[1] Physical activity also plays an important role in the prevention of obesity and enhancement of immunosurveillance. Nonetheless, this meta-analysis indicates that physical activity does not have a major impact on prostate cancer.

D. C. Nieman, DrPH

Reference

1. Friedenreich CM, Thune I. A review of physical activity and prostate cancer risk. *Cancer Causes Control.* 2001;12:461-475.

Aerobic Exercise as a Therapy Option for Migraine: A Pilot Study

Darabaneanu S, Overath CH, Rubin D, et al (Univ Clinic of Kiel, Germany; et al)
Int J Sports Med 32:455-460, 2011

Exercise is assumed to have a positive effect on migraine. However, none of the few studies on this topic can prove the expected positive influence of exercise. Therefore, the aim of this pilot study was to develop a training program suitable for migraine patients and to examine its effect on migraine. 16 patients were examined. 8 migraine patients completed a 10-week aerobic running exercise program consisting of 3 workouts per week. The program was developed by sports scientists especially to increase the fitness level. Physical fitness, i.e., physical working capacity, was assessed using a PWC 150 test. There was also a control group of 8 patients without any special physical training. Migraine patients of the exercise group showed both a reduction in the number of migraine days per month (p = 0.048) and the intensity of the attacks (p = 0.028). An increase in fitness level resulted in a lowered stress level. Stress strategies like "displacement activity" (r = −0.715; p = 0.046), "looking for self-affirmation" (r = −0.742; p = 0.035) and "feelings of aggression" (r = −0.802; p = 0.017) were reduced. Increasing the level of fitness (PWC 150) is one predictor for migraine improvement (r = 0.409, p = 0.031). Aerobic exercise which leads to a better fitness level is an alternative therapy method for migraine (Fig 4).

▶ Severe migraine can be a serious disability for some patients, although its causes are poorly defined. It is sometimes considered as a tension headache, and this would point toward the possible therapeutic value of physical activity, particularly if such activity were to be undertaken in relaxing surroundings. Others have suggested that vigorous exercise may be helpful because it raises

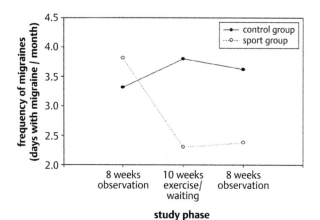

FIGURE 4.—Migraine days of exercise and control group over the 3 study phases (phase 1 = 8 weeks observation, phase 2 = 10 weeks exercise training, phase 3 = 8 weeks observation). (Reprinted from Darabaneanu S, Overath CH, Rubin D, et al. Aerobic exercise as a therapy option for migraine: a pilot study. *Int J Sports Med.* 2011;32:455-460, with permission from Georg Thieme Verlag KG Stuttgart.)

an individual's pain threshold. Perhaps in part because the mode of physical activity is an important variable in the release of tension, previous reports on the value of physical activity have given conflicting results.[1-5] This small-scale matched-controlled trial showed a statistically significant benefit (fewer attacks per month, less intense pain; Fig 4) after a 10-week program of aerobic exercise (30 min of jogging in the aerobic intensity zone 3 times per week), with benefit greatest in those individuals who developed the largest increment of physical work capacity at a heart rate of 150 beats per minute and showed an associated reduction in 1 simple estimate of stress level. The big issue when evaluating the therapeutic use of exercise in conditions such as migraine is that it is not possible to blind patients as to their group assignment. However, even if some of the benefit is finally shown to be a placebo effect, there are other health dividends that patients realize from an increase in their aerobic fitness, and a program such as that reported here seems a useful adjuvant or alternative to pharmaceutical treatment for persistent migraine.

R. J. Shephard, MD (Lond), PhD, DPE

References

1. Dittrich SM, Günther V, Franz G, Burtscher M, Holzner B, Kopp M. Aerobic exercise with relaxation: influence on pain and psychological well-being in female migraine patients. *Clin J Sport Med.* 2008;18:363-365.
2. Fitterling JM, Martin JE, Gramling S, Cole P, Milan MA. Behavioral management of exercise training in vascular headache patients: an investigation of exercise adherence and headache activity. *J Appl Behav Anal.* 1988;21:9-19.
3. Grimm L, Douglas D, Hanson P. Aerobic training in the prophylaxis of migraine. *Med Sci Sports Exerc.* 1981;13:98.
4. Köseoglu E, Akboyraz A, Soyuer A, Ersoy AO. Aerobic exercise and plasma beta endorphin levels in patients with migrainous headache without aura. *Cephalalgia.* 2003;23:972-976.
5. Narin SO, Pinar L, Erbas D, Oztürk V, Idiman F. The effects of exercise and exercise-related changes in blood nitric oxide level on migraine headache. *Clin Rehabil.* 2003;17:624-630.

The Relationship Between Physical Activity and Brain Responses to Pain in Fibromyalgia
McLoughlin MJ, Stegner AJ, Cook DB (Univ of Wisconsin-Madison)
J Pain 12:640-651, 2011

The relationship between physical activity and central nervous system mechanisms of pain in fibromyalgia (FM) is unknown. This study determined whether physical activity was predictive of brain responses to experimental pain in FM using functional magnetic resonance imaging (fMRI). Thirty-four participants (n = 16 FM; n = 18 Control) completed self-report and accelerometer measures of physical activity and underwent fMRI of painful heat stimuli. In FM patients, positive relationships ($P < .005$) between physical activity and brain responses to pain were observed in the dorsolateral prefrontal cortex, posterior cingulate cortex, and the posterior insula, regions implicated in pain regulation. Negative relationships ($P < .005$) were found for the primary sensory and superior parietal cortices, regions implicated in the sensory aspects of pain. Greater physical activity was significantly ($P < .05$) associated with decreased pain ratings to repeated heat stimuli for FM patients. A similar nonsignificant trend was observed in controls. In addition, brain responses to pain were significantly ($P < .005$) different between FM patients categorized as low active and those categorized as high active. In controls, positive relationships ($P < .005$) were observed in the lateral prefrontal, anterior cingulate, and superior temporal cortices and the posterior insula. Our results suggest an association between measures of physical activity and central nervous system processing of pain.

Perspective.—Our data suggest that brain responses to pain represent a dynamic process where perception and modulation co-occur and that physical activity plays a role in balancing these processes. Physically active FM patients appear to maintain their ability to modulate pain while those who are less active do not.

▶ McLoughlin and colleagues used functional magnetic resonance imaging (fMRI) to evaluate the relationship between physical activity and central nervous system (CNS) processing of nociceptive signals in women with fibromyalgia (FM) and controls. Altered CNS processing of pain signals may be responsible for the widespread pain that is characteristic of FM. Exercise is an efficacious treatment for FM, but patients are reluctant to increase physical activity because they fear exacerbation of pain. The evidence suggests that decreased physical activity increases FM symptoms, and these symptoms further depress physical activity. To better comprehend the mechanisms whereby exercise mitigates FM pain, the authors exposed women with FM and controls to painful heat stimuli while undergoing brain fMRI. CNS activity in regions of the brain involved with the sensory dimensions of pain and pain modulation was measured. The participants completed self-reported physical activity questionnaires (International Physical Activity Questionnaire) and wore an accelerometer for 7 days prior to the fMRI. The central hypothesis was that both self-reported and objectively measured physical activity would be negatively related to brain activity in areas involved in sensory dimensions of pain, and positively related to areas involved in pain modulation. The FM patients were further divided into 2 groups of high and low activity per self-report. The primary finding was greater pain regulation capacity in FM patients who were more physically active. When compared with physically inactive FM patients, active FM patients reported less pain intensity across the spectrum of pain stimuli, greater responses in brain regions associated with pain modulation, and lower responses in regions associated with pain sensation. Because of the cross-sectional study design, it is unclear if physical activity changed the brain activity responses to pain in FM patients. An exercise intervention study would be needed to determine if exercise training can alter CNS-mediated pain modulation and symptom severity in women with FM.

C. M. Jankowski, PhD

The Relationship Between Physical Activity and Brain Responses to Pain in Fibromyalgia

McLoughlin MJ, Stegner AJ, Cook DB (Univ of Wisconsin-Madison)
J Pain 12:640-651, 2011

The relationship between physical activity and central nervous system mechanisms of pain in fibromyalgia (FM) is unknown. This study determined whether physical activity was predictive of brain responses to experimental pain in FM using functional magnetic resonance imaging (fMRI). Thirty-four participants (n = 16 FM; n = 18 Control) completed self-report and accelerometer measures of physical activity and underwent fMRI of painful heat stimuli. In FM patients, positive relationships ($P < .005$) between physical activity and brain responses to pain were observed in the dorsolateral prefrontal cortex, posterior cingulate cortex, and the posterior insula, regions implicated in pain regulation. Negative relationships ($P < .005$) were found for the primary sensory and superior parietal cortices, regions implicated in the sensory aspects of pain. Greater physical activity was significantly ($P < .05$) associated with decreased pain ratings to repeated heat stimuli for FM patients. A similar nonsignificant trend was observed in controls. In addition, brain responses to pain were significantly ($P < .005$) different between FM patients categorized as low active and those categorized as high active. In controls, positive relationships ($P < .005$) were observed in the lateral prefrontal, anterior cingulate, and superior temporal cortices and the posterior insula. Our results suggest an association between measures of physical activity and central nervous system processing of pain.

Perspective.—Our data suggest that brain responses to pain represent a dynamic process where perception and modulation co-occur and that physical activity plays a role in balancing these processes. Physically active FM patients appear to maintain their ability to modulate pain while those who are less active do not (Fig 1).

▶ The etiology of fibromyalgia remains obscure, but there is growing evidence that 1 factor in this condition is an altered processing of pain signals,[1,2] with altered spinal levels of some of the biochemical substrates of pain perception such as substance P and serotonin.[3,4] Patients with fibromyalgia are often reluctant to increase their physical activity for fear of worsening symptoms, although exercise is one consistently successful form of therapy.[5] The mechanism of benefit is also unclear, but one possibility might be an effect of physical activity upon brain responses to painful stimuli. McLoughlin and colleagues thus examined cross-sectional relationships between subjective (questionnaire) and objective (accelerometer) measures of habitual physical activity and cerebral responses to a standard painful heat stimulus (43°-49°C). Their subjects were all women, so the responses of male patients (who typically have higher pain thresholds) remain to be evaluated; moreover, none had concurrent chronic fatigue syndrome, and even the most active were taking relatively little exercise. Functional MRIs of their patients showed that physical

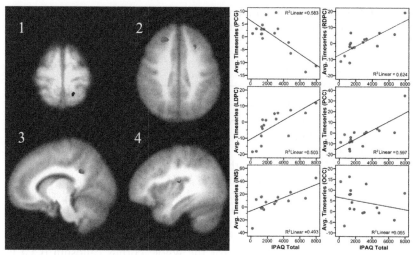

FIGURE 1.—Brain regions showing significant associations between self-reported physical activity and responses to heat pain in FM patients. A negative correlation was found in the post-central gyrus, extending into the superior parietal cortex (image 1). Positive correlations were found in the left and right dorsolateral prefrontal cortex (image 2), posterior cingulate cortex (image 3), and the mid to posterior insula (image 4). Images shown are with voxel-wise threshold set a $P = .005$ and cluster size thresholding at 200 mm^3. Functional timeseries data (average cluster values) for each individual were extracted and are shown plotted against physical activity values with the corresponding r-squared values. (Reprinted from McLoughlin MJ, Stegner AJ, Cook DB. The relationship between physical activity and brain responses to pain in fibromyalgia. *J Pain*. 2011;12:640-651, with permission from the American Pain Society.)

activity elicited a positive response in parts of the brain concerned with the regulation of pain and a negative response in areas related to the sensory appreciation of pain (Fig 1). These data suggest that relatively modest amounts of physical activity can have a useful therapeutic effect in fibromyalgia, although this needs to be verified experimentally.

R. J. Shephard, MD (Lond), PhD, DPE

References

1. Clauw DJ. Fibromyalgia: an overview. *Am J Med*. 2009;122:S3-S13.
2. Staud R. Evidence of involvement of central neural mechanisms in generating fibromyalgia pain. *Curr Rheumatol Rep*. 2002;4:299-305.
3. Russell IJ, Vaeroy H, Javors M, Nyberg F. Cerebrospinal fluid biogenic amine metabolites in fibromyalgia/fibrositis syndrome and rheumatoid arthritis. *Arthritis Rheum*. 1992;35:550-556.
4. Schwarz MJ, Späth M, Müller-Bardorff H, Pongratz DE, Bondy B, Ackenheil M. Relationship of substance P, 5-hydroxyindole acetic acid and tryptophan in serum of fibromyalgia patients. *Neurosci Lett*. 1999;259:196-198.
5. Busch AJ, Schachter CL, Overend TJ, Peloso PM, Barber KA. Exercise for fibromyalgia: a systematic review. *J Rheumatol*. 2008;35:1130-1144.

Fractional anisotropy and mean diffusivity in the corpus callosum of patients with multiple sclerosis: the effect of physiotherapy

Ibrahim I, Tintera J, Skoch A, et al (Inst for Clinical and Experimental Medicine, Prague; Czech Republic; et al)
Neuroradiology 53:917-926, 2011

Introduction.—Modulation of neurodegeneration by physical activity is an active topic in contemporary research. The purpose of this study was to investigate changes in the brain's microstructure in multiple sclerosis (MS) after facilitation physiotherapy.

Methods.—Eleven patients with MS were examined using motor and neuropsychological testing and multimodal MRI at the beginning of the study, with second baseline measurement after 1 month without any therapy, and after a 2-month period of facilitation physiotherapy. Eleven healthy controls were examined at the beginning of the study and after 1 month. Fractional anisotropy (FA), mean diffusivity (MD), axial diffusivity (λ_{ax}), and radial diffusivity (λ_{rad}) were calculated for the whole corpus callosum (CC) in the midsagittal slice of T1 W 3D MPRAGE spatially normalized images. Data were analyzed using linear mixed-effect models, paired, and two-sample tests.

Results.—At the baseline, patients with MS showed significantly lower values in FA ($p<0.001$), and significantly higher values in MD ($p<0.001$), λ_{ax} ($p=0.003$), and λ_{rad} ($p<0.001$) compared to control subjects. The FA, MD, λ_{ax}, and λ_{rad} did not change between the first and second baseline examinations in either group. Differences 2 months after initiating facilitation physiotherapy were in FA, MD, and in λ_{rad} significantly higher than differences in healthy controls ($p<0.001$ for FA, $p=0.02$ for MD, and $p=0.002$ for λ_{rad}). In MS patients, FA in the CC significantly increased ($p<0.001$), MD and λ_{rad} significantly decreased ($p=0.014$ and $p=0.002$), and thus approached the values in healthy controls.

Conclusion.—The results of the study show that facilitation physiotherapy influences brain microstructure measured by DTI.

▶ This is a small yet important study that illustrates benefits of physiotherapy in patients with relapsing-remitting multiple sclerosis (MS) (who were able to ambulate at least 200 m with 2 canes). The study does have several weaknesses. First, the type of physiotherapy that was used was called *facilitation physiotherapy*. It is unclear as to what exactly this was, although the authors describe this as applying sensorimotor stimuli (such as adaptive resistance, verbal command, and maximal stretching prior to movement) in various functional positions. It would be important to have a better description as to what exactly this entailed so that the program could be replicated. Second, there is not much information about the controls (who these were, and how were they selected). Third, it is unclear as to the validity of the counting of lesions. Notwithstanding these weaknesses, the study proposes that physiotherapy influences brain microstructure, and there was a nonsignificant trend toward improvement in function (characterized by the EDSS—expanded disability status scale). The implication is that this type of facilitation physiotherapy may induce neuroplasticity and possibly promote functional improvement—something that definitely warrants further study.

D. E. Feldman, PT, PhD

Sensorimotor network in cervical dystonia and the effect of botulinum toxin treatment: A functional MRI study
Opavský R, Hluštík P, Otruba P, et al (Palacký Univ and Univ Hosp, Olomouc, Czech Republic)
J Neurol Sci 306:71-75, 2011

Background.—The evidence suggests that the origin of primary dystonia is at least partly associated with widespread dysfunction of the basal ganglia and cortico—striato—thalamo—cortical circuits. The aim of the study was to assess the sensorimotor activation pattern outside the circuits controlling the affected body part in cervical dystonia, as well as to determine task-related activation changes induced by botulinum toxin type A (BoNT-A) treatment.

Methods.—Seven patients suffering from cervical dystonia and nine healthy controls were examined with functional MRI during skilled hand motor task; the examination was repeated 4 weeks after BoNT-A application to dystonic neck muscles.

Results.—Functional MRI data demonstrated overall reduced extent of hand movement-related cortical activation but greater magnitude of blood oxygenation level dependent signal change in the contralateral secondary somatosensory cortex in patients compared to controls. Effective BoNT-A treatment led to reduced activation of the ipsilateral supplementary motor area and dorsal premotor cortex in patients. The patients' post-treatment sensorimotor maps showed significantly smaller basal ganglia activation compared to controls.

Conclusions.—These results provide imaging evidence that abnormalities in sensorimotor activation extend beyond circuits controlling the affected body parts in cervical dystonia. The study also supports observations that BoNT-A effect has a correlate at central nervous system level, and such effect may not be limited to cortical and subcortical representations of the treated muscles.

▶ Focal dystonias can severely impact an individual's quality of life by interfering with coordinated activity and the ability to participate in recreational sport activity. Dystonia is usually inherited and is characterized as a disorder of muscle tone where, in some cases, severe involuntary contortions of affected muscle groups, whole limbs, or trunk occur. Cervical dystonia is a form of focal dystonia affecting muscles in the neck resulting in a sustained rotation of the head, or a head tilt, in a specific direction often referred to as *torticollis*. While still inconclusive, the prevailing thought is that primary dystonia such as this one reflects sensorimotor dysfunction with aberrant activity in basal ganglia and the considerable cerebral circuitry forming the cortico-striatal-thalamo-cortical circuit.[1] Disordered, dysfunctional sensorimotor integration seems to be crucial to the development of dystonia and is not specific to the affected body part or muscle group.[2] Opavský and colleagues used exactly this observation to assess sensorimotor activation patterns during performance of a skilled hand task in patients with cervical dystonia compared with healthy controls. In addition, they compared the patterns of activation in patients with cervical dystonia before and after treatment with botulinum toxin type A (BoNT-A), a common form of management in individuals with spasticity. The hand task used was one of a pattern of finger movements performed with the hand ipsilateral to the direction of deviation of the head specific to the patients and was performed with the eyes closed while the subject lay supine in the magnet. In normal subjects, this task activates extensive cortical areas, including primary motor and sensory areas as well as higher-order processing areas of both frontal and parietal lobes together with activation of cerebellum and basal ganglia. Interestingly, patients with cervical dystonia showed reduced diffuse activation but over activity in a higher-processing area of contralateral parietal lobe named the *parietal operculum*. In patients after BoNT-A, activity in the internal segment of the globus pallidus of the basal ganglia was reduced and more so ipsilaterally than contralaterally. Moreover, there was a posttreatment effect in the reduction of activity in higher-processing areas of the motor frontal lobe. Overall, this study is important in the detection of defective sensorimotor integration and abnormal sensory processing that is more widespread than in areas specifically related to affected body parts.[3] Related to this is the important finding that treatment with BoNT-A has both peripheral and central effects.

V. Galea, PhD

References

1. Obermann M, Yaldizli O, de Greiff A, et al. Increased basal-ganglia activation performing a non-dystonia-related task in focal dystonia. *Eur J Neurol.* 2008;8: 831-838.
2. Obermann M, Vollrath C, deGreiff A, et al. Sensory disinhibition on passive movement in cervical dystonia. *Mov Disord.* 2010;25:2627-2633.
3. Tanji J. New concepts of the supplementary motor area. *Curr Opin Neurobiol.* 1996;6:782-787.

Bilateral somatosensory cortex disinhibition in complex regional pain syndrome type I
Lenz M, Höffken O, Stude P, et al (Ruhr-Universität Bochum, Germany)
Neurology 77:1096-1101, 2011

Objective.—In a previous study, we found bilateral disinhibition in the motor cortex of patients with complex regional pain syndrome (CRPS). This finding suggests a complex dysfunction of central motor-sensory circuits. The aim of our present study was to assess possible bilateral excitability changes in the somatosensory system of patients with CRPS.

Methods.—We measured paired-pulse suppression of somatosensory evoked potentials in 21 patients with unilateral CRPS I involving the hand. Eleven patients with upper limb pain of nonneuropathic origin and 21 healthy subjects served as controls. Innocuous paired-pulse stimulation of the median nerve was either performed at the affected and the unaffected hand, or at the dominant hand of healthy controls, respectively.

Results.—We found a significant reduction of paired-pulse suppression in both sides of patients with CRPS, compared with control patients and healthy control subjects.

Conclusion.—These findings resemble our findings in the motor system and strongly support the hypothesis of a bilateral complex impairment of central motor-sensory circuits in CRPS I.

▶ The phenomenon of neuropathic pain, that is, chronic pain arising from abnormal neural activity secondary to disease, injury, or dysfunction of the nervous system, is a complex one. Neuropathic pain tends to persist without ongoing disease and may manifest in various forms, for example, as a painful phantom limb. A particularly intervention-resistant form of neuropathic pain is a condition termed *complex regional pain syndrome* (CRPS) that may manifest after trauma (sometimes a mild innocuous trauma) or surgical procedures. Patients so affected have frank motor sensory disturbances, hyperalgesia to touch or temperature, dysfunction of the autonomic nervous system, limb edema, and deep somatic pain. While any part of the body might be involved, the structure most often involved is the upper limb. In this study, Lenz and coworkers followed up on previous work indicating bilateral disinhibition of the motor cortex in patients with CRPS1, a form of CRPS in which there is no nerve injury.[1] They postulated that the bilateral increased activation in the motor cortex may also be reflected in the somatosensory cortex and used a technique termed paired-pulse suppression of somatosensory-evoked potentials (SEPs) to investigate whether the somatosensory cortex of patients with CRPS1 of the hand exhibited decreased somatosensory paired-pulse suppression compared with patients with nonneuropathic pain and healthy controls. SEPs are evoked potentials observed using electroencephalogram-type electrodes applied over the human somatosensory cortex and in this study were evoked via stimulation of the median nerve at the wrist. The paired-pulse suppression paradigm involves the application of 2 asynchronous stimuli with the expectation that the second stimulus is significantly reduced. The actual outcome is the ratio of the second stimulus to the first stimulus. In all cases, patients with CRPS1 had higher ratios (indicating reduced paired-pulse suppression) than either the nonneuropathic pain patients or healthy subjects. This was clearly not a normal reaction to chronic pain. In addition, CRPS1 patients exhibited this disinhibition bilaterally, so that the effect was observed for both affected and unaffected sides and was not related to pain intensity or duration of illness, indicating that the sensation of pain was not driving the bilateral motor-sensory dysfunction. Collectively, these authors may have unearthed a consequence of the disease process or, more importantly, a predisposition to development of the disease. The fact that some patients with similar traumatic incidents or surgical procedures go on to develop this condition has been and continues to be a confounding aspect of this disease. This bilateral motor-sensory involvement should be of interest to clinicians concerned with management of patients with this disease.

V. Galea, PhD

Reference

1. Schwenkreis P, Janssen F, Rommel O, et al. Bilateral motor cortex disinhibition in complex regional pain syndrome (CRPS) type I of the hand. *Neurology.* 2003;61: 515-519.

Adaptation of motor function after spinal cord injury: novel insights into spinal shock
Boland RA, Lin CS-Y, Engel S, et al (Neuroscience Res Australia, Sydney, New South Wales; Univ of New South Wales, Sydney, Australia; Prince of Wales Hosp, Sydney, New South Wales, Australia)
Brain 134:495-505, 2011

The mechanisms underlying spinal shock have not been clearly defined. At present, clinical assessment remains the mainstay to describe progression through spinal shock following traumatic spinal cord injury. However, nerve excitability studies in combination with conventional nerve conduction and clinical assessments have the potential to investigate spinal shock at the level of the peripheral axon. Therefore, peripheral motor axon excitability was prospectively and systematically evaluated in more than 400 studies of 11 patients admitted to hospital after traumatic spinal cord injury, with cord lesions above T9 (nine cervical, two thoracic). Recordings commenced within 15 days of admission from the median nerve to abductor pollicis brevis in the upper limb and the common peroneal nerve to tibialis anterior in both lower limbs, and were continued until patient discharge from hospital. Excitability was assessed using threshold tracking techniques and recordings were compared with data from healthy controls. In addition, concurrent clinical measures of strength, serum electrolytes and nerve conduction were collected. High threshold stimulus–response relationships were apparent from the early phase of spinal shock that coincided with depolarization-like features that reached a peak on Day 16.9 (± 2.7 standard error) for the common peroneal nerve and Day 11.8 (± 2.0 standard error) for the median nerve. Overall, changes in the common peroneal nerve were of greater magnitude than for the median nerve. For both nerves, the most significant changes were in threshold electrotonus, which was 'fanned in', and during the recovery cycle superexcitability was reduced ($P < 0.001$). However, refractoriness was increased only for the common peroneal nerve ($P < 0.05$). Changes in the spinal injured cohort could not be explained on the basis of an isolated common peroneal nerve palsy. By the time patients with spinal injury were discharged from hospital between

Days 68 and 215, excitability for upper and lower limbs had returned towards normative values, but not for all parameters. Electrolyte levels and results for nerve conduction studies remained within normal limits throughout the period of admission. Contrary to prevailing opinion, these data demonstrate that significant changes in peripheral motor axonal excitability occur early during spinal shock, with subsequent further deterioration in axonal function, before recovery ensues.

▶ The processes underlying spinal cord shock immediately following spinal cord injury remain quite complex and have yet to be clearly established. Clinically, spinal cord shock is described initially as a period of flaccid paralysis, loss of voluntary movement, and reduced tendon reflexes. In later spinal cord shock, patients are described as transitioning from this period of flaccidity to a condition of hyperexcitability and hyperreflexia. Initially, these changes are attributed to the disconnection of the spinal cord from descending drive and consequent reductions in spinal motor neuron pool excitability, while later changes are attributed to alterations in central input in the balance of excitatory and inhibitory drive. Interestingly the condition of peripheral axons is not taken into consideration during this period of initiation and transition of spinal shock.[1] Boland and coworkers intricately and expertly address the condition of the peripheral nerve axons in this publication. Specifically, they examined the onset and progression of peripheral axonal changes in both the median nerve and common peroneal nerve (CPN) using a novel combination of conventional clinical assessments, nerve conduction studies, and precise nerve excitability techniques.[2] Data were collected from the time of onset of the acute phase of spinal cord shock until discharge. The most interesting finding from this study was that although there were no significant differences in repeated nerve conduction studies of either median or CPN, there were definite changes in axonal excitability as measured by stimulus-response curves, current-threshold relationships (which measure the rectifying properties of axonal membranes), threshold electrotonus (a recording of changes in threshold from axons at the areas of the nodes of Ranvier and from intermodal axonal membranes), and recovery cycles, which provide an indicator of absolute and relative refractory periods as well as the ranges of nerve excitability. The evidence presented in this article contributes significantly to the state of knowledge regarding spinal shock by showing that peripheral nerve axons are affected both in the acute and during the transitional phase.[3] This challenges conventional wisdom that the peripheral nerves are in some sort of "state of hibernation," as the authors point out. The implications of these findings become important to rehabilitation of patients with spinal cord injury, particularly in those protocols using peripheral electrical stimulation to artificially activate muscle in the absence of the voluntary drive following spinal cord injury.

V. Galea, PhD

References

1. Boland RA, Bostock H, Kiernan MC. Plasticity of lower limb motor axons after cervical cord injury. *Clin Neurophysiol.* 2009;120:204-209.

2. Kiernan MC, Burke D, Andersen KV, Bostock H. Multiple measures of axonal excitability: a new approach in clinical testing. *Muscle Nerve.* 2000;23:399-409.
3. Lin CS, Macefield VG, Elam M, Wallin BG, Engel S, Kiernan MC. Axonal changes in spinal cord injured patients distal to the site of injury. *Brain.* 2007;130:985-994.

Aquatic Therapy Versus Conventional Land-Based Therapy for Parkinson's Disease: An Open-Label Pilot Study

Vivas J, Arias P, Cudeiro J (Univ of A Coruña, Spain)
Arch Phys Med Rehabil 92:1202-1210, 2011

Objectives.—To assess and compare 2 different protocols of physiotherapy (land or water therapy) for people with Parkinson's disease (PD) focused on postural stability and self-movement, and to provide methodological information regarding progression within the program for a future larger trial.

Design.—Randomized, controlled, open-label pilot trial.

Setting.—Outpatients, Parkinson's disease Center of Ferrol-Galicia (Spain).

Participants.—Individuals (N = 11) with idiopathic PD in stages 2 or 3 according to the Hoehn and Yahr Scale completed the investigation (intervention period plus follow-up).

Interventions.—After baseline evaluations, participants were randomly assigned to a land-based therapy (active control group) or a water-based therapy (experimental group). Participants underwent individual sessions for 4 weeks, twice a week, for 45 minutes per session. Both interventions were matched in terms of exercise features, which were structured in stages with clear objectives and progression criteria to pass to the next phase.

Main Outcome Measures.—Participants underwent a first baseline assessment, a posttest immediately after 4 weeks of intervention, and a follow-up assessment after 17 days. Evaluations were performed OFF-dose after withholding medication for 12 hours. Functional assessments included the Functional Reach Test (FRT), the Berg Balance Scale (BBS), the UPDRS, the 5-m walk test, and the Timed Up and Go test.

Results.—A main effect of both therapies was seen for the FRT. Only the aquatic therapy group improved in the BBS and the UPDRS.

Conclusions.—In this pilot study, physiotherapy protocols produced improvement in postural stability in PD that was significantly larger after aquatic therapy. The intervention protocols are shown to be feasible and seem to be of value in amelioration of postural stability—related impairments in PD. Some of the methodological aspects detailed here can be used to design larger controlled trials.

▶ This small randomized controlled trial merits attention for several reasons. The study uses standardized protocols in individualized contexts. The exercise program is oriented according to the International Classification of Functioning, and progression criteria were clearly delineated and followed. The presentation of exercise programs for both the land-based and aquatic-based programs enable better understanding of the actual programs as well as the possibility of replicating this study on a larger basis. The investigators chose 3 main areas that are relevant to Parkinson disease: trunk mobility, balance, and task orientation. They used objective outcome variables: functional reach distance, Berg Balance Score (BBS), objective gait measures (turn time, velocity, cadence, and step amplitude), Timed Up and Go, and Unified Parkinson's Disease Rating scale (UPDRS). The results indicate that both land and water therapy were beneficial, although only improvement in functional reach test was statistically significant. There was an advantage for aquatic therapy over land therapy in terms of balance (BBS) and UPDRS. Although a larger trial is needed, I applaud this study in terms of its detailed procedure descriptions, which make it easier to understand exactly what exercise interventions were done. This type of detail would benefit many other studies that comprise exercise and rehabilitation interventions.

D. E. Feldman, PT, PhD

Critical neural substrates for correcting unexpected trajectory errors and learning from them
Mutha PK, Sainburg RL, Haaland KY (NM VA Healthcare System, Albuquerque; Pennsylvania State Univ)
Brain 134:3644-3658, 2011

Our proficiency at any skill is critically dependent on the ability to monitor our performance, correct errors and adapt subsequent movements so that errors are avoided in the future. In this study, we aimed to dissociate the neural substrates critical for correcting unexpected trajectory errors and learning to adapt future movements based on those errors. Twenty stroke patients with focal damage to frontal or parietal regions in the left or right brain hemispheres and 20 healthy controls performed a task in which a novel mapping between actual hand motion and its visual feedback was introduced. Only patients with frontal damage in the right hemisphere failed to correct for this discrepancy during the ongoing movement. However, these patients were able to adapt to the distortion such that their movement direction on subsequent trials improved. In contrast, only patients with parietal damage in the left hemisphere showed a clear deficit in movement adaptation, but not in online correction. Left frontal or right parietal damage did not adversely impact upon either process. Our findings thus identify, for the first time, distinct and lateralized neural substrates critical for correcting unexpected errors during ongoing movements and error-based movement adaptation (Figs 2 and 5).

▶ Acquisition of skill is ultimately dependent on the ability to correct errors and then learn from them. We monitor our performance, correct those errors, and then adapt to the task so that those errors are not repeated. Mutha, Sainburg, and Haaland extend on an impressive body of work to show for the first time that the left and right cortical hemispheres are distinctly lateralized in processes

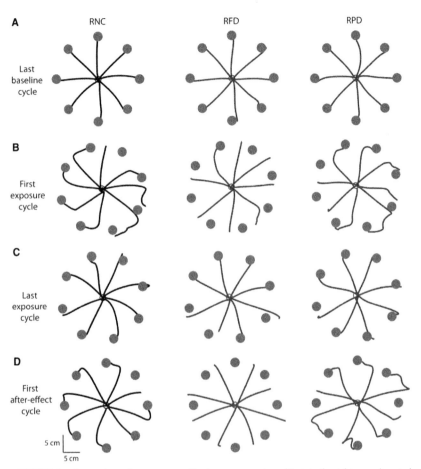

FIGURE 2.—Comparison of movement profiles for representative subjects in the right normal controls (RNC, black), and right frontal damage (RFD) and right parietal damage (RPD, grey) groups. (**A**) Last eight trials (last cycle) of the baseline session; (**B**) First cycle of movements following exposure to the visuomotor rotation (exposure session). (**C**) Last cycle of movements of the exposure session and (**D**) first cycle of the after-effect session when the visuomotor rotation was removed. (Reprinted from Mutha PK, Sainburg RL, Haaland KY. Critical neural substrates for correcting unexpected trajectory errors and learning from them. *Brain.* 2011;134:3644-3658, with permission of the Guarantors of Brain, Oxford University Press.)

subserving motor control and learning. A popular probe used for investigation of these processes by sensorimotor neuroscientists consists of novel and unpredictable perturbations of a "reaching to a horizontal target" movement. Using this paradigm, one may observe both movement corrections and adaptation to the novel perturbation. In this particular study, Mutha and colleagues recruited patients with either right or left frontal lobe lesions, right or left parietal lobe lesions, and healthy controls and asked the patients to perform these tasks with their ipsilesional (and therefore relatively unaffected) side to investigate the specialized abilities of these cortical areas. Healthy controls performed the

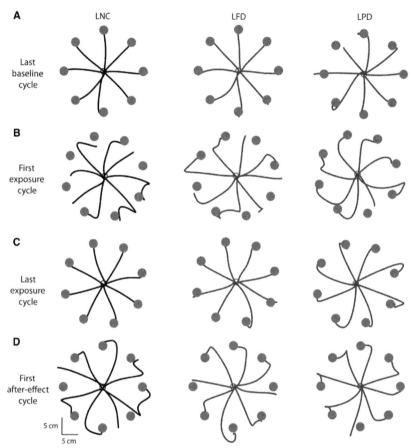

FIGURE 5.—Comparison of movement profiles for representative subjects in the left normal controls (LNC, black), and groups with left frontal damage (LFD) and left parietal damage (LPD, grey). (A) Last eight trials (last cycle) of the baseline session. (B) First cycle of movements following exposure to the visuomotor rotation (exposure session). (C) Last cycle of movements of the exposure session and (D) first cycle of the after-effect session when the visuomotor rotation was removed. (Reprinted from Mutha PK, Sainburg RL, Haaland KY. Critical neural substrates for correcting unexpected trajectory errors and learning from them. *Brain.* 2011;134:3644-3658, with permission of the Guarantors of Brain, Oxford University Press.)

tasks with either their right or left side. The type of perturbation used was a fairly common visuomotor rotation in which motion of the subject-controlled cursor is dissociated from the actual direction of hand motion. Acquisition (via a motion capture system) of the hand trajectory to the target yields considerable information, and in this case, the outcomes were initial direction error, hand path curvature, and final position error. The experimental protocol consisted of a series of baseline cycles of horizontal reaching to 8 different targets placed in a circle where cursor and hand motion are congruent, a series of test cycles in which a 30° visuomotor rotation of the cursor was induced, thereby dissociating the cursor and hand, and a series of cycles in which the perturbation was removed and the cursor and hand were once again congruent or, in the authors' words, "veridical." The latter cycles are designed to determine whether adaptation to the perturbation had taken place; if so, the observer will notice the presence of "after-effects." Based on previous work, the expectation was that the left parietal cortex is crucial for adaptation to the perturbed condition, whereas the right frontal cortex is instrumental for correction of movement errors until learning has taken place because such patients with focal lesions in these areas should show related deficits.

Figs 2 and 5 are good representations of the task protocol and show the performance of representative subjects from the healthy control, frontal lobe damage, and parietal lobe damage groups. Results were consistent with the investigator expectations in that patients with right frontal lobe lesions had difficulty correcting errors during the movement; however, performance over cycles showed that they were able to learn from those errors. In contrast, patients with left parietal lobe lesions were able to correct errors during the movement; however, they clearly showed deficits in movement adaptation. The authors go on to point out that error correction circuitry must also include the basal ganglia, citing other work in which patients with basal ganglia pathology (Huntington's disease) were unable to make online corrections. One of the most interesting findings from this study is the hemispheric distinction between error correction and learning from errors (in this case, visuomotor errors) to adapt subsequent movements to the perturbation. The left parietal cortex in fact seems to influence the performance of either arm used. Motor control and learning of a novel task is dependent on these interactions. This study is tremendously informative to those concerned with exercise prescription in patients with neurological damage because knowledge of this nature will be informative to the design of targeted rehabilitation protocols and possibly informative as to whether patients with certain types of neurological damage will respond to a particular intervention.

V. Galea, PhD

Arm Motor Control as Predictor for Hypertonia After Stroke: A Prospective Cohort Study
de Jong LD, Hoonhorst MH, Stuive I, et al (Ctr for Rehabilitation, Zwolle, The Netherlands; Univ of Groningen, The Netherlands)
Arch Phys Med Rehabil 92:1411-1417, 2011

Objectives.—To analyze the development of hypertonia in the hemiparetic elbow flexors, and to explore the predictive value of arm motor control on hypertonia in a cohort of first-ever stroke survivors in the first 6 months poststroke.

Design.—A prospective cohort study.

Setting.—A cohort of stroke survivors from a large, university-affilliated hospital in The Netherlands.

Participants.—Patients (N = 50) with first-time ischemic strokes and initial arm paralysis who were admitted to a stroke unit.

Interventions.—Not applicable.

Main Outcome Measures.—At 48 hours, 10 to 12 days, 3 and 6 months poststroke, hypertonia and arm motor control were assessed using the Modified Ashworth Scale and the Fugl-Meyer Assessment arm score.

Results.—The incidence rate of hypertonia reached its maximum before the third month poststroke (30%). Prevalence was 42% at 3 and 6 months. Participants with poor arm motor control at 48 hours poststroke were 13 times more likely to develop hypertonia in the first 6 months poststroke than those with moderate to good arm motor control. These results were not confounded by the amount of arm function training received.

Conclusions.—Hypertonia develops in a large proportion of patients with stroke, predominantly within the first 3 months poststroke. Poor arm motor control is a risk factor for the development of hypertonia.

▶ Hypertonia is often misrepresented as spasticity and should correctly be defined as increased resistance to passive stretch.[1,2] This situation manifests quite commonly in individuals after they have experienced a cerebral vascular accident or stroke. The prevailing thought is that the signs of hypertonia are caused by the hyperexcitability of spinal motor neurons due to the variable loss of descending drive from corticomotoneurons affected by the stroke. In this article, de Jong and collaborators performed serial measurements of both hypertonia, using a subjective measurement instrument called the Modified Ashworth Scale, and a functional measure of upper limb function using the 66-arm function items from the Fugl-Meyer Assessment scale. One of their objectives was to look at the incidence and prevalence of hypertonia over 4 time points during the first 6 months after stroke. In addition, they were also concerned with influence of upper limb motor control and time on the development of hypertonia, as this situation rarely develops right away after stroke. Given that those individuals who experience stroke present with variable functional loss, the authors were also interested in the predictive power of the extent of early upper limb control on the subsequent development of hypertonia. This is an important study to the readers of this volume because knowledge of existing hypertonia in individuals who participate in community activities after stroke will have unique limitations, especially to the affected hemiparetic arm. It should be said that there is at least 1 considerable limitation to this study in that the investigators only looked at the commonly affected elbow flexors for the presence of hypertonia and not within any other muscle group. This study is novel in that this is the first time that elbow flexor hypertonia has been recorded over time during the first 6 months following a stroke in first-time stroke survivors. They were careful to select participants with previous stroke to remove the confounder of existing hypertonia and contracture. A Fugl-Meyer score of 18 or less 48 hours after stroke was the cutoff for identifying those with poor motor control, and these individuals were 13 times as likely to develop hypertonia, usually by 3 months after, than their higher-functioning cohorts. Hypertonia itself (defined as a Modified Ashworth Score of $+1$) reached a maximum before the third month after stroke, and 42% of the participants ($n = 50$) had hypertonia at 3 and 6 months. Knowledge of the presence of hypertonia and the consequent contracture that will develop if the patient continues to display learned nonuse of that arm after stroke is imperative to the health practitioner concerned with rehabilitation or activity involvement in these individuals because of the impact on quality of life a nonfunctional limb will have on that patient. If nothing else, concerned effort should be made to prevent or at least decrease the development of contracture through passive and active range-of-motion exercise.

V. Galea, PhD

References

1. Pandyan AD, Price CI, Rodgers H, Barnes MP, Johnson GR. Biomechanical examination of a commonly used measure of spasticity. *Clin Biomech (Bristol, Avon).* 2001;16:859-865.
2. Pandyan AD, Price CI, Barnes MP, Johnson GR. A biomechanical investigation into the validity of the Modified Ashworth Scale as a measure of elbow spasticity. *Clin Rehabil.* 2003;17:290-293.

Attention Deficit Hyperactivity Disorder and the Athlete: An American Medical Society for Sports Medicine Position Statement
Putukian M, Kreher JB, Coppel DB, et al (Princeton Univ, NJ; Massachusetts General Hosp for Children, Boston; Univ of Washington, Seattle; et al)
Clin J Sport Med 21:392-401, 2011

Attention deficit hyperactivity disorder (ADHD) is an important issue for the physician taking care of athletes since ADHD is common in the athletic population, and comorbid issues affect athletes of all ages. The health care provider taking care of athletes should be familiar with making the diagnosis of ADHD, the management of ADHD, and how treatment medications impact exercise and performance. In this statement, the term "Team Physician" is used in reference to all healthcare providers that take care of athletes. These providers should understand the side effects of medications, regulatory issues regarding stimulant medications, and indications for additional testing. This position statement is not intended to be a comprehensive review of ADHD, but rather a directed review of the core issues related to the athlete with ADHD (Table 1).

▶ I do not recall seeing a single case of attention-deficit disorder (ADD) during my medical training, and the topic was certainly not discussed in either my pediatric or medical textbooks. The *Diagnostic and Statistical Manual of Mental Disorders* (DSM-II) of 1968 first noted a "Hyperkinetic Reaction of Childhood." The DSM-III termed the condition as "ADD with or without hyperactivity," and in the revised DSM-III-R of 1987 this was changed to attention-deficit/hyperactivity disorder (ADHD). Now, it is supposedly the most common psychiatric disorder of childhood, affecting 3% to 5% of children worldwide and 4% to 8% of US children, possibly with an even greater prevalence among participants in aggressive sports.[1-3] Why has this condition emerged? Is it simply a reflection of reduced discipline in home and school, or the aggressive marketing efforts of those selling Ritalin? One sociologist described it as "no more than the medicalization of deviant behavior."[4] However, the American Medical Society for Sports

TABLE 1.—Traits Common to Athletes With ADHD Without Treatment

Poor attention span
Difficulty initiating or completing tasks in activities they find boring or nonengaging
Too much attention to novel situations
Difficulty waiting one's turn
Increased risk-taking behaviors
Inability to manage own time
Difficulties with unstructured time
Lack of organizational skills
Common co-morbidities: anxiety, depression, disruptive behavior, learning disorders, substance abuse
  disorders, and psychotic disorders

Medicine has now considered the issue of sufficient importance to prepare a consensus position statement, underlying the various likely problems when the children concerned participate in sports (Table 1). Interestingly, some authors have suggested that sport participation can mitigate the symptoms of inattention and impulsivity.[5,6] Athletes with a diagnosis of ADHD may encounter problems not only from the condition itself but also from the stimulant medications that are prescribed for its control, particularly appetite suppression, difficulties in the development of muscle mass, and poor thermoregulation. At higher levels of competition, the drugs are also banned by most antidoping agencies.

R. J. Shephard, MD (Lond), PhD, DPE

References

1. Rowland AS, Lesesne CA, Abramowitz AJ. The epidemiology of attention-deficit/hyperactivity disorder (ADHD): a public health view. *Ment Retard Dev Disabil Res Rev.* 2002;8:162-170.
2. Harel EH, Brown WD. Attention deficit hyperactivity disorder in elementary school children in Rhode Island: associated psychosocial factors and medications used. *Clin Pediatr (Phila).* 2003;42:497-503.
3. Barbaresi WJ, Katusic SK, Colligan RC, et al. How common is attention-deficit/hyperactivity disorder? Incidence in a population-based birth cohort in Rochester, Minn. *Arch Pediatr Adolesc Med.* 2002;156:217-224.
4. Parrillo VN. *Encyclopedia of Social Problems.* Thousand Oaks, CA: Sage; 2008. 63.
5. Etscheidt MA, Ayllon T. Contingent exercise to decrease hyperactivity. *J Child Adolesc Psychother.* 1987;4:192-198.
6. Molloy GN. Chemicals, exercise and hyperactivity: a short report. *Int J Disabil Dev Educ.* 1989;36:57-61.

Community-Associated Methicillin-Resistant *Staphylococcus aureus* Survival on Artificial Turf Substrates

Waninger KN, Rooney TP, Miller JE, et al (Temple Univ School of Medicine, Philadelphia, PA; Temple Univ, Philadelphia, PA; Delaware Valley College, Doylestown, PA)
Med Sci Sports Exerc 43:779-784, 2011

Objective.—Artificial turf has been suggested as a risk factor for community-associated methicillin-resistant *Staphylococcus aureus* (CA-MRSA).

This is an experimental study looking at survival of CA-MRSA on artificial turf.

Methods.—MRSA strain USA-300-0114 was grown as either planktonic cells or biofilms in liquid cultures of beef heart infusion broth overnight at 37°C. Beakers containing ProGrass (Pittsburgh, PA) turf were inoculated at the dirt interface with either $\sim 5 \times 10^7$ planktonic bacteria or with biofilms. The inoculum included varying nutrient conditions consisting of spent medium, saline, or 5% mucin. The beakers were incubated at 37°C in ambient air. The main outcome measure was the number of surviving colony-forming units determined by plating on mannitol salt agar.

Results.—Survival was biphasic with a colony-forming unit drop from $\sim 5 \times 10^7$ to $\sim 5 \times 10^5$ after the first week followed by survival of between 10^4 and 10^3 bacteria until termination of the experiment (20–50 d). Survival was dependent on nutrients, and washed cells survived less than 1 d. Mucin could serve as a nutrient source and slightly increased surviving numbers to 10^4–10^5 bacteria. Biofilm formation did not influence survival.

Conclusions.—CA-MRSA survivability on artificial turf surfaces is dependent on the availability of nutrients. These results suggest that CA-MRSA could survive on artificial turf in significant numbers for 1 wk, and lower numbers for at least 1 month, if supplied with appropriate

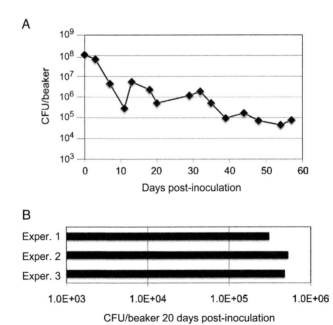

FIGURE 2.—CA-MRSA survives in high numbers on turf in the presence of mucin. The minimum level of detection is 1000 CFU. (Reprinted from Waninger KN, Rooney TP, Miller JE, et al. Community-associated methicillin-resistant *Staphylococcus aureus* survival on artificial turf substrates. *Med Sci Sports Exerc.* 2011;43:779-784, with permission from the American College of Sports Medicine.)

nutrients. Outdoor environmental conditions may affect these findings (Fig 2).

▶ Methicillin-resistant *Staphylococcus aureus* is an increasing clinical problem both in outpatients and on hospital wards[1,2] due in part to an excessive and inappropriate prescription of antibiotics and in part to the widespread use of antibiotics by agribusiness. Athletes may have some increase in risk of developing such problems, in part because of frequent superficial injuries and suppression of immune function during periods of intensive training.[3-5] A further possible issue is repeated visits to tourist-class hotels, where proscription of the use of and/or resistance to insecticides such as DDT has led to widespread infestation with bedbugs (*Cimex lectularius*).[6] The report of Waninger and associates demonstrates that methicillin-resistant staphylococci (and presumably other microorganisms can survive on artificial turf for some weeks if the surface of the turf is contaminated with mucin (Fig 2). However, as artificial turf manufacturers allege, the survival of the microorganisms is probably reduced substantially by higher environmental temperatures and exposure to ultraviolet light.[7] There is at least a similar risk with other playing surfaces, including natural turf and wrestling mats, and it is important to adhere closely to National College Athletic Association guidelines for the cleaning and disinfecting of playing surfaces and athletic gear.

R. J. Shephard, MD (Lond), PhD, DPE

References

1. Creel AM, Durham SH, Benner KW, Alten JA, Winkler MK. Severe invasive community-associated methicillin-resistant *Staphylococcus aureus* infections in previously healthy children. *Pediatr Crit Care Med.* 2009;10:323-327.
2. Lindenmayer JM, Schoenfeld S, O'Grady R, Carney JK. Methicillin-resistant *Staphylococcus aureus* in a high school wrestling team and the surrounding community. *Arch Intern Med.* 1998;158:895-899.
3. Benjamin HJ, Nikore V, Takagishi J. Practical management: community-associated methicillin-resistant *Staphylococcus aureus* (CA-MRSA): the latest sports epidemic. *Clin J Sport Med.* 2007;17:393-397.
4. Kirkland EB, Adams BB. Methicillin-resistant *Staphylococcus aureus* and athletes. *J Am Acad Dermatol.* 2008;59:494-502.
5. Kuehnert MJ, Kruszon-Moran D, Hill HA, et al. Prevalence of *Staphylococcus aureus* nasal colonization in the United States, 2001–2002. *J Infect Dis.* 2006; 193:172-179.
6. Lowe CF, Romney MG. Bedbugs as vectors for drug-resistant bacteria. *Emerg Infect Dis.* 2011;17:1132-1134.
7. McNitt AS. Survival of *Staphylococcus aureus* on synthetic turf. http://cropsoil. psu.edu/mcnitt/staph/index.cfm. Accessed May 12, 2011.

8 Environmental Factors

Impact of heat and pollution on oxidative stress and CC16 secretion after 8 km run
Gomes EC, Stone V, Florida-James G (Edinburgh Napier Univ, UK)
Eur J Appl Physiol 111:2089-2097, 2011

To investigate the acute effect of a hot, humid and ozone-polluted (O_3) environment on lung inflammation and oxidative tress of runners performing 8 km time trial run. Using a single-blinded randomized design, 10 male athletes (mean $\dot{V}O_{2max}$ max=64.4 $mlO_2\,kg^{-1}\,min^{-1}$, SD = 4.4) took part in a time trial run in four different environmental conditions: $20°C + 50\%$ relative humidity (rh) (Control); $20°C + 50\%$ rh + 0.10 ppm O_3 (Control + O_3); $31°C + 70\%$ rh (Heat); $31°C + 70\%$ rh + 0.10 ppm O_3 (Heat + O_3). Blood samples and nasal lavage were collected post-exercise and analyzed for inflammatory, epithelial damage and oxidative stress markers. Data were analyzed using repeated measures ANOVA with Tukey's post hoc test. A significant increase in CC16 concentration ($P < 0.05$) and GSH/protein concentration ($P < 0.05$) in the upper respiratory airways was observed following the 8 km run in the Heat + O_3 trial compared with the control trial. There were no differences in the neutrophil counts between trials. No differences were observed for the other antioxidants analyzed. A hot, humid and ozone-polluted environment (0.1 ppm) elicits an early epithelial damage and antioxidant protection process in the upper respiratory airways of athletes immediately after performing 8 km time trial run (Fig 2).

▶ Commonly encountered ambient urban concentrations of ozone[1] have long been known to have adverse effects on exercise performance.[2-4] One factor leading to impaired performance is injury to the lung epithelium, with an associated increase in permeability of the lung—epithelial barrier. This can be detected as an increase in blood and airway levels of Clara cell protein (CC16).[5] The study of Gomes and associates was based on a simulated 8-km run performed on a laboratory treadmill. It found no increase of CC16 with exposure to either ozone alone (0.10 ppm) or heat alone (31°C, 70% relative humidity), but a combination of the two adverse environments increased airway concentrations of both CC16 and antioxidants in nasal washings (Fig 2). There

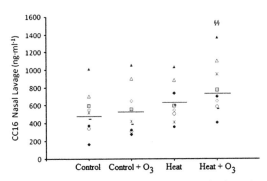

FIGURE 2.—Individual nasal lavage CC16 concentration. Mean value for each trial is represented by *lines.* §§ Significantly different from Control trial ($P = 0.03$). (Reprinted from Gomes EC, Stone V, Florida-James G. Impact of heat and pollution on oxidative stress and CC16 secretion after 8 km run. *Eur J Appl Physiol.* 2011;111:2089-2097, Copyright 2011, with kind permission of Springer Science+ Business Media.)

was also a 9–10% decrease in average running speed over the 8 km. Plainly, those who are organizing urban competitions need to consider not only the likely levels of ozone pollution but also interactions between the effects of ozone and a hot and humid environment. Outdoor concentrations of ozone are highest during and immediately after periods of bright sunshine, and exposure can thus be reduced by running in the early morning and late evening.

R. J. Shephard, MD (Lond), PhD, DPE

References

1. Baldasano JM, Valera E, Jiménez P. Air quality data from large cities. *Sci Total Environ.* 2003;307:141-165.
2. Folinsbee LJ, Silverman F, Shephard RJ. Exercise responses following ozone exposure. *J Appl Physiol.* 1975;38:996-1001.
3. Gibbons SI, Adams WC. Combined effects of ozone exposure and ambient heat on exercising females. *J Appl Physiol.* 1984;57:450-456.
4. Gong H Jr, Bradley PW, Simmons MS, Tashkin DP. Impaired exercise performance and pulmonary function in elite cyclists during low-level ozone exposure in a hot environment. *Am Rev Respir Dis.* 1986;134:726-733.
5. Blomberg A, Mudway I, Svensson M, et al. Clara cell protein as a biomarker for ozone-induced lung injury in humans. *Eur Respir J.* 2003;22:883-888.

Light-Induced Changes of the Circadian Clock of Humans: Increasing Duration is More Effective than Increasing Light Intensity
Dewan K, Benloucif S, Reid K, et al (The Baylor College of Medicine, Houston, TX; Northwestern Univ Feinberg School of Medicine, Chicago, IL)
Sleep 34:593-599, 2011

Study Objectives.—To evaluate the effect of increasing the intensity and/ or duration of exposure on light-induced changes in the timing of the circadian clock of humans.

Design.—Multifactorial randomized controlled trial, between and within subject design.

Setting.—General Clinical Research Center (GCRC) of an academic medical center.

Participants.—56 healthy young subjects (20-40 years of age).

Interventions.—Research subjects were admitted for 2 independent stays of 4 nights/3 days for treatment with bright or dim-light (randomized order) at a time known to induce phase delays in circadian timing. The intensity and duration of the bright light were determined by random assignment to one of 9 treatment conditions (duration of 1, 2, or 3 hours at 2000, 4000, or 8000 lux).

Measurements and Results.—Treatment-induced changes in the dim light melatonin onset (DLMO) and dim light melatonin offset (DLMOff) were measured from blood samples collected every 20-30 min throughout baseline and post-treatment nights. Comparison by multi-factor analysis of variance (ANOVA) of light-induced changes in the time of the circadian melatonin rhythm for the 9 conditions revealed that changing the duration of the light exposure from 1 to 3 h increased the magnitude of light-induced delays. In contrast, increasing from moderate (2,000 lux) to high (8,000 lux) intensity light did not alter the magnitude of phase delays of the circadian melatonin rhythm.

Conclusions.—Results from the present study suggest that for photo-therapy of circadian rhythm sleep disorders in humans, a longer period of moderate intensity light may be more effective than a shorter exposure period of high intensity light (Table 1).

▶ There have been suggestions that exposure to bright light can facilitate the adaptation of an athlete to a new time zone. This is physiologically plausible, given that the light/dark cycle is the primary synchronizing signal for the circadian pacemaker, and bright light also has a direct alerting effect.[1] Exposure during the late afternoon and early part of the night delays the pacemaker, and exposure early in the morning advances the pacemaker. However, there is little agreement in the literature on the optimal intensity or duration of illumination. Authors have advocated levels ranging from 2500 to 12 000 lux, with exposure durations ranging from 20 minutes to 4 or more hours. The intensity of illumination is a particularly critical variable, because to achieve intensities greater than 4000 lux, it is necessary for an athlete to keep in close proximity to the source of light.[2,3] The present study compared exposures of 1 to

TABLE 1.—Delay in the Melatonin Rhythm Following 1, 2, or 3 Hours of Light Exposure

Duration of Light (Hours)	N	DLMO 50% (Hours ± SD)**	DLMOff 50% (Hours ± SD)
1	18	−0.17 ± 1.06	−0.37 ± 0.92
2	22	−0.88 ± 1.05	−0.45 ± 0.85
3	16	−1.46 ± 1.67	−0.94 ± 1.41

**P = 0.01.

3 hours at 2000, 4000, or 8000 lux, with melatonin levels indicating the phase shift achieved over a single night of exposure. Increasing the duration of exposure from 1 to 3 hours was the most effective tactic (Table 1), with 3 hours of illumination giving a circadian shift of more than 1 hour in a single night. However, for most classes of competition, it remains debatable whether athletes will want to spend 3 hours sitting under a very bright light to achieve a 1-hour shift of biological rhythms, particularly when other adaptive tactics such as the timing of meals and training sessions can induce at least some of this same response.

R. J. Shephard, MD (Lond), PhD, DPE

References

1. Cajochen C. Alerting effects of light. *Sleep Med Rev.* 2007;11:453-464.
2. Eastman CI, Liu L, Fogg LF. Circadian rhythm adaptation to simulated night shift work: effect of nocturnal bright-light duration. *Sleep.* 1995;18:399-407.
3. Smith MR, Eastman CI. Phase delaying the human circadian clock with blue-enriched polychromatic light. *Chronobiol Int.* 2009;26:709-725.

Low prevalence of exercise-associated hyponatremia in male 100 km ultra-marathon runners in Switzerland
Knechtle B, Knechtle P, Rosemann T (Gesundheitszentrum St Gallen, Switzerland; Univ of Zurich, Switzerland)
Eur J Appl Physiol 111:1007-1016, 2011

We investigated the prevalence of exercise-associated hyponatremia (EAH) in 145 male ultra-marathoners at the '100-km ultra-run' in Biel, Switzerland. Changes in body mass, urinary specific gravity, haemoglobin, haematocrit, plasma [Na$^+$], and plasma volume were determined. Seven runners (4.8%) developed asymptomatic EAH. Body mass, haematocrit and haemoglobin decreased, plasma [Na$^+$] remained unchanged and plasma volume increased. Δ body mass correlated with both post race plasma [Na$^+$] and Δ plasma [Na$^+$]. Δ plasma volume was associated with post race plasma [Na$^+$]. The athletes consumed 0.65 (0.30) L/h; fluid intake correlated significantly and negatively ($r = -0.50, p < 0.0001$) to race time. Fluid intake was neither associated with post race plasma [Na$^+$] nor with Δ plasma [Na$^+$], but was related to Δ body mass. To conclude, the prevalence of EAH was low at ~5% in these male 100 km ultra-marathoners. EAH was asymptomatic and would not have been detected without the measurement of plasma [Na$^+$] (Fig 2).

▶ A recent article claimed that nefarious commercial influences arising from the sale of "sports drinks" had sought to hide problems arising from overingestion of fluid during long-distance events, leading to an "epidemic" of exercise-associated hyponatremia (EAH).[1] A lead article in a previous edition of the YEAR BOOK,[2] however, cautioned that hype might exceed the extent of problems from hyponatremia,[2] and a more recent review[3] concluded that although there

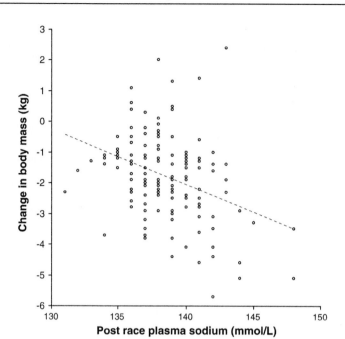

FIGURE 2.—The change in body mass was significantly and negatively associated with post race plasma [Na⁺] in the 145 finishers ($r = -0.35$, $p < 0.0001$). (Reprinted from Knechtle B, Knechtle P, Rosemann T. Low prevalence of exercise-associated hyponatremia in male 100 km ultra-marathon runners in Switzerland. *Eur J Appl Physiol.* 2011;111:1007-1016, with kind permission of Springer Science+Business Media.)

were undoubtedly occasional incidents of EAH, the prevalence of this condition was insufficient to meet usually accepted criteria of an epidemic, and evidence of a commercial conspiracy to encourage an excessive intake of fluid was far from convincing. Most of the published cases have been asymptomatic, or "biochemical" cases of EAH, with a plasma sodium in the range 130 to 135 mE/L, a zone where apparently abnormal post-race figures could reflect interindividual variation among a large pool of runners and/or the substantial measurement error of field tests of plasma sodium.[4] Problems are much more likely during ultramarathon than marathon events, because competitors have a longer period to absorb fluids, and a disturbance of fluid balance is more likely if conditions are cool or cold. Data from the Biel ultramarathon are thus of interest. In this event, 2 of 145 competitors were hypernatremic, and 7 had a biochemical hyponatremia, but none developed any symptoms; moreover, at least 5 of the 7 with apparent EAH fell within the measurement error of the i-STAT device (133-134 mE/L, Fig 2). The runners were offered fluid at 17 drinking stations, but their average intake (650 mL/h) matched the recommended fluid intake, corresponding to expected peak rate of fluid absorption in an exercising subject.[5] The data of Knechtle et al. are reassuring, although 2 notes of caution should be added: The runners were experienced (inexperience is one factor contributing to EAH), and no information was obtained on the use of nonsteroidal anti-inflammatory drugs (which can modify renal function[6]).

R. J. Shephard, MD (Lond), PhD, DPE

References

1. Noakes TD. Changes in body mass alone explain almost all of the variance in the serum sodium concentrations during prolonged exercise. Has commercial influence impeded scientific endeavour? *Br J Sports Med.* 2011;45:475-477.
2. Shephard RJ. Hype or hyponatremia. In: Shephard RJ, Cantu RC, Feldman DE, et al., eds. *Year Book of Sports Medicine, 2007.* Philadelphia, PA: Elsevier/Mosby; 2007:19-28.
3. Shephard RJ. Suppression of information on the prevalence and prevention of exercise-associated hyponatraemia? *Br J Sports Med.* 2011;45:1238-1242.
4. Erickson KA, Wilding P. Evaluation of a novel point-of-care system, the i-STAT portable clinical analyzer. *Clin Chem.* 1993;39:283-287.
5. Kavanagh T, Shephard RJ. Maintenance of hydration in "post-coronary" marathon runners. *Br J Sports Med.* 1975;9:129-135.
6. Reid SA, Speedy DB, Thompson JM, et al. Study of hematological and biochemical parameters in runners completing a standard marathon. *Clin J Sport Med.* 2004; 14:344-353.

Exercise-associated hyponatremia: the influence of pre-exercise carbohydrate status combined with high volume fluid intake on sodium concentrations and fluid balance

Hubing KA, Bassett JT, Quigg LR, et al (Texas Christian Univ, Fort Worth; et al)
Eur J Appl Physiol 111:797-807, 2011

To evaluate the effect of hydration and carbohydrate (CHO) status on plasma sodium, fluid balance, and regulatory factors (IL-6 & ADH) during and after exercise; 10 males completed the following conditions: low CHO, euhydrated (fluid intake = sweat loss) (LCEH); low CHO, dehydrated (no fluid) (LCDH); high CHO, euhydrated (HCEH); and high CHO, dehydrated (HCDH). Each trial consisted of 90-min cycling at 60% VO_2 max in a 35°C environment followed by 3-h rehydration (RH). During RH, subjects received either 150% of sweat loss (LCDH & HCDH) or an additional 50% of sweat loss (LCEH and HCEH). Blood was analyzed for glucose, IL-6, ADH, and Na^+. Post-exercise Na^+ was greater ($p < 0.001$) for LCDH and HCDH (141.7 + 0.72 and 141.6 + 0.4 mM) versus LCEH and HCEH (136.4 + 0.6 and 135.9 + 0.3 mM). Post-exercise IL-6 was similar in all conditions, and postexercise ADH was greater ($p = 0.01$) in dehydrated versus euhydrated conditions. The rate of urine production was greater in HCEH (7.59 + 3.0 mL/min) compared to all other conditions (3.86 + 2.2, 5.29 + 3.1, and 2.96 + 1.1 mL/min for LCDH, LCEH, and HCDH, respectively). Despite CHO and hydration manipulations, no regulatory effects of IL-6 and ADH on plasma [Na^+] were observed. With euhydration during exercise and additional fluid consumed during recovery, a high-CHO status increased urinary output during recovery, and it decreased the frequency of hyponatremia (Na^+ <135 mM). Therefore,

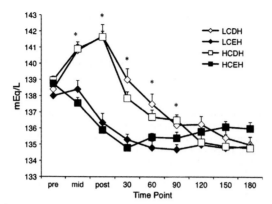

FIGURE 1.—Plasma sodium responses (mean ± SE). *Asterisks* indicate that LCEH and HCEH conditions are significantly different from HCDH and LCDH conditions at the time points indicated. ($p < 0.05$). (Reprinted from Hubing KA, Bassett JT, Quigg LR, et al. Exercise-associated hyponatremia: the influence of pre-exercise carbohydrate status combined with high volume fluid intake on sodium concentrations and fluid balance. *Eur J Appl Physiol.* 2011;111:797-807, Copyright 2011 with kind permission of Springer Science+Business Media.)

a high-CHO status may provide some protection against exercise-associated hyponatremia (Fig 1).

▶ Much has been written about hyponatremia,[1] possibly too much relative to the prevalence of this condition in sports events.[2] There are undoubtedly some cases, particularly in ultra-endurance and triathlon races, held under cold and wet conditions, and at least 8 fatalities have been reported. But the exact numbers of affected athletes have been clouded by the imprecision of field estimates of serum sodium, symptoms that are readily confused with effects of heat stress, and vast discrepancies between the numbers with biochemical and clinical hyponatremia. The main cause of this condition is an excessive intake of fluid, whether water or a sports drink with a low sodium ion content. However, most runners find it difficult to ingest more than about 600 mL of fluid per hour while they are running, and under typical North American race conditions this does not compensate for fluid lost in sweating. Possibly, the problem arises from overenthusiastic provision of fluids in the emergency tent. But there have also been suggestions that other mechanisms may make certain individuals more vulnerable to a low plasma sodium level, particularly an unusually high secretion of antidiuretic hormone (ADH).[3] The cytokine interleukin-6 (IL-6) may also be implicated, because it stimulates the release of ADH,[4] and IL-6 concentrations are usually increased during prolonged exercise as muscle glycogen is depleted.[5] The study of Hubing and associates thus compared responses in subjects who had followed a high hydration and carbohydrate (CHO) (8 g/kg body mass) or low CHO (0.5 kg/kg) diet for 2 days prior to a 90-minute cycle ergometer ride at 60% of maximal oxygen intake under hot conditions. Carbohydrate supplements did not appear to influence ADH, IL-6, or plasma sodium levels (Fig 1). However, the study does show the rapid decrease of sodium concentrations during the postrace period, regardless of whether the excess of fluid is ingested during exercise or during the recovery period. In assessing fluid requirements during and after prolonged exercise, it is important to take into account not only changes in body mass but also water released during glycogen metabolism.

R. J. Shephard, MD (Lond), PhD, DPE

References

1. Noakes TD, Sharwood K, Speedy D, et al. Three independent biological mechanisms cause exercise-associated hyponatremia: evidence from 2,135 weighed competitive athletic performances. *Proc Natl Acad Sci U S A.* 2005;102:18550-18555.
2. Shephard RJ. Hype or hyponatremia? Year Book of Sports Medicine, 2007. In: Shephard RJ, et al., eds. Philadelphia, PA: Elsevier/Mosby; 2007:19-28.
3. Armstrong LE, Curtis WC, Hubbard RW, Francesconi RP, Moore R, Askew EW. Symptomatic hyponatremia during prolonged exercise in heat. *Med Sci Sports Exerc.* 1993;25:543-549.
4. Siegel AJ. Exercise-associated hyponatremia: role of cytokines. *Am J Med.* 2006; 119:S74-S78.
5. Febbraio MA, Pedersen BK. Muscle-derived interleukin-6: mechanisms for the activation and possible biological roles. *FASEB J.* 2002;16:1335-1347.

Tear Fluid Osmolarity as a Potential Marker of Hydration Status
Fortes MB, Diment BC, Di Felice U, et al (Bangor Univ, Gwynedd, UK; et al)
Med Sci Sports Exerc 43:1590-1597, 2011

It has been suggested that tear fluid is isotonic with plasma, and plasma osmolality (P_{osm}) is an accepted, albeit invasive, hydration marker. Our aim was to determine whether tear fluid osmolarity (T_{osm}) assessed using a new, portable, noninvasive, rapid collection and measurement device tracks hydration.

Purpose.—This study aimed to compare changes in T_{osm} and another widely used noninvasive marker, urine specific gravity (USG), with changes in P_{osm} during hypertonic—hypovolemia.

Methods.—In a randomized order, 14 healthy volunteers exercised in the heat on one occasion with fluid restriction (FR) until 1%, 2%, and 3% body mass loss (BML) and with overnight fluid restriction until 08:00 h the following day, and on another occasion with fluid intake (FI). Volunteers were rehydrated between 08:00 and 11:00 h. T_{osm} was assessed using the TearLab™ osmolarity system.

Results.—P_{osm} and USG increased with progressive dehydration on FR ($P < 0.001$). T_{osm} increased significantly on FR from 293 ± 9 to 305 ± 13 mOsm·L^{-1} at 3% BML and remained elevated overnight (304 ± 14 mOsm·L^{-1}; $P < 0.001$). P_{osm} and T_{osm} decreased during exercise on FI and returned to preexercise values the following morning. Rehydration restored P_{osm}, USG, and T_{osm} to within preexercise values. The mean correlation between T_{osm} and P_{osm} was $r = 0.93$ and that between USG and Posm was $r = 0.72$.

Conclusions.—T_{osm} increased with dehydration and tracked alterations in P_{osm} with comparable utility to USG. Measuring T_{osm} using the

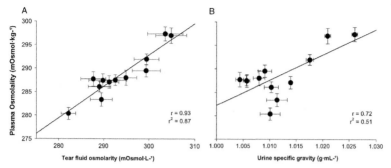

FIGURE 3.—Scatter plots depicting the relationship between mean plasma osmolality and mean tear fluid osmolarity (A) and mean plasma osmolality and mean USG (B) during fluid intake and fluid restriction (both trials pooled into one data set). Both correlations are significant ($P < 0.01$). *Solid line* represents the regression line. (Reprinted from Fortes MB, Diment BC, Di Felice U, et al. Tear fluid osmolarity as a potential marker of hydration status. *Med Sci Sports Exerc.* 2011;43:1590-1597, with permission from the American College of Sports Medicine.)

TearLab™ osmolarity system may offer sports medicine practitioners, clinicians, and research investigators a practical and rapid hydration assessment technique (Fig 3).

▶ The monitoring of dehydration during an athletic event is normally based on careful weighing, measurements of urine specific gravity, and (in case of doubt) field measurements of plasma sodium. A rapidly responding commercial device has now been developed for determining the osmolarity of tear fluid. Fortes and colleagues contend that not only does it yield rapid and highly reproducible results (a within-subject coefficient of variation of 2.8%), but also the findings correlate closely with plasma osmolarity (Fig 3). In my view, there are a number of important limitations to this claim, particularly in the athletic context. On theoretical grounds, it is not clear that tear fluid is a direct plasma filtrate,[1] and indeed, the relative proportion of various electrolytes sometimes differs between plasma and tear samples.[2] To produce dehydration, Fortes et al had their test subjects exercise on a cycle ergometer in an environmental chamber under closely regulated conditions (a dry bulb temperature of 33°C and a relative humidity of 50%). However, during a normal athletic competition, athletes would be exposed to varying amounts of wind plus a relative air movement created by cycling or other forms of body displacement, and such air currents would surely change the volume and osmolarity of the tear fluid. Moreover, these changes would be exacerbated by day-to-day differences in moisture content of the ambient air, by lacrimogenic air pollutants, and even by the emotions of competition. It might be worthwhile to conduct a field trial of tear fluid analyses versus plasma sodium determinations, but I am fairly confident that the latter would remain the procedure of choice.

R. J. Shephard, MD (Lond), PhD, DPE

References

1. Tiffany JM. Tears in health and disease. *Eye (Lond).* 2003;17:923-926.

2. Ubels JL, Williams KK, Lopez Bernal D, Edelhauser HF. Evaluation of effects of a physiologic artificial tear on the corneal epithelial barrier: electrical resistance and carboxyfluorescein permeability. *Adv Exp Med Biol.* 1994;350:441-452.

Optimising the Acquisition and Retention of Heat Acclimation

Daanen HAM, Jonkman AG, Layden JD, et al (TNO Defence, Soesterberg, The Netherlands; et al)
Int J Sports Med 32:822-828, 2011

Heat acclimation (HA) often starts in a moderately hot environment to prevent thermal overload and stops immediately prior to athletic activities. The aims of this study were 1) to establish whether acclimation to a moderately hot climate is sufficient to provide full acclimation for extreme heat and 2) to investigate the physiological responses to heat stress during the HA decay period. 15 male subjects exercised for 9 consecutive days at 26°C Wet Bulb Globe Temperature (WBGT) and 3 days at 32°C WBGT on a cycle ergometer for up to 2 h per day and repeated the exercise 3, 7 and 18 days later in 26°C WBGT. Rectal temperature (T_{re}) and heart rate (HR) were measured during 60 min of steady state exercise (~45% of maximum oxygen uptake). During days 1—9, end-exercise T_{re} was reduced from 38.7 ± 0.1 to a plateau of 38.2 ± 0.1°C (p < 0.05), HR was reduced from 156 ± 10 to 131 ± 11 bpm (p < 0.05). No changes in HR and T_{re} occurred during the 3 days in the very hot environment. However, T_{re} during rest and exercise were significantly lower by 0.4—0.5°C after HA compared with day 9, suggesting that heat acclimation did not decay but resulted in further favourable adaptations (Table 2).

▶ Heat acclimatization is a relatively slow process, and to maximize adjustments, both physiologic and psychological, it is necessary for athletes to live on site in the hot environment rather than undergo physiologic acclimation in an environmental chamber in their home country.[1,2] To avoid unnecessarily long periods of residence at the competitive site, it is important for those managing athletes to know just how rapidly such adaptation is acquired and lost. There is general agreement that the development of acclimatization seems about 75% complete at 5 days, and little further adaptation is seen at 10 days.[3] However, the rate of decay of acclimatization is more controversial, estimates varying from a few days to a month[4] (Table 2). The study of Daanen and associates suggests that after full adaptation to moderate heat (exercising for 100 min/d at a wet bulb globe temperature 26°C for 9 days), adaptive responses are not further enhanced by a further 3 days of exercising in extreme heat (wet bulb globe temperature 32°C). However, that additional adaptation becomes apparent after withdrawal of the stimulus, as with a period of heavy training; in other words, heat adaptations need some form of tapering. This would perhaps explain some of the variability in the apparent rate of decay of acclimatization. One obvious weakness in the study is that, having underscored the difference between acclimatization and acclimation, the subjects were

TABLE 2.—Change in Rectal Temperature (°C) Related to the Number of Days After Full Heat Acclimation

Study	Acclimation Days	Days After HA	dTre-Rest (°C)	dTre-Exercise (°C)	Remarks
Adam et al., 1960	12	2			acclimated group was much better after 2 days than non-acclimated group
This study	12	3	−0.3	−0.4	
Pandolf et al., 1977	9	3		−0.16	
Saat et al., 2005	14	5		0.01	0.11 when daily exercise in cold after HA
Wyndham & Jacobs, 1957	12	6		0.39	mouth in stead of rectal, midway work
Pandolf et al., 1977	9	6		0.09	
Williams et al., 1967	16	7	0.27	0.33	for winter
Weller et al., 2007	10	12	0	−0.04	
Pandolf et al., 1977	9	12		0.14	
Williams et al., 1967	16	14	0.1	0.49	for winter
Pandolf et al., 1977	9	18		0.03	
Williams et al., 1967	16	21	0.27	0.61	for winter
Weller et al., 2007	10	26	0.05	0.03	

Editor's Note: Please refer to original journal article for full references.

exposed to a daily period of 100 minutes in a climatic chamber rather than life in a hot natural environment. Studies are needed in which athletes train for 9 to 12 days in a hot natural environment and then taper their efforts either by cutting back on their training or moving to an air-conditioned environment.

R. J. Shephard, MD (Lond), PhD, DPE

References

1. Glossary of terms for thermal physiology. Second edition. Revised by the commission for thermal physiology of the international union of physiological sciences (IUPS Thermal Commission). *Pflugers Arch.* 1987;410:567-587.
2. Milne CJ, Shaw MT. Travelling to China for the Beijing 2008 Olympic Games. *Br J Sports Med.* 2008;42:321-326.
3. Pandolf KB. Time course of heat acclimation and its decay. *Int J Sports Med.* 1998; 19:S157-S160.
4. Weller AS, Linnane DM, Jonkman AG, Daanen HA. Quantification of the decay and re-induction of heat acclimation in dry-heat following 12 and 26 days without exposure to heat stress. *Eur J Appl Physiol.* 2007;102:57-66.

Does summer in a humid continental climate elicit an acclimatization of human thermoregulatory responses?

Bain AR, Jay O (Univ of Ottawa, Ontario, Canada)
Eur J Appl Physiol 111:1197-1205, 2011

Many thermal physiologists follow the conventional wisdom that physiological heat adaptations occur in the summer for people living in a humid continental climate (e.g. Central Canada, North-eastern and Mid-western United States and Eastern Europe); therefore experimentation across seasons is often avoided. However, since modern behavioral adaptations, such as air conditioning, are accessible and commonplace, it is not clear whether such physiological adjustments actually do occur. It was hypothesized that despite warm weather, residing in a humid continental climate throughout a summer will not elicit any significant physiological heat adaptations since the environmental stimulus for such adjustments will be mitigated by behavioral adaptations. Eight young healthy male volunteers cycled at 60% VO2max for 90-min in a temperate environment before (mid-May) and at the end of (start of September) summer. Core temperature [measured in the esophagus (T_{es}), rectum (T_{re}) and aural canal (T_{au})], mean skin temperature (T_{sk}), forearm skin blood flow (SkBf), upper back sweat rate (LSR) and heart rate (HR) were measured throughout exercise. Weekly activity logs and a lifestyle questionnaire were also administered throughout the summer months. No significant differences between pre- and end-summer were observed throughout exercise for T_{es} ($p = 0.565$), T_{re} ($p = 0.350$), T_{au} ($p = 0.261$), T_{sk} ($p = 0.955$), SkBf ($p = 0.112$), LSR ($p = 0.394$) or HR ($p = 0.343$). Likewise, the thermosensitivity and Tes at the onset threshold for LSR ($p = 0.177$, $p = 0.512$) and SkBf ($p = 0.805$, $p = 0.556$) were also not significantly different. The apparent lack of heat acclimatization could be due to frequent air-conditioning use and an avoidance of outdoor activity during the hottest times of day but may also be due to a lack of environmental stimulus (Fig 3).

▶ Athletes from a temperate region usually find themselves at a substantial disadvantage if they must compete in a hot and humid climate. Such individuals can achieve substantial physiological acclimation by exercising (or even sitting) in a heated climatic chamber daily for a couple of weeks,[1] but the classical view is that they will reach a more complete acclimatization by living in the new, warmer environment for a comparable time. A corollary of this argument is that in the summer months, athletes who have been living in a continental climate should not require heat acclimatization before competition. However, there has been

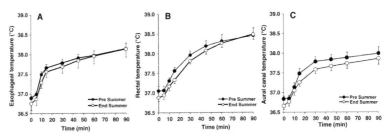

FIGURE 3.—Core temperature measurements throughout 90-min of exercise for pre-summer (*black*) and end-summer (*white*) in the esophagus (a), rectum (b) and aural canal (c). *Error bars* indicate standard error. (Reprinted from Bain AR, Jay O. Does summer in a humid continental climate elicit an acclimatization of human thermoregulatory responses? *Eur J Appl Physiol.* 2011;111:1197-1205, Copyright 2011, with kind permission of Springer Science+Business Media.)

little experimental evidence to support this viewpoint, and indeed one study of highly trained runners in the northeast of the United States saw no differences in physiological responses between spring and summer training.[2] Bain and Jay evaluated this issue further, testing a small group of young men living in Ottawa, Ontario; their subjects performed 90 minutes of moderate cycle ergometer exercise (60% of maximal oxygen intake) during the last 2 weeks of May (following a month when daily peak temperatures had been in the range of 17° to 18° C) and during the first 2 weeks of September (following a month when peak temperatures had been 25° to 26° C, and humidex values had frequently exceeded 35° C). There was little evidence of heat acclimation (as shown by core temperatures or rates of skin blood flow) at the end of the summer (Fig 3). Bain and Jay suggested that currently, city dwellers have little exposure to summer heat; all of their subjects worked in an air-conditioned environment, and 4 of the 8 also had air-conditioning at home. Moreover, most of their daily physical activity was undertaken either in air-conditioned facilities or during the evening (when thermal conditions had moderated). Plainly, in developed societies, it is no longer possible to assume that a period of summer weather will ensure adequate heat adaptation for athletes.

R. J. Shephard, MD (Lond), PhD, DPE

References

1. Taylor NA. Challenges to temperature regulation when working in hot environments. *Ind Health*. 2006;44:331-344.
2. Armstrong LE, Hubbard RW, DeLuca JP, Christensen EL. Heat acclimatization during summer running in the northeastern United States. *Med Sci Sports Exerc*. 1987;19:131-136.

Changes in Copeptin and Bioactive Vasopressin in Runners With and Without Hyponatremia

Hew-Butler T, Hoffman MD, Stuempfle KJ, et al (Oakland Univ, Rochester, MI; Univ of California Davis Med Ctr, Sacramento; Gettysburg College, Gettysburg, PA; et al)
Clin J Sport Med 21:211-217, 2011

Objective.—To evaluate changes in both the N-terminal (arginine vasopressin; AVP) and C-terminal (copeptin) fragments of the vasopressin prohormone before, during, and after an ultramarathon race and to assess vasopressin and copeptin concentrations in runners with and without hyponatremia.

Design.—Observational study.

Setting.—Three trials (2 sodium balance and 1 hyponatremia treatment) in 2 separate approximately 160-km footraces [Western States Endurance Run (WSER) and Javelina Jundred Mile Race (JJ100)].

Participants.—Six hyponatremic and 20 normonatremic runners; 19 finishers with 7 completing 100 km.

Main Outcome Measures.—Plasma AVP ($[AVP]_p$), copeptin ([copeptin]$_p$), sodium ($[Na^+]_p$), and protein (%plasma volume change; %PV) concentrations.

Results.—In the WSER Sodium Trial, a 3-fold prerace to postrace increase in both $[AVP]_p$ (0.7 ± 0.4 to 2.7 ± 1.9 pg/mL; $P < 0.05$) and [copeptin]$_p$ (10.3 ± 12.5 to 28.2 ± 16.3 pmol/L; nonsignificant) occurred, despite a 2 mEq/L decrease in $[Na^+]_p$ (138.7 ± 2.3 to 136.7 ± 1.6 mEq/L; NS). A significant correlation was noted between $[AVP]_p$ and [copeptin]$_p$ postrace ($r = 0.82$; $P < 0.05$). In the WSER Treatment Trial, despite the presence of hyponatremia pretreatment versus posttreatment ($[Na^+]_p = 130.3$ vs 133.5 mEq/L, respectively), both $[AVP]_p$ (3.2 vs 2.1 pg/mL) and [copeptin]$_p$ (22.5 vs 24.9 pmol/L) were well above the detectable levels. A significant correlation was noted between $[AVP]_p$ and [copeptin]$_p$ 60 minutes after treatment ($r = 0.94$; $P < 0.05$). In the JJ100 Sodium Trial, significant correlations were found between [copeptin]$_p$ change and %PV change ($r = -0.34$; $P < 0.05$) and between $[AVP]_p$ change and $[Na^+]_p$ change ($r = 0.39$; $P < 0.05$) but not vice-versa.

Conclusions.—[Copeptin]$_p$ seems to be a reliable surrogate of stimulated $[AVP]_p$ during exercise. Nonosmotic vasopressin stimulation occurs during ultradistance running. [Copeptin]$_p$ may better reflect chronic (% PV) vasopressin secretion under conditions of endurance exercise (Fig 2).

▶ Symptomatic exercise-associated hyponatremia is quite rare, and although ingestion of an excessive volume of fluid is an important underlying cause, there have also been suggestions that in at least some of the affected individuals, there is an inappropriate and excessive secretion of antidiuretic hormone during very prolonged exercise.[1-3] This has been a rather difficult issue to explore

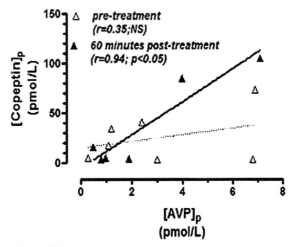

FIGURE 2.—Plasma AVP versus copeptin concentrations pretreatment and posttreatment with 100 mL of 3% NaCl in 6 hyponatremic WSER runners. (Reprinted from Hew-Butler T, Hoffman MD, Stuempfle KJ, et al. Changes in copeptin and bioactive Vasopressin in runners with and without hyponatremia. *Clin J Sport Med.* 2011;21:211-217, with permission from Lippincott Williams & Wilkins.)

experimentally, since bioactive arginine vasopressin (AVP) has a very short half-life (10-20 min), and requires a moderately large sample of plasma (0.5-1.0 mL) that may be difficult to collect during or immediately following a race. Copeptin, the C-terminal fragment of the vasopressin prohormone, has recently been proposed as a surrogate indicator of AVP secretion.[4-6] Copeptin can be analyzed in 50-µL samples of either plasma or serum, and specimens can be stored at room temperature for as long as 7 days with a change in concentration < 20%. The analytic procedure remains fairly time consuming, although it demands hours rather than the days needed to assay AVH.[4,5] To obtain subjects who would develop hyponatremia, Hew-Butler and associates studied a small group of runners during ultralong (160 km) foot races. Postrace, a moderately close correlation was found between AVH and copeptin concentrations under both normonatremic and hyponatremic conditions (Fig 2). Both AVP and copeptin tended to increase over the 160-km course (2- to 3-fold and 3- to 4-fold, respectively), with AVP representing a short-term and copeptin a longer-term stimulus to an increase of plasma volume. It remains to be seen how far either of these measurements will become clinically useful in identifying individuals who are at increased risk of hyponatremia during ultralong distance races.

R. J. Shephard, MD (Lond), PhD, DPE

References

1. Hew-Butler T, Jordaan E, Stuempfle KJ, et al. Osmotic and nonosmotic regulation of arginine vasopressin during prolonged endurance exercise. *J Clin Endocrinol Metab.* 2008;93:2072-2078.
2. Hew-Butler T, Ayus JC, Kipps C, et al. Statement of the second international exercise-associated hyponatremia consensus development conference, New Zealand, 2007. *Clin J Sport Med.* 2008;18:111-121.
3. Siegel AJ, Verbalis JG, Clement S, et al. Hyponatremia in marathon runners due to inappropriate arginine vasopressin secretion. *Am J Med.* 2007;120:461.e11-461.e17.
4. Morgenthaler NG, Struck J, Jochberger S, Dünser MW. Copeptin: clinical use of a new biomarker. *Trends Endocrinol Metab.* 2008;19:43-49.
5. Morgenthaler NG, Struck J, Alonso C, Bergmann A. Assay for the measurement of copeptin, a stable peptide derived from the precursor of vasopressin. *Clin Chem.* 2006;52:112-119.
6. Jochberger S, Morgenthaler NG, Mayr VD, et al. Copeptin and arginine vasopressin concentrations in critically ill patients. *J Clin Endocrinol Metab.* 2006; 91:4381-4386.

Factors Associated With a Self-Reported History of Exercise-Associated Muscle Cramps in Ironman Triathletes: A Case—Control Study
Shang G, Collins M, Schwellnus MP (Univ of Cape Town, South Africa)
Clin J Sport Med 21:204-210, 2011

Objective.—Exercise-associated muscle cramping (EAMC) is a common medical condition in endurance athletes. The exact cause of and risk factors for EAMC are still being investigated. The main objective of this study was to investigate factors that are associated with a self-reported history of EAMC in Ironman triathletes.

Design.—Case–control study.

Setting.—Field study at an international Ironman Triathlon.

Participants.—Triathletes participating in an Ironman Triathlon were recruited as subjects.

Assessment of Risk Factors.—A previously validated prerace questionnaire was completed by 433 subjects who were divided into subjects who reported a history of EAMC (EAMC group = 216) and those who no reported history of EAMC (CON group = 217).

Main Outcome Measures.—Training, anthropometric, injury and performance, and other variables that were related to the history of EAMC.

Results.—Compared with the CON group, triathletes in the EAMC group were significantly taller and heavier, had faster Ironman race times despite being of similar caliber (past personal best times), and predicted and achieved a faster overall time during the Ironman Triathlon. There was an association among a positive family history for EAMC, a history of tendon and/or ligament injuries, and a selfreported history of EAMC.

Conclusions.—There is evidence from this study that a history of EAMC is associated with (1) exercising at a higher intensity during a race that may result in premature muscle fatigue, (2) an inherited risk (positive family history), and (3) a history of tendon and/or ligament injury (Table 6).

▶ Exercise-associated muscle cramps (EAMC) have traditionally been regarded as an expression of heat exposure, dehydration, and electrolyte disturbance (particularly sodium depletion).[1-3] They were traditionally seen in the stokers of coal-fired boilers ("stokers' cramps"); however, the evidence supporting a role for heat exposure is not very strong in the case of long-distance athletes.[4] Symptoms are particularly common during and following Ironman triathlon competition.[5] Thus, Shang and associates made a case-control comparison between those triathlon participants who had a history of EAMC (n = 216) and an equal number of competitors (n = 217) who did not suffer from cramps. Significant differences in the questionnaire responses of the EAMC group were a slightly higher intensity of effort during the swimming and cycling legs of the race, a positive family history (37% vs 16%), and a history of tendon or ligament injury (Table 6); the information on injuries and family history is of course open to

TABLE 6.—Regression Analysis for the Determination of Independent Risk Factors EAMC in Ironman Triathletes

	Level of Effect	Estimate ± Standard Error	Wald Statistic	P
Height, cm	—	0.049 ± 0.017	8.60	0.003
Age, y	—	0.024 ± 0.015	2.64	0.104
Overall time, min	—	−0.003 ± 0.001	4.11	0.043
History of tendon and ligament injury	Yes	−0.329 ± 0.144	5.21	0.022
Family history EAMC	Yes	0.493 ± 0.143	11.84	0.001
History of tendon and ligament injury × family history EAMC	—	−0.125 ± 0.143	0.76	0.382

EAMC, exercise-associated muscle cramping.

"recall bias." Cramping occurred in localized muscle groups that had been involved in the event, the duration of the spasm was usually short (4—5 minutes), and symptoms were commonly relieved by stretching. These various observations tend to support the alternative, nonthermal hypothesis that the cause of the cramps is "altered neuromuscular control" secondary to muscle fatigue.[4]

R. J. Shephard, MD (Lond), PhD, DPE

References

1. Bergeron MF. Muscle cramps during exercise—is it fatigue or electrolyte deficit. *Curr Sports Med Rep.* 2008;7:S50-S55.
2. Armstrong LE, Casa DJ, Millard-Stafford M, Moran DS, Pyne SW, Roberts WO. ACSM position stand. Exertional heat illness during training and competition. *Med Sci Sports Exerc.* 2007;39:556-572.
3. Eichner ER. The role of sodium in 'heat cramping'. *Sports Med.* 2007;37:368-370.
4. Schwellnus MP. Cause of exercise associated muscle cramps (EAMC)—altered neuromuscular control, dehydration or electrolyte depletion? *Br J Sports Med.* 2009;43:401-408.
5. Dallam GM, Jonas S, Miller TK. Medical considerations in triathlon competition: recommendations for triathlon organisers, competitors and coaches. *Sports Med.* 2005;35:143-161.

Neck Cooling and Running Performance in the Heat: Single versus Repeated Application

Tyler CJ, Sunderland C (Roehampton Univ, London, UK; Nottingham Trent Univ, UK)
Med Sci Sports Exerc 43:2388-2395, 2011

Purpose.—This study aimed to evaluate the effect of sustained neck cooling during time trial running in a hot environment.

Methods.—Seven nonacclimated, familiarized males completed three experimental 90-min preloaded time trials in the heat (30.4°C ± 0.1°C and 53% ± 2% relative humidity). During one of the trials, the, participants wore a cooling collar from the start (CC); in another, they wore a collar from the start which was replaced at 30-min intervals (CC$_{replaced}$); and in the last trial, they wore no collar (NC). Participants ran for 75 min at 60% $\dot{V}O_{2max}$ and then performed a 15-min time trial blinded from the distance ran. Distance ran, rectal temperature, neck skin temperature, HR, fluid loss and consumption, peripheral lactate, glucose, dopamine, serotonin and cortisol, RPE, thermal sensation, and feeling scales were recorded. Significance was set *a priori* at the $P < 0.05$ level.

Results.—Participants ran further in CC (2779 ± 299 m) compared with NC (2597 ± 291 m, $P = 0.007$; $d = 0.67$) and in CC$_{replaced}$ (2776 ± 331 m) compared with NC ($P = 0.008$; $d = 0.62$). There was no difference in the distance covered in CC compared with that in CC$_{replaced}$ ($P = 0.998$). The collar lowered neck temperature ($P < 0.001$) and the thermal sensation of the neck region ($P < 0.001$) but had no effect on any of the other physiological, endocrinological, or perceptual variables.

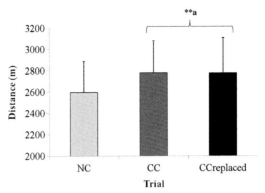

FIGURE 1.—Mean ± SD distances covered during the 15-min time trials in the NC, CC, and CC$_{replaced}$ trials. **$P < 0.01$. [a]Compared to NC. Main effect of trial ($P = 0.003$). (Reprinted from Tyler CJ, Sunderland C. Neck cooling and running performance in the heat: single versus repeated application. *Med Sci Sports Exerc.* 2011;43:2388-2395, with permission from the American College of Sports Medicine.)

Conclusions.—Cooling the surface of the neck improves time trial performance in a hot environment without altering physiological or neuro-endocrinological responses. Maintenance of a lower neck temperature via the replacement of a CC has no additional benefit to an acute cooling intervention (Fig 1).

▶ Because the effectiveness of cooling interventions may be dependent on the difference between the amount of cooling and thermal strain experienced, this study aimed to test whether there was an advantage to cooling the neck via replacement of a cooling neck collar to maintain the cool temperature, versus no replacement of the neck collar, versus wearing no collar (ie, no neck cooling whatsoever). The main outcome was time trial performance. Participants ran farther distances (over 90 minutes) when wearing a neck collar versus no collar; performance was improved by approximately 7%. However, there was no difference between the cooling collar placed at the beginning of the run and having the cooling collar replaced at 30 and 60 minutes to try and maintain the cold temperature (Fig 1). The authors raise the question as to whether the neck is, in fact, the optimal site for cooling with respect to perceived thermal state. They also caution that wearing a cooling collar may enable participants to withstand higher levels of heat and cardiovascular strain, which may present certain risks for safety. They also suggest that collar replacement may have provided a false signal in that participants initially adopted a faster pace but were unable to sustain that pace. The message for the practitioner is that cooling the neck improves trial performance in a hot environment but replacement of the neck collar provides no additional benefit.

D. E. Feldman, PT, PhD

Passive flooding of paranasal sinuses and middle ears as a method of equalisation in extreme breath-hold diving

Germonpré P, Balestra C, Musimu P (Centre for Hyperbaric Oxygen Therapy, Brussels, Belgium; Divers Alert Network (DAN) Europe Res Division, Belgium)
Br J Sports Med 45:657-659, 2011

Breath-hold diving is both a recreational activity, performed by thousands of enthusiasts in Europe, and a high-performance competitive sport. Several 'disciplines' exist, of which the 'no-limits' category is the most spectacular: using a specially designed heavy 'sled,' divers descend to extreme depths on a cable, and then reascend using an inflatable balloon, on a single breath. The current world record for un-assisted descent stands at more than 200 m of depth. Equalising air pressure in the paranasal sinuses and middle-ear cavities is a necessity during descent to avoid barotraumas. However, this requires active insufflations of precious air, which is thus unavailable in the pulmonary system. The authors describe a diver who, by training, is capable of allowing passive flooding of the sinuses and middle ear with (sea) water during descent, by suppressing protective (parasympathetic) reflexes during this process. Using this technique, he performed a series of extreme-depth breath-hold dives in June 2005, descending to 209 m of sea water on one breath of air.

▶ Competitive breath-hold diving is a dangerous pursuit, with many medical hazards. Seawater has a pressure greater than 20 atmospheres at a depth of 200 m, and differences of pressure between the circulation and various body cavities become particularly hazardous, sometimes inducing hemorrhages in both the lungs (a "pulmonary squeeze") and the sinuses.[1] As the breath-hold is prolonged, there is no longer sufficient air to allow equalization of pressures. This brief case report describes a 36-year-old diver who succeeded in diving to 209 m without problem; he claims that by not wearing a nose clip, he learned a technique of allowing seawater to enter his nasal sinuses and eustachian tubes, thus providing a counterpressure and preventing injury. It is difficult to verify this during a dive, but in support of his claim, MRIs obtained "in the dry" show that he was able to fill the sinuses and eustachian tubes when water was insufflated into the nostrils. Although there are some advantages to this new approach, there are also risks. The water is contaminated at many of the sites used for breath-hold diving, and there is thus a risk of sinus and middle-ear infections.[2] Frequent exposure to fresh or salt water may also predispose to degeneration of the middle ear mucosa and the development of external ear osteomas.[3,4] Furthermore, it is likely that most divers would require prolonged training to overcome the normal reactions of sneezing and/or discomfort associated with the entry of water under high pressure.

R. J. Shephard, MD (Lond), PhD, DPE

References

1. Fitz-Clarke JR. Adverse events in competitive breath-hold diving. *Undersea Hyperb Med.* 2006;33:55-62.

2. Goldstein NA, Mandel EM, Kurs-Lasky M, Rockette HE, Casselbrant ML. Water precautions and tympanostomy tubes: a randomized, controlled trial. *Laryngoscope*. 2005;115:324-330.
3. Silver FM, Orobello PW Jr, Mangal A, Pensak ML. Asymptomatic osteomas of the middle ear. *Am J Otol*. 1993;14:189-190.
4. Hurst W, Bailey M, Hurst B. Prevalence of external auditory canal exostoses in Australian surfboard riders. *J Laryngol Otol*. 2004;118:348-351.

Venous and Arterial Bubbles at Rest after No-Decompression Air Dives

Ljubkovic M, Dujic Z, Møllerløkken A, et al (Univ of Split School of Medicine, Croatia, Norway; Norwegian Univ of Science and Technology, Trondheim, Norway)
Med Sci Sports Exerc 43:990-995, 2011

Purpose.—During SCUBA diving, breathing at increased pressure leads to a greater tissue gas uptake. During ascent, tissues may become supersaturated, and the gas is released in the form of bubbles that typically occur on the venous side of circulation. These venous gas emboli (VGE) are usually eliminated as they pass through the lungs, although their occasional presence in systemic circulation (arterialization) has been reported and it was assumed to be the main cause of the decompression sickness. The aims of the present study were to assess the appearance of VGE after air dives where no stops in coming to the surface are required and to assess their potential occurrence and frequency in the systemic circulation.

Methods.—Twelve male divers performed six dives with 3 d of rest between them following standard no-decompression dive procedures: 18/60, 18/70, 24/30, 24/40, 33/15, and 33/20 (the first value indicates depth in meters of sea water and the second value indicates bottom time in minutes). VGE monitoring was performed ultrasonographically every 20 min for 120 min after surfacing.

Results.—Diving profiles used in this study produced unexpectedly high amounts of gas bubbles, with most dives resulting in grade 4 (55/69 dives) on the bubble scale of 0–5 (no to maximal bubbles). Arterializations of gas bubbles were found in 5 (41.7%) of 12 divers and after 11 (16%) of 69 dives. These VGE crossovers were only observed when a large amount of bubbles was concomitantly present in the right valve of the heart.

Conclusions.—Our findings indicate high amounts of gas bubbles produced after no-decompression air dives based on standardized diving protocols. High bubble loads were frequently associated with the crossover of VGE to the systemic circulation. Despite these findings, no acute decompression-related pathology was detected.

▶ The development of bubbles on the right side of the heart following a dive has generally been regarded as of no great clinical significance, because it is anticipated that the bubbles will disappear as the blood passes through the pulmonary capillaries. On the other hand, bubbles found on the left side of the heart have a potential to pass as emboli into the cerebral circulation, causing neurological manifestations of decompression sickness. Passage of bubble from the right to the left side of the heart has commonly been associated with a patent foramen ovale and a rise of right ventricular pressure.[1,2] A crossover of bubbles occurred in 5 of the 12 divers studied by Ljubkovic et al, even though only 1 member of the group had evidence of a patent foramen ovale (tested by trans-thoracic echocardiography, using agitated saline as a contrast agent). This finding supports a recent suggestion by the same authors that bubbles can pass from the pulmonary to the arterial circulation by some route other than the foramen ovale, perhaps through intrapulmonary arterio-venous shunts, or even the pulmonary capillaries.[3] Two other points in this study deserve emphasis: The bubbles occurred despite careful adherence to Norwegian diving tables, and no symptoms of decompression sickness were observed despite the bubbles seen on the left side of the heart. This last observation may give divers a false sense of security; symptoms may well have been seen if the number of subjects who developed left ventricular bubbles had been larger than 5. Even if it is confirmed that left-sided bubbles do not commonly lead to decompression sickness, it is desirable to avoid this phenomenon, because it can also lead to acute endothelial dysfunction,[4] a problem diminished if not abolished by the administration of antioxidants before the dive.[5]

R. J. Shephard, MD (Lond), PhD, DPE

References

1. Moon RE, Camporesi EM, Kisslo JA. Patent foramen ovale and decompression sickness in divers. *Lancet.* 1989;1:513-514.
2. Wilmshurst PT, Byrne JC, Webb-Peploe MM. Relation between interatrial shunts and decompression sickness in divers. *Lancet.* 1989;2:1302-1306.
3. Ljubkovic M, Marinovic J, Obad A, Breskovic T, Gaustad SE, Dujic Z. High incidence of venous and arterial gas emboli at rest after trimix diving without protocol violations. *J Appl Physiol.* 2010;109:1670-1674.
4. Nossum V, Hjelde A, Brubakk AO. Small amounts of venous gas embolism cause delayed impairment of endothelial function and increase polymorphonuclear neutrophil infiltration. *Eur J Appl Physiol.* 2002;86:209-214.
5. Obad A, Palada I, Valic Z, et al. The effects of acute oral antioxidants on diving-induced alterations in human cardiovascular function. *J Physiol.* 2007;578:859-870.

Endurance exercise immediately before sea diving reduces bubble formation in scuba divers
Castagna O, Brisswalter J, Vallee N, et al (Naval Med Inst (IMNSSA-Toulon), France; Univ of Nice Sophia Antipolis, France)
Eur J Appl Physiol 111:1047-1054, 2011

Previous studies have observed that a single bout of exercise can reduce the formation of circulating bubbles on decompression but, according to different authors, several hours delay were considered necessary between the end of exercise and the beginning of the dive. The objective of this study was to evaluate the effect of a single bout of exercise taken immediately before a dive on bubble formation. 24 trained divers performed open-sea dives to 30 msw depth for 30 min followed by a 3 min stop at 3 msw, under two conditions: (1) a control dive without exercise before (No-Ex), (2) an experimental condition in which subjects performed an exercise before diving (Ex). In the Ex condition, divers began running on a treadmill for 45 min at a speed corresponding to their own ventilatory threshold 1 h before immersion. Body weight, total body fluid volume, core temperature, and volume of consumed water were measured. Circulating bubbles were graded according to the Spencer scale using a precordial Doppler every 30 min for 90 min after surfacing. A single submaximal exercise performed immediately before immersion significantly reduces

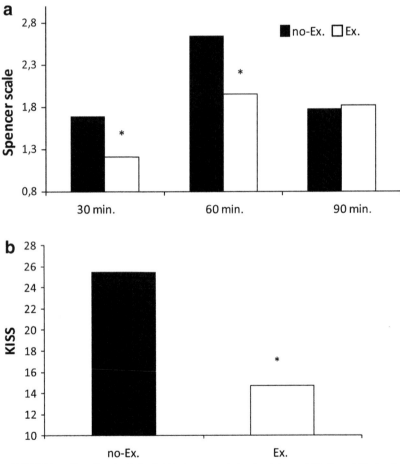

FIGURE 3.—a Post-dive circulating bubble Spencer scale (medians) detected 30, 60, and 90 min after surfacing for all divers in both conditions. *Significant difference between conditions, $p < 0.01$. b Post-dive circulating bubble detection (KISS) for all divers in both conditions. *Significant difference between conditions, $p < 0.01$. (Reprinted from Castagna O, Brisswalter J, Vallee N, et al. Endurance exercise immediately before sea diving reduces bubble formation in scuba divers. *Eur J Appl Physiol.* 2011;111:1047-1054, Copyright 2011, with kind permission of Springer Science+Business Media.)

bubble grades ($p < 0.001$). This reduction was correlated not only to sweat dehydration, but also to the volume of water drunk at the end of the exercise. Moderate dehydration seems to be beneficial at the start of the dive whereas restoring the hydration balance should be given priority during decompression. This suggests a biphasic effect of the hydration status on bubble formation (Fig 3).

▶ Previous authors have suggested that exercising either 2 hours[1,2] or 24 hours[3] before diving can reduce bubble formation during decompression. However, in some situations (particularly in military diving), it may not be possible to allow such a long predive interval. In contrast to these observations, animal studies of electrically induced exercise and a human study of knee-bend squats[4] carried out immediately before submersion suggested a deleterious effect of exercise. The observations of Castagna et al relate to 2 dives to a depth of 30 meters, held for 30 minutes, with subjects serving as their own controls. In one trial, the dive was performed without prior activity, but in the second, vigorous submaximal aerobic exercise was performed from 60 to 15 minutes before the dive; in the latter trial, subjects showed a substantially lower incidence of bubble formation as measured by Doppler scanning carried out every 30 minutes for 90 minutes after surfacing. Bubble scores were assessed on the Spencer scale and converted to a linearized Kisman integrated severity score for purposes of statistical analysis (Fig 3). The bubble scores were negatively correlated with the individual's fluid loss during exercise, and the authors suggest that dehydration reduced blood volume and thus perfusion of tissues where inert gases normally accumulate during a dive. Conversely, the bubble score was also reduced by rehydration and probable improvement of tissue perfusion following the exercise bout. One alternative explanation that needs to be explored is a possible beneficial effect of exercise via endothelial nitric oxide production[5]; unfortunately, the investigation of Castagna et al did not include measurements of nitric oxide production. Nevertheless, the observed benefit from the exercise bout was sufficiently large to merit further study.

R. J. Shephard, MD (Lond), PhD, DPE

References

1. Blatteau JE, Boussuges A, Gempp E, et al. Haemodynamic changes induced by submaximal exercise before a dive and its consequences on bubble formation. *Br J Sports Med.* 2007;41:375-379.
2. Jurd KM, Tacker JC. The effect of pre-dive exercise mode on post-décompression venous gas enboli. In: Ross JA, ed. Proceedings of the 35th Annual Meeting of the European Underwater and Baromedical Society; August 25th-28th, 2009; Aberdeen, Scotland, 106–107.
3. Dujic Z, Duplancic D, Marinovic-Terzic I, et al. Aerobic exercise before diving reduces venous gas bubble formation in humans. *J Physiol.* 2004;555:637-642.
4. Dervay JP, Powell MR, Butler B, Fife CE. The effect of exercise and rest duration on the generation of venous gas bubbles at altitude. *Aviat Space Environ Med.* 2002;73:22-27.
5. Wisløff U, Richardson RS, Brubakk AO. Exercise and nitric oxide prevent bubble formation: a novel approach to the prevention of decompression sickness? *J Physiol.* 2004;555:825-829.

Ultrasound lung "comets" increase after breath-hold diving

Lambrechts K, Germonpré P, Charbel B, et al (Environmental & Occupational Physiology Laboratory, Brussels, Belgium)
Eur J Appl Physiol 111:707-713, 2011

The purpose of the study was to analyze the ultrasound lung comets (ULCs) variation, which are a sign of extra-vascular lung water. Forty-two healthy individuals performed breath-hold diving in different conditions: dynamic surface apnea; deep variable-weight apnea and shallow, face immersed without effort (static maximal and non-maximal). The number of ULCs was evaluated by means of an ultrasound scan of the chest, before and after breath-hold diving sessions. The ULC score increased significantly from baseline after dynamic surface apnea ($p = 0.0068$), after deep breath-hold sessions ($p = 0.0018$), and after static maximal apnea ($p = 0.031$). There was no statistically significant difference between the average increase of ULC scores after dynamic surface apnea and deep breath-hold diving. We, therefore, postulate that extravascular lung water accumulation may be due to other factors than (deep) immersion alone, because it occurs during dynamic surface apnea as well. Three mechanisms may be responsible for this. First, the immersion-induced hydrostatic pressure gradient applied on the body causes a shift of peripheral venous blood towards the thorax. Second, the blood pooling effect found during the diving response Redistributes blood to the pulmonary vascular bed. Third, it is possible that the intense involuntary diaphragmatic contractions occurring during the "struggle phase" of the breath-hold can also produce a blood shift from the pulmonary capillaries to the pulmonary alveoli. A combination of these factors may explain the observed increase in ULC scores in deep, shallow maximal and shallow dynamic apneas, whereas shallow non-maximal apneas seem to be not "ULC provoking".

▶ Lung comets, as seen on ultrasound, are widely accepted as a sign of extra-vascular accumulation of water and edema in the lungs.[1,2] Leakage is thought to be caused by either an excessive pulmonary capillary pressure or a change in permeability of the pulmonary capillaries,[3] often associated with the use of SCUBA equipment or the external pressures encountered during deep breath-hold diving. However, the present observations show that an equal number of comets can develop when engaged in prolonged breath-holding in shallow water. A variety of factors seem responsible, including external water pressure, the diving response, Valsalva maneuvers to clear the ears, and struggling during the final stage of a breath-hold. From the clinical viewpoint, there may be concomitant increases in pulmonary arterial pressure, diminished left ventricular contractility, and increased release of B-type natriuretic peptides,[4] suggesting significant cardiopulmonary strain. Moreover, if dives are repeated, extravascular lung water and pulmonary arterial pressures remain elevated, implying a potential for a cumulative risk of pulmonary edema.[5]

R. J. Shephard, MD (Lond), PhD, DPE

References

1. Picano E, Frassi F, Agricola E, Gligorova S, Gargani L, Mottola G. Ultrasound lung comets: a clinically useful sign of extravascular lung water. *J Am Soc Echocardiogr.* 2006;19:356-363.
2. Frassi F, Pingitore A, Cialoni D, Picano E. Chest sonography detects lung water accumulation in healthy elite apnea divers. *J Am Soc Echocardiogr.* 2008;21: 1150-1155.
3. West JB, Mathieu-Costello O. Stress failure of pulmonary capillaries as a limiting factor for maximal exercise. *Eur J Appl Physiol Occup Physiol.* 1995;70:99-108.
4. McDonagh TA, Holmer S, Raymond I, Luchner A, Hildebrant P, Dargie HJ. NT-proBNP and the diagnosis of heart failure: a pooled analysis of three European epidemiological studies. *Eur J Heart Fail.* 2004;6:269-273.
5. Marinovic J, Ljubkovic M, Obad A, et al. Assessment of extravascular lung water and cardiac function in trimix SCUBA diving. *Med Sci Sports Exerc.* 2010;42: 1054-1061.

The contribution of haemoglobin mass to increases in cycling performance induced by simulated LHTL

Garvican LA, Pottgiesser T, Martin DT, et al (Australian Inst of Sport, Belconnen, Canberra; Univ Hosp of Freiburg, Germany; et al)

Eur J Appl Physiol 111:1089-1101, 2011

We sought to determine whether improved cycling performance following 'Live High-Train Low' (LHTL) occurs if increases in haemoglobin mass (Hb_{mass}) are prevented via periodic phlebotomy during hypoxic exposure. Eleven, highly trained, female cyclists completed 26 nights of simulated LHTL (16 h day^{-1}, 3000 m). Hb_{mass} was determined in quadruplicate before LHTL and in duplicate weekly thereafter. After 14 nights, cyclists were pair-matched, based on their Hb_{mass} response (ΔHb_{mass}) from baseline, to form a response group (Response, n = 5) in which Hb_{mass} was free to adapt, and a Clamp group (Clamp, n = 6) in which ΔHb_{mass} was negated via weekly phlebotomy. All cyclists were blinded to the blood volume removed. Cycling performance was assessed in duplicate before and after LHTL using a maximal 4-min effort (MMP_{4min}) followed by a ride time to exhaustion test at peak power output (T_{lim}). VO_{2peak} was established during the MMP_{4min}. Following LHTL, Hb_{mass} increased in Response (mean ± SD, 5.5 ± 2.9%). Due to repeated phlebotomy, there was no ΔHb_{mass} in Clamp ($-0.4 ± 0.6\%$). VO_{2peak} increased in Response (3.5 ± 2.3%) but not in Clamp (0.3 ± 2.6%). MMP_{4min} improved in both the groups (Response 4.5 ± 1.1%, Clamp 3.6 ± 1.4%) and was not different between groups ($p = 0.58$). T_{lim} increased only in Response, with Clamp substantially worse than Response (-37.6%; 90% CL -58.9 to -5.0, $p = 0.07$). Our novel findings, showing an $\sim$4% increase in MMP_{4min} despite blocking an $\sim$5% increase in Hb_{mass}, suggest that accelerated erythropoiesis is not the sole mechanism by which LHTL improves performance. However, increases in Hb_{mass} appear to influence

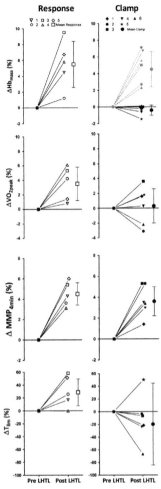

FIGURE 3.—Individual and mean ($\pm$ SD) changes (%) in Hb_{mass} (both actual in *black* and theoretical in *grey*), VO_{2peak}, MMP_{4min}, and T_{lim} following 26 nights of live high train low. All values are backtransformed from log-data effects compared with baseline ($\pm$ SD). (Reprinted from Garvican LA, Pottgiesser T, Martin DT, et al. The contribution of haemoglobin mass to increases in cycling performance induced by simulated LHTL. *Eur J Appl Physiol.* 2011;111:1089-1101, Copyright 2011, with kind permission of Springer Science+Business Media.)

the aerobic contribution to high-intensity exercise which may be important for subsequent high-intensity efforts (Fig 3).

▶ Living high, training low[1] has become an important ritual for many endurance athletes who have cherished the belief that the altitude-induced increase in hemoglobin level of 5% or more translates directly into an increased maximal oxygen intake and thus competitive performance. Laboratory findings do indeed suggest that a 1-g increase of hemoglobin mass leads to a 4 mL/min gain in maximal oxygen intake.[2,3] There is also little doubt that living high, training low improves endurance performance, but the specific role of the increment in hemoglobin level has not been tested previously. Garvican and associates carefully matched a small group of female cyclists in terms of their initial hemoglobin response to a regimen of spending > 14 h/d at a simulated 3000 m and training at 600 m. After 26 days, they then carried out a blinded phlebotomy to restore the sea-level hemoglobin values in one-half of the athletes, although other aspects of the regimen remained unchanged. Although the peak oxygen intake decreased in the group whose hemoglobin was clamped in this manner, their maximal power output over a single 4-minute test remained closely matched with that of the group whose hemoglobin remained elevated (the response group, Fig 3). Nevertheless, endurance of a subsequent all-out test was impaired in the clamped group, probably because they ran up a larger oxygen debt during the initial 4-minute test. Garvican et al suggest that because hemoglobin levels did not increase in the clamp group, they likely enhanced alternative, anaerobic pathways that sustained them through at least the first 4 minutes of activity (although they remained at a disadvantage in a situation in which repeated bouts of anaerobic activity were required). Further study of the nature of these ancillary mechanisms may help in enhancing the performance of endurance athletes. One limitation of the study is that because of antidoping regulations, the authors were unable to make good the decrease of plasma volume immediately following phlebotomy. However, they argued that this was not a serious weakness, because with adequate fluid intake, plasma volumes should have normalized within 24 hours.

R. J. Shephard, MD (Lond), PhD, DPE

References

1. Levine BD, Stray-Gundersen J. "Living high-training low": effect of moderate-altitude acclimatization with low-altitude training on performance. *J Appl Physiol*. 1997;83:102-112.
2. Gledhill N, Warburton D, Jamnik V. Haemoglobin, blood volume, cardiac function, and aerobic power. *Can J Appl Physiol*. 1999;24:54-65.
3. Schmidt W, Prommer N. Impact of alterations in total hemoglobin mass on VO$_2$max. *Exerc Sport Sci Rev*. 2010;38:68-75.

Index Measured at an Intermediate Altitude to Predict Impending Acute Mountain Sickness

Modesti PA, Rapi S, Paniccia R, et al (Univ of Florence, Italy; et al)
Med Sci Sports Exerc 43:1811-1818, 2011

Purpose.—Acute mountain sickness (AMS) is a neurological disorder that may be unpredictably experienced by subjects ascending at a high altitude. The aim of the present study was to develop a predictive index, measured at an intermediate altitude, to predict the onset of AMS at a higher altitude.

Methods.—In the first part, 47 subjects were investigated and blood withdrawals were performed before ascent, at an intermediate altitude

(3440 m), and after acute and chronic exposition to high altitude (Mount Everest Base Camp, 5400 m (MEBC1 and MEBC2)). Parameters independently associated to the Lake Louise scoring (LLS) system, including the self-reported and the clinical sections, and coefficients estimated from the model obtained through stepwise regression analysis were used to create a predictive index. The possibility of the index, measured after an overnight stay at intermediate altitude (Gnifetti hut, 3647 m), to predict AMS (defined as headache and LLS ≥ 4) at final altitude (Capanna Margherita, 4559 m), was then investigated in a prospective study performed on 44 subjects in the Italian Alps.

Results.—During the expedition to MEBC, oxygen saturation, hematocrit, day of expedition, and maximum velocity of clot formation were selected as independently associated with LLS and were included in the predictive index. In the Italian Alps, subjects with a predictive index value ≥ 5.92 at an intermediate altitude had an odds ratio of 8.1 (95% confidence limits = 1.7–38.6, sensitivity = 85%, specificity = 59%) for developing AMS within 48 h of reaching high altitude.

Conclusion.—In conclusion, a predictive index combining clinical and hematological parameters measured at an intermediate step on the way to the top may provide information on impending AMS (Table 2).

▶ It would certainly be helpful to know who is likely to develop mountain sickness; at very high altitudes, weather conditions may make immediate evacuation difficult. However, if a vulnerable individual is identified at a base camp, preventive medication can be taken, and if the symptoms do not abate within 1 to 2 days, their ascent can be aborted.[1] Arterial oxygen saturation has been the only previously recognized marker.[2] Modesti and associates collected markers of pending acute mountain sickness at 3340 m and they then developed a multivariate equation based on oxygen saturation, hematocrit, day of expedition, and a point of care estimate of maximum velocity of clot formation (Table 2) to predict the probability of adverse responses at 5400 m. They tested this equation on a second group of subjects (average age 40 years, history of severe mountain sickness, and exclusion criterion) who were studied at slightly different altitudes (3647 and 4559 m). The markers obtained at 3647 m had quite a high likelihood of predicting those who would manifest headache and

TABLE 2.—Multivariate Modeling of LLS During the HIGHCARE Expedition (Stepwise Multiple Regression Analysis)

Selected Variable	B Coefficient	95% CL	P
O$_2$ saturation (%)	−0.174	−0.21 to −0.14	0.000
Hematocrit (%)	−0.050	−0.09 to −0.01	0.027
Days (*n*)	−0.074	−0.12 to −0.03	0.002
MAXV (mm·min^{-1})	0.077	0.02 to 0.14	0.013

Variables included in the model: age, sex, body mass index, day of expedition, atmospheric pressure, CT, CFT, MCF, α angle, MAXV, hematocrit, systolic and diastolic pressure, HR, respiratory rate, pulmonary artery pressure, oxygen saturation, epinephrine and norepinephrine, with LLS as dependent variable.
Multiple *r* = 0.714.

a Lake Louise score[3] of 4 (based on the response to 5 questions [headache, gastrointestinal symptoms, dizziness, lassitude or fatigue, and sleeping difficulty] each one rating from 0 to 3), with an odds ratio of 8.1, a sensitivity of 85%, and a specificity of 59%. Nevertheless, the 15% of false-negative results offers a continuing challenge to improvement of the prediction equation.

R. J. Shephard, MD (Lond), PhD, DPE

References

1. Schoene RB. Illnesses at high altitude. *Chest.* 2008;134:402-416.
2. Burtscher M, Flatz M, Faulhaber M. Prediction of susceptibility to acute mountain sickness by SaO2 values during short-term exposure to hypoxia. *High Alt Med Biol.* 2004;5:335-340.
3. Roach RC, Bärtsch P, Hackett PH, Oelz O, et al. The Lake Louise acute mountain sickness scoring system. In: Sutton JR, Houston CS, Coates G, eds. *Hypoxia and Molecular Medicine.* Burlington, VT: Queen City Printers; 1993:272-274.

Sea-Level Assessment of Dynamic Cerebral Autoregulation Predicts Susceptibility to Acute Mountain Sickness at High Altitude
Cochand NJ, Wild M, Brugniaux JV, et al (Cardiff Univ, UK; Univ of Wales, Swansea, UK; Univ of Glamorgan, Pontypridd, UK)
Stroke 42:3628-3630, 2011

Background and Purpose.—Dynamic cerebral autoregulation is impaired in subjects who develop acute mountain sickness (AMS), a neurological disorder characterized by headache. The present study examined if the normoxic sea-level measurement of dynamic cerebral autoregulation would predict subsequent susceptibility to AMS during rapid ascent to terrestrial high altitude.

Methods.—A dynamic cerebral autoregulation index was determined in 18 subjects at sea level from continuous recordings of middle cerebral artery blood flow velocity (Doppler ultrasonography) and arterial blood pressure (finger photoplethysmography) after recovery from transiently induced hypotension. Six hours after passive ascent to 3800 m (Mt Elbrus, Russia), the Lake Louise and Environmental Symptoms Cerebral Symptoms questionnaires were used to assess AMS.

Results.—AMS scores increased markedly at high-altitude (Lake Louise: +3±2 points, $P=0.001$ and Environmental Symptoms Cerebral Symptoms: +0.6±0.9 points, $P=0.0003$ versus sea level). Inverse relationships were observed between the sea-level autoregulation index score and the high-altitude-induced increases in the Lake Louise ($r=-0.62$, $P=0.007$) and Environmental Symptoms Cerebral Symptoms ($r=-0.78$, $P=0.01$) scores. One subject with a history of high-altitude pulmonary and cerebral edema presented with the lowest sea-level autoregulation index score (3.7 versus group: 6.2±1.0 points) and later developed high-altitude cerebral edema at 4800 m during the summit bid.

Conclusions.—These findings suggest that a lower baseline autoregulation index may be considered a potential risk factor for AMS. This laboratory measurement may prove a useful screening tool for the expedition doctor when considering targeted pharmacological prophylaxis in individuals deemed "AMS-susceptible."

▶ The recent observation of a relationship between the capacity for dynamic cerebral autoregulation (as determined in this study by measurements of arterial blood pressure and cerebral artery flow before and after occlusion of flow to the thighs) and acute mountain sickness (AMS),[1,2] although not always observed,[1] suggests that a study of this parameter may offer an index of risk of AMS before beginning a climb. The sample size used in the present investigation was quite small (n = 18), and a nonparametric method was thus chosen to analyze the data. The findings suggested that some 60% of the variance in symptoms of AMS could be explained by the cerebral autoregulatory index. In other words, the person who had difficulty buffering a sudden change of arterial pressure was at greater risk of cerebral hyperperfusion and thus AMS. One objection to the present observations is that adoption of the thigh exclusion technique evaluated the cerebral blood flow response to sudden hypotension, although at high altitudes, the response to a hypoxia-induced hypertension would be more relevant. There remains scope for further studies on a larger group of subjects, using alternative measures of cerebral autoregulation.

R. J. Shephard, MD (Lond), PhD, DPE

References

1. Subudhi AW, Panerai RB, Roach RC. Effects of hypobaric hypoxia on cerebral autoregulation. *Stroke.* 2010;41:641-646.
2. Bailey DM, Evans KA, James PE, et al. Altered free radical metabolism in acute mountain sickness: implications for dynamic cerebral autoregulation and blood-brain barrier function. *J Physiol.* 2009;587:73-85.

9 Special Considerations: Children, Women, the Elderly, and Special Populations

Physical activity in Ontario preschoolers: prevalence and measurement issues

Obeid J, Nguyen T, Gabel L, et al (McMaster Univ and McMaster Children's Hosp, Hamilton, Ontario, Canada)

Appl Physiol Nutr Metab 36:291-297, 2011

Early childhood is a critical period for the development of active living behaviours; however, very little is known about the physical activity levels of preschoolers from Canada. The objectives of this study were to (*i*) examine physical activity in a sample of Ontario preschoolers by using high-frequency accelerometry to determine activity and step counts; (*ii*) assess the relationship between step counts and physical activity; (*iii*) examine the influence of epoch length or sampling interval on physical activity; and (*iv*) compare measured physical activity to existing recommendations. Thirty 3- to 5-year-old children wore accelerometers to monitor habitual physical activity in 3-s epochs over a 7-day period. Preschoolers engaged in an average of 220 min of daily physical activity, 75 min of which were spent in moderate-to-vigorous physical activity (MVPA), and they accumulated 7529 ± 1539 steps·day^{-1}. Preschoolers who engaged in more MVPA also took more steps on a daily basis ($r = 0.81$, $p < 0.001$). Compared with a 3-s epoch, sampling intervals of 15, 30, and 60 s resulted in an average of 2.9, 9.0, and 16.7 missed minutes of MVPA per day, respectively. All 30 preschoolers met the National Association for Sport and Physical Education recommendation of at least 120 min of total physical activity per day for preschool-age children. Our data highlight important methodological considerations when measuring physical activity in preschoolers and the need for preschool-specific physical activity guidelines for Canadian children.

▶ Being the father of 2 young children, I really enjoyed reading this article and could certainly relate to its findings. The early years are a critical period for the development of active living behaviors and the development of fundamental movement and motor skills. Society has traditionally thought of the early years as being a time of life when children are naturally active enough and, therefore, quite healthy. However, recent evidence suggests that preschool age children may not be engaging in as much physical activity as people think.

The authors of this study measured physical activity in a relatively small sample of 3- to 5-year-olds over a 7-day period using accelerometers—small motion sensors worn on the hip. The accelerometers that they used measured physical activity continuously over the 7 days in 3-second intervals. Thus, 21 600 distinct 3-second pieces of information on physical activity and motion were obtained and analyzed for each participant! On average, the preschool children in this study accumulated 144 minutes per day of light-intensity physical activity and 75 minutes per day of moderate-to-vigorous physical activity (MVPA). Interestingly, the physical activity levels were almost identical in boys and girls. Conversely, in the later childhood and adolescent years, boys are far more active than girls. Another key finding of the study was that about 50% of the MVPA that the preschool children participated in occurred in 3-second intervals. In fact, had the authors used a 60-second accelerometer sampling frame, which is the traditional approach used in the adult physical activity literature, 71% of the MVPA would not have been recorded as MVPA. This finding highlights the fact that we cannot approach measuring or prescribing physical activity in children, particularly young children, using the same approaches we use in adults. Physically active adults tend to accumulate their MVPA in bouts lasting several minutes or more in duration, whereas children's activity patterns are extremely sporadic. So, while I like to go for a single long run in the afternoon, my kids, who get as much or more MVPA as I do, are up and down like a yo-yo.

I. Janssen, PhD

Promoting Fundamental Movement Skill Development and Physical Activity in Early Childhood Settings: A Cluster Randomized Controlled Trial
Jones RA, Riethmuller A, Hesketh K, et al (Univ of Wollongong, New South Wales, Australia; Deakin Univ, Melbourne, Victoria, Australia)
Pediatr Exerc Sci 23:600-615, 2011

The aim of this study was to assess the feasibility, acceptability and potential efficacy of a physical activity program for preschool children. A 20-week, 2-arm parallel cluster randomized controlled pilot trial was conducted. The intervention comprised structured activities for children and professional development for staff. The control group participated in usual care activities, which included designated inside and outside playtime. Primary outcomes were movement skill development and objectively measured physical activity. At follow-up, compared with children in the control group, children in the intervention group showed greater improvements in movement skill proficiency, with this improvement statically significant for overall movement skill development (adjust diff. = 2.08,

95% CI 0.76, 3.40; Cohen's d = 0.47) and significantly greater increases in objectively measured physical activity (counts per minute) during the preschool day (adjust diff. = 110.5, 95% CI 33.6, 187.3; Cohen's d = 0.46). This study demonstrates that a physical activity program implemented by staff within a preschool setting is feasible, acceptable and potentially efficacious.

▶ The early years are a critical time for the development of physical activity behaviors and movement skills. Unfortunately, many young children do not engage in sufficient activity and consequently have poorly developed movement skills. In developed countries, most children in their early years spend a large proportion of their time on weekdays in a childcare setting such as a preschool, daycare, or nursery. These childcare settings therefore have an important role to play in fostering physical activity and movement skill development in children in their early years. This novel study set out to develop a physical activity program that could be used within the early childhood setting.

The summary movement skill development score increased by 3.8 units (12.7-16.5) in the intervention group and by 1.7 units (13.0-14.6) in the control group. The effect size (Cohen's d) for this difference was 0.47, which is small to modest. Physical activity levels also increased to a greater extent in the intervention group than in the control group. As this was a pilot study of 97 preschool children, caution should be used when interpreting the findings. Nonetheless, the findings do suggest that a physical activity program can be implemented by staff within a childcare setting, and thus such programs can be beneficial to the physical activity and movement skill development.

I. Janssen, PhD

Recommended aerobic fitness level for metabolic health in children and adolescents: a study of diagnostic accuracy

Adegboye ARA, Anderssen SA, Froberg K, et al (Copenhagen Univ Hosp, Denmark; Norwegian School of Sport Sciences, Oslo, Norway; Univ of Southern Denmark, Odense, Denmark; et al)
Br J Sports Med 45:722-728, 2011

Objective.—To define the optimal cut-off for low aerobic fitness and to evaluate its accuracy to predict clustering of risk factors for cardiovascular disease in children and adolescents.

Design.—Study of diagnostic accuracy using a cross-sectional database.

Setting.—European Youth Heart Study including Denmark, Portugal, Estonia and Norway.

Participants.—4500 schoolchildren aged 9 or 15 years.

Main Outcome Measure.—Aerobic fitness was expressed as peak oxygen consumption relative to bodyweight ($mlO_2/min/kg$).

Results.—Risk factors included in the composite risk score (mean of z-scores) were systolic blood pressure, triglyceride, total cholesterol/HDL-cholesterol ratio, insulin resistance and sum of four skinfolds.

14.5% of the sample, with a risk score above one SD, were defined as being at risk. Receiver operating characteristic analysis was used to define the optimal cut-off for sex and age-specific distribution. In girls, the optimal cut-offs for identifying individuals at risk were: 37.4 mlO$_2$/min/kg (9-year-old) and 33.0 mlO$_2$/min/kg (15-year-old). In boys, the optimal cut-offs were 43.6 mlO$_2$/min/kg (9-year-old) and 46.0 mlO$_2$/min/kg (15-year-old). Specificity (range 79.3–86.4%) was markedly higher than sensitivity (range 29.7–55.6%) for all cut-offs. Positive predictive values ranged from 19% to 41% and negative predictive values ranged from 88% to 90%. The diagnostic accuracy for identifying children at risk, measured by the area under the curve (AUC), was significantly higher than what would be expected by chance (AUC >0.5) for all cut-offs.

Conclusions.—Aerobic fitness is easy to measure, and is an accurate tool for screening children with clustering of cardiovascular risk factors. Promoting physical activity in children with aerobic fitness level lower than the suggested cut-points might improve their health.

▶ Data from aerobic fitness tests have been used to create national and international percentiles for aerobic fitness scores for boys and girls of all ages. These percentiles are based on the fitness level of the population rather than the fitness level that is needed to achieve good health. Thus, aerobic fitness percentiles have a limited utility for the clinical scenario as a screening tool for the pediatric population. This study used analysis of receiver operating characteristics to define the optimal health-based aerobic fitness cutoffs for low, or unhealthy, aerobic fitness levels. Such cutoffs could potentially be used as a risk stratification tool to identify children at increased health risk based on their fitness and therefore in special need of physical activity counseling.

In girls, the optimal Vo$_2$max cutoffs that were identified in this study were 37 ml/kg/min in 9-year-old children and 33 ml/kg/min in 15-year-old children. The corresponding cutoffs in boys were 44 ml/kg/min and 46 ml/kg/min, respectively. The sensitivity of these cutoffs was very good (around 80%), meaning that the proportion of actual positives, which would be correctly identified with fitness testing, is high. Conversely, the specificity of the cutoffs was low (around 30%), meaning that the proportion of negatives correctly identified as such with fitness testing is low. Because regular aerobic exercise is not harmful for children and can reduce their risk of chronic disease, it is far more important for the cutoffs to have a high sensitivity than a high specificity. Future research is needed to develop health-related aerobic fitness cutoffs for a wider age spectrum.

I. Janssen, PhD

Physical Activity and Performance at School: A Systematic Review of the Literature Including a Methodological Quality Assessment
Singh A, Uijtdewilligen L, Twisk JWR, et al (VU Univ Med Ctr, Amsterdam, the Netherlands)
Arch Pediatr Adolesc Med 166:49-55, 2012

Objective.—To describe the prospective relationship between physical activity and academic performance.

Data Sources.—Prospective studies were identified from searches in PubMed, PsycINFO, Cochrane Central, and Sportdiscus from 1990 through 2010.

Study Selection.—We screened the titles and abstracts for eligibility, rated the methodological quality of the studies, and extracted data.

Main Exposure.—Studies had to report at least 1 physical activity or physical fitness measurement during childhood or adolescence.

Main Outcome Measures.—Studies had to report at least 1 academic performance or cognition measure during childhood or adolescence.

Results.—We identified 10 observational and 4 intervention studies. The quality score of the studies ranged from 22% to 75%. Two studies were scored as high quality. Methodological quality scores were particularly low for the reliability and validity of the measurement instruments. Based on the results of the best-evidence synthesis, we found evidence of a significant longitudinal positive relationship between physical activity and academic performance.

Conclusions.—Participation in physical activity is positively related to academic performance in children. Because we found only 2 high-quality studies, future high-quality studies are needed to confirm our findings. These studies should thoroughly examine the dose-response relationship between physical activity and academic performance as well as explanatory mechanisms for this relationship.

▶ Participation in physical activity has been linked to improved brain function and cognition and may improve academic performance within the pediatric population. However, increasing pressures to improve academic success have led to a reduction in the time and resources devoted to physical education and other physical activities within schools. That is, more time has been devoted to subjects such as mathematics and reading at the expense of physical activity. While several studies have examined the link between physical activity and academic performance, this literature has been inconclusive. This article attempted to address this issue by performing a systematic review with a special focus on the longitudinal relationship between general physical activity and academic performance.

Unfortunately, 12 of the 14 studies included in the systematic review, or 86% of the total, were not rated as being of a high methodologic quality. The 2 high-quality studies included in the systematic review both suggest that being active is positively related to improved academic performance in children. Furthermore, the synthesis of evidence based on all 14 studies found strong evidence of a significant positive relationship between physical activity and academic performance.

In my opinion, it is a pity that most school children in North America receive less than 1 hour of classroom physical education or activity each week. It is a pity that, at least within my home province, physical education is not a requirement past grade 9. I hope the findings of this systematic review can be used as an effective promotional tool to stress the need for more physical activity in schools to parents, teachers, and school administrators.

I. Janssen, PhD

The association between school-based physical activity, including physical education, and academic performance: A systematic review of the literature
Rasberry CN, Lee SM, Robin L, et al (Ctrs for Disease Control and Prevention, Atlanta, GA; et al)
Prev Med 52:S10-S20, 2011

Objective.—The purpose of this review is to synthesize the scientific literature that has examined the association between school-based physical activity (including physical education) and academic performance (including indicators of cognitive skills and attitudes, academic behaviors, and academic achievement).

Method.—Relevant research was identified through a search of nine electronic databases using both physical activity and academic-related search terms. Forty-three articles (reporting a total of 50 unique studies) met the inclusion criteria and were read, abstracted, and coded for this synthesis. Findings of the 50 studies were then summarized.

Results.—Across all the studies, there were a total of 251 associations between physical activity and academic performance, representing measures of academic achievement, academic behavior, and cognitive skills and attitudes. Slightly more than half (50.5%) of all associations examined were positive, 48% were not significant, and 1.5% were negative. Examination of the findings by each physical activity context provides insights regarding specific relationships.

Conclusion.—Results suggest physical activity is either positively related to academic performance or that there is not a demonstrated relationship between physical activity and academic performance. Results have important implications for both policy and schools.

▶ One option for increasing the level of physical activity among children is to ensure that a large part of the required daily dose of exercise is provided through an hour of vigorous physical education. School boards are sometimes reluctant to agree to such an initiative on the grounds that students must learn an ever-growing volume of scientific material; they argue that educational standards will be compromised if an hour is taken from academic curricular time on each school day. There is growing experimental evidence, however, to reassure school administrators on this point. During the 1970s, we conducted a substantial 6-year quasi-experimental study with a sample of 546 primary school students from the Province of Quebec.[1-3] Experimental students received an additional hour of specialist-taught physical education per day throughout their 6 years in primary school, and control students were drawn from the preceding and succeeding classes in the same schools. Although the academic teaching of the experimental students was reduced by some 14%, they gained significantly higher marks than control students in both mathematics and English language classes. Recent reviews[4,5] have confirmed a positive response to added physical education. The study of Rasberry et al is from an entire issue of *Preventive Medicine* allocated to this topic. It offers an extensive systematic review, based on articles published between 1985 and 2008. The 50 studies that were included in the analysis examined both physical education and extracurricular sports activities, and adopted broadly ranging criteria of educational attainment (graduation or drop-out rates, performance on standardized tests, grade point average, years of school completed, time on task, attentiveness, school attendance, and disciplinary problems). The findings should perhaps be discounted somewhat because of the tendency of journals to publish studies showing positive findings rather than an absence of response, but nevertheless there seems no reason why studies that found an adverse effect of physical education should be denied publication. The overwhelming number of articles with a positive or neutral conclusion thus further reinforces the view that a substantial amount of curricular time can be allocated to physical education without impairing a child's learning. The mechanism of any benefit is less clear; there may be effects on the brain (as suggested by several recent studies of exercise and cognition in the elderly), but other possibilities include a boosting of self-esteem, a calming of the hyperactive child, an arousal of the sleepy child, or simply a break from the classroom and more preparation time for overworked academic teachers.

R. J. Shephard, MD (Lond), PhD, DPE

References

1. Volle M, Tisal H, LaBarre R, et al. Influence d'un programme expérimental d'activités physiques integré à l'école primaire sur le developpement de quelques eléments psychomoteurs. In: Lavallée H, Shephard RJ, eds. *Child Growth & Development*. Trois Rivières, Canada: Univ. de Québec à Trois Rivières; 1982: 201-222.
2. Shephard RJ, Volle M, Lavallée H, et al. Required physical activity and academic grades: a controlled study. In: Ilmarinen J, Valimaki I, eds. *Children and Sport*. Berlin: Springer Verlag; 1984:58-63.
3. Shephard RJ. Curricular physical activity and academic performance. *Pediatr Exerc Sci*. 1997;9:113-126.
4. Trudeau F, Shephard RJ. Physical education, school physical activity, school sports and academic performance. *Int J Behav Nutr Phys Act*. 2008;5 10.1186/1479–5868-5-10, http://www.ijbnpa.org/content/5/1/10.
5. Trudeau F, Shephard RJ. Relationships of physical activity to brain health and the academic performance of schoolchildren. *Am J Lifestyle Med*. 2010;4:138-150.

Fluid Replacement Requirements for Child Athletes
Rowland T (Baystate Med Ctr, Springfield, MA)
Sports Med 41:279-288, 2011

Thermoregulatory responses to exercise differ in prepubertal athletes compared with their adult counterparts. It is important, therefore, to consider fluid requirements specific to this age group to prevent risks of dehydration and diminished sports performance. Relative to their body size, children demonstrate lower sweat water losses during exercise than adults. Nonetheless, percentage levels of incurred dehydration are similar in pre- and postpubertal athletes. Moreover, voluntary (*ad libitum*) drinking volumes in children in respect to their body size are comparable or greater than those of adults. Given an adequate opportunity to drink during exercise, volume intake driven by thirst should be expected to prevent significant levels of dehydration in child athletes. The amount can be calculated conservatively as an hourly fluid intake of 13 mL/kg (6 mL/lb) bodyweight. Equally important is post-exercise fluid replenishment (approximately 4 mL/kg 2 mL/lb for each hour of exercise) to avoid initiating subsequent exercise bouts in a dehydrated state. Choice of fluid should be dictated by taste preference, since volume of intake, rather than fluid content, is the most critical issue in child athletes. Since children may lack motivation for proper fluid intake behaviours, the responsibility falls to coaches and parents to assure that young athletes receive appropriate hydration during and after exercise bouts (Table 2).

▶ Dr Rowland presents evidence dispelling the myth that thermoregulation is impaired in children compared with adults. Although sweat rates in prepubertal children are lower than those of adults, particularly in males, relative dehydration in response to exertion in hot laboratory conditions are equivalent in children and adults. Prepubertal child athletes (age 8 to 13 years) are likely to consume

TABLE 2.—Recommended Minimal Fluid Intake During and Following Exercise in Child Athletes. Values During Exercise are 'per Hour' and Based on 75% of Expected Sweat Fluid Loss. Recommendations After Exercise Indicate Supplementary Volume Required to Fully Compensate for Deficits Incurred During Exercise

Bodyweight		Fluid Replacement During Exercise		Replacement After Exercise[a]	
kg	lb	mL/h	oz/h	mL/h of Prior Exercise	oz/h of Prior Exercise
22.7	50	300	10	100	4
27.2	60	360	12	130	4
31.8	70	420	14	138	5
36.3	80	480	16	150	5
40.8	90	540	18	162	6
45.4	100	600	20	175	6
49.9	110	660	22	184	6
54.4	120	720	24	194	7
59.0	130	780	26	200	7

[a]In addition to normal fluid intake.

sufficient fluids ad libitum during exercise to prevent dehydration, if fluids are made available, and the importance of consuming fluids is emphasized by adult supervisors. Children are less likely than adults to overconsume water during extended exercise and induce hyponatremia. Fluids that are appealing to children should be provided throughout practices and competition. Water, flavored water, or sports drinks can be consumed for hydration; children who sweat heavily or lose excess sodium, as evidenced by white salt residue on clothing, may benefit from drinks with added sodium. Because the sodium concentration of sweat is lower in children than adults, children are less likely to become hyponatremic. Carbohydrate-enriched sports drinks may enhance performance in children competing in endurance events lasting over an hour, but the research is limited. Carbonated beverages and juices should be avoided during exercise because they can slow gastric emptying and cause gastrointestinal upset. The most unpredictable aspect of keeping child athletes hydrated is their drinking behavior during competitions. Because children can be distracted by the intensity of competition, it is even more important to emphasize fluid intake before, during, and after a competitive event. Complete rehydration prior to the next competition or training session is important to preventing dehydration during subsequent activity. Changes in body weight during physical exertion under hot and humid conditions can be used to monitor dehydration. The recommendation is for children to drink 480 mL (16 oz) for each 0.5 kg (1 lb) of weight lost during an athletic event or workout. Recommended minimal fluid intakes during and following exercise are provided for child athletes relative to body weight (Table 2). This article will guide physicians, coaches, parents, and others who supervise child athletes to provide fluids and monitor drinking behavior during practices and competitions.

C. M. Jankowski, PhD

Skeletal Age and Age Verification in Youth Sport
Malina RM (Univ of Texas at Austin)
Sports Med 41:925-947, 2011

Problems with accurate chronological age (CA) reporting occur on a more or less regular basis in youth sports. As a result, there is increasing discussion of age verification. Use of 'bone age' or skeletal age (SA) for the purpose of estimating or verifying CA has been used in medicolegal contexts for many years and also in youth sport competitions. This article reviews the concept of SA, and the three most commonly used methods of assessment. Variation in SA within CA groups among male soccer players and female artistic gymnasts is evaluated relative to the use of SA as a tool for verification of CA. Corresponding data for athletes in several other sports are also summarized. Among adolescent males, a significant number of athletes will be identified as older than a CA cutoff because of advanced skeletal maturation when they in fact have a valid CA. SA assessments of soccer players are comparable to MRI assessments of epiphyseal-diaphyseal union of the distal radius in under-17 soccer players. Both

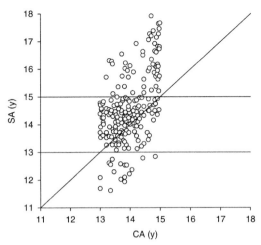

FIGURE 1.—Distributions of skeletal (SA) and chronological ages (CA) in youth soccer players 13–14 years of age. Drawn from data reported in Malina et al.[63] *Editor's Note*: Please refer to original journal article for full references. (Reprinted from Malina RM. Skeletal age and age verification in youth sport. *Sports Med*. 2011;41:925-947, with permission from Adis Data Information BV.)

protocols indicate a relatively large number of false negatives among youth players aged 15–17 years. Among adolescent females, a significant number of age-eligible artistic gymnasts will be identified as younger than the CA cutoff because of later skeletal maturation when in fact they have a valid CA. There is also the possibility of false positives-identifying gymnasts as younger than the CA cutoff because of late skeletal maturation when they have a valid CA. The risk of false negatives and false positives implies that SA is not a valid indicator of CA (Fig 1).

▶ There are many areas of sport in which precise age classification is important to both safety and fair competition. However, competitors in international events may come from countries that do not have birth certificates, and, in at least a few instances, there have been suspicions that such documents have been falsified.[1] Some authors have thus suggested that the answer is for on-site determination of the age of athletes using biological markers,[2,3] and this approach has been tried in some soccer and cricket events. Available methods of age determination include genital inspection (where there are issues of privacy), radiographic determinations of skeletal age (where exposure to radiation may be criticized), inspection of teeth (applicable over a limited age range), and (where multiple observations are available) the estimation of height velocity. Although grouped information (eg, a comparison between gymnasts and sedentary children) may be informative, as with many biological tests, individual variation is such that these markers are of little help in confirming the age of a particular athlete (Fig 1).[4,5] The only recourse seems to rely on the honesty of the participants, and, sadly, this cannot always be assured.

R. J. Shephard, MD (Lond), PhD, DPE

References

1. Macur J. China stripped of gymnastics medal. *New York Times.* 2010 Apr 28, http://www.nytimes.com/2010/04/29/sports/olympics/29gymnast.html. Accessed November 22, 2011.
2. Tritrakarn A, Tansuphasiri V. Roentgenographic assessment of skeletal ages of Asian junior youth football players. *J Med Assoc Thai.* 1991;74:459-464.
3. Dvorak J, George J, Junge A, Holder J. Application of MRI of the wrist for age determination in international U-17 soccer competitions. *Br J Sports Med.* 2007; 41:497-500.
4. Engebretsen L, Steffen K, Bahr R, et al. The International Olympic Committee consensus statement on age determination in high-level young athletes. *Br J Sports Med.* 2010;44:476-484.
5. Liversidge HM, Smith BH, Maber M. Bias and accuracy of age estimation using developing teeth in 946 children. *Am J Phys Anthropol.* 2010;143:545-554.

Habitual Levels of Vigorous, But Not Moderate or Light, Physical Activity Is Positively Related to Cortical Bone Mass in Adolescents

Sayers A, Mattocks C, Deere K, et al (Univ of Bristol, UK; Univ of Bath, UK)

J Clin Endocrinol Metab 96:E793-E802, 2011

Context.—The intensity of habitual physical activity (PA) needed to affect skeletal development in childhood is currently unclear.

Objective.—To examine associations between light PA, moderate PA, and vigorous PA (as assessed by accelerometry), and tibial cortical bone mass (BMC_C) as measured by peripheral quantitative computed tomography.

Design/Setting.—Cross-sectional analysis based on the Avon Longitudinal Study of Parents and Children.

Participants.—A total of 1748 boys and girls (mean age 15.5 yr) participated in the study.

Outcome Measures.—We measured BMC_C, cortical bone mineral density, periosteal circumference, and endosteal circumference by tibial peripheral quantitative computed tomography.

Results.—Multivariable models, adjusted for height and other activity levels, indicated vigorous PA was positively related to BMC_C ($P = 0.0001$). There was little evidence of a relationship with light PA or moderate PA (both $P \geq 0.7$). In path analyses, the relationship between vigorous PA and BMC_C [0.082(95% confidence interval [CI]: 0.037, 0.128), $P = 0.0004$] (SD change per doubling of vigorous PA) was minimally attenuated by adjusting for body composition [0.070 (95% CI: 0.026, 0.115), $P = 0.002$]. In analyses adjusted for body composition, the relationship between vigorous PA and BMC_C was explained by the periosteal circumference pathway [0.043 (95% CI: 0.004, 0.082), $P = 0.03$] and the endosteal circumference adjusted for periosteal circumference pathway [0.031 (95% CI: 0.011, 0.050), $P = 0.002$], while there was little contribution from the cortical bone mineral density pathway ($P = 0.3$).

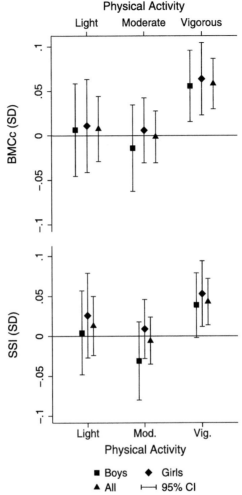

FIGURE 1.—The association of light, moderate, and vigorous activity on BMC_C (*top*) and SSI (*bottom*), adjusted for age, height, average recording time, and other levels of exercise intensity in boys (n = 778) and girls (n = 970). *y* axis represent β coefficients with 95% confidence limits, expressed as SD change in pQCT variable per SD increase in light activity and per doubling in moderate or vigorous activity. BMC_C, *P* values for light activity P(ALL) = 0.68 (B = 0.81, G = 0.68), for moderate activity P(ALL) = 0.93 (B = 0.57, G = 0.75), and for vigorous activity P(ALL) = 0.00001 (B = 0.007, G = 0.002). SSI, *P* values for light activity P(ALL) = 0.49 (B = 0.87, G = 0.33), for moderate activity P(ALL) = 0.69 (B = 0.21, G = 0.64), and for vigorous activity P(ALL) = 0.003 (B = 0.06, G = 0.01). No evidence of any sex differences were observed for light, moderate, or vigorous PA (*P* = 0.2 in all instances). B, Boys; G, girls. (Reprinted from Sayers A, Mattocks C, Deere K, et al. Habitual levels of vigorous, but not moderate or light, physical activity is positively related to cortical bone mass in adolescents. *J Clin Endocrinol Metab.* 2011;96:E793-E802, Copyright 2011, with permission from The Endocrine Society.)

Conclusions.—Vigorous day-to-day PA is associated with indices of BMC_C and geometry in adolescents, whereas light or moderate PA has no detectable association. Therefore, promoting PA in childhood is unlikely to benefit skeletal development unless high-impact activities are also increased (Fig 1).

▶ This cross-sectional study addresses the dose response of weight-bearing physical activity on bone quality in adolescents. Weight-bearing physical activity has been positively associated with bone mineral accrual in children, although less is known about the dose of activity needed to achieve bone benefits. The repeated exposure of the skeleton to mechanical strain from ground reaction forces during weight-bearing activity is the mechanistic underpinning of a potential dose-response effect of exercise on lower extremity bones during growth. The health implications of reaching peak bone density and bone strength during growth include preventing or delaying osteoporosis and fracture later in life. Most of the previous studies of physical activity and bone health in children have relied on dual-energy x-ray absorptiometry (DXA), which measures 2-dimensional (areal) bone density. The peripheral quantitative computed tomography (pQCT) technology provides more specific 3-dimensional measures of cortical and trabecular bone area that can be used to derive an index of bone strength. This investigation included pQCT measures of cortical bone in the right midtibia and physical activity measured by accelerometry in more than 1400 boys and girls aged 15.5 years. The adolescents were categorized into light, moderate, or vigorous physical activity intensity categories using well-accepted cut points of accelerometer counts. Because body composition is a determinant of bone quality, DXA was used to measure total body fat and lean tissue mass. The main finding of the study was that vigorous physical activity, as opposed to lower intensity levels, was more strongly associated with greater cortical bone area, bone content, and strain index in girls and boys (Fig 1). This result suggests that, in late puberty, a threshold exists in skeletal response when exercise intensity increases from the level of brisk walking to jogging (above and below 6 kcal/kg/h). At the higher intensity of physical activity, the concomitant increase in lean mass and loss of fat mass offset changes in cortical bone. The recommendation to exercise more vigorously for bone health benefits may conflict with the message to be more active at any level to prevent obesity in youth. However, given that the mean (± SD) duration of vigorous activity was 4.3 ± 5.8 min/d and 2.2 ± 3.7 min/d in boys and girls, respectively, short blasts of vigorous activity could have important benefits to the bone health of adolescents.

C. M. Jankowski, PhD

Habitual Levels of Vigorous, But Not Moderate or Light, Physical Activity Is Positively Related to Cortical Bone Mass in Adolescents
Sayers A, Mattocks C, Deere K, et al (Univ of Bristol, UK; Univ of Bath, UK)
J Clin Endocrinol Metab 96:E793-E802, 2011

Context.—The intensity of habitual physical activity (PA) needed to affect skeletal development in childhood is currently unclear.

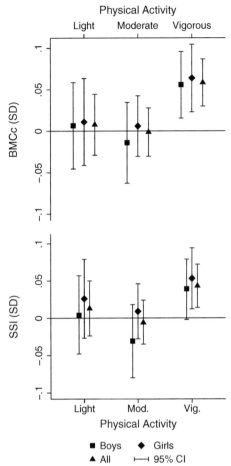

FIGURE 1.—The association of light, moderate, and vigorous activity on BMC_C (*top*) and SSI (*bottom*), adjusted for age, height, average recording time, and other levels of exercise intensity in boys ($n = 778$) and girls ($n = 970$). y axis represent β coefficients with 95% confidence limits, expressed as SD change in pQCT variable per SD increase in light activity and per doubling in moderate or vigorous activity. BMC_C, P values for light activity $P(ALL) = 0.68$ ($B = 0.81$, $G = 0.68$), for moderate activity $P(ALL) = 0.93$ ($B = 0.57$, $G = 0.75$), and for vigorous activity $P(ALL) < 0.00001$ ($B = 0.007$, $G = 0.002$). SSI, P values for light activity $P(ALL) = 0.49$ ($B = 0.87$, $G = 0.33$), for moderate activity $P(ALL) = 0.69$ ($B = 0.21$, $G = 0.64$), and for vigorous activity $P(ALL) = 0.003$ ($B = 0.06$, $G = 0.01$). No evidence of any sex differences were observed for light, moderate, or vigorous PA ($P \geq 0.2$ in all instances). B, Boys; G, girls. (Reprinted from Sayers A, Mattocks C, Deere K, et al. Habitual levels of vigorous, but not moderate or light, physical activity is positively related to cortical bone mass in adolescents. *J Clin Endocrinol Metab.* 2011;96:E793-E802, Copyright 2011, with permission from The Endocrine Society.)

Objective.—To examine associations between light PA, moderate PA, and vigorous PA (as assessed by accelerometry), and tibial cortical bone mass (BMC_C) as measured by peripheral quantitative computed tomography.

Design/Setting.—Cross-sectional analysis based on the Avon Longitudinal Study of Parents and Children.

Participants.—A total of 1748 boys and girls (mean age 15.5 yr) participated in the study.

Outcome Measures.—We measured BMC_C, cortical bone mineral density, periosteal circumference, and endosteal circumference by tibial peripheral quantitative computed tomography.

Results.—Multivariable models, adjusted for height and other activity levels, indicated vigorous PA was positively related to BMC_C ($P = 0.0001$). There was little evidence of a relationship with light PA or moderate PA (both $P \geq 0.7$). In path analyses, the relationship between vigorous PA and BMC_C [0.082 (95% confidence interval [CI]: 0.037, 0.128), $P = 0.0004$] (SD change per doubling of vigorous PA) was minimally attenuated by adjusting for body composition [0.070 (95% CI: 0.026, 0.115), $P = 0.002$]. In analyses adjusted for body composition, the relationship between vigorous PA and BMC_C was explained by the periosteal circumference pathway [0.043 (95% CI: 0.004, 0.082), $P = 0.03$] and the endosteal circumference adjusted for periosteal circumference pathway [0.031 (95% CI: 0.011, 0.050), $P = 0.002$], while there was little contribution from the cortical bone mineral density pathway ($P = 0.3$).

Conclusions.—Vigorous day-to-day PA is associated with indices of BMC_C and geometry in adolescents, whereas light or moderate PA has no detectable association. Therefore, promoting PA in childhood is unlikely to benefit skeletal development unless high-impact activities are also increased (Fig 1).

▶ Approximately 98% of the adult bone mineral content is deposited by age 20 years, and this process is affected by both genetic and lifestyle factors.[1] Osteoporosis is viewed as a pediatric health issue, and increasing attention is being focused on the influence of physical activity on bone mass during adolescence. In this large cohort of 15-year-old boys and girls, habitual levels of vigorous activity were positively related to tibial cortical bone mass after multivariate adjustment. As summarized in Fig 1, this association was not detected in adolescents engaging in light or moderate physical activity. Thus, mechanical strain is an important factor in higher levels of bone mass in growing boys and girls.

D. C. Nieman, DrPH

Reference

1. U.S. Department of Health and Human Services. *Bone Health and Osteoporosis: A Report of the Surgeon General.* Rockville, MD: HHS, Office of the Surgeon General; 2004.

Levels of Physical Activity That Predict Optimal Bone Mass in Adolescents: The HELENA Study

Gracia-Marco L, on behalf of the HELENA Study Group (Univ of Zaragoza, Spain; et al)
Am J Prev Med 40:599-607, 2011

Background.—Physical activity is necessary for bone mass development in adolescence. There are few studies quantifying the associations between physical activity and bone mass in adolescents.

Purpose.—To assess the relationship between moderate-to-vigorous physical activity (MVPA) and vigorous physical activity (VPA) and bone mass in adolescents.

Methods.—Bone mass was measured by dual-energy X-ray absorptiometry and physical activity by accelerometers in 380 healthy Spanish adolescents (189 boys, aged 12.5−17.5 years) from the HELENA−CSS (2006−2007). Subjects were classified according to the recommended amount of MVPA (<60 minutes or ≥60 minutes of MVPA/day). Receiver operating characteristic curve analysis was applied to calculate the relationship between physical activity and bone mass.

Results.—Less than 41 and 45 minutes of MVPA/day are associated with reduced bone mass at the trochanter and femoral neck. More than 78 minutes of MVPA/day is associated with increased bone mineral density (BMD) at the femoral neck. Regarding VPA, more than 28 minutes/day for the hip and intertrochanter and more than 32 minutes/day for the femoral neck are associated with increased BMD.

Conclusions.—The recommended amount of physical activity (minutes/day) seems insufficient to guarantee increased bone mass. With some minutes of VPA/day, bone adaptations could be obtained at different bone sites (Table 4).

▶ In terms of an optimum amount of physical activity, bone has been thought a relatively exigent tissue; in old people, activity levels of up to 9000 steps per day are associated with progressively lower risks of osteopenia.[1] The standard physical activity recommendations for children and adolescents from both US and Canadian authorities are more demanding than those for adults: 60 or more minutes of moderate to vigorous physical activity per day, with at least 3 of these days including activities to improve bone and muscle strength.[2,3] However, this article shows little difference of bone mineral content or bone density (as assessed by dual-energy x-ray absorptiometry) between adolescents taking greater or less than 60 minutes of physical activity per day (Table 4). One factor contributing to this departure from expectation is that many of the epidemiologic studies setting the optimal duration of physical activity have relied on questionnaires. For various reasons, this approach exaggerates the true amount of activity that has been taken in almost all age groups.[4,5] In children, time spent listening to the gym teacher, changing, showering and even traveling to sports facilities tends to be included in the estimated total of active time. The daily intake of calcium was a little low in the girls studied by Gracia-Marco and colleagues.

TABLE 4.—Time of MVPA and VPA to Predict High (+2 SD) BMC and BMD

	Minutes/day	AUC (CI)	Sensitivity	Specificity	OMR (%)[a]	PPV (%)[a]	NPV (%)[a]	PLR[a]	NLR[a]	A[a]
MVPA										
BMC										
Whole body	41	0.562 (0.419, 0.705)	0.909	0.270	—	—	—	—	—	—
Hip	57	0.643 (0.501, 0.786)	0.778	0.537	—	—	—	—	—	—
Lumbar spine	73	0.581 (0.392, 0.770)	0.545	0.759	—	—	—	—	—	—
Hip scan										
Trochanter	41	0.591 (0.45, 0.732)	0.909	0.290	—	—	—	—	—	—
Intertrochanter	57	0.541 (0.369, 0.714)	0.667	0.534	—	—	—	—	—	—
Femoral neck	78	0.544 (0.340, 0.747)	0.444	0.825	—	—	—	—	—	—
BMD										
Whole body	44	0.566 (0.373, 0.76)	0.889	0.331	—	—	—	—	—	—
Hip	78	0.673 (0.497, 0.848)	0.500	0.824	—	—	—	—	—	—
Lumbar spine	82	0.442 (0.168, 0.717)	0.333	0.849	—	—	—	—	—	—
Hip scan										
Trochanter	53	0.475 (0.293, 0.657)	0.600	0.479	—	—	—	—	—	—
Intertrochanter	46	0.664 (0.509, 0.818)	0.889	0.263	—	—	—	—	—	—
Femoral neck	78	0.835** (0.735, 0.936)	0.643	0.586	63.33	87.66	26.45	1.55	0.61	0.23
VPA										
BMC										
Whole body	23	0.609 (0.447, 0.771)	0.545	0.668	—	—	—	—	—	—
Hip	19	0.692* (0.557, 0.828)	0.583	0.608	60.77	4.52	97.87	1.49	0.68	0.19
Lumbar spine	22	0.632 (0.435, 0.829)	0.727	0.648	—	—	—	—	—	—
Hip scan										
Trochanter	28	0.665 (0.513, 0.818)	0.545	0.778	—	—	—	—	—	—
Intertrochanter	19	0.576 (0.411, 0.741)	0.777	0.574	—	—	—	—	—	—
Femoral neck	27	0.608 (0.408, 0.809)	0.555	0.757	—	—	—	—	—	—
BMD										
Whole body	38	0.567 (0.349, 0.786)	0.333	0.898	—	—	—	—	—	—
Hip	28	0.802** (0.666, 0.937)	0.667	0.794	79.23	4.82	99.35	3.24	0.42	0.46
Lumbar spine	38	0.477 (0.188, 0.765)	0.333	0.896	—	—	—	—	—	—

(Continued)

TABLE 4. (*continued*)

	Minutes/day	AUC (CI)	Sensitivity	Specificity	OMR (%)[a]	PPV (%)[a]	NPV (%)[a]	PLR[a]	NLR[a]	A[a]
Hip scan										
Trochanter	24	0.514 (0.309, 0.719)	0.500	0.683	—	—	—	—	—	—
Intertrochanter	28	**0.741** (0.578, 0.908)	0.556	0.795	78.97	6.02	98.70	2.71	0.56	0.35
Femoral neck	32	**0.889** (0.813, 0.964)	0.667	0.846	84.36	6.35	99.39	4.34	0.39	0.51

Note: Boldface indicates significance.

A, Youden index; AUC, area under the curve (ROC analysis); BMC, bone mineral content; BMD, bone mineral density; MVPA, moderate-to-vigorous physical activity; NLR, negative likelihood ratio; NPV, negative predictive value; OMR, overall misclassification rate; PLR, positive likelihood ratio; PPV, positive predictive value; VPA, vigorous physical activity.

[a]Only significant results are shown.

*p<0.05.

**p≤0.01

Objective measurements of physical activity were obtained (7-day counts recorded by a uniaxial accelerometer). Such figures are much more reliable than questionnaire data, although they also may be unreliable if a child spends much time on a bicycle. A second factor is that bone health depends on the type of physical activity that is taken as well as the total amount,[6] and unfortunately the uniaxial accelerometer gives no indication of activity type. Even assuming that the current findings are confirmed by further research, there may remain cardiovascular and other metabolic reasons for recommending that children continue to take at least 60 minutes of physical activity per day. However, it seems necessary to weigh all questionnaire-based recommendations against more objective data.

R. J. Shephard, MD (Lond), PhD, DPE

References

1. Park H, Park S, Shephard RJ, Aoyagi Y. Objectively measured physical activity and calcaneal bone health in older Japanese adults: longitudinal data from the Nakanojo Study. International Congress on Physical Activity Monitoring; 2011; Glasgow, Scotland.
2. U.S. DHHS. Key guidelines for children and adolescents. www.health.gov/PAGuidelines/. Accessed May 23, 2011.
3. Janssen I. Physical activity guidelines for children and youth. *Can J Public Health*. 2007;98:S109-S121.
4. Hagströmer M, Bergman P, De Bourdeaudhuij I, et al. Concurrent validity of a modified version of the International Physical Activity Questionnaire (IPAQ-A) in European adolescents: the HELENA study. *Int J Obes (Lond)*. 2008;32:S42-S48.
5. Bassett DR Jr. Validity and reliability issues in objective monitoring of physical activity. *Res Q Exerc Sport*. 2000;71:S30-S36.
6. Vicente-Rodríguez G. How does exercise affect bone development during growth? *Sports Med*. 2006;36:561-569.

Differential Effects of Intraventricular Hemorrhage and White Matter Injury on Preterm Cerebellar Growth
Tam EWY, Miller SP, Studholme C, et al (Univ of California San Francisco; et al)
J Pediatr 158:366-371, 2011

Objective.—To hypothesize that detailed examination of early cerebellar volumes in time would distinguish differences in cerebellar growth associated with intraventricular hemorrhage (IVH) and white matter injury in preterm infants.

Study Design.—Preterm newborns at the University of California San Francisco (n = 57) and the University of British Columbia (n = 115) were studied with serial magnetic resonance imaging scans near birth and again at near term-equivalent age. Interactive semi-automated tools were used to determine volumes of the cerebellar hemispheres.

Results.—Adjusting for supratentorial brain injury, cerebellar hemorrhage, and study site, cerebellar volume increased 1.7 cm³/week postmenstrual age (95% CI, 1.6-1.7; P < .001). More severe supratentorial IVH was associated with slower growth of cerebellar volumes ($P < .001$). Volumes by 40 weeks were 1.4 cm^3 lower in premature infants with grade 1 to 2 IVH and 5.4 cm^3 lower in infants with grade 3 to 4 IVH. The same magnitude of decrease was found between ipsilateral and contralateral IVH. No association was found with severity of white matter injury ($P = .3$).

Conclusions.—Early effects of decreased cerebellar volume associated with supratentorial IVH in either hemisphere may be a result of concurrent cerebellar injury or direct effects of subarachnoid blood on cerebellar development.

▶ Alterations in cerebellar development and function have been implicated in various neurologic disorders of infancy and childhood. The cerebellum starts to develop from 4 weeks after conception with development going on up to 2 years postnatally.[1] Prematurely born infants are at particular risk for deficits in sensorimotor coordination, cognitive dysfunction, and adverse behavioral outcomes.[2] The objective of this study was to investigate the association between brain injury happening above the tentorium cerebelli (supratentorial injury) and cerebellar volume. The presence of supratentorial intraventricular hemorrhage (IVH) correlated with decreased cerebellar volume as measured by magnetic resonance imaging (MRI) scanning and 3-dimensional tracings of the cerebellar hemispheres.[3] Importantly, a slowing of cerebellar growth occurred in those infants with severe IVH as measured using serial MRI scans near birth and again at near term equivalent age. The decrease in cerebellar volume and its adverse effect on cerebellar growth was not associated with white matter injury in contrast to results from other studies. The authors proposed 3 different mechanisms for this impairment in cerebellar growth in the presence of IVH. The first mechanism may be caused by a diaschisis (a disconnection) of fiber tracts after a significant injury of the supratentorial parenchyma. These authors found that cerebellar growth was impaired bilaterally with a negative correlation between IVH severity and bilateral impaired cerebellar growth. Another suggestion for mechanism was the presence of bilateral cerebellar injury as a result of concurrent injury during the onset of IVH. In addition, a third (favored) mechanism was the presence of circulating blood products in the cerebrospinal fluid that would impair cerebellar growth. These are compelling results from the standpoint that the period of premature birth from 24 to 37 weeks of gestational age is known to be a time when the cerebellum undergoes rapid growth and maturation. Significant clinical implications ensue as a consequence of this impairment in growth of the cerebellum. The results of this study are important in that they highlight risk factors that in the past were unknown. The decrease in cerebellar volume and ensuing adverse effects on cerebellar growth are informative from the perspective of targeted, informed therapies possibly ameliorating the effects of this condition during that time of rapid cerebellar development.

V. Galea, PhD

References

1. Limperopoulos C, Soul JS, Gauvreau K, et al. Late gestation cerebellar growth is rapid and impeded by premature birth. *Pediatrics.* 2005;115:688-695.

2. Volpe JJ. Cerebellum of the premature infant: rapidly developing, vulnerable, clinically important. *J Child Neurol.* 2009;24:1085-1104.
3. Partridge SC, Mukherjee P, Berman JI, et al. Tractography-based quantitation of diffusion tensor imaging parameters in white matter tracts of preterm newborns. *J Magn Reson Imaging.* 2005;22:467-474.

No Proprioceptive Deficits in Autism Despite Movement-Related Sensory and Execution Impairments

Fuentes CT, Mostofsky SH, Bastian AJ (Johns Hopkins School of Medicine, Baltimore, MD)

J Autism Dev Disord 41:1352-1361, 2011

Autism spectrum disorder (ASD) often involves sensory and motor problems, yet the proprioceptive sense of limb position has not been directly assessed. We used three tasks to assess proprioception in adolescents with ASD who had motor and sensory perceptual abnormalities, and compared them to age- and IQ-matched controls. Results showed no group differences in proprioceptive accuracy or precision during active or passive tasks. Both groups showed (a) biases in elbow angle accuracy that varied with joint position, (b) improved elbow angle precision for active versus passive tasks, and (c) improved precision for a fingertip versus elbow angle estimation task. Thus, a primary proprioceptive deficit may not contribute to sensorimotor deficits in ASD. Abnormalities may arise at later sensory processing stages.

▶ Somatosensation is vital to our successful interaction with our environment. Individuals with autism spectrum disorder (ASD) experience poor social interaction and exhibit repetitive behaviors and interests with excessive focus on details. It has been suggested that these symptoms may be consequences of impairment in the usage and processing of sensory information to generate movements to interact with others and engage within their environment. We receive information from our muscles, ligaments, and tendons through various receptors, collectively forming our proprioceptive system. This system crucially conveys ongoing information related to kinesthesia—our sense of body position and movement. The study by Fuentes and colleagues is yet another excellent investigation from the laboratory of Dr Amy Bastian at Johns Hopkins University.[1] The authors rightly point out that systematic examination of proprioception is sorely lacking in studies on children with ASD. Furthermore, studies are equivocal in informing us of whether these differences in sensory processing among individuals with ASD are at the receptor level at the periphery, changes in afferent flow to spinal cord and up, or at the level of cortical processing.[2] The objective, therefore, was to establish whether adolescents (n = 12) were different from controls in their peripheral proprioceptive systems or whether this aspect of somatosensory information is received, processed, and neutrally integrated with motor (efferent) information. Despite significant differences from the control subjects (n = 12) in motor and sensory function using established scales, such as the "Revised Physical and Neurological Examination for Subtle (Motor) Signs (PANESS) and Adolescent/Adult Sensory Profile, where participants with ASD showed significant motor and sensory processing impairments, they found no significant differences in performance of a passive task, in which participants had to match elbow angle, nor in an active task, in which subjects had to match a target representing the position of their forearm by actively rotating the elbow. This was true for both proprioceptive accuracy (difference in elbow angle between displayed and actual angle in degrees) and precision (standard deviation of the perceived angle across trials). An interesting observation was that there was also no difference in a task in which subjects had to match the position of their right fingertip using a joystick with their left hand (this was similar to the passive elbow matching task). Collectively, this was an indicator that peripheral proprioceptors were conveying the correct information. One must then ask why was there such a discrepancy between the tests of motor function and sensory processing and the passive positioning tasks used to test proprioception? Furthermore, their improved proprioceptive precision on active versus passive elbow angle matching tasks is indicative of their ability to glean additional positional information from efference copies of motor commands, implying that adolescents with ASD have the ability to form internal models of motor control. In other words, individuals with ASD have the ability to combine efferent (motor) with afferent information to which is a hallmark of formation of internal models of motor control to form more precise sensory estimates. These unexpected observations have been previously reported from this laboratory, and it begs the question of how this can be so when formation of internal models has been linked to normal cerebellar function, which is not normal in ASD. Taken with the evidence of disruptions in cortical and cerebellar connectivity in ASD, one must presume that there are ASD-associated differences in cortical organization that may surface when tasks are more complex and challenging. On the other hand, the finding that proprioceptive systems are functioning well in ASD—at least at the peripheral level—bodes well for interventions targeting motor control deficits and improvements in complex skill acquisition.

V. Galea, PhD

References

1. Gidley Larson JC, Bastian AJ, Donchin O, Shadmehr R, Mostofsky SH. Acquisition of internal models of motor tasks in children with autism. *Brain.* 2008;131:2894-2903.
2. Haswell CC, Izawa J, Dowell LR, Mostofsky SH, Shadmehr R. Representation of internal models of action in the autistic brain. *Nat Neurosci.* 2009;12:970-972.

Disrupted Neural Synchronization in Toddlers with Autism
Dinstein I, Pierce K, Eyler L, et al (Univ of California San Diego, La Jolla; et al)
Neuron 70:1218-1225, 2011

Autism is often described as a disorder of neural synchronization. However, it is unknown how early in development synchronization abnormalities emerge and whether they are related to the development of early autistic behavioral symptoms. Here, we show that disrupted synchronization is evident in the spontaneous cortical activity of naturally sleeping toddlers with autism, but not in toddlers with language delay or typical development. Toddlers with autism exhibited significantly weaker interhemispheric synchronization (i.e., weak "functional connectivity" across the two hemispheres) in putative language areas. The strength of synchronization was positively correlated with verbal ability and negatively correlated with autism severity, and it enabled identification of the majority of autistic toddlers (72%) with high accuracy (84%). Disrupted cortical synchronization, therefore, appears to be a notable characteristic of autism neurophysiology that is evident at very early stages of autism development.

▶ Early detection of neurodevelopmental disorders such as autism is becoming a significant area of study for neurodevelopmental neuroscientists. Largely because of the potential for early (novel) intervention at times before potentially irreversible changes in cortical function take place. Early identification of autism is difficult because autism is one on a spectrum of disorders that may manifest in many different ways. In fact, no child on the spectrum of autism spectrum disorders is the same. More frequently, autism has been described as a disorder of neural synchronization, specifically interhemispheric synchronization, between systems that belong to a specific functional system, such as the motor or visual system. Recent data point to the possibility that autism arises from the development of abnormal neural networks with irregular synaptic connectivity and abnormal neural synchronization, which could explain the social and behavioral symptoms, such as language delay, observed in children with autism. In this publication, Dinstein and colleagues took advantage of the fact that reliable fMRI data of interhemispheric synchronization can be acquired during sleep,[1] thereby rendering the opportunity to measure synchronization in typically developing toddlers as well as in toddlers with language delay and, importantly, in another group of toddlers with autism.[2] Typically, functionally related cortical areas show temporally correlated neural activation patterns even without the presence of task-related activity, such as in rest and sleep. Strong synchronization, such as that found in corresponding contralateral cortical locations, is even found in newborn infants. The results of this study are compelling, because the authors were also able to include severely affected toddlers with autism that is not often possible when task-related activity is necessary. Overall, toddlers with autism showed significantly weaker interhemispheric synchronization than in typically developing toddlers or in toddlers with language delay. More importantly, this disruption in synchronization was not global but rather specific to the inferior frontal gyrus and the superior temporal gyrus areas associated with language production and comprehension, respectively.[3] Also notable was the strong association between autism severity and weak interhemispheric synchronization. These findings are compelling because they are promising of an early diagnostic tool that can be used in toddlers. The fact that this fMRI data acquisition and quantification were available during natural sleep provides an exciting possibility for pediatric neurologists and occupational and physiotherapists for early identification and thereby opens doors for early intervention. Researchers do make the assumption that underlying pathological mechanisms that give rise to the disruption in synchronization during sleep also disrupt it during wakefulness and would disrupt normal perception and possibly motor behavior. This early biological marker of abnormal neural connectivity is an exciting development for future management of children with autism.

V. Galea, PhD

References

1. Raichle ME. Two views of brain function. *Trends Cogn Sci.* 2010;14:180-190.
2. Zweigenbaum L, Bryson S, Lord C, et al. Clinical assessment and management of toddlers with suspected autism spectrum disorder: insights from studies of high-risk infants. *Pediatrics.* 2009;123:1383-1391.
3. Anderson JS, Druzgal TJ, Froehlich A, et al. Decreased interhemispheric functional connectivity in autism. *Cereb Cortex.* 2011;21:1134-1146.

Gait patterns in children with autism

Calhoun M, Longworth M, Chester VL (Univ of New Brunswick, Fredericton, Canada)
Clin Biomech 26:200-206, 2011

Background.—Very few studies have examined the gait patterns of children with autism. A greater awareness of movement deviations could be beneficial for treatment planning. The purpose of this study was to compare kinematic and kinetic gait patterns in children with autism versus age-matched controls.

Methods.—Twelve children with autism and twenty-two age-matched controls participated in the study. An eight camera motion capture system and four force plates were used to compute joint angles and joint kinetics during walking. Parametric analyses and principal component analyses were applied to kinematic and kinetic waveform variables from the autism (n = 12) and control (n = 22) groups. Group differences in parameterization values and principal component scores were tested using one-way ANOVAs and Kruskal–Wallis tests.

Findings.—Significant differences between the autism and control group were found for cadence, and peak hip and ankle kinematics and kinetics. Significant differences were found for three of the principal component scores: sagittal ankle moment principal component one, sagittal ankle angle principal component one, and sagittal hip moment principal component two. Results suggest that children with autism demonstrate reduced plantarflexor moments and increased dorsiflexion angles, which may be associated with hypotonia. Decreased hip extensor moments were found for the autism group compared to the control group, however, the clinical significance of this result is unclear.

Interpretation.—This study has identified several gait variables that were significantly different between autism and control group walkers.

This is the first study to provide a comprehensive analysis of gait patterns in children with autism.

▶ Interest and attention to the variety of motor symptoms demonstrated in children with autism spectrum disorder (ASD) is happily increasing. Clearly, persons with autism generally exhibit impairments in communication and social interaction and from a very early age. Knowledge of the sensory-motor consequences of this disorder has the potential to be very informative to the treatment protocols used in this particular pediatric population. For example, children with ASD often exhibit hypotonia and gross motor delay. Calhoun and coworkers have carried out an examination of gait in children with autism and for the first time have reported a detailed 3-dimensional kinematic and kinetic analysis of these children in comparison with age-matched typically developing controls. Interestingly, cadence was the only one temporal-spatial parameter that was statistically different between the 2 groups. Both parametric and principal component analyses of all the gait variables revealed that the only significant differences lay in the sagittal plane ankle angles and moments. Children with autism had reduced plantarflexor moments during the stance phase of the gait cycle with a reduction in peak ankle plantarflexion angle and an increase in peak dorsiflexion angle. Although the authors indicate within the text that the latter was significant, this was not so identified in the tabled and graphed data. There is also some inconsistency in that ankle power was not different between the groups. Some of the results could be explained by the hypotonia identified in 33% of their study sample; however, this is not sufficiently addressed in the discussion. Studies such as this one are a significant challenge not only because of the character of the population involved, but also because there is such heterogeneity in the population of children with ASD, thereby obliging one to question the generalizability of these results and the usefulness to clinicians working with this population.

V. Galea, PhD

Brain growth across the life span in autism: Age-specific changes in anatomical pathology
Courchesne E, Campbell K, Solso S (Univ of California, San Diego)
Brain Res 1380:138-145, 2011

Autism is marked by overgrowth of the brain at the earliest ages but not at older ages when decreases in structural volumes and neuron numbers are observed instead. This has led to the theory of age-specific anatomic abnormalities in autism. Here we report age-related changes in brain size in autistic and typical subjects from 12 months to 50 years of age based on analyses of 586 longitudinal and cross-sectional MRI scans. This dataset is several times larger than the largest autism study to date. Results demonstrate early brain overgrowth during infancy and the toddler years in autistic boys and girls, followed by an accelerated rate of decline in size and perhaps degeneration from adolescence to late middle age in this disorder. We theorize that underlying these age-specific changes in anatomic abnormalities in autism, there may also be age-specific changes in gene expression, molecular, synaptic, cellular, and circuit abnormalities. A peak age for detecting and studying the earliest fundamental biological underpinnings of autism is prenatal life and the first three postnatal years. Studies of the older autistic brain may not address original causes but are essential to discovering how best to help the older aging autistic person. Lastly, the theory of age-specific anatomic abnormalities in autism has broad implications for a wide range of work on the disorder including the design, validation, and interpretation of animal model, lymphocyte gene expression, brain gene expression, and genotype/CNV-anatomic phenotype studies.

▶ The changes in brain growth in people with autism were investigated from a very large data set of 586 longitudinal and cross-sectional magnetic resonance imaging (MRI) scans in individuals from infancy to age 50. This important and wide-sweeping work is seminal in the support of age-specific anatomic abnormalities in the brain structure of those afflicted with this condition. Three different periods of pathologic brain development emerged from these studies. Firstly, there is a brief period of abnormally accelerated brain overgrowth from early in postnatal life and extending into young childhood (ages 2—4). This is followed by a period of abnormally slow and, in some cases, arrested growth that exists between young and older childhood and extends into preadolescence. Finally, the lifespan evidence from this study unearths a premature and accelerated rate of decline in brain size as the individual develops into adolescence and continues until they reach later middle age. The first period of rapid overgrowth is of interest in that the neural defects that cause this overgrowth may point to the neural basis of autism and is in fact the earliest known indicator of the original biological events. The normal child's brain develops and grows more slowly during this period. Changes in brain growth during this time are reflective of functional activity that is modeled and guided through experience and learning. In fact, slower growth, particularly of the frontal lobes, has been associated with higher abilities in long-term outcome studies. The overgrowth in the autistic brain is not reflective of experience and learning but of abnormal cortical neural and laminar connectivity and organization. The authors go on to point to the possibility that this abnormal acceleration of growth may trigger a remodeling phase in which there is an attempt by the system to prune excess axonal connections and neurons leading to the secondary slowing and arrested growth evidenced in that phase observed in older childhood and preadolescence. The degeneration then seen as the child moves into adolescence and adulthood appears in several manifestations of neuroinflammatory processes, such as cortical thinning and atrophy and abnormal increases in cerebrospinal fluid volumes. Clearly, the anatomic pathology changes with age and should prompt those concerned with the care and management of the autistic child, adolescent, and adult to take note and to investigate both behavioral[1] and pharmacologic interventions that improve the patient's quality of life and well being. Lastly, the theory of age-specific brain structure abnormalities in autism will be instrumental in the development and interpretation of animal models to study the disease and studies of brain gene expression.

V. Galea, PhD

Reference

1. Shaw P, Greenstein D, Lerch J, et al. Intellectual ability and cortical development in children and adolescents. *Nature.* 2006;440:676-679.

Physical Activity and Body Mass: Changes in Younger versus Older Postmenopausal Women
Sims ST, Larson JC, Lamonte MJ, et al (Stanford Univ, CA; Fred Hutchinson Cancer Res Ctr, Seattle, WA; Univ at Buffalo, NY; et al)
Med Sci Sports Exerc 44:89-97, 2012

Purpose.—The study's purpose was to investigate the relationship of sedentary (≤ 100 MET·min·wk^{-1}), low (>100–500 MET·min·wk^{-1}), moderate (>500–1200 MET·min·wk^{-1}), and high (>1200 MET·min·wk^{-1}) habitual physical activity with body weight, body mass index, and measures of fat distribution (waist-to-hip ratio) in postmenopausal women by age decades.

Methods.—A prospective cohort study of 58,610 postmenopausal women age 50–79 yr weighed annually during 8 yr at one of 40 US clinical centers was analyzed to determine the relationship of high versus low habitual physical activity with changes in body weight and fat distribution by age group.

Results.—Among women age 50–59 yr, there was significant weight loss in those expending >500–1200 MET·min·wk^{-1} (coefficient = −0.30, 95% confidence interval = −0.53 to −0.07) compared with the group expending ≤ 100 MET·min·wk^{-1}. Among women age 70–79 yr, higher physical activity was associated with less weight loss (coefficient = 0.34, 95% confidence interval = 0.04–0.63). Age at baseline significantly modified the association between physical activity and total weight change, whereas baseline body mass index did not.

Conclusions.—High habitual physical activity is associated with less weight gain in younger postmenopausal women and less weight loss in older postmenopausal women. These findings suggest that promoting physical activity among postmenopausal women may be important for managing body weight changes that accompany aging.

▶ Weight gain early in menopause contributes to increased risk for cardiovascular disease and diabetes, whereas weight loss in women aged 70 and older is associated with increased risk of frailty. The role of physical activity on body weight and fat distribution change over 3 decades was investigated by Sims et al in 58 000 postmenopausal women. Baseline weekly habitual physical activity was determined from self-report. Body weight, body mass index (BMI), and waist-to-hip ratio (WHR) were measured at baseline and over approximately 8 years of follow-up. Body weight and BMI increased in 50- to 59-year-olds (age at study entry), remained stable in women aged 60 to 69 years, and decreased in 70- to 79-year-olds. However, when analyzed by level of physical activity, interesting age group trends emerged. Body weight and BMI were better maintained in 70- to 79-year-old women who reported greater than 1200 MET-min/week of physical activity compared with less active women. After adjusting for numerous demographic, dietary, and lifestyle covariates, a trend ($P = .08$) was found for moderate to higher levels of physical activity (> 500–1200 MET-min/week) to attenuate weight gain in all age groups combined. Weight gain was significantly attenuated in women aged 50 to 59 years, whereas weight gain was greater in 70- to 79-year-olds expending more than 500 MET-min/week compared with the respective sedentary age group. A loss of fat mass in younger women and preservation of lean mass in older women were implied, but not measured. Physical activity did not attenuate the age-associated increase in WHR, suggesting that central adiposity is an effect of aging per se. An energy expenditure of more than 500 to 1200 MET-min/week is in line with the current public health recommendations for adults to exercise at a moderate intensity for 150 min per week.

C. M. Jankowski, PhD

Motor planning and control in autism. A kinematic analysis of preschool children
Forti S, Valli A, Perego P, et al (I.R.C.C.S. "Eugenio Medea" – Ass. La Nostra Famiglia v. Don Luigi Monza, Bosisio Parini (LC), Italy)
Res Autism Spectr Disord 5:834-842, 2011

Kinematic recordings in a reach and drop task were compared between 12 preschool children with autism without mental retardation and 12 gender and age-matched normally developing children. Our aim was to investigate whether motor anomalies in autism may depend more on a planning ability dysfunction or on a motor control deficit. Planning and control processes were separately investigated by examining kinematic recordings divided into primary movement- (planning-based) and corrective submovement- (control-based) phases.

Despite longer movement durations, participants with autism were as accurate in their movements as normally developing children were and showed a preserved movement structure. No differences were observed for the initial movement phases for hand velocity, accuracy and inter-trial variability.

Our main finding was that of a group difference in proximity of the target, at transition from planning-based to control-based movement guidance. At primary movement conclusion, the normally developing children had already reduced velocity and begun orienting their hands for ball drop. Also, they tended to terminate movements within the same movement unit that had transported the hand into the target box. Compared to this group, participants with autism reached this stage with less preparation: their speed was significantly higher, wrist inclination reduced and they showed further movement units after entering the box over the vast majority of trials. These additional movement units were presumed to represent late control-based spatial adjustments. Hence, our data support the hypothesis that children with autism have a greater need for corrective submovements.

We provide evidence that motor anomalies in autism might be determined either by a disruption in planning-control integration, or by a limited planning process capacity, as participants with autism might have been able to plan only the very beginning of the movement, leaving its final phases to further planning on the fly, with important consequences on movement time optimization.

▶ The capacity for motor planning in individuals with autism has been investigated in young adults and adolescents and older children. The publication by Forti and colleagues is important in that they report on the capacity for motor planning and motor control in a much younger age group, preschool children with autism (all age younger than 5 years) compared with gender- and age-matched typically developing preschoolers. In this article, the authors probe the issue of motor planning—motor control dichotomy by designing a simple reach and grasp task, consisting of reaching and grasping a ball and then lifting that ball up to a Plexiglass box with a hole and placing it within the hole. The task was simple enough in that higher-level functioning was not required, thereby ensuring that all participants could complete the task. Additionally, kinematic analysis allowed for acquisition and identification of planning-based movements and control-based movements. In a visually guided task such as this, a motor program is generated through initial planning processes with the program being appropriate to the intended action.[1] The motor control phase would encompass the execution of the task. Control processes would compare the actual movement with the motor plan and errors with respect to the target. Glazebrook et al[2] hypothesized that young adults with autism likely experience dysfunctional motor planning processes resulting in inappropriate timing and specification of muscle forces necessary to the initial aspects of reaching—the part of the task requiring the capacity for motor planning. Conversely, preschoolers with autism were not different from their typically developing counterparts in the movement planning phase, with the exception that movement duration was twice as long than in the controls and that this difference could not only be accounted for by IQ. Of interest to the readers of this volume was the significant difference in the amount of submovements observed in the autism group. Participants with autism showed at least 1 if not several adjustments/corrections, indicating that this group had difficulty with the planning to control transition. Typically developing preschoolers basically completed the task within the first movement phase with very little need for adjustments observed in only 17 of 120 trials. Why is this significant? Essentially, the children with autism from this study showed less capacity for transitions from planning-based to control-based movement guidance in disagreement with the earlier studies on young adults with autism by Glazebrook et al.[2] The tasks used were different, and one might speculate that if transitions from planning to control are dysfunctional in children younger than 5 years, the observations in the young adult might not be reflective of an additive effect that now disrupts motor planning as well. In another vein, these observations may also be hampered by the inherent heterogeneity in individuals with autism and the difficulty in recruiting and assessing participants on the full range of the spectrum, in other words, both high- and low-functioning children with autism.[3]

Note from associate editor: It is unfortunate that errors in the data within the different tables reported in this publication were not corrected before publication. This is one of the few studies out there in which a task such as this has been tested in preschoolers, and for that reason it was deemed worthwhile for inclusion.

V. Galea, PhD

References

1. Glover S. Separate visual representations in the planning and control of action. *Behav Brain Sci.* 2004;27:3-78.
2. Glazebrook CM, Elliott D, Lyons J. A kinematic analysis of how young adults with and without autism plan and control goal-directed movements. *Motor Control.* 2006;10:244-264.
3. Fabbri-Destro M, Cattaneo L, Boria S, Rizzolatti G. Planning actions in autism. *Exp Brain Res.* 2009;192:521-525.

Brief Report: Further Evidence of Sensory Subtypes in Autism
Lane AE, Dennis SJ, Geraghty ME (The Ohio State Univ, Columbus)
J Autism Dev Disord 41:826-831, 2011

Distinct sensory processing (SP) subtypes in autism have been reported previously. This study sought to replicate the previous findings in an independent sample of thirty children diagnosed with an Autism Spectrum Disorder. Model-based cluster analysis of parent-reported sensory functioning (measured using the Short Sensory Profile) confirmed the triad of sensory subtypes reported earlier. Subtypes were differentiated from each other based on degree of SP dysfunction, taste/smell sensitivity and vestibular/ proprioceptive processing. Further elucidation of two of the subtypes was also achieved in this study. Children with a primary pattern of sensory-based inattention could be further described as sensory seekers or non-seekers. Children with a primary pattern of vestibular/proprioceptive dysfunction were also differentiated on movement and tactile sensitivity (Fig 1).

▶ The heterogeneity of presentation of dysfunctional sensory behaviors in children with autism is an area of concern in the design of appropriate and targeted intervention strategies. This study follows and builds on an earlier (2010) publication by Lane[1] and coauthors in the identification of sensory processing subtypes in children with autism disorder. Using a parent self-report tool (the Short Sensory Profile, or SSP), with responses based on a 5-point Likert scale (bounded with "never responds in this manner" and "always" etc.) and then a model-based cluster analysis of the SSP z scores, 5 clusters of

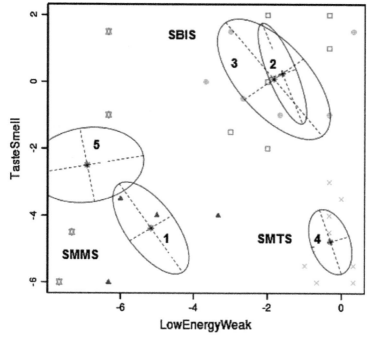

FIGURE 1.—Model-based cluster analysis result. (Reprinted from Lane AE, Dennis SJ, Geraghty ME. Brief report: further evidence of sensory subtypes in autism. *J Autism Dev Disord.* 2011;41:826-831, with permission from Springer Science+Business Media, LLC.)

sensory-processing subtypes became evident. Of particular importance to readers of the YEAR BOOK were the clusters in which the "Low Energy/Weak" domain scores were definitely atypical, such as clusters 1 and 5 (see Fig 1). This domain pertains to the tendency of underresponsiveness to vestibular and proprioceptive sensation and includes items that ask parents about the child's ability for exercise (eg, "seems to have weak muscles," has poor endurance and tires easily, needs to support self while moving"). Concurrent and closely associated with this domain were the domains dealing with tactile and taste/smell sensitivity. Of interest was the observation that the participants in cluster 5 showed greater dysfunction in tactile and movement sensitivity than all other participants. Given recent information on the movement planning difficulties (see the commentary on Forti et al in this volume), it is consistent that these children would be unwilling to challenge their proprioceptive and vestibular systems. In fact, in this publication, the authors describe children within this cluster as being "gravitationally insecure" with a certain dislike of falling, having their feet leave the ground, and being upside down—a very popular maneuver by children playing on monkey bars found on most playgrounds. Publications such as this one by Lane and colleagues provide excellent questions for researchers concerned with the underlying mechanisms of autism and other neurodevelopmental dysfunctions such as developmental coordination disorder because it is only recently that developmental neuroscientists are tackling the difficult neurophysiological and biomechanical consequences of autism. These studies are necessary because they supplement and clarify the self-report-based studies that reveal these sensory processing difficulties and provide further bases for sensory-based targeted interventions, as also suggested by Lane and coauthors. Observation of dysfunction in sensory processing may also provide another biological marker, allowing for earlier identification of autism and autism spectrum disorders because these processes manifest in early childhood.

V. Galea, PhD

Reference

1. Lane AE, Young RL, Baker AE, Angley MT. Sensory processing subtypes in autism: association with adaptive behavior. *J Autism Dev Disord.* 2010;40:112-122.

Neural signatures of autism

Kaiser MD, Hudac CM, Shultz S, et al (Yale School of Medicine, New Haven, CT)

Proc Natl Acad Sci U S A 107:21223-21228, 2010

Functional magnetic resonance imaging of brain responses to biological motion in children with autism spectrum disorder (ASD), unaffected siblings (US) of children with ASD, and typically developing (TD) children has revealed three types of neural signatures: (*i*) state activity, related to the state of having ASD that characterizes the nature of disruption in brain circuitry; (*ii*) trait activity, reflecting shared areas of dysfunction in US and children with ASD, thereby providing a promising neuroendophenotype to facilitate efforts to bridge genomic complexity and disorder heterogeneity; and (*iii*) compensatory activity, unique to US, suggesting a neural system—level mechanism by which US might compensate for an increased genetic risk for developing ASD. The distinct brain responses to biological motion exhibited by TD children and US are striking given the identical behavioral profile of these two groups. These findings offer far-reaching implications for our understanding of the neural systems underlying autism.

▶ Our understanding of neural systems underlying autism spectrum disorder (ASD) is far from adequate and is woefully incomplete. ASD is a developmental disorder that becomes evident during the first year of life. Of note is the tremendous heterogeneity of this disorder, leading clinicians to use the mantra, "If you have seen 1 child with ASD, you have seen 1 child with ASD!" Kaiser and coworkers contribute a significant step forward in this work through the identification of 3 types of neural signatures, as revealed by functional MRI, in children with ASD, unaffected siblings of children with ASD, and typically developing children. Previous neuroimaging studies in adults and older children with ASD have shown abnormal activity, in response to biologic motion, in the posterior superior temporal sulcus, which is an area of the brain supporting social interaction. In this study, the authors compared brain activation to point-light displays of human motion with that to scrambled motion, given that visual sensitivity to people's movements is fundamental to adaptive social engagement and interaction. Moreover, visual sensitivity to biologic motion is an ontogenetically early-emerging mechanism. Point-light displays are videos created by placing lights on parts of a moving person, usually on major joints or segments, and then filming them in the dark while they are moving. State activity, defined as "activity related to the state of having ASD that characterizes the nature of disruption in brain circuitry," was observed in children with ASD as young as 4 years, who showed dysfunctional activity in the right amygdala, right posterior superior temporal sulcus, bilateral fusiform gyri, left ventrolateral prefrontal cortex, and left ventromedial prefrontal cortex, as in adults with ASD. Trait activity is defined as "that activity reflecting shared areas of dysfunction in unaffected siblings and children with ASD." The observations related to trait activity are particularly important regarding first-order relatives of children with ASD, although the majority were unrelated probands, that is, they were not related to the children with ASD in the ASD group. Interestingly, the unaffected siblings were rigorously screened on various scales of social responsiveness and adaptive behavior scales and thus were behaviorally indistinguishable from the group of typically developing children. It is this trait activity that promises to provide what the authors call a neuroendophenotype aiding in the bridging of the gene-behavior gap and to contribute to the search for pathophysiological mechanisms of this devastating disorder. This article is of interest to readers of the YEAR BOOK because it will extend the knowledge of those who work with children with ASD, possibly in the area of developing exercise-related interventions. These children do not learn the same way as typically developing children and exhibit dysfunctional motor coordination.

V. Galea, PhD

Sensory Processing in Autism: A Review of Neurophysiologic Findings
Marco EJ, Hinkley LBN, Hill SS, et al (Univ of California, San Francisco)
Pediatr Res 69:48R-54R, 2011

Atypical sensory-based behaviors are a ubiquitous feature of autism spectrum disorders (ASDs). In this article, we review the neural underpinnings of sensory processing in autism by reviewing the literature on neurophysiological responses to auditory, tactile, and visual stimuli in autistic individuals. We review studies of unimodal sensory processing and multisensory integration that use a variety of neuroimaging techniques, including electroencephalography (EEG), magnetoencephalography (MEG), and functional MRI. We then explore the impact of covert and overt attention on sensory processing. With additional characterization, neurophysiologic profiles of sensory processing in ASD may serve as valuable biomarkers for diagnosis and monitoring of therapeutic interventions for autism and reveal potential strategies and target brain regions for therapeutic interventions.

▶ The search for neurophysiological biomarkers for diagnosis of autism spectrum disorder (ASD) is important to the early detection of this disorder and for implementation of early intervention and management. The problem is compounded by the significant heterogeneity of the presentation; however, besides the definite impairment in communication and social interaction exhibited by most persons on the autism spectrum, sensory behavioral differences from typically developing children are common. Children with ASD often show atypical (quite distressed) responses to seemingly innocuous auditory stimuli, such as a running vacuum cleaner. Marco and coworkers contribute an excellent review of the current literature on abnormal unimodal stimuli (auditory, visual, and tactile) as well as both low- and high-level multisensory integration. This is an important article for clinicians working with children and adults with ASD because of the insights to management of these deficits in unimodal sensory processing and multisensory integration provide. Of interest are the atypical behavioral responses to tactile stimulation, which usually manifest as a hypersensitivity to stimuli in this domain. One might also ask how proprioception is affected in these individuals because abnormal cerebellar activity has been implicated in both unimodal and multisensory integration processing in ASD. Unfortunately, tactile sensation has been largely overlooked in the research literature, and studies on proprioceptive function do not seem to exist at all. These deficits point toward the ever-increasing evidence of motor dyscoordination in children with ASD, which then becomes yet another factor that compounds their inability to interact within their peer groups and integrate into society. As these authors conclude, an understanding of basic sensory procession in ASD is an important undertaking. Of particular interest is whether these deficits in sensory processing, which manifest as either a hyper- or a hyposensitivity, are a primary feature of this disorder or are the result of learned behaviors. This can be investigated through studies of infant siblings of children with ASD. Of significance to the readers of the YEAR BOOK is the knowledge gained through the careful characterization of sensory behaviors so that treatment is appropriate to the child and is effective to that child's particular sensory behavioral phenotype.

V. Galea, PhD

Spectrum of neurodevelopmental disabilities in children with cerebellar malformations
Bolduc M-E, Du Plessis AJ, Sullivan N, et al (McGill Univ, Montreal, Quebec, Canada; Children's Hosp Boston and Harvard Med School, MA; et al)
Dev Med Child Neurol 53:409-416, 2011

Aim.—Advances in perinatal care and neuroimaging techniques have increased the detection of cerebellar malformations (CBMs) in the fetus and young infant. As a result, this has necessitated a greater understanding of the neurodevelopmental consequences of CBMs on child development. The aim of this study was to delineate the impact of CBMs on long-term neurodevelopmental outcomes.

Method.—We conducted a cross-sectional study and systematically iden- tified children with CBMs born between December 2000 and December 2006. We then performed follow-up magnetic resonance imaging studies, neurologic examination, and standardized neurodevelopmental outcome testing (Mullen Scales of Early Learning, Vineland Adaptive Behavior Scale, Child Behavior Checklist, Modified Checklist for Autism in Toddlers, and the Pediatric Quality of Life Inventory).

Results.—Our sample comprised 49 children (29 males, 20 females; mean age, 28.4mo, SD 16.4) with a CBM. Infants with evidence of acquired fetal or neonatal brain injury, intracranial birth trauma, inherited metabolic disease, or major pre- or postnatal cerebral ischemia were excluded. Our findings highlight that children with CBMs experience a high prevalence of neurologic, developmental, and functional disabilities including motor, cognitive, language, and social—behavioral deficits, as well as poor quality of life. The associated supratentorial anomalies, chromosomal findings, and malformations affecting the cerebellar vermis were significant indepen- dent predictors of neurodevelopmental disabilities in young children with CBMs. The associated supratentorial anomalies and chromosomal findings were also predictive of global developmental delay ($p=0.01$), cognitive impairment ($p=0.03$), gross and fine motor delay ($p=0.02$ and $p=0.01$ respectively), and positive screening for autism spectrum disorder ($p=0.01$). Additionally, malformations affecting the cerebellar vermis were significant independent predictors of expressive language ($p=0.04$) and gross motor delays ($p=0.02$).

Interpretation.—Developmental surveillance and early intervention programs should be an integral part of the long-term follow-up of survi- vors of CBM.

▶ Studies reporting on the quality of life in children with cerebellar malformations are rare, and those that do exist tend to be plagued by poor design and outcome determination. This study by Bolduc and colleagues is part of a cross-sectional study of children born at term with cerebellar malformations and is the first of its kind to evaluate health-related quality of life in these children. Participants were identified through an electronic search of a magnetic resonance image data- base and had an antenatal or neonatal diagnosis of various cerebellar malforma- tions; the families of these patients were then approached for inclusion in the study. Extensive testing was performed in the form of standard neurologic exam- inations of oculomotor, motor, and sensory function as well as measurement of head circumference and developmental and functional measures such as the Mullen Scales of Early Learning and the Peabody Developmental Motor Scale; health-related quality of life was measured using a parent proxy instrument, the Pediatric Quality of Life Inventory, and finally measures of social-behavioral indices, the Child Behavior Checklist and the Modified Checklist for Autism in Toddlers.[1] Testing took place at 1 time point between ages 1 and 6 years. Of particular importance to those interested in the impact of cerebellar damage to behavior and motor/sensory function is the impact of the various diagnostic groups of cerebellar malformation as well as the impact on social and behavioral dysfunction in those children with vermal malformations.[2,3] The vermis forms the midline of the cerebellum and connects the cerebellar hemispheres. These authors report that malformations involving the vermis were the ones mostly associated with greater developmental disabilities, such as cognitive, gross motor, and language impairments. A vast spectrum of neurologic impairment as well as developmental and social-behavioral dysfunction represented a considerable impact on the quality of life of these children. The impact of this diagnosis on the child and family's quality of life necessitates targeted early intervention programs that will hopefully ameliorate this situation.

V. Galea, PhD

References

1. Boddaert N, Klein O, Ferguson N, et al. Intellectual prognosis of the Dandy-Walker malformation in children: the importance of vermian lobulation. *Neuroradiology.* 2003;45:320-324.
2. Bolduc ME, Limperopoulos C. Neurodevelopmental outcomes in children with cerebellar malformations: a systematic review. *Dev Med Child Neurol.* 2009;51: 256-267.
3. Limperopoulos C, Robertson RL, Estroff JA, et al. Diagnosis of inferior vermian hypoplasia by fetal magnetic resonance imaging: potential pitfalls and neurodevelopmental outcome. *Am J Obstet Gynecol.* 2006;194:1070-1076.

Statistically characterizing intra- and inter-individual variability in children with Developmental Coordination Disorder
King BR, Harring JR, Oliveira MA, et al (Univ of Maryland, College Park)
Res Dev Disabil 32:1388-1398, 2011

Previous research investigating children with Developmental Coordination Disorder (DCD) has consistently reported increased intra- and inter-individual variability during motor skill performance. Statistically characterizing this variability is not only critical for the analysis and interpretation of behavioral data, but also may facilitate our understanding of the processes underlying DCD. Thus, the primary purpose of this research was to demonstrate the utility of a flexible statistical technique, a random coefficient model (RCM), that characterizes the increased intra- and inter-individual variability in children with and without DCD. We analyzed data from a sensorimotor adaptation task during which participants executed discrete aiming movements under conditions of rotated visual feedback. To highlight the advantages of this statistical approach, we contrasted the results from the RCM with those from a traditionally employed general linear model (GLM). The RCM revealed differences between the two groups of children that the GLM did not detect; and, characterized trajectories of change for each individual. The RCM provides researchers an opportunity to probe behavioral deficits at the *individual* level and may provide new insights into the behavioral heterogeneity in children with DCD.

▶ Recent evidence points to the existence of several subtypes of a condition collectively called developmental coordination disorder (DCD). Those interested in the mechanisms underlying these deficits are hampered in their studies by the considerable between-subject variability encountered in this population. Too often, the result, using traditional statistical general linear models (GLM), is no significant differences between DCD and typically developing (TD) children in various motor tasks. The work by King and collaborators offers alternate statistical paradigms that allow for statistical treatment of both average change in the population of interest and, more importantly, a subject-specific change that is unique to each individual. To demonstrate the utility of this statistical treatment, they tested the performance of TD children and children with DCD on a discrete aiming movement task using a visuomotor "distortion" protocol. Briefly, the child is asked to execute aiming movement to 3 different visual targets located 9 cm from a central start position. The hand is hidden from vision with visual feedback of the movement being provided on a computer monitor. This experimental setup then allows for distortion of the visual feedback of the hand displacement, which, in this case, was rotated 60° clockwise to the veridical trajectory. The child must then adapt their hand movement to hit the target. The variable of interest in this type of sensorimotor adaptation task is the root mean squared error (RMSE) between the actual movement and the straight line from the start to the target position. Errors in both motor planning and control are reflected in the RMSE with higher values of this variable reflecting progressively poorer performance. The RMSE is an excellent outcome measure for this population because it is thought to reflect errors in both motor planning and execution (control), both of which are deficient in children with DCD. This publication contains an excellent explanation and application of a random coefficient model (RCM), including some excellent resources for those interested in adopting this statistical technique. One significant benefit is the ability of this model to handle missing data in the repeated measures/longitudinal design as opposed to the problem with GLM, where the entire participant would have to be deleted because of missing data points. In addition, the variance/covariance structure within an RCM does not have to meet the assumption of constancy across observations (variance) or any 2 observations (covariance). This assumption is often violated with longitudinal data when using general linear models. The task in question revealed two rates of adaptation to the visuomotor distortion, and so a double exponential was used for this data set. Use of the RCM revealed that the number of children with DCD were decreased in the slow adaptation rate and also exhibited considerable between-subject variability with 2 of the DCD participants performing considerably worse than the TD children and others performing considerably better than the TD and other children in the DCD group. These statistical techniques are useful when determining various child groups' responses to an exercise intervention and would also be useful in the possible identification of responder subtypes.

V. Galea, PhD

Annual Research Review: Development of the cerebral cortex: implications for neurodevelopmental disorders

Rubenstein JLR (Univ of California at San Francisco)
J Child Psychol Psychiatry 52:339-355, 2011

The cerebral cortex has a central role in cognitive and emotional processing. As such, understanding the mechanisms that govern its development and function will be central to understanding the bases of severe neuropsychiatric disorders, particularly those that first appear in childhood. In this review, I highlight recent progress in elucidating genetic, molecular and cellular mechanisms that control cortical development. I discuss basic aspects of cortical developmental anatomy, and mechanisms that regulate cortical size and area formation, with an emphasis on the roles of fibroblast growth factor (Fgf) signaling and specific transcription factors. I then examine how specific types of cortical excitatory projection neurons are generated, and how their axons grow along stereotyped pathways to their targets. Next, I address how cortical inhibitory (GABAergic) neurons are generated, and point out the role of these cells in controlling cortical plasticity and critical periods. The paper concludes with an examination of four possible developmental mechanisms that could contribute to some forms of neurodevelopmental disorders, such as autism.

▶ Autism spectrum disorder (ASD) has become one of the most studied neurodevelopmental disorders. The central role of the cerebral cortex in cognitive and emotional processing is intricately studied in this review by Rubenstein from the perspective of aspects of both cortical anatomical development and the mechanisms that regulate cortical size, a factor known to be increased in patients with ASD, and the behavioral consequences of such deficits in molecular programming of growth and development. Of interest to the readers of this volume are the significant deficits in cortical pathways contributing to normal sensorimotor development, pathways that support motor control and motor learning, and pathways, such as the prefrontal-tectal-cerebellar and the cortical-basal ganglia circuitry, that support the development of goal-directed movement. Within this excellent review, one also finds new information as to the importance of the cerebellum in aspects of cognitive function. Given that the typical cortical growth and identity of developing structures in the brain are regulated through the secretion of a family of molecules called morphogens and that this is a dose-dependent mechanism, one is tempted to speculate about the contribution of deficits in dosage to other disorders of childhood, such as developmental coordination disorder and other motor learning issues that have been identified in childhood. This review provides excellent background information for those clinicians concerned with the development of motor function and the ability to engage in sport and exercise during childhood and adolescence.

V. Galea, PhD

Exclusive breastfeeding duration and cardiorespiratory fitness in children and adolescents

Labayen I, Ruiz JR, Ortega FB, et al (Univ of the Basque Country, Vitoria, Spain; Karolinska Institutet, Huddinge, Sweden; et al)
Am J Clin Nutr 95:498-505, 2012

Background.—Breastfeeding has been associated with a protective effect against cardiovascular disease. Higher cardiorespiratory fitness during childhood is associated with healthier cardiovascular profile later in life.

Objectives.—The objective was to examine the association of exclusive breastfeeding duration with fitness in children and adolescents and to test the role of body composition and sociodemographic factors in this relation.

Design.—At the time of the study, exclusive breastfeeding duration was reported by mothers and grouped into 4 categories: exclusively formula fed or breastfed for <3, 3–6, or >6 mo. Fitness was determined by a maximal cycle-ergometer test in 1025 children (aged 9.5 ± 0.4 y) and in 971 adolescents (aged 15.5 ± 0.5 y) from Estonia and Sweden.

Results.—Longer duration of breastfeeding was associated with higher fitness regardless of confounders [+5.1% L/min; country, sex, age, pubertal status, and BMI (adjusted $P < 0.001$) or fat mass and fat-free mass (FFM) (+3.3%; adjusted $P < 0.001$)]. Further adjustment for birth weight, physical activity, and maternal educational level did not change the results ($P = 0.001$). The results were consistent in children and adolescents with low ($P < 0.001$) or high ($P = 0.013$) FFM, in nonoverweight ($P < 0.001$) or overweight ($P = 0.002$) children and adolescents, in offspring of nonoverweight ($P < 0.001$) or overweight ($P = 0.003$) mothers, in mothers with a low ($P = 0.004$) or high ($P < 0.001$) educational level, and in participants born within upper ($P = 0.001$), middle ($P = 0.017$), or lower ($P = 0.007$) tertiles of birth weight.

Conclusions.—Longer exclusive breastfeeding has a beneficial effect on cardiorespiratory fitness in children and adolescents. Because early infant-feeding patterns are potentially modifiable, a better understanding of the possible programming effect of exclusive breastfeeding on cardiorespiratory fitness is of public health interest (Table 1).

▶ Nutrition during early life is plainly very important to the health of the developing child, although 2 previous studies[1,2] have found little influence of the duration of breastfeeding on physical fitness during childhood and adolescence. Because cardiorespiratory fitness is usually expressed in units of milliliter per kilogram minutes, the most obvious way in which fitness might be affected would be by a greater development of body fat in the bottle-fed babies. The data of Labayen and associates do show an almost significant trend in this sense, and, although the units of relative aerobic power (mL/[kg·min]) show benefit to those who were breastfed, the absolute values (L/min) do not. However, the most striking trend, again nonsignificant, is a trend to a much greater lean tissue mass in those breast fed for more than 6 months (Table 1), an observation in keeping with the previously observed greater long jump in those who were breast fed

TABLE 1.—Patterns of Exclusive Breastfeeding Duration in Swedish and Estonian Children and Adolescents

| | Estonian | | Swedish | |
| | Children ($n = 508$) | Adolescents ($n = 458$) | Children ($n = 517$) | Adolescents ($n = 513$) |
Duration of breastfeeding	%		%	
Exclusively formula-fed	16.7	21.7	12.0	13.0
Breastfed				
<3 mo	60.2	50.2	31.1	36.0
3-6 mo	13.9	18.4	38.9	32.7
>6 mo	9.2	9.7	18.0	18.3

for a long period.[1] Other possible biological mechanisms include suggestions that breast milk contains substances lacking in infant formulae, such as long-chain polyunsaturated fatty acids, trophic substances, hormones, and specific nutrients.[3,4] Nevertheless, it is difficult to exclude confounding factors, particularly as the mothers who engaged in prolonged breastfeeding seem to have come from a lower socioeconomic stratum. There seems scope for further study of this interesting issue.

R. J. Shephard, MD (Lond), PhD, DPE

References

1. Artero EG, Ortega FB, España-Romero V, et al. Longer breastfeeding is associated with increased lower body explosive strength during adolescence. *J Nutr.* 2010; 140:1989-1995.
2. Wennlöf AH, Yngve A, Sjöström M. Sampling procedure, participation rates and representativeness in the Swedish part of the European Youth Heart Study (EYHS). *Public Health Nutr.* 2003;6:291-299.
3. Forsyth JS. Do LCPUFAs influence cardiovascular function in early childhood? *Adv Exp Med Biol.* 2009;646:59-63.
4. Koletzko B, von Kries R, Closa R, et al. Can infant feeding choices modulate later obesity risk? *Am J Clin Nutr.* 2009;89:1502S-1508S.

Who is really at risk? Identifying risk factors for subthreshold and full syndrome eating disorders in a high-risk sample

Jacobi C, Fittig E, Bryson SW, et al (Technische Universität Dresden, Germany; Washington Univ Saint Louis, MO; Stanford Univ School of Medicine, CA)
Psychol Med 41:1939-1949, 2011

Background.—Numerous longitudinal studies have identified risk factors for the onset of most eating disorders (EDs). Identifying women at highest risk within a high-risk sample would allow for focusing of preventive resources and also suggests different etiologies.

Method.—A longitudinal cohort study over 3 years in a high-risk sample of 236 college-age women randomized to the control group of a prevention trial for EDs. Potential risk factors and interactions between risk factors were assessed using the methods developed previously. Main outcome measures were time to onset of a subthreshold or full ED.

Results.—At the 3-year follow-up, 11.2% of participants had developed a full or partial ED. Seven of 88 potential risk factors could be classified as independent risk factors, seven as proxies, and two as overlapping factors. Critical comments about eating from teacher/coach/siblings and a history of depression were the most potent risk factors. The incidence for participants with either or both of these risk factors was 34.8% (16/46) compared to 4.2% (6/144) for participants without these risk factors, with a sensitivity of 0.75 and a specificity of 0.82.

Conclusions.—Targeting preventive interventions at women with high weight and shape concerns, a history of critical comments about eating weight and shape, and a history of depression may reduce the risk for EDs.

▶ This prospective 3-year longitudinal cohort study of a high-risk sample of college women identified 7 independent risk factors, 7 proxies, and 2 overlapping factors, with relatively high specificity and sensitivity for predicting development of subthreshold or full-syndrome eating disorders (EDs) in 11.2% of this population. This incidence is similar to that reported in other cross-sectional studies using *Diagnostic and Statistical Manual of Mental Disorders* (Fourth Revision) definitions of anorexia nervosa, bulimia nervosa, and binge ED (BED) as well as syndromes not otherwise specified.

High-risk status was determined by using a cutoff score on the Weight Concerns Scale (WCS), and exact definitions and research methods for identifying risk and etiology factors were employed. Prebaseline measures were assessed retrospectively and baseline measures prospectively at 1, 2, and 3 years. Case definition was with the Eating Disorder Examination (EDE) interview, adapted to include the diagnostic criteria for BED.

Of importance, prebaseline comments about eating and about weight and shape by either teacher or coach were related significantly and positively to ED onset. A history of depression was also significant. At baseline, the Eating Concern scale of the Eating Disorder Examination Questionnaire, level of compensatory behaviors, and number of alcohol drinks in a week predicted ED onset.

The results of this study suggest that a 2-step screening process (first, using the WCS to identify women with high weight and shape concerns; second, further screening for history of negative comments about eating and/or depression) might be theoretically useful to pick up women most at risk for development of subthreshold and full-syndrome ED in select populations. In the setting of athletic teams, such a tool could easily be incorporated into the preparticipation physical examination, and this approach could also aid in targeting preventative measures for those at highest risk.

C. Lebrun, MDCM, MPE, CCFP, Dip Sport Med, FACSM

Associations Between Disordered Eating, Menstrual Dysfunction, and Musculoskeletal Injury Among High School Athletes

Thein-Nissenbaum JM, Rauh MJ, Carr KE, et al (Univ of Wisconsin School of Medicine and Public Health, Madison; Rocky Mountain Univ of Health Professions, Provo, UT; et al)
J Orthop Sports Phys Ther 41:60-69, 2011

Study Design.—Retrospective cohort study.

Objectives.—To determine the prevalence of, and association between, disordered eating (DE), menstrual dysfunction (MD), and musculoskeletal injury (MI) among high school female athletes.

Background.—Female athlete triad (Triad) syndrome is the interrelatedness of DE, MD, and low bone mass. Few studies have examined 2 or more Triad components simultaneously, or their relationship to injury, among female high school athletes.

Methods.—The subject sample consisted of 311 female high school athletes competing on 33 interscholastic high school teams during the 2006-2007 school year. Athletes completed the Eating Disorder Examination Questionnaire (EDE-Q) and Healthy Wisconsin High School Female Athletes Survey (HWHSFAS). Athletes were classified by sport type as aesthetic (AES), endurance (END), or team/anaerobic (T/A).

Results.—Of those surveyed, 35.4% reported DE, 18.8% reported MD, and 65.6% reported sustaining a sports-related musculoskeletal injury during the current sports season. Athletes reporting DE were twice as likely to be injured compared to those reporting normal eating behaviors (odds ratio [OR], 2.3; 95% confidence interval [CI]: 1.4, 4.0). Multivariate logistic regression analyses revealed that athletes who reported a history of DE (OR, 2.1; 95% CI: 1.1, 3.9) or prior injury (OR, 5.1; 95% CI: 2.9, 8.9) were more likely to be injured during the sports season.

Conclusion.—A high prevalence of DE and MD exists among high school female athletes. Additionally, athletes with DE were over 2 times more likely to sustain a sports-related injury during a sports season. Screening and intervention programs designed to identify and decrease the prevalence of DE should be implemented with high school females.

Level of Evidence.—Prognosis, level 2b (Table 5).

▶ Thein-Nissenbaum and colleagues fill a gap in understanding the association of 2 components of the female athlete triad (Triad)—disordered eating and menstrual dysfunction—with musculoskeletal injuries among high school athletes. The physiologic underpinning of these associations could be low energy availability that compromises the integrity of cellular activities necessary to maintain musculoskeletal function, repair, and recovery from injury. The outcomes were obtained from questionnaires pertaining to eating habits, menstrual cycle history, and injury history over a season of sport participation by approximately 300 female high school athletes. Aesthetic (eg, cheerleading, gymnastics), endurance (eg, basketball, cross country), and team/anaerobic (eg, volleyball, track and field) sports were included. The main finding was a 2-fold greater incidence of overuse and

TABLE 5.—Injury Incidence and Crude Odds Ratios by Disordered Eating (DE) Status

Variable	n	Overuse Injury Incidence (%)	OR	95% CI	Traumatic Injury Incidence (%)	OR	95% CI	Overall Injury Incidence (%)	OR	95% CI
Aesthetic										
Normal	24	66.7	1.0	Reference	37.5	1.0	Reference	66.7	1.0	Reference
DE*	17	88.2	3.8	0.7, 20.6	41.2	1.2	0.3, 4.2	94.1	8.0	0.9, 71.6
Endurance										
Normal	56	51.8	1.0	Reference	32.1	1.0	Reference	62.5	1.0	Reference
DE*	33	60.6	1.4	0.6, 3.4	48.5	2.0	0.8, 4.8	81.8	2.7	1.0, 7.6
Team/anaerobic										
Normal	121	48.8	1.0	Reference	20.7	1.0	Reference	56.2	1.0	Reference
DE*	60	70.0	2.5†	1.3, 4.7	23.3	1.2	0.6, 2.5	70.0	1.8	0.9, 3.5
Total										
Normal	201	51.7	1.0	Reference	25.9	1.0	Reference	59.2	1.0	Reference
DE*	110	70.0	2.2†	1.3, 3.6	33.6	1.5	0.9, 2.4	77.3	2.3†	1.4, 4.0

Abbreviations: CI, confidence interval (upper and lower bounds); DE, disordered eating; OR, odds ratio.
*DE defined as a mean score of 4.0 or higher on the dietary restraint, weight concern, or shape concern subscales of the EDE-Q or having a mean global score of greater than 4.0 on the EDE-Q, or having a pathologic behavior).
†Odds ratio for injury is significantly greater for DE group when compared to the reference group, as CI does not include 1 ($P \leq .05$).

traumatic musculoskeletal injuries in athletes who reported disordered eating (Table 5). The classification of an injury included those injuries that were not reported to a coach or trainer and injuries that did not cause a missed practice or competition. Some interesting secondary findings were that 38% of athletes who sustained an injury did not report it, and, of these athletes, 16% feared that reporting the injury would limit their participation in the sport. Menstrual disorder was defined as < 9 cycles in the previous year or lack of menstruation by age 15. Menstrual disorder was not significantly associated with injury, but this finding comes with the caveat that menstrual cycle irregularities are prevalent within the first 5 years after menarche, so "regular" menstrual cycles are not necessarily normal among high school athletes. A follow-up study that includes circulating sex hormone levels would shed more light on the relation of menstrual disorder and musculoskeletal injuries. The greater prevalence in female than male athletes of injuries such as spondylolysis, patellofemoral pain, chronic exertional compartment syndrome, and anterior cruciate ligament injury points to mechanisms that could be mediated by sex hormones. The revised definition of the female athlete triad is the interrelatedness of energy availability, menstrual function, and bone mineral density.[1] Although this study was underway before the revised Triad was published, it remains relevant because so little is known about the early onset or warning signs of the Triad.

C. M. Jankowski, PhD

Reference

1. Nattiv A, Loucks AB, Manore MM, Sanborn CF, Sundgot-Borgen J, Warren MP. American College of Sports Medicine position stand. The female athlete triad. *Med Sci Sports Exerc.* 2007;39:1867-1882.

Cardiovascular Consequences of Ovarian Disruption: A Focus on Functional Hypothalamic Amenorrhea in Physically Active Women
O'Donnell E, Goodman JM, Harvey PJ (Univ of Toronto, Ontario, Canada)
J Clin Endocrinol Metab 96:3638-3648, 2011

Context.—Evidence indicates that hypoestrogenemia is linked with accelerated progression of atherosclerosis. Premenopausal women presenting with ovulatory disruption due to functional hypothalamic amenorrhea (FHA) are characterized by hypoestrogenemia. One common and reversible form of FHA in association with energy deficiency is exercise-associated amenorrhea (EAA).

Evidence Acquisition.—Articles were found via PubMed search for both original and review articles based on peer review publications between 1974 and 2011 reporting on cardiovascular changes in women with FHA, with emphasis placed on women with EAA.

Evidence Synthesis.—Despite participation in regular exercise training, hypoestrogenic women with EAA demonstrate paradoxical changes in cardiovascular function, including endothelial dysfunction, a known permissive factor for the progression and development of atherosclerosis. Such alterations suggest that the beneficial effects of regular exercise training on vascular function are obviated in the face of hypoestrogenemia. The long-term cardiovascular consequences of altered vascular function in response to ovulatory disruption in women with EAA remain to be determined. Retrospective data, however, suggest premature development and progression of coronary artery disease in older premenopausal women reporting a history of hypothalamic ovulatory disruption. Importantly, in women with EAA, estrogen therapy, folic acid supplementation without change in menstrual status, and resumption of menses restores endothelial function. In this review, we focus on the influence of hypoestrogenemia in association with energy deficiency in mediating changes in cardiovascular function in women with EAA, including endothelial function, regional blood flow, lipid profile, and autonomic control of blood pressure, heart rate, and baroreflex sensitivity. The influence of exercise training is also considered.

Conclusion.—With the premenopausal years typically considered to be cardioprotective in association with normal ovarian function, ovarian disruption in women with EAA is of importance. Further investigation of the short-term, and potentially long-term, cardiovascular consequences of hypoestrogenemia in women with EAA is recommended (Fig 2, Table 1).

▶ It is commonly accepted that hypoestrogenism due to ovarian disruption and functional hypothalamic amenorrhea has important implications for both short-term and long-term bone health. It is less well recognized that there are also many potential cardiovascular consequences. Prior to menopause, women have a much lower incidence of coronary artery disease than age-matched men, largely because of the beneficial effects of endogenous estrogen. This is because of the protective effects on myriad multifaceted mechanisms, including endothelial,

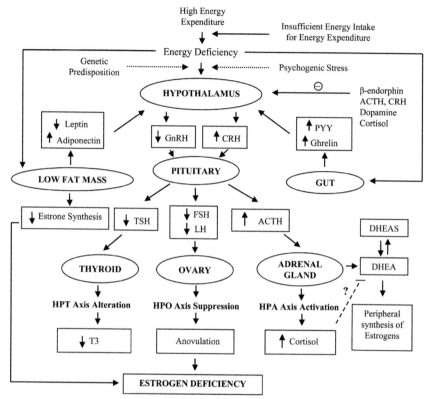

FIGURE 2.—Metabolic consequences of EAA. HPO, Hypothalamic-pituitary-ovarian; DHEA-S, DHEA sulfate. HPA, Hypothalamic-pituitary-adrenal; HPO, hypothalamic-pituitary-ovarian; HPT, hypothalamic-pituitary-thyroid; PYY, peptide YY. (Reprinted from O'Donnell E, Goodman JM, Harvey PJ. Cardiovascular consequences of ovarian disruption: a focus on functional hypothalamic amenorrhea in physically active women. *J Clin Endocrinol Metab.* 2011;96:3638-3648, Copyright 2011, with permission from The Endocrine Society.)

myocardial, neurohumoral, vascular, and metabolic factors. For example, amenorrhea has been associated with impaired bioactivity of nitric oxide, endothelial dysfunction, and altered lipid profile, all of which contribute to premature initiation and accelerated progression of atherosclerosis.[1,2] It has also been established that it is the low energy availability, not the stress of exercise, that disrupts the hypothalamic-pituitary axis in these women.[3] It is therefore important to balance regular aerobic exercise training with maintenance of energy balance and optimal estrogen levels in these young athletic women to prevent any untoward cardiovascular sequelae.

This well-referenced article reviews the current literature about the complex interactions of metabolic alterations (Fig 2) and known or potential clinical consequences (Table 1) occurring as a result of exercise-associated amenorrhea. It discusses the role of regular aerobic exercise training and suggests future areas

TABLE 1.—Mechanisms of Action and Known or Potential Clinical Consequences of Altered Cardiovascular Function in Hypoestrogenic Premenopausal Women with EAA

Physiological Outcome	Mechanisms of Action	Known or Potential Clinical Consequences
Endothelial dysfunction	Estrogen deficiency leading to impaired NO bioavailability. Role of metabolic or psychogenic stress unclear.	ED is a permissive factor in the development and progression of atherogenesis. Not yet known whether women with EAA are at increased risk of premature development of CAD.
Lowered regional blood flow	Estrogen deficiency leading to impaired NO bioavailability. Role of metabolic or psychogenic stress unclear.	CV consequences of lowered regional blood flow in women with EAA are unclear.
Increased regional vascular resistance	Counter-mechanism to help defend/ regulate blood pressure in the face of lowered SBP? Role of estrogen deficiency and metabolic or psychogenic stress unclear.	Increased peripheral vascular resistance is associated with increased arterial stiffness. Not yet known whether women with EAA demonstrate altered arterial stiffness.
Lowered resting SBP	Potentially favorable adaptation to caloric restriction? Role of estrogen deficiency or metabolic stress unclear.	Low "normal" resting blood pressure is favorable to vascular structure and function. However, hypotension may result in orthostatic intolerance. Orthostatic intolerance in women with EAA has not yet been investigated.
Lowered resting HR	Potentially favorable adaptation to caloric restriction? Role of estrogen deficiency or metabolic stress unclear.	Low resting HR is associated with favorable autonomic tone. Altered autonomic function has not yet been confirmed in women with EAA.
Altered lipid profile and increased lipid peroxidation potential	Conflicting influence of elevated LDLc and HDLc on endothelial function unclear. Decreased antioxidant status and/or increased prooxidant status in the face of estrogen deficiency? Role of metabolic stress unclear.	Elevated LDLc negatively, and elevated HDLc positively, influence vascular function. Lipid peroxidation is implicated in the pathogenesis of atherosclerotic vascular disease. Not yet known whether altered lipid profile and/or "potential" to lipid peroxidation contributes to vascular dysfunction in women with EAA.

CV, Cardiovascular; ED, endothelial dysfunction; HR, heart rate; SBP, systolic blood pressure.

for research. It is a must-read for any clinicians and scientists interested in this field.

C. Lebrun, MDCM, MPE, CCFP, Dip Sport Med, FACSM

References

1. Rickenlund A, Eriksson MJ, Schenck-Gustafsson K, Hirschberg AL. Amenorrhea in female athletes is associated with endothelial dysfunction and unfavorable lipid profile. *J Clin Endocrinol Metab.* 2005;90:1354-1359.
2. Hoch AZ, Jurva JW, Staton MA, et al. Athletic amenorrhea and endothelial dysfunction. *WJM.* 2007;106:301-306.
3. Loucks AB, Verdun M, Heath EM. Low energy availability, not stress of exercise, alters LH pulsatility in exercising women. *J Appl Physiol.* 1998;84:37-46.

Bone Quality and Muscle Strength in Female Athletes with Lower Limb Stress Fractures

Schnackenburg KE, MacDonald HM, Ferber R, et al (Univ of Calgary, Alberta, Canada; Univ of British Columbia, Vancouver)
Med Sci Sports Exerc 43:2110-2119, 2011

Purpose.—Lower limb stress fractures (SF) have a high prevalence in female athletes of running-related sports. The purpose of this study was to investigate bone quality, including bone microarchitecture and strength, and muscle strength in athletes diagnosed with SF.

Methods.—Female athletes with lower limb SF (SF subjects, $n = 19$, 18–45 yr, premenopausal) and healthy female athletes (NSF subjects, $n = 19$) matched according to age, sport, and weekly training volume were recruited. Bone microarchitecture of all participants was assessed using high-resolution peripheral quantitative computed tomography at two skeletal sites along the distal tibia of the dominant leg. Bone strength and load distribution between cortical and trabecular bone was estimated by finite element analysis. Using dual-energy x-ray absorptiometry, areal bone mineral density (aBMD) at the hip, femoral neck, and spine was measured. Muscle torque (knee extension, plantarflexion, eversion/inversion) was assessed (Biodex dynamometer) as a measure of lower leg muscle strength.

Results.—SF subjects, after adjusting for body weight, had thinner tibia compared with NSF subjects as indicated by a lower tibial cross-sectional area (-7.8%, $P = 0.02$) and higher load carried by the cortex as indicated by finite element analysis (4.1%, $P = 0.02$). Further site-specific regional analysis revealed that, in the posterior region of the tibia, SF subjects had lower trabecular BMD (-19.8%, $P = 0.02$) and less cortical area (-5.2%, $P = 0.02$). The SF group exhibited reduced knee extension strength (-18.3%, $P = 0.03$) compared with NSF subjects.

Conclusions.—These data suggest an association of impaired bone quality, particularly in the posterior region of the distal tibia, and decreased muscle strength with lower limb SF in female athletes.

▶ This is a fascinating cross-sectional study of regional bone quality in the distal tibia, comparing female athletes with documented stress fractures (SFs) of the lower limb with a matched control group without SF. It presents a novel investigation using newly developed techniques such as 3-dimensional high-resolution peripheral quantitative computed tomography (HR-pQCT) and associated finite element analysis (FEA), as well as a customized regional analysis method to examine spatial variation by quadrants (Fig 2 in the original article). As would be expected, the subjects with SF had thinner tibia with lower cross-sectional area than the subjects with navicular SF, but results also showed that they had a higher load carried by the cortex, as determined by the sophisticated methods of FEA. Interestingly, as well, a total of 10 out of 19 of these premenopausal subjects aged 18 to 45 years (6 with SF and 4 without) were found to have bone mineral density (BMD) measurements in lumbar spine in the osteopenic range! This speaks to an underlying problem with development and maintenance of optimal BMD in this group of active women, who, by the nature of their weight-bearing sporting activities, should have BMD values from 5% to 15% higher than normal for their age group. Also of note in this study, the bone microarchitecture in the tibia was not assessed at the site of the actual SF, as has been done previously by other investigators.[1] Another group has also used pQCT to assess the cortical density of the midtibia in adolescent girls and boys.[2] As explained by the authors, this limitation was because of the actual technique used (HR-pQCT), which was able to provide other useful information with 3-dimensional analysis. Functional muscle testing indicated significantly lower knee extension muscle torque. Although a causal relationship cannot be determined with such cross-sectional data, these findings suggest that both bone quality and muscle strength (both of which are potentially modifiable) are factors in SF in this population.

C. Lebrun, MDCM, MPE, CCFP, Dip Sport Med, FACSM

References

1. Popp KL, Hughes JM, Smock AJ, et al. Bone geometry, strength, and muscle size in runners with a history of stress fracture. *Med Sci Sports Exerc.* 2009;41:2145-2150.
2. Cooper DML, Ahamed Y, Macdonald HM, McKay HA. Characterising cortical density in the mid-tibia: intra-individual variation in adolescent girls and boys. *Br J Sport Med.* 2008;42:690-695.

Exercise During Pregnancy, Maternal Prepregnancy Body Mass Index, and Birth Weight
Fleten C, Stigum H, Magnus P, et al (Norwegian Inst of Public Health, Oslo, Norway)
Obstet Gynecol 115:331-337, 2010

Objective.—To estimate the direct associations between exercise during pregnancy and offspring birth weight and between maternal prepregnancy body mass index (BMI) and birth weight. Furthermore, we estimated the indirect association between maternal BMI and birth weight, explained by exercise during pregnancy.

Methods.—This study included pregnant women and their offspring recruited from 1999 to 2006 in the Norwegian Mother and Child Cohort Study, conducted by the Norwegian Institute of Public Health. Linear regression analyses were based on exposure data from two self-administered questionnaires during pregnancy and birth weight data from the Medical Birth Registry of Norway.

Results.—The study included 43,705 pregnancies. The median exercise frequency during the first 17 weeks of gestation was six times per month and four times per month thereafter until week 30. Mean maternal prepregnancy BMI was 24 kg/m^2, and mean birth weight of the offspring was 3,677 g. The adjusted direct association between exercise and birth weight was a 2.9-g decrease in birth weight per unit increase in exercise (one time per month). In contrast, the adjusted direct association between

BMI and birth weight was a 20.3-g increase in birth weight for a one-unit increase in BMI (1 kg/m), and the indirect association explained by exercise was only a 0.3-g increase in birth weight.

Conclusion.—Exercise during pregnancy has a minor impact on birth weight, whereas maternal prepregnancy BMI has a larger influence. Thus, we suggest that health care professionals should focus on normalizing the BMI of women in fertile ages.

▶ This is one of few large-scale studies investigating associations between maternal exercise during pregnancy and birth weight of the offspring. Exercise training during pregnancy had a minor impact on birth weight, with body mass index having a larger influence. Thus, health care professionals should focus on preventing or treating overweight and obesity in fertile women to lower the odds of large-birth-weight offspring. As long as exercise during pregnancy is believed by the clinician to be safe in all aspects for the fetus and the pregnant woman and there are no contraindications, exercise during pregnancy should be recommended for the health of the mothers in accordance with the current guidelines.[1]

D. C. Nieman, DrPH

Reference

1. Davies GA, Wolfe LA, Mottola MF, MacKinnon C; Society of Obstetricians and Gynecologists of Canada, SOGC Clinical Practice Obstetrics Committee. Joint SOGC/CSEP clinical practice guideline: exercise in pregnancy and the postpartum period. *Can J Appl Physiol.* 2003;28:330-341.

Strength training stops bone loss and builds muscle in postmenopausal breast cancer survivors: a randomized, controlled trial
Winters-Stone KM, Dobek J, Nail L, et al (Oregon Health & Science Univ, Portland; et al)
Breast Cancer Res Treat 127:447-456, 2011

Targeted exercise training could reduce risk factors for fracture and obesity-related diseases that increase from breast cancer treatment, but has not been sufficiently tested. We hypothesized that progressive, moderate-intensity resistance + impact training would increase or maintain hip and spine bone mass, lean mass and fat mass and reduce bone turnover compared to controls who participated in a low-intensity, non-weight bearing stretching program. We conducted a randomized, controlled trial in 106 women with early stage breast cancer who were >1 year post-radiation and/or chemotherapy, ≥50 years of age at diagnosis and postmenopausal, free from osteoporosis and medications for bone loss, resistance and impact exercise naïve, and cleared to exercise by a physician. Women were randomly assigned to participate in 1 year of thrice-weekly progressive, moderate-intensity resistance + impact (jump) exercise or in a similar frequency and length control program of progressive, low-intensity stretching. Primary endpoints were bone mineral density (BMD; g/cm^2) of the hip and spine and whole body bone-free lean and fat mass (kg) determined by DXA and biomarkers of bone turnover—serum osteocalcin (ng/ml) and urinary deoxypyrodiniline cross-links (nmol/mmolCr). Women in the resistance + impact training program preserved BMD at the lumbar spine (0.47 vs. −2.13%; $P = 0.001$) compared to controls. The resistance + impact group had a smaller increase in osteocalcin (7.0 vs. 27%, $P = 0.03$) and a larger decrease in deoxypyrodinoline (−49.9 vs. −32.6%, $P = 0.06$) than controls. Increases in lean mass from resistance + impact training were greatest among women currently taking aromatase inhibitors compared to controls not on this therapy ($P = 0.01$). Our combined program of resistance + impact exercise reduced risk factors for fracture among postmenopausal breast cancer survivors (BCS) and may be particularly relevant for BCS on aromatase

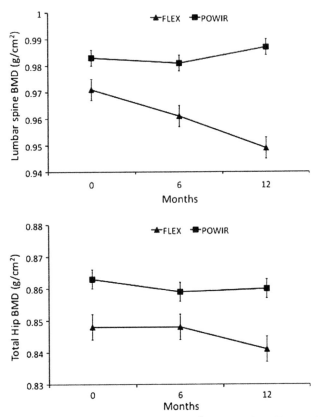

FIGURE 2.—Pattern of changes in spine and hip BMD (g/cm^2) in FLEX and POWIR across the 12-month intervention for participants with complete data sets for all time points. (Reprinted from Winters-Stone KM, Dobek J, Nail L, et al. Strength training stops bone loss and builds muscle in postmenopausal breast cancer survivors: a randomized, controlled trial. *Breast Cancer Res Treat.* 2011;127:447-456, with permission from Springer Science+Business Media, LLC.)

inhibitors (AIs) because of the additional benefit of exercise on muscle mass that could reduce falls (Fig 2).

▶ Breast cancer survivors are more likely to experience a bone fracture than their age-matched peers because of accelerated bone loss and bone turnover imparted by chemotherapy, chemotherapy-induced menopause, and aromatase inhibitor treatment. The American College of Sports Medicine[1] recommends bone loading exercises for the prevention of bone loss in women. Winters-Stone and colleagues took this approach in an exercise training intervention aimed at maintaining body mass index (BMD) in breast cancer survivors who had completed chemo- or radiotherapy at least 1 year earlier, did not have osteoporosis, and were not participating in resistance exercise regularly. Women were randomly assigned to 12-month resistance and impact exercise (POWIR) or a flexibility training (control) group with stratification by adjuvant hormone therapy or aromatase inhibitors versus neither treatment, and aerobic activity at study entry ($\geq$90 vs $\leq$90 min/wk). The POWIR intervention included progressive intensity resistance exercise and jumps performed with weighted vests 3 times a week with 2 supervised and 1 home-based exercise session. Over 12 months, women in the flexibility group lost 2% of baseline lumbar spine BMD, while the bone loading group maintained BMD (Fig 2). The divergence of BMD between groups was evident at 6 months. The use of aromatase inhibitors or SERMs did not modify the effects of bone loading exercise on lumbar spine BMD. The changes in hip BMD were not significantly different between the 2 groups. The authors suggest that hip remodeling may take different types of loading than presented in POWIR or a longer time to manifest in postmenopausal women. The increases in lean tissue and fat mass were not significantly different between exercise groups. However, use of aromatase inhibitors was associated with a larger increase in lean tissue mass within the bone loading group, perhaps because of a relative hyperandrogenicity. Adherence to the POWIR intervention was 57% of total sessions attended, 76% for supervised sessions, and 23% for home sessions. There were no injuries or adverse events and no worsening of upper extremity lymphedema, regardless of training group. The combined resistance exercise and bone loading intervention maintained lumbar spine BMD, independently of adjuvant and antihormonal therapies, and was well tolerated in postmenopausal breast cancer survivors.

C. M. Jankowski, PhD

Reference

1. Kohrt WM, Bloomfield SA, Little KD, Nelson ME, Yingling VR. American College of Sports Medicine Position Stand: physical activity and bone health. *Med Sci Sports Exerc.* 2004;36:1985-1996.

Hormonal Responses to Resistance Exercise during Different Menstrual Cycle States

Nakamura Y, Aizawa K, Imai T, et al (Tsukuba Univ of Technology, Ibaraki, Japan; The Univ of Tokyo, Japan; Univ of Tsukuba, Ibaraki, Japan; et al)
Med Sci Sports Exerc 43:967-973, 2011

Purpose.—To investigate the effect of menstrual cycle states on ovarian and anabolic hormonal responses to acute resistance exercise in young women.

Methods.—Eight healthy women (eumenorrhea; EM) and eight women with menstrual disorders including oligomenorrhea and amenorrhea (OAM) participated in this study. The EM group performed acute resistance exercises during the early follicular (EF) and midluteal (ML) phases, and the OAM group performed the same exercises. All subjects performed three sets each of lat pull-downs, leg curls, bench presses, leg extensions, and squats at 75%–80% of one-repetition maximum with a 1-min rest between sets. Blood samples were obtained before exercise, immediately after, 30 min after, and 60 min after the exercise.

Results.—In the EM group, resting serum levels of estradiol and progesterone in the ML phase were higher than those in the EF phase and higher than those in the OAM group. Serum estradiol and progesterone in the ML phase increased after the exercise but did not change in the EF phase or in the OAM group. In contrast, resting levels of testosterone in the OAM group were higher than those in both the ML and EF phases of the EM group. After the exercise, serum growth hormone increased in both the ML and EF phases but did not change in the OAM group.

Conclusions.—The responses of anabolic hormones to acute resistance exercise are different among the menstrual cycle states in young women. Women with menstrual disturbances with low estradiol and progesterone serum levels have an attenuated anabolic hormone response to acute resistance exercise, suggesting that menstrual disorders accompanying low ovarian hormone levels may affect exercise-induced change in anabolic hormones in women.

▶ Resistance exercise–induced anabolic hormone changes are different between men and women, but the hormonal responses to exercise are also modified by ovarian systems in women. In addition to the known effects of menstrual dysfunction on bone health, as well as cardiovascular risk factors, there may also be implications for exercise training–induced skeletal muscular adaptation. This study examined 8 women with eumenorrhea (EM) and 8 women with menstrual disorders, including oligomenorrhea and amenorrhea (OAM), and looked at the responses of anabolic hormones (growth hormone, testosterone, dehydroepiandrosterone sulfate), cortisol, and the female reproductive hormones (estradiol and progesterone) to a standardized acute resistance exercise protocol. In a randomized order, the EM group performed the exercises during the early follicular phase (days 4-7 of the menstrual cycle) and the midluteal phase (ML; 7-10 days after ovulation), while the OAM group participated in the exercise series on an arbitrary day. Cycle phases were confirmed by measurement of serum estradiol and progesterone levels. Change in whole blood lactate did not differ between the groups, suggesting that exercise intensity was similar. The results were interesting and somewhat complicated, but the authors have discussed their findings in comparison with those of other investigators. Most striking was the GH response to the resistance exercise: this was different between menstrual cycle phases, being higher in the ML phase, when estradiol is higher. This is concordant with similar research in postmenopausal women, where greater GH responses to exercise have been shown in those receiving hormone replacement therapy compared with those without treatment. There was no change in the level of growth hormone (GH) in the women with menstrual disorders. The clinical significance of this particular study is that differences in hypothalamic-pituitary function between women with menstrual disorders and women with EM (and also during different phases of the menstrual cycle in this latter group) appear to alter GH responses to resistance exercise. The implications are that both menstrual cycle phase and menstrual status may influence response to training, specifically skeletal muscular adaptation in response to anabolic hormones. This remains to be studied in a more elite athletic population and also in women taking oral contraceptives.

C. Lebrun, MDCM, MPE, CCFP, Dip Sport Med, FACSM

Short-Term, Light- to Moderate-Intensity Exercise Training Improves Leg Muscle Strength in the Oldest Old: A Randomized Controlled Trial

Serra-Rexach JA, Bustamante-Ara N, Hierro Villarán M, et al (Hospital General Universitario Gregorio Marañón, Madrid, Spain; Universidad Europea de Madrid, Spain; Residencia Los Nogales-Pacífico, Madrid, Spain; et al)
J Am Geriatr Soc 59:594-602, 2011

Objectives.—To assess the effects of an 8-week exercise training program with a special focus on light- to moderate-intensity resistance exercises (30—70% of one repetition maximum, 1RM) and a subsequent 4-week training cessation period (detraining) on muscle strength and functional capacity in participants aged 90 and older.

Design.—Randomized controlled trial performed during March to September 2009.

Setting.—Geriatric nursing home.

Participants.—Forty nonagenarians (90—97) were randomly assigned to an intervention or control group (16 women and 4 men per group).

Intervention.—Eight-week muscle strength exercise intervention focused on lower limb strength exercises of light to moderate intensity.

Measurements.—Primary outcome: 1RM leg press. Secondary outcomes: handgrip strength, 8-m walk test, 4-step stairs test, Timed Up and Go test, and number of falls.

Results.—A significant group by time interaction effect ($P=.02$) was observed only for the 1RM leg press. In the intervention group, 1RM leg press increased significantly with training by 10.6 kg [95% confidence interval (CI) = 4.1–17.1 kg; $P = .01$]. Except for the mean group number of falls, which were 1.2 falls fewer per participant in the intervention (95% CI = 0.0–3.0; $P = .03$), no significant training effect on the secondary outcome measures was found.

Conclusion.—Exercise training, even of short duration and light to moderate intensity, can increase muscle strength while decreasing fall risk in nonagenarians (Fig 2).

▶ The take-home message of this study is that you're never too old to gain the benefits of resistance exercise. Nonagenarians residing in an assisted-living facility and in stable health had a significant increase in leg strength after 8 weeks of resistance exercise. The main focus of the training was on leg strength (leg press), but training also included upper body exercises. Exercise intensity progressed from 30% to 70% of the estimated initial 1 repetition maximum (1RM). The control group engaged in the light stretching and range of motion exercises 5 days per week; this activity was part of the daily routine of the facility. The strength gains did not translate to significant improvements in functional performance, although walk and timed up-and-go speed increased in exercisers. The study may have been underpowered for functional outcomes. A unique feature of this study was the 4-week follow-up phase to ascertain the maintenance of performance following the supervised intervention. Although strength tended to decline in the exercise group following cessation of training, it remained greater than that of the control group over the same time (Fig 2). It is possible that less-frequent sessions of supervised exercise would be sufficient to maintain greater strength over the long term while keeping programmatic costs down.

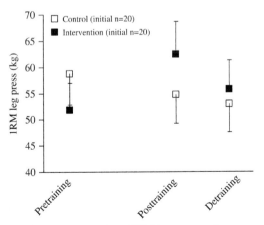

FIGURE 2.—Results of one-repetition maximum (1RM) leg press according to group. Data are means ± standard errors of the mean. Twenty, 19, and 16 participants in each group were evaluated before and after training and after detraining, respectively. *P*-values for group, time, and group by time interaction effect were .89, .22, and .02, respectively. *$P = .01$ for the pre-versus posttraining comparison within the intervention group. The range for 1RM leg press in the total study population was 15.0–122.0 kg. (Reprinted from Serra-Rexach JA, Bustamante-Ara N, Hierro Villarán M, et al. Short-term, light- to moderate-intensity exercise training improves leg muscle strength in the oldest old: a randomized controlled trial. *J Am Geriatr Soc.* 2011;59:594-602, with permission from the American Geriatrics Society, John Wiley and Sons.)

The number of falls reported in the exercise group was significantly less than that of the controls, which is an important health and health care outcome for this population. To enhance the safety of the exercise intervention, each fitness specialist supervised no more than 3 residents at one time. The safety and feasibility of this intervention for the oldest old was demonstrated by the absence of exercise-related adverse events and 75% adherence to the exercise intervention.

C. M. Jankowski, PhD

Serum 25-Hydroxyvitamin D and Physical Function in Older Adults: The Cardiovascular Health Study All Stars

Houston DK, Tooze JA, Davis CC, et al (Wake Forest School of Medicine, Winston Salem, NC; et al)
J Am Geriatr Soc 59:1793-1801, 2011

Objectives.—To examine the association between 25-hydroxyvitamin D (25(OH)D) and physical function in adults of advanced age.

Design.—Cross-sectional and longitudinal analysis of physical function over 3 years of follow-up in the Cardiovascular Health Study All Stars.

Setting.—Forsyth County, North Carolina; Sacramento County, California; Washington County, Maryland; and Allegheny County, Pennsylvania.

Participants.—Community-dwelling adults aged 77 to 100 (N = 988).

Measurements.—Serum 25-hydroxyvitamin D (25(OH)D), Short Physical Performance Battery (SPPB), and grip and knee extensor strength assessed at baseline. Mobility disability (difficulty walking half a mile or up 10 steps) and activities of daily living (ADLs) disability were assessed at baseline and every 6 months over 3 years of follow-up.

Results.—Almost one-third (30.8%) of participants were deficient in 25(OH)D (<20 ng/mL). SPPB scores were lower in those with deficient 25(OH)D (mean (standard error) 6.53 (0.24)) than in those with sufficient 25(OH)D (≥30 ng/mL) (7.15 (0.25)) after adjusting for sociodemographic characteristics, season, health behaviors, and chronic conditions ($P = .006$). Grip strength adjusted for body size was also lower in those with deficient 25(OH)D than in those with sufficient 25(OH)D (24.7 (0.6) kg vs 26.0 (0.6) kg, $P = .02$). Participants with deficient 25(OH)D were more likely to have prevalent mobility (OR = 1.44, 95% confidence interval (CI)) = 0.96–2.14) and ADL disability (OR = 1.51, 95% CI = 1.01–2.25) at baseline than those with sufficient 25(OH)D. Furthermore, participants with deficient 25(OH)D were at greater risk of incident mobility disability over 3 years of follow-up (hazard ratio = 1.56, 95% CI = 1.06–2.30).

Conclusion.—Vitamin D deficiency was common and was associated with poorer physical performance, lower muscle strength, and prevalent mobility and ADL disability in community-dwelling older adults. Moreover, vitamin D deficiency predicted incident mobility disability (Table 2).

▶ One benefit of regular physical activity that is often overlooked in elderly patients is an increased intake of food and, thus, a reduced risk of developing

TABLE 2.—Hydroxyvitamin D (25(OH)D) Status and Physical Performance: Cardiovascular Health Study All Stars

Physical Performance	<20.0	25(OH)D, ng/mL 20.0–29.9 Least Squares Mean (Standard Error)	≥30.0	P for Trend
SPPB score (range: 0–12)				
N	293	339	322	—
Model 1	6.12 (0.18)‡	6.62 (0.19)*	7.09 (0.20)	<.001
Model 2	6.53 (0.24)†	6.87 (0.24)	7.15 (0.25)	.006
3-m gait speed score (range: 0–4)				
N	296	345	323	—
Model 1	2.61 (0.08)†	2.71 (0.08)*	2.89 (0.09)	.006
Model 2	2.80 (0.10)	2.81 (0.10)	2.91 (0.11)	.24
Standing balance score (range: 0–4)				
N	302	349	328	—
Model 1	2.37 (0.08)‡	2.67 (0.08)	2.82 (0.09)	<.001
Model 2	2.49 (0.12)†	2.73 (0.11)	2.81 (0.12)	.003
Chair stand score (range: 0–4)				
N	303	353	329	—
Model 1	1.09 (0.07)*	1.15 (0.07)*	1.32 (0.08)	.01
Model 2	1.19 (0.10)	1.23 (0.10)	1.36 (0.10)	.08
3 m gait speed, m/s				
N	263	315	302	—
Model 1	0.73 (0.01)†	0.75 (0.01)*	0.78 (0.02)	.003
Model 2	0.75 (0.02)	0.75 (0.02)	0.77 (0.02)	.18

Model 1 adjusted for age, sex, race, education, field center, and season.
Model 2 adjusted for variables in Model 1 plus body mass index, walking for physical activity, smoking, alcohol use, creatinine, depression, cognition, diabetes mellitus, osteoporosis, and cardiovascular disease.
SPPB = Short Physical Performance Battery.
*$P < .05$.
†$P < .01$.
‡$P < .001$ from 25(OH)D ≥30.0 ng/mL.

deficiencies of vitamins and micronutrients. In the case of people living in northern climates, a shortage of vitamin D is a particular hazard during the winter months, when those who are inactive tend to remain indoors. Vitamin D is important in the prevention of osteoporosis, but it may also be linked in some way to the prevention of diabetes, hypertension, and osteoarthritis.[1] The subjects studied by Houston et al were in the age range (77–100 years) in which physical activity patterns have a substantial impact on dietary intake, and, as in the elderly individuals tested during the US National Health & Examination Survey of 2000-2004,[2] about a third of those examined had less than the minimum desirable serum 2.5 hydroxy vitamin D of 20 ng/mL. Further, the percentage of patients with deficiencies was greater in the winter (35%) than in the summer months (24%). Others, also, have linked low serum vitamin D levels and poor muscle strength.[3-6] The cross-sectional associations that Houston et al demonstrated between a low serum vitamin D level and poor scores for a short physical performance test battery, muscle force per kilogram of body mass, mobility, and ability to perform the activities of daily living (Table 2) do not necessarily imply that vitamin D has a direct role in sustaining physical function. The association could have arisen in the opposite sense, because of the influence of limited physical activity upon food consumption. The relationship between a low initial vitamin D level and incident disability over a 3-year follow-up points a little more strongly toward a causal role, although, again, a low initial level of physical activity may have hastened the onset of disability. The critical study proving that the administration of vitamin D supplements slows the onset of disability has yet to be done.[7]

R. J. Shephard, MD (Lond), PhD, DPE

References

1. Holick MF. Vitamin D deficiency. *N Engl J Med.* 2007;357:266-281.
2. Looker AC, Pfeiffer CM, Lacher DA, Schleicher RL, Picciano MF, Yetley EA. Serum 25-hydroxyvitamin D status of the US population: 1988-1994 compared with 2000-2004. *Am J Clin Nutr.* 2008;88:1519-1527.
3. Mowé M, Haug E, Bøhmer T. Low serum calcidiol concentration in older adults with reduced muscular function. *J Am Geriatr Soc.* 1999;47:220-226.
4. Bischoff HA, Stahelin HB, Urscheler N, et al. Muscle strength in the elderly: its relation to vitamin D metabolites. *Arch Phys Med Rehabil.* 1999;80:54-58.
5. Zamboni M, Zoico E, Tosoni P, et al. Relation between vitamin D, physical performance, and disability in elderly persons. *J Gerontol A Biol Sci Med Sci.* 2002;57: M7-M11.
6. Dhesi JK, Bearne LM, Moniz C, et al. Neuromuscular and psychomotor function in elderly subjects who fall and the relationship with vitamin D status. *J Bone Miner Res.* 2002;17:891-897.
7. Annweiler C, Schott AM, Berrut G, Fantino B, Beauchet O. Vitamin D-related changes in physical performance: a systematic review. *J Nutr Health Aging.* 2009;13:893-898.

Serum 25-Hydroxyvitamin D and Physical Function in Older Adults: The Cardiovascular Health Study All Stars

Houston DK, Tooze JA, Davis CC, et al (Wake Forest School of Medicine, Winston-Salem, NC; et al)
J Am Geriatr Soc 59:1793-1801, 2011

Objectives.—To examine the association between 25-hydroxyvitamin D (25(OH)D) and physical function in adults of advanced age.

Design.—Cross-sectional and longitudinal analysis of physical function over 3 years of follow-up in the Cardiovascular Health Study All Stars.

Setting.—Forsyth County, North Carolina; Sacramento County, California; Washington County, Maryland; and Allegheny County, Pennsylvania.

Participants.—Community-dwelling adults aged 77 to 100 (N = 988).

Measurements.—Serum 25-hydroxyvitamin D 25(OH)D), Short Physical Performance Battery (SPPB), and grip and knee extensor strength assessed at baseline. Mobility disability (difficulty walking half a mile or up 10 steps) and activities of daily living (ADLs) disability were assessed at baseline and every 6 months over 3 years of follow-up.

Results.—Almost one-third (30.8%) of participants were deficient in 25(OH)D (<20 ng/mL). SPPB scores were lower in those with deficient 25(OH)D (mean (standard error) 6.53 (0.24)) than in those with sufficient 25(OH)D (≥30 ng/mL) (7.15 (0.25)) after adjusting for sociodemographic characteristics, season, health behaviors, and chronic conditions ($P = .006$).

Grip strength adjusted for body size was also lower in those with deficient 25(OH)D than in those with sufficient 25(OH)D (24.7 (0.6) kg vs 26.0 (0.6) kg, $P = .02$). Participants with deficient 25(OH)D were more likely to have prevalent mobility (OR = 1.44, 95% confidence interval (CI)) = 0.96−2.14) and ADL disability (OR = 1.51, 95% CI = 1.01−2.25) at baseline than those with sufficient 25(OH)D. Furthermore, participants with deficient 25(OH)D were at greater risk of incident mobility disability over 3 years of follow-up (hazard ratio = 1.56, 95% CI = 1.06−2.30).

Conclusion.—Vitamin D deficiency was common and was associated with poorer physical performance, lower muscle strength, and prevalent mobility and ADL disability in community-dwelling older adults. Moreover, vitamin D deficiency predicted incident mobility disability (Fig 1).

▶ This is an insightful prospective epidemiologic study that showed vitamin D deficiency was common in older individuals (Fig 1) and was associated with lower physical performance and muscle strength and increased disability in community-dwelling adults of advanced age. An adult in a bathing suit experiencing slight pinkness in the skin the next day obtains the equivalent of 10 000 to 25 000 IU vitamin D.[1] Few foods naturally contain vitamin D, and important sources are cod liver oil, canned fish, salmon, sun-dried shitake mushrooms, and fortified milk and juices. Adults should consume 600 IU/d vitamin D, with an upper limit of 4000 IU/d. The vitamin D receptor is found in most tissues of the body, and vitamin D has been linked to wide-ranging biological effects, including improved calcium absorption and bone health, blood vessel growth, muscle function, immune function, and insulin production. Low serum vitamin D levels are associated with numerous health conditions, such as the metabolic syndrome, obesity, colon cancer (and perhaps breast cancer), infection,

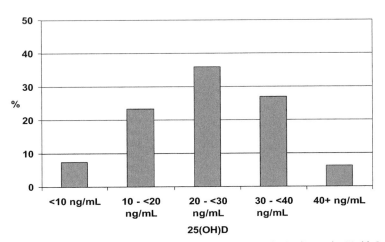

FIGURE 1.—Distribution of 25-Hydroxyvitamin D (25(OH)D) Levels: Cardiovascular Health Study All Stars. (Reprinted from Houston DK, Tooze JA, Davis CC, et al. Serum 25-hydroxyvitamin D and physical function in older adults: the cardiovascular health study all stars. *J Am Geriatr Soc.* 2011;59: 1793-1801. Reprinted with permission from 2011, Copyright the Authors, The American Geriatrics Society, John Wiley and Sons.)

autoimmunity, falls, fractures, and age-related decline in cognitive function.[2] In recent decades, there has been increased awareness of the impact of vitamin D on muscle function.[3] In the early 20th century, athletes and coaches felt that ultraviolet rays had a positive impact on athletic performance, and evidence is accumulating to support this view. Both cross-sectional and longitudinal studies support a functional role for vitamin D in muscle, and the discovery of the vitamin D receptor in muscle tissue provides a mechanistic pathway for understanding the role of vitamin D within muscle. Studies in athletes have found that vitamin D status is variable and is dependent on outdoor training time (during peak sunlight), skin color, and geographic location.[4]

D. C. Nieman, DrPH

References

1. Holick MF, Binkley NC, Bischoff-Ferrari HA, et al; Endocrine Society. Evaluation, treatment, and prevention of vitamin D deficiency: an Endocrine Society clinical practice guideline. *J Clin Endocrinol Metab.* 2011;96:1911-1930.
2. Bouvard B, Annweiler C, Sallé A, et al. Extraskeletal effects of vitamin D: facts, uncertainties, and controversies. *Joint Bone Spine.* 2011;78:10-16.
3. Hamilton B. Vitamin D and human skeletal muscle. *Scand J Med Sci Sports.* 2010; 20:182-190.
4. Bartoszewska M, Kamboj M, Patel DR. Vitamin D, muscle function, and exercise performance. *Pediatr Clin North Am.* 2010;57:849-861.

Increased Average Longevity among the "Tour de France" Cyclists

Sanchis-Gomar F, Olaso-Gonzalez G, Corella D, et al (Univ of Valencia, Spain)
Int J Sports Med 32:644-647, 2011

It is widely held among the general population and even among health professionals that moderate exercise is a healthy practice but long term high intensity exercise is not. The specific amount of physical activity necessary for good health remains unclear. To date, longevity studies of elite athletes have been relatively sparse and the results are somewhat conflicting. The Tour de France is among the most gruelling sport events in the world, during which highly trained professional cyclists undertake high intensity exercise for a full 3 weeks. Consequently we set out to determine the longevity of the participants in the Tour de France, compared with that of the general population. We studied the longevity of 834 cyclists from France (n = 465), Italy (n = 196) and Belgium (n = 173) who rode the Tour de France between the years 1930 and 1964. Dates of birth and death of the cyclists were obtained on December 31ˢᵗ 2007. We calculated the percentage of survivors for each age and compared them with the values for the pooled general population of France, Italy and Belgium for the appropriate age cohorts. We found a very significant increase in average longevity (17%) of the cyclists when compared with the general population. The age at which 50% of the general population died was 73.5 vs. 81.5 years in Tour de France participants. Our major finding is that repeated very intense exercise prolongs life span in well trained

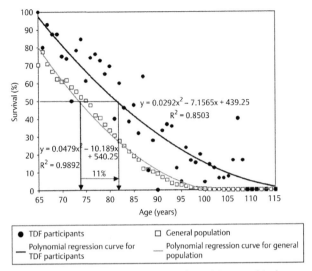

FIGURE 2.—Percentage of survival related to age in TdF participants and in the general population. Persons born between 1892 and 1942 have been studied. Average life span of TdF participants is higher (p = 0.004; 17.5%) than the general population of the same country in which the cyclists were born. The age at which 50% of the general population died was 73.5 vs. 81.5 years in TdF participants, i.e., 11% increase. (Reprinted from Sanchis-Gomar F, Olaso-Gonzalez G, Corella D, et al. Increased average longevity among the "Tour de France" cyclists. *Int J Sports Med.* 2011;32:644-647, with permission from Georg Thieme Verlag KG Stuttgart.)

practitioners. Our findings underpin the importance of exercising without the fear that becoming exhausted might be bad for one's health (Fig 2).

▶ In 2008, Chakravarty et al[1] reported that participation in long-term running and other vigorous exercise among older adults was associated with less disability and lower mortality over 2 decades of follow-up. This study goes one step further, indicating that even a history of extremely intense and prolonged exercise training is associated with reduced mortality and enhanced life expectancy (Fig 2). The authors admit that a strong selection bias exists in this analysis but argue that in the data from Ruiz et al,[2] the association between athletic endeavor and increased life expectancy is not biased by genetic selection. Elite athletes are also lean, tend not to smoke, and have other favorable lifestyle habits that predict lowered risk of disease. Nonetheless, these data on Tour de France athletes at the very least do not support the fear of some clinicians that extreme exercise predicts early mortality.

D. C. Nieman, DrPH

References

1. Chakravarty EF, Hubert HB, Lingala VB, Fries JF. Reduced disability and mortality among aging runners: a 21-year longitudinal study. *Arch Intern Med.* 2008;168: 1638-1646.
2. Ruiz JR, Morán M, Arenas J, Lucia A. Strenuous endurance exercise improves life expectancy: it's in our genes. *Br J Sports Med.* 2011;45:159-161.

Cardiorespiratory fitness in aging men and women: the DR's EXTRA study

Hakola L, Komulainen P, Hassinen M, et al (Kuopio Res Inst of Exercise Medicine, Finland)
Scand J Med Sci Sports 21:679-687, 2011

The aim of the study was to describe the levels and to create reference values of cardiorespiratory fitness, expressed as maximal oxygen consumption (VO_{2max}), maximal metabolic equivalents (METs) and maximal workload in aging men and women. We measured VO_{2max} directly by a breath-by-breath method during a maximal exercise stress test on a bicycle ergometer with a linear workload increase of 20 W/min in a representative population sample of 672 men and 677 women aged 57–78 years. We presented the age and sex-specific categories of cardiorespiratory fitness (very low, low, medium, high and very high) based on variable distribution and non-linear regression models of VO_{2max}, maximal METs and maximal workload. The linear age-related decrement of VO_{2max} was −0.047 L/min/year (−2.3%) and −0.404 mL/kg/min/year (−1.6%) in men and −0.027 L/min/year (−1.9%) and −0.328 mL/kg/min/year (−1.6%) in women. After exclusion of diseased individuals, the rate of VO_{2max} decrement remained similar. The number of chronic diseases (0, 1, 2 or ≥3) was inversely associated with VO_{2max} in men (*P*<0.001) and women (*P*<0.001). The present study provides clinically useful reference values of cardiorespiratory fitness for primary and secondary prevention purposes in aging people (Fig 4).

▶ In this study, VO_{2max} was measured in more than 1200 women and men aged 57-78 years. The rationale for the article was to establish reference values for

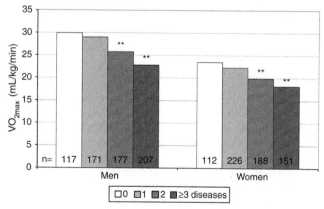

FIGURE 4.—Maximal oxygen uptake (mL/kg/min) according to the number of diseases in men and women. Bars represent the number of diseases. Diseases include cardiovascular disease, pulmonary disease, joint disease, diabetes or impaired glucose regulation, metabolic syndrome and cancer. Two and ≥ 3 diseases: diagnosis from two/at least three groups of diseases, respectively. **P<0.001 for difference using non-diseased as reference group and adjusting for age (univariate analysis of variance, Bonferroni's *post hoc* test). (Reprinted from Hakola L, Komulainen P, Hassinen M, et al. Cardiorespiratory fitness in aging men and women: the DR's EXTRA study. *Scand J Med Sci Sports.* 2011;21:679-687, with permission from John Wiley & Sons A/S.)

VO_{2max} using a standard bicycle ergometer test protocol and thereby promote the use of maximal cardiorespiratory testing in clinical practice. The data presented are baseline measures from the Dose Responses to Exercise Training randomized controlled trial of the health effects of regular physical activity and diet in older adults being conducted in Finland. In this cross-sectional analysis, lower VO_{2max} was associated with older age, prevalent chronic disease, high waist circumference, low levels of moderate to vigorous physical activity, and the use of β-blockers in men and women. In men, smoking also contributed to lower VO_{2max}. With increasing age, there was a faster decline in VO_{2max} in men compared with women. This could be attributed to a higher VO_{2max} in men than women in middle age but could also be a sex-specific indicator of impending loss of functional independence or onset of frailty in older men. There was a stair-step relation between the number of chronic diseases and reduced VO_{2max} (Fig 4); moderate to vigorous physical activity slightly weakened this association. The presence of 1 chronic disease was not associated with lower VO_{2max} with 1 interesting exception: women with metabolic syndrome had 17% lower VO_{2max} than women without chronic disease. Given the prevalence of metabolic syndrome among older women, clinicians should be aware of the co-occurrence of reduced cardiorespiratory fitness. An important test administration tip for clinicians was provided in this article: small increments in workload not only allow for more precise acquisition of VO_{2max}, but also may overcome some of the effects of localized, lower-extremity muscle fatigue in older adults unaccustomed to bicycling. This article provides clinicians with sex-specific categories of VO_{2max}, maximal metabolic equivalents, and maximal workload in 2-year increments for middle-aged and older adults.

C. M. Jankowski, PhD

Atrophy of the lower limbs in elderly women: is it related to walking ability?

Ikezoe T, Mori N, Nakamura M, et al (Kyoto Univ, Japan)
Eur J Appl Physiol 111:989-995, 2011

This study investigated the relationship between walking ability and age-related muscle atrophy of the lower limbs in elderly women. The subjects comprised 20 young women and 37 elderly women who resided in nursing homes or chronic care institutions. The elderly subjects were divided into three groups according to their walking ability. The muscle thickness of the following ten lower limb muscles were measured by B-mode ultrasound: the gluteus maximus, gluteus medius, gluteus minimus, psoas major, rectus femoris, vastus lateralis, vastus intermedius, biceps femoris, gastrocnemius and soleus. Compared to the young group, muscle thicknesses of all muscles except the soleus muscle were significantly smaller in all the elderly groups. There were no significant differences between the fast- and slow-walking groups in the thickness of any muscle. In the dependent elderly group, noticeable muscle atrophy was observed in the quadriceps femoris muscle. The results of this study suggest that the elderly who are capable of locomotion,

TABLE 5.—Differences in the *t* Score Between Muscles in the Elderly Groups

	Fast Walking	Slow Walking	Dependent
Gluteus maximus	−3.13 ± 1.16[a]	−3.19 ± 1.39	−5.09 ± 0.79[b]
Gluteus medius	−1.37 ± 0.74	−1.42 ± 0.68	−2.28 ± 0.40
Gluteus minimus	−1.01 ± 0.65	−1.08 ± 0.67	−1.51 ± 0.28
Psoas major	−3.84 ± 1.41[b]	−3.22 ± 0.72[b]	−4.37 ± 1.04[c]
Rectus femoris	−1.82 ± 1.07	−2.22 ± 1.60	−5.55 ± 0.42[d]
Vastus lateralis	−2.47 ± 1.22	−3.04 ± 0.96	−5.70 ± 0.41[d]
Vastus intermedius	−1.75 ± 1.64	−2.62 ± 1.42	−5.10 ± 0.76[b]
Biceps femoris	−3.80 ± 1.06[b]	−3.96 ± 0.78[b]	−5.17 ± 0.94[b]
Gastrocnemius	−2.40 ± 1.18	−2.50 ± 1.74	−4.01 ± 0.76[c]
Soleus	−0.76 ± 1.40	−1.22 ± 0.81	−2.77 ± 1.07

Values are expressed as means ± the standard deviation (SD).
[a]Significant difference with soleus and gluteus minimus.
[b]Significant difference with soleus, gluteus minimus and gluteus medius.
[c]Significant difference with gluteus minimus and gluteus medius.
[d]Significant difference with soleus, gluteus minimus, gluteus medius and gastrocnemius.

regardless of their walking speed, show a moderate degree of age-related atrophy, while those who do not walk exhibit more severe atrophy, especially in the quadriceps femoris muscle (Table 5).

▶ We have previously demonstrated a strong relationship between objective pedometer/accelerometer measurements of the amount of daily physical activity undertaken by an elderly person and evidence of sarcopenia.[1] Muscle mass was assessed by dual-beam x-ray absorptiometry, and the association was closer for the legs than for the arms; 65- to 85-year-old individuals who walked 7000 to 8000 steps per day or took 15 to 20 minutes per day of exercise were likely to remain above the sarcopenia threshold. Ikezoe et al.'s article adds to this study by making 2-dimensional ultrasound estimates of the size of individual muscles in the lower limb and relating these to an alternative assessment of physical activity (a 3-level classification of the individual's habitual walking speed). Two points emerge from this new investigation. The big difference is not between fast and slow walkers, but rather between those who walk (irrespective of speed) and those who do not. The largest difference related to dependency is seen in the quadriceps, with the smallest difference in the soleus and the deep muscles around the hip joint (mainly type I, postural muscle fibers) (Table 5). Although it seems likely that inactivity played a causal role in the loss of muscle tissue, longitudinal studies are still required to establish causality.

R. J. Shephard, MD (Lond), PhD, DPE

Reference

1. Park H, Park S, Shephard RJ, et al. Yearlong physical activity and sarcopenia in older adults: the Nakanojo Study. *Eur J Appl Physiol.* 2010;109:953-961.

Arterial Stiffness, Physical Function, and Functional Limitation: The Whitehall II Study

Brunner EJ, Shipley MJ, Witte DR, et al (Univ College London, UK)
Hypertension 57:1003-1009, 2011

Arterial stiffness has been proposed as an indicator of vascular aging. We aimed to examine this concept by analyzing associations of arterial stiffness with age, subjective and objective measures of physical functioning, and self-reported functional limitation. We measured aortic pulse wave velocity by applanation tonometry among 5392 men and women aged 55 to 78 years. Arterial stiffness was strongly associated with age (mean difference [SE] per decade: men, 1.37 m/s [0.06 m/s]; women: 1.39 m/s [0.10 m/s]). This association was robust to individual and combined adjustment for pulse pressure, mean arterial pressure, antihypertensive treatment, and chronic disease. Participants took an 8.00-ft (2.44-m) walking speed test, a spirometry lung function test, and completed health functioning and (instrumental) activities of daily living questionnaires. Associations of stiffness and blood pressure with physical function scores scaled to SD of 10 were compared. One-SD higher stiffness was associated with lower walking speed (coefficient [95% CI]: -0.96 [-1.29 to -0.64] m/s) and physical component summary score (-0.91 [-1.21 to -0.60]) and poorer lung function (-1.23 [-1.53 to -0.92] L) adjusted for age, sex, and ethnic group. Pulse pressure and mean arterial pressure were linked inversely only with lung function. Associations of stiffness with functional limitation were robust to multiple adjustment, including pulse pressure and chronic disease. In conclusion, the concept of vascular aging is reinforced by the observation that arterial stiffness is a robust correlate of physical functioning and functional limitation in early old age. The nature of the link between arterial stiffness and quality of life in older people merits attention (Table 3).

▶ The growing availability of instruments for measuring pulse wave velocity and thus arterial distensibility has increased interest in this aspect of human aging. Loss of distensibility provides a measure of an increased risk of both cardiovascular and all-cause mortality,[1] and it has been linked to objective estimates of habitual activity in elderly populations.[2] There is some disagreement as to the arterial region that is most affected by changes in distensibility; in both our observations[2] and those of Tanaka et al,[3] the greatest changes of pulse wave velocity were seen in the central vessels, possibly reflecting a decrease of elastin and an increase of collagen in the vessel walls as well as their impregnation with calcium. However, others have reported that the changes affect the peripheral muscular vessels as well.[4] In this study, Brunner et al measured only the carotid-femoral velocity, a measure of central arterial stiffness. Their report is based on an extensively studied group of British civil servants that began in 1985, when the participants were 35 to 55 years of age. At the time of this report, those tested had an average age of 65 years. As might be anticipated from the studies of Aoyagi et al,[2] loss of distensibility was associated with a reduced walking speed, SF-36 questionnaire responses suggesting a loss of physical function, and self reports

TABLE 3.—Association of Pulse Wave Velocity, Blood Pressure Measures, and Chronic Disease With Standardized Physical Function Scores in Those Seen at the Clinical Examination

Independent Measures	Walking Speed (N=5286) Coefficient (95% CI)*	P	SF-36 Physical Component Summary Score (N=5227) Coefficient (95% CI)*	P	Lung Function (N=4234) Coefficient (95% CI)*	P
Pulse wave velocity	-0.96 (-1.29 to -0.64)	<0.001	-0.91 (-1.21 to -0.60)	<0.001	-1.23 (-1.53 to -0.92)	<0.001
Pulse pressure	-0.08 (-0.37 to 0.21)	0.58	0.25 (-0.05 to 0.55)	0.11	-0.80 (-1.11 to -0.50)	<0.001
Mean arterial pressure	-0.20 (-0.47 to 0.08)	0.16	0.26 (-0.02 to 0.55)	0.07	-0.47 (-0.76 to -0.17)	0.002
Antihypertensive treatment (yes vs no)	-1.96 (-2.53 to -1.39)	<0.001	-3.27 (-3.85 to -2.68)	<0.001	-1.60 (-2.18 to -1.03)	<0.001
Chronic disease†	-1.80 (-2.50 to -1.10)	<0.001	-3.10 (-3.83 to -2.37)	<0.001	-2.06 (-2.78 to -1.33)	<0.001
Pulse wave velocity, fully adjusted‡	-0.67 (-1.06 to -0.24)	<0.001	-0.70 (-1.09 to -0.31)	<0.001	-0.72 (-1.11 to -0.33)	<0.001

SF indicates short form. All of the models are adjusted for age, sex, and ethnic group. Analytic samples were restricted to those with observed physical function outcomes.
*Regression coefficients of functioning scores were scaled to SD=10, per 1-SD change in pulse wave velocity, pulse pressure, and mean arterial pressure.
†Chronic disease was defined as prevalent stroke, myocardial infarction, or diabetes mellitus.
‡Fully adjusted model is adjusted for age, sex, ethnic group, mean arterial pressure, heart rate, antihypertensive treatment, and chronic disease.

of problems with the activities of daily living as well as with poor lung function as assessed by a portable spirometer (Table 3). Moreover, association with these losses of function was weakened only slightly by adjusting for a number of important covariates, including pulse pressure, mean arterial pressure, use of hypertensive medications, and the presence of chronic disease. These observations underline the importance of maintaining vascular health during the aging process, and they point out the need for long-term studies of the association between habitual physical activity and arterial distensibility.[2]

R. J. Shephard, MD (Lond), PhD, DPE

References

1. Vlachopoulos C, Aznaouridis K, Stefanadis C. Prediction of cardiovascular events and all-cause mortality with arterial stiffness: a systematic review and meta-analysis. *J Am Coll Cardiol.* 2010;55:1318-1327.
2. Aoyagi Y, Park H, Kakiyama T, Park S, Yoshiuchi K, Shephard RJ. Yearlong physical activity and regional stiffness of arteries in older adults: the Nakanojo study. *Eur J Appl Physiol.* 2010;109:455-464.
3. Tanaka H, Dinenno FA, Monahan KD, Clevenger CM, DeSouza CA, Seals DR. Aging, habitual exercise, and dynamic arterial compliance. *Circulation.* 2000; 102:1270-1275.
4. Yamada S, Inaba M, Goto H, et al. Associations between physical activity, peripheral atherosclerosis and bone status in healthy Japanese women. *Atherosclerosis.* 2006;188:196-202.

Translating Weight Loss and Physical Activity Programs Into the Community to Preserve Mobility in Older, Obese Adults in Poor Cardiovascular Health
Rejeski WJ, Brubaker PH, Goff DC Jr, et al (Wake Forest Univ, Winston-Salem, NC; Wake Forest Univ School of Medicine, Winston-Salem, NC; et al)
Arch Intern Med 171:880-886, 2011

Background.—Limitations in mobility are common among older adults with cardiovascular and cardiometabolic disorders and have profound effects on health and well-being. With the growing population of older adults in the United States, effective and scalable public health approaches are needed to address this problem. Our goal was to determine the effects of a physical activity and weight loss intervention on 18-month change in mobility among overweight or obese older adults in poor cardiovascular health.

Methods.—The study design was a translational, randomized controlled trial of physical activity (PA) and weight loss (WL) on mobility in overweight or obese older adults with cardiovascular disease (CVD) or at risk for CVD. The study was conducted within the community infrastructure of Cooperative Extension Centers. Participants were randomized to 1 of 3 interventions: PA, WL + PA, or a successful aging (SA) education control arm. The primary outcome was time to complete a 400-m walk in seconds (400MWT).

Results.—A significant treatment effect ($P = .002$) and follow-up testing revealed that the WL + PA group improved their 400MWT (adjusted mean

[SE], 323.3 [3.7] seconds) compared with both PA (336.3 [3.9] seconds; $P = .02$) and SA (341.3 [3.9] seconds; $P < .001$). Participants with poorer mobility at baseline benefited the most ($P < .001$).

Conclusion.—Existing community infrastructures can be effective in delivering lifestyle interventions to enhance mobility in older adults in poor cardiovascular health with deficits in mobility; attention should be given to intervening on both weight and sedentary behavior since weight loss is critical to long-term improvement in mobility.

Trial Registration.—clinicaltrials.gov Identifier: NCT00119795.

▶ As summarized in Fig 1 in the original article, the combination of weight loss and physical activity improved walking mobility in older, diseased, obese adults. Physical activity alone was insufficient to improve walking speed over the entire 1.5-year length of this study. The 400-m walk test is a useful measure of mobility in older adults, with a slow time predicting increased morbidity, disability, cardiovascular disease, and mortality.[1]

D. C. Nieman, DrPH

Reference

1. Newman AB, Simonsick EM, Naydeck BL, et al. Association of long-distance corridor walk performance with mortality, cardiovascular disease, mobility limitation, and disability. *JAMA*. 2006;295:2018-2026.

Effects of Whole-Body Vibration Training on Different Devices on Bone Mineral Density

Von Stengel S, Kemmler W, Bebenek M, et al (Inst of Med Physics Univ of Erlangen-Nueremberg, Germany)
Med Sci Sports Exerc 43:1071-1079, 2011

Purpose.—Whole-body vibration (WBV) is a new nonpharmacological approach to counteract osteoporosis. However, the specific vibration protocol to most effectively reduce osteoporotic risk has not been reported. In the ELVIS II (Erlangen Longitudinal Vibration Study II) trial, we determined the effect of different WBV devices on bone mineral density (BMD) and neuromuscular performance.

Methods.—A total of 108 postmenopausal women (65.8 ± 3.5 yr) were randomly allocated to 1) rotational vibration training (RVT), i.e., 12.5 Hz, 12 mm, three sessions per week, for 15 min, including dynamic squat exercises; 2) vertical vibration training (VVT), i.e., 35 Hz, 1.7 mm, as above; and 3) a wellness control group (CG), i.e., two blocks of 10 low-intensity gymnastics sessions. BMD was measured at the hip and lumbar spine at baseline and after 12 months of training using dual-energy X-ray absorptiometry. Maximum isometric leg extension strength and leg power were determined using force plates.

Results.—A BMD gain at the lumbar spine was observed in both vibration VT groups (RVT = +0.7% $\pm$ 2.2%, VVT = +0.5% $\pm$ 2.0%), which was significant compared with the CG value (-0.4% ± 2.0%) for RVT ($P = 0.04$) and borderline nonsignificant for VVT ($P = 0.08$). In the neck region, no significant treatment effect occurred. Neck BMD values tended to increase in both VT groups (RVT = $+0.3\%$ ± 2.7%, VVT = $+1.1\%$ ± 3.4%) and remained stable in CG (-0.0% ± 2.1%). Both VT groups gained maximum leg strength (RVT = $+27\%$ ± 22%, VVT = $+24\%$ ± 34%) compared with CG ($+6\%$ ± 20%, $P = 0.000$), whereas power measurements did not reach the level of significance ($P = 0.1$).

Conclusions.—WBV training is effective for reducing the risk for osteoporosis by increasing lumbar BMD and leg strength.

▶ Both osteoporosis and falls in elderly women can lead to hip, vertebral, and other fractures, with significant morbidity and often resulting mortality. Weight-bearing exercise is known to positively affect bone mineral density (BMD), and strength training in the elderly can also improve neuromuscular function and proprioception, decreasing the risk for falls. The challenge always is how to engage these patients in the appropriate exercise regime and maintain compliance. Sometimes coexisting medical conditions also preclude strenuous conventional exercise, but, frequently, people are just unwilling and/or not motivated to follow such a program.

Whole-body vibration (WBV) has been suggested as an alternative method of mechanical loading of bone, although the optimal frequency, amplitude, duration, and other factors remain to be determined. This study made use of 2 different commercially marketed high-intensity WBV devices (rotational vs vertical) and examined the effect of specific WBV training (3 weekly sessions of 15 minutes each) on BMD and fall-related neuromuscular performance, in comparison with a control wellness group who did sham exercise. The vibration plate-specific settings were selected to result in the same acceleration. After a year, repeat dual-energy x-ray absorptiometry showed significant gains in BMD in the lumbar spine in the rotational group, whereas the effect in the vertically vibrating group was borderline nonsignificant. In contrast to some other studies, hip BMD was not affected, but WBV increased maximum leg strength by about 25% in both vibration training groups. The addition of video guidance (with a DVD player) for the training programs, in addition to initial supervision by certified instructors, increased compliance, and, therefore, such an approach might be both feasible and attractive, with high potential for large-scale implementation in different institutions. However, as noted in the conclusions, further study is needed to determine the differential effect of various devices or vibration protocols and to identify the critical variables and most effective programs in humans.

C. Lebrun, MDCM, MPE, CCFP, Dip Sport Med, FACSM

Physical Activity and Cognition in Women With Vascular Conditions

Vercambre M-N, Grodstein F, Manson JE, et al (Mutuelle Generale de l'Education Nationale, Paris, France; Harvard Med School, Boston, MA; Harvard School of Public Health, Boston, MA)
Arch Intern Med 171:1244-1250, 2011

Background.—Individuals with vascular disease or risk factors have substantially higher rates of cognitive decline, yet little is known about means of maintaining cognition in this group.

Methods.—We examined the relation between physical activity and cognitive decline in participants of the Women's Antioxidant Cardiovascular Study, a cohort of women with prevalent vascular disease or at least 3 coronary risk factors. Recreational physical activity was assessed at baseline (October 1995 through June 1996) and every 2 years thereafter. Between December 1998 and July 2000, a total of 2809 women 65 years or older underwent a cognitive battery by telephone interview, including 5 tests of global cognition, verbal memory, and category fluency. Tests were administered 3 additional times over 5.4 years. We used multivariable-adjusted general linear models for repeated measures to compare the annual rates of cognitive score changes across levels of total physical activity and energy expended in walking, as assessed at Women's Antioxidant Cardiovascular Study baseline.

Results.—We found a significant trend ($P < .001$ for trend) toward decreasing rates of cognitive decline with increasing energy expenditure. Compared with the bottom quintile of total physical activity, significant differences in rates of cognitive decline were observed from the fourth quintile ($P = .04$ for the fourth quintile and $P < .001$ for the fifth quintile), or the equivalent of daily 30-minute walks at a brisk pace. This was equivalent to the difference in cognitive decline observed for women who were 5 to 7 years younger. Regularly walking for exercise was strongly related to slower rates of cognitive decline ($P = .003$ for trend).

Conclusion.—Regular physical activity, including walking, was associated with better preservation of cognitive function in older women with vascular disease or risk factors.

▶ As summarized in Fig 1 in the original article, higher levels of physical activity were linked to reduced cognitive decline in older women with vascular disease or coronary risk factors. Exercise may have several beneficial effects over time, including preservation of neuronal structures by stimulating brain-derived neurotrophic factor, neuronal growth, blood vessel health, and lowered inflammation. There is increasing evidence that exercise training preserves cognition in both healthy and unhealthy older adults.[1]

D. C. Nieman, DrPH

Reference

1. Sofi F, Valecchi D, Bacci D, et al. Physical activity and risk of cognitive decline: a meta-analysis of prospective studies. *J Intern Med.* 2011;269:107-117.

Activity Energy Expenditure and Incident Cognitive Impairment in Older Adults

Middleton LE, Manini TM, Simonsick EM, et al (Sunnybrook Health Sciences Centre, Toronto, Ontario, Canada; Univ of Florida, Gainesville; Natl Inst on Aging, Bethesda, MD; et al)
Arch Intern Med 171:1251-1257, 2011

Background.—Studies suggest that physically active people have reduced risk of incident cognitive impairment in late life. However, these studies are limited by reliance on self-reports of physical activity, which only moderately correlate with objective measures and often exclude activity not readily quantifiable by frequency and duration. The objective of this study was to investigate the relationship between activity energy expenditure (AEE), an objective measure of total activity, and incidence of cognitive impairment.

Methods.—We calculated AEE as 90% of total energy expenditure (assessed during 2 weeks using doubly labeled water) minus resting metabolic rate (measured using indirect calorimetry) in 197 men and women (mean age, 74.8 years) who were free of mobility and cognitive impairments at study baseline (1998-1999). Cognitive function was assessed at baseline and 2 or 5 years later using the Modified Mini-Mental State Examination. Cognitive impairment was defined as a decline of at least 1.0 SD (9 points) between baseline and follow-up evaluations.

Results.—After adjustment for baseline Modified Mini-Mental State Examination scores, demographics, fat-free mass, sleep duration, self-reported health, and diabetes mellitus, older adults in the highest sex-specific tertile of AEE had lower odds of incident cognitive impairment than those in the lowest tertile (odds ratio, 0.09; 95% confidence interval, 0.01-0.79). There was also a significant dose response between AEE and incidence of cognitive impairment ($P = .05$ for trend over tertiles).

Conclusions.—These findings indicate that greater AEE may be protective against cognitive impairment in a dose-response manner. The significance of overall activity in contrast to vigorous or light activity should be determined.

▶ This article, along with a companion article in the same issue of the *Archives of Internal Medicine*,[1] joins a substantial chorus of investigators[2-5] who have suggested that regular physical activity can help to prevent the cognitive decline normally associated with a combination of extreme old age and atherosclerosis. The interpretation of data has often been complicated by reliance on questionnaire assessments of physical activity, which are notoriously unreliable in the elderly. But in the study reported here, energy expenditures were measured accurately by the doubly labeled water technique; the only disadvantage of this approach (apart from its cost) is that it yields an average figure for energy expenditure over a 2-week period, without indicating whether this was accumulated through long periods of light activity or shorter periods of vigorous exercise. It is difficult to examine the direction of relationships in humans using direct experiments, and often the studies of cognitive decline have relied on the demonstration of statistically significant correlations between reported activity and some assessment of mental status, leaving the possibility that mental deterioration caused a drop in physical activity rather than the converse. However, Middleton and associates followed a substantial sample of seniors, all of whom were shown to be free of either cognitive problems or impairment of mobility at the outset of their 5-year study. When the most active individuals were compared with the least active tercile over this period, the odds ratio of a decline in cognitive state favoring the more active group was very impressive (mean, 0.09; range, 0.01-0.79). Potential explanations of benefit include an increase of arousal, a stimulation of systemic blood pressure and thus of cerebral perfusion, increased concentrations of neurotransmitters and neurotrophins (the latter encouraging the formation of new neural synapses), and long-term hippocampal potentiation.[6] The study of Vercambre et al[1] was based on questionnaire assessments of the volume of physical activity in women with known vascular conditions; it also demonstrated a slower cognitive decline in the most active individuals.

R. J. Shephard, MD (Lond), PhD, DPE

References

1. Vercambre M-N, Grodstein F, Manson JE, Stampfer MJ, Kang JH. Physical activity and cognition in women with vascular conditions. *Arch Intern Med.* 2011;171:1244-1250.
2. Larson EB, Wang L, Bowen JD, et al. Exercise is associated with reduced risk for incident dementia among persons 65 years of age and older. *Ann Intern Med.* 2006;144:73-81.
3. Laurin D, Verreault R, Lindsay J, MacPherson K, Rockwood K. Physical activity and risk of cognitive impairment and dementia in elderly persons. *Arch Neurol.* 2001;58:498-504.
4. Rockwood K, Middleton L. Physical activity and the maintenance of cognitive function. *Alzheimers Dement.* 2007;3:S38-S44.
5. Rovio S, Kåreholt I, Helkala EL, et al. Leisure-time physical activity at midlife and the risk of dementia and Alzheimer's disease. *Lancet Neurol.* 2005;4:705-711.
6. Shephard RJ, Trudeau F. Relationships of physical activity to brain health and the academic performance of Schoolchildren. *Am J Lifestyle Med.* 2009;4:138-150.

Exergaming and Older Adult Cognition: A Cluster Randomized Clinical Trial

Anderson-Hanley C, Arciero PJ, Brickman AM, et al (Union College, Schenectady, NY; Columbia Univ, NY; et al)
Am J Prev Med 42:109-119, 2012

Background.—Dementia cases may reach 100 million by 2050. Interventions are sought to curb or prevent cognitive decline. Exercise yields cognitive benefits, but few older adults exercise. Virtual reality—enhanced exercise or "exergames" may elicit greater participation.

Purpose.—To test the following hypotheses: (1) stationary cycling with virtual reality tours ("cybercycle") will enhance executive function and clinical status more than traditional exercise; (2) exercise effort will explain improvement; and (3) brain-derived neurotrophic growth factor (BDNF) will increase.

Design.—Multi-site cluster randomized clinical trial (RCT) of the impact of 3 months of cybercycling versus traditional exercise, on cognitive function in older adults. Data were collected in 2008–2010; analyses were conducted in 2010–2011.

Setting/Participants.—102 older adults from eight retirement communities enrolled; 79 were randomized and 63 completed.

Interventions.—A recumbent stationary ergometer was utilized; virtual reality tours and competitors were enabled on the cybercycle.

TABLE 2.—Neuropsychologic and Physiologic Outcomes After 3 Months of Exercise (Intent-to-Treat Analysis)[a]

	Mean Difference From Baseline (95% CI)		
	Cybercycle ($n=38$)	Control Bike ($n=41$)	p-value (df)[b]
PRIMARY COGNITIVE OUTCOMES			
Executive function			
Color Trails Difference (2-1) (s)	−15.94 (−16.21, 15.66)	9.74 (9.48, 10.00)	0.007 (1, 73)
Stroop C (s)	−6.59 (−6.67, −6.51)	0.56 (0.49, 0.64)	0.05 (1, 73)
Digits Backward (sum score)	0.36 (0.34, 0.38)	−0.83 (−0.85, −0.82)	0.03 (1, 73)
SECONDARY COGNITIVE OUTCOMES[c]			
Attention			
LDST (sum score)	0.79 (0.62, 0.95)	0.73 (0.57, 0.89)	0.95 (1, 72)
Verbal fluency			
COWAT (sum score)	3.51 (2.77, 4.25)	2.33 (1.62, 3.03)	0.63 (1, 73)
Categories (sum score)	−0.03 (0.11, −0.18)	1.18 (1.32, 1.04)	0.22 (1, 73)
Verbal memory (immediate)			
RAVLT (sum 5 trials score)	−0.73 (−1.27, −0.19)	0.85 (0.33, 1.37)	0.50 (1, 73)
RAVLT immediate recall (score)	0.77 (0.60, 0.94)	0.06 (−0.10, 0.22)	0.32 (1, 73)
Verbal memory (delayed)			
RAVLT delayed recall (score)	0.71 (0.62, 0.79)	0.10 (0.01, 0.18)	0.43 (1, 73)
Fuld delayed recall (score)	0.15 (0.13, 0.17)	0.39 (0.37, 0.41)	0.61 (1, 73)
Visuospatial skill			
Figure copy (sum score)	3.27 (3.56, 2.98)	3.69 (3.97, 3.40)	0.81 (1, 72)
Clock (sum score)	0.07 (0.07, 0.07)	−0.19 (−0.19, −0.19)	0.45 (1, 72)
Visuospatial memory (delayed)			
Figure delayed recall (score)	0.07 (0.22, −0.08)	1.66 (1.80, 1.52)	0.28 (1, 72)
Motor function			
Pegboard dominant hand (s)	10.61 (8.64, 12.57)	6.13 (4.22, 8.03)	0.56 (1, 72)
Pegboard nondominant hand (s)	7.76 (5.86, 9.65)	13.79 (11.95, 15.63)	0.36 (1, 72)
PHYSIOLOGIC OUTCOMES			
Weight (kg)	−0.63 (−0.75, −0.52)	−0.04 (−0.15, 0.07)	0.24 (1, 72)
BMI	−0.26 (−0.29, −0.23)	−0.03 (−0.06, 0.00)	0.26 (1, 67)
Fat mass (kg)	−1.04 (−0.95, −1.13)	−0.76 (−0.67, −0.84)	0.50 (1, 72)
Lean mass (kg)	0.39 (0.31, 0.47)	0.56 (0.48, 0.63)	0.65 (1, 72)
Abdominal fat (%)	−1.79 (−1.97, −1.61)	−0.94 (−1.11, −0.78)	0.32 (1, 66)
Leg extension 60° (s^{-1})	−2.96 (−3.00, −2.92)	11.09 (11.05, 11.13)	0.04 (1, 71)
Leg flex 60° (s^{-1})	−2.79 (−3.26, −2.31)	5.70 (5.25, 6.15)	0.07 (1, 71)
Insulin (uU/mL)	2.75 (2.39, 3.12)	1.53 (1.16, 1.90)	0.46 (1, 67)
Glucose (mM/L)	−0.09 (−0.01, −0.16)	−0.06 (0.01, −0.13)	0.90 (1, 68)

COWAT, Controlled Oral Word Association Test; LDST, Letter Digit Symbol Test; RAVLT, Rey Auditory Verbal Learning Test.
[a]Marginal mean differences and CIs reported, based on repeated measures ANCOVA controlling for age and education.
[b]For ANCOVA, repeated measures, group X time; the first df in parentheses refers to the effect (group X time) and the second refers to the error term.
[c]No significant changes expected given prior research literature.

Main Outcome Measures.—Executive function (Color Trails Difference, Stroop C, Digits Backward); clinical status (mild cognitive impairment; MCI); exercise effort/fitness; and plasma BDNF.

Results.—Intent-to-treat analyses, controlling for age, education, and cluster randomization, revealed a significant group X time interaction for composite executive function ($p=0.002$). Cybercycling yielded a medium effect over traditional exercise ($d=0.50$). Cybercyclists had a 23% relative risk reduction in clinical progression to MCI. Exercise effort and fitness were comparable, suggesting another underlying mechanism. A significant group X time interaction for BDNF ($p=0.05$) indicated enhanced neuroplasticity among cybercyclists.

Conclusions.—Cybercycling older adults achieved better cognitive function than traditional exercisers, for the same effort, suggesting that simultaneous cognitive and physical exercise has greater potential for preventing cognitive decline.

Trial Registration.—This study is registered at Clinicaltrials.gov NCT01167400 (Table 2).

▶ There is growing evidence that regular physical activity can help to slow the loss of cognitive skills that is associated with aging.[1-3] The problem is keeping people involved in their exercise programs. Some 50 years ago, I suggested to the Ontario Science Museum a system in which people could sit watching television as long as they pedaled a cycle ergometer with sufficient vigor. Recently, gadgets that combine exercise with simulated environments have become increasingly popular as a means of sustaining exercise motivation.[4] In the study of Anderson-Hanley and associates, the benefits of the new equipment relative to conventional cycle ergometry were meager; many potential outcomes were tested (Table 2), but only 1 test (the Color Trails Difference) showed a really significant difference. Two other tests apparently showed borderline gains, but because the authors did not apply a Bonferroni correction, statistical significance could have arisen simply from the making of multiple comparisons. Further, the amount of exercise performed over the 3-month period did not differ between the normal and the enhanced cycle ergometer, so that if there was any benefit from virtual reality, additional exercise was not the key factor. My conclusion must be that the virtual reality cycle is an expensive and apparently unnecessary gimmick and that it offers little benefit to most people. My suggestion to the average senior would be that rather than investing in a virtual reality cycle, why not take a walk in the real surroundings of the countryside?

R. J. Shephard, MD (Lond), PhD, DPE

References

1. Larson EB. Physical activity for older adults at risk for Alzheimer disease. *JAMA.* 2008;300:1077-1079.
2. Chang M, Jonsson PV, Snaedal J, et al. The effect of midlife physical activity on cognitive function among older adults: AGES—Reykjavik Study. *J Gerontol A Biol Sci Med Sci.* 2010;65:1369-1374.
3. Scarmeas N, Luchsinger JA, Schupf N, et al. Physical activity, diet, and risk of Alzheimer disease. *JAMA.* 2009;302:627-637.

4. Annesi JJ, Mazas J. Effects of virtual reality-enhanced exercise equipment on adherence and exercise-induced feeling states. *Percept Mot Skills.* 1997;85: 835-844.

Cardiorespiratory Fitness as a Predictor of Dementia Mortality in Men and Women

Liu R, Sui X, Laditka JN, et al (Natl Inst of Environmental Health Sciences, Research Triangle Park, NC; Univ of South Carolina, Columbia; Univ of North Carolina at Charlotte; et al)
Med Sci Sports Exerc 44:253-259, 2012

There is evidence that physical activity may reduce the risk of developing Alzheimer disease and dementia. However, few reports have examined the physical activity–dementia association with objective measures of physical activity. Cardiorespiratory fitness (hereafter called fitness) is an objective reproducible measure of recent physical activity habits.

Purpose.—We sought to determine whether fitness is associated with lower risk for dementia mortality in women and men.

Methods.—We followed 14,811 women and 45,078 men, age 20–88 yr at baseline, for an average of 17 yr. All participants completed a preventive health examination at the Cooper Clinic in Dallas, TX, during 1970–2001. Fitness was measured with a maximal treadmill exercise test, with results expressed in maximal METs. The National Death Index identified deaths through 2003. Cox proportional hazards models were used to examine the association between baseline fitness and dementia mortality, adjusting for age, sex, examination year, body mass index, smoking, alcohol use, abnormal ECGs, and health status.

Results.—There were 164 deaths with dementia listed as the cause during 1,012,125 person-years of exposure. Each 1-MET increase in fitness was associated with a 14% lower adjusted risk of dementia mortality (95% confidence interval (CI) = 6%–22%). With fitness expressed in tertiles, adjusted hazard ratios (HRs) for those in the middle- and high-fitness groups suggest their risk of dementia mortality was less than half that of those in the lowest fitness group (HR = 0.44, CI = 0.26–0.74 and HR = 0.49, CI = 0.26–0.90, respectively).

Conclusions.—Greater fitness was associated with lower risk of mortality from dementia in a large cohort of men and women (Fig 1).

▶ The increase in Alzheimer disease (AD)- and dementia-related mortality has become a major public health concern. Epidemiologic evidence suggests that physical activity may decrease the risk of AD, but the findings vary greatly in part because of the methods used for measuring physical activity. Rather than estimate physical activity, Liu and colleagues measured cardiorespiratory fitness (CRF) from maximal treadmill exercise test performance in more than 14 000 women and 45 000 men (mean ± SD age 43 ± 10 years) and then classified the participants by tertile of CRF (low-medium-high). The primary outcome

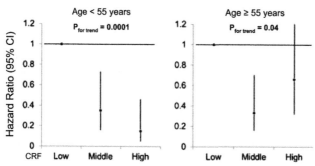

FIGURE 1.—Multivariate-adjusted total dementia mortality HRs (and 95% CIs), by CRF level and age groups. The number of individuals and total dementia deaths in the low-, middle-, and high-CRF groups were 16,518 and 37, 15,369 and 11, and 19,573 and 5, respectively, among those age <55 yr and 5336 and 83, 1949 and 12, and 1144 and 13, respectively, among those age ≥55 yr. (Reprinted from Liu R, Sui X, Laditka JN, et al. Cardiorespiratory fitness as a predictor of dementia mortality in men and women. *Med Sci Sports Exerc.* 2012;44:253-259, with permission from the American College of Sports Medicine.)

was death attributed to AD or vascular dementia over 17 years of follow-up, on average. Significantly fewer total dementia and vascular-dementia related deaths, but not AD deaths, occurred in the middle- and high-fitness groups compared with the low-fitness group. Persons in the middle- and high-fitness categories had a 73% and 69% lower mortality risk for vascular dementia, respectively, compared with the low-fitness group. Vascular dementia mortality risk was reduced by 18% for each 1-MET increase in fitness. When the cohort was divided by age (< 55 or ≥55 years), a strong gradient trend for decreased dementia mortality risk with increasing CRF was found in the younger group (Fig 1). In the older participants, the high CRF level did not confer additional dementia mortality reduction, but this could be attributed to fewer cases in this tertile. In the young and older groups, the middle CRF category was associated with a 60% decreased risk of total dementia mortality. Fitness may protect against dementia through a variety of mechanisms acting directly on the brain or by lowering the risk of other conditions, such as cardiovascular disease and diabetes that are related to cognitive decline.

C. M. Jankowski, PhD

Does cerebral oxygenation affect cognitive function during exercise?

Ando S, Kokubu M, Yamada Y, et al (Kyoto Prefectural Univ of Medicine, Japan; Kyoto Univ, Japan)
Eur J Appl Physiol 111:1973-1982, 2011

This study tested whether cerebral oxygenation affects cognitive function during exercise. We measured reaction times (RT) of 12 participants while they performed a modified version of the Eriksen flanker task, at rest and while cycling. In the exercise condition, participants performed the cognitive task at rest and while cycling at three workloads [40, 60, and 80% of peak oxygen uptake ($\dot{V}O_2$)]. In the control condition, the workload was fixed at 20 W. RT was divided into premotor and motor components based on surface electromyographic recordings. The premotor component of RT (premotor time) was used to evaluate the effects of acute exercise on cognitive function. Cerebral oxygenation was monitored during the cognitive task over the right frontal cortex using near-infrared spectroscopy. In the exercise condition, we found that premotor time significantly decreased during exercise at 60% peak $\dot{V}O_2$ relative to rest. However, this improvement was not observed during exercise at 80% peak $\dot{V}O_2$. In the control condition, premotor time did not change during exercise. Cerebral oxygenation during exercise at 60% peak $\dot{V}O_2$ was not significantly different from that at rest, while cerebral oxygenation substantially decreased during exercise at 80% peak $\dot{V}O_2$. The present results suggest that an improvement in cognitive function occurs during moderate exercise, independent of cerebral oxygenation (Fig 4).

▶ Although it is now widely agreed that regular physical activity can slow the aging of cognitive function, various potential mechanisms continue to be widely debated. One frequent suggestion has been that physical activity elevates the systemic blood pressure, and this, at least temporarily, augments cerebral blood flow. However, the study of Ando and associates appears to negate this possibility. The study participants performed a visual reaction task, and prefrontal cerebral function was inferred from the premovement component of total reaction time. This component was enhanced relative to control (exercise at 20% of aerobic

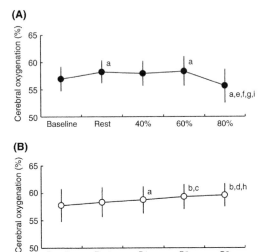

(A)

(B)

FIGURE 4.—erebral oxygenation in the exercise (a) and control (b) conditions. Data are expressed as mean ± SD. [a]$P < 0.05$, [b]$P < 0.001$ versus values at the baseline; [c]$P < 0.05$, [d]$P < 0.01$ versus [e]$P < 0.001$ versus values at rest; [f]$P < 0.001$ versus value at 40%; [g]$P < 0.001$ versus value at 60%; [h]$P < 0.05$ versus value at B1; [i]$P < 0.001$ versus value in the control condition. (Reprinted from Ando S, Kokubu M, Yamada Y, et al. Does cerebral oxygenation affect cognitive function during exercise? *Eur J Appl Physiol.* 2011;111:1973-1982, Copyright 2011, with kind permission of Springer Science+Business Media.)

power) when on the experimental days subjects were exercising for 6 minutes on a cycle ergometer at 60% (but not at 80%) of their maximal aerobic power. Nevertheless, near infrared spectroscopy measurements over the forehead (with subtraction of cutaneous flows as inferred from a superficial probe) suggested that the blood flow to the cerebral tissues was unchanged at 60% and appreciably decreased at 80% of aerobic power (Fig 4). This finding is somewhat surprising and merits checking because there may have been day-to-day differences in positioning of the superficial probes. Physiologists have long contended that cerebral perfusion depends largely on blood pressure rather than cerebral vasodilatation and that flows should rise during exercise. Nevertheless, it is conceivable that the drop in arterial Pco_2 associated with prolonged exercise[1] may have been enough to restrict cerebral blood flow despite the concomitant increase in blood pressure; unfortunately the study did not measure changes in $Paco_2$. Greater cerebral arousal and hormonal changes are other factors that could possibly explain the faster reaction times observed during moderate exercise.

R. J. Shephard, MD (Lond), PhD, DPE

Reference

1. Nybo L, Secher NH. Cerebral perturbations provoked by prolonged exercise. *Prog Neurobiol.* 2004;72:223-261.

Independent and Combined Effects of Calcium-Vitamin D₃ and Exercise on Bone Structure and Strength in Older Men: An 18-Month Factorial Design Randomized Controlled Trial

Kukuljan S, Nowson CA, Sanders KM, et al (Deakin Univ, Victoria, Australia; Univ of Melbourne, Geelong Victoria, Australia; et al)
J Clin Endocrinol Metab 96:955-963, 2011

Context.—Exercise and calcium-vitamin D are independently recognized as important strategies to prevent osteoporosis, but their combined effects on bone strength and its determinants remain uncertain.

Objective.—To assess whether calcium-vitamin D₃ fortified milk could enhance the effects of exercise on bone strength, structure, and mineral density in middle-aged and older men.

Design, Setting, Participants.—An 18-month factorial design randomized controlled trial in which 180 men aged 50—79 years were randomized to the following: exercise + fortified milk; exercise; fortified milk; or controls. Exercise consisted of progressive resistance training with weight-bearing impact activities performed 3 d/week. Men assigned to fortified milk consumed 400 ml/d of 1% fat milk containing 1000 mg/d calcium and 800 IU/d vitamin D₃.

Main Outcome Measures.—Changes in bone mineral density (BMD), bone structure, and strength at the lumbar spine (LS), proximal femur, mid-femur, and mid-tibia measured by dual energy x-ray absorptiometry and/or quantitative computed tomography.

Results.—There were no exercise-by-fortified milk interactions at any skeletal site. Main effect analysis showed that exercise led to a 2.1% (95% confidence interval, 0.5—3.6) net gain in femoral neck section modulus, which was associated with an approximately 1.9% gain in areal BMD and cross-sectional area. Exercise also improved LS trabecular BMD [net gain 2.2% (95% confidence interval, 0.2—4.1)], but had no effect on mid-femur or mid-tibia BMD, structure, or strength. There were no main effects of the fortified milk at any skeletal site.

Conclusion.—A community-based multi-component exercise program successfully improved LS and femoral neck BMD and strength in healthy older men, but providing additional calcium-vitamin D3 to these replete men did not enhance the osteogenic response.

▶ Exercise is needed to stimulate bone modeling and remodeling, and calcium is an important substrate for bone mineralization. However, these findings indicate that weight lifting and weight-bearing impact exercise, but not extra calcium and vitamin D, were effective for improving bone mineral density in the femur and lumbar spine areas of older men. The diets of the subjects were sufficient to provide all the calcium needed for exercise-induced improvements in bone density. The exercise program was demanding: 3 nonconsecutive days per week for 18 months, with each session lasting 60 to 75 minutes and consisting of a 5- to 10-minute warm up and cool down involving stationary cycling and stretching, 6 to 8 moderate- to high-intensity progressive resistance training exercises, and 3 moderate-impact, weight-bearing exercises (eg, jumping off 15- and 30-cm benches).

D. C. Nieman, DrPH

Addressing Secondary Prevention of Osteoporosis in Fracture Care: Follow-up to "Own the Bone"
Edwards BJ, Koval K, Bunta AD, et al (Northwestern Univ, Chicago, IL; Dartmouth-Hitchcock Med Ctr, Lebanon, NH)
J Bone Joint Surg Am 93:e87.1-e87.7, 2011

The majority of the 1.8 million individuals who sustain a fracture annually in the United States have osteopenia or osteoporosis, yet <15% of these patients subsequently receive treatment for osteoporosis. A prospective cohort study was conducted to assess the effect of two different interventions on the rate of osteoporosis treatment in patients with a fragility fracture. Patients who were fifty years of age or older and were hospitalized for the treatment of a fragility fracture at either of two academic institutions were eligible for inclusion in the study. The intervention at one hospital involved immediate care for osteoporosis, including initiation of pharmacologic therapy during hospitalization. The intervention at the other hospital involved delayed care, including recommendations for osteoporosis counseling, bone-mineral density testing, and potential treatment for osteoporosis that were communicated to the primary care physician after the patient was discharged from the hospital. Patients were surveyed by telephone six months after the fracture, and their medical and pharmacy records were reviewed to verify the osteoporosis treatment that they had received. The mean age was 73 ± 10 years in the immediate-care group and 74 ± 12 years in the delayed-care group. Eighty percent of the patients were women. Sixty-five percent of the patients in each group completed the telephone interview six months after the fracture, and most had seen their primary care physician and undergone bone-mineral density testing. The rate of bone-mineral density testing was 92% in the immediate-care group compared with 76% in the delayed-care group. Both immediate and delayed care for osteoporosis resulted in a significant increase in the treatment rate compared with the baseline rate of 0% (p < 0.001). However, the primary care physician had initiated osteoporosis therapy by six months after the fracture in only 30% of the patients in the delayed-care group compared with a treatment rate of 67% in the immediate-care group (p < 0.001). Limitations of the study include the possibility that the findings resulted from a difference between the two study centers rather than between the two strategies. In addition, because of the academic and integrated nature of the medical systems at which the study was conducted, the findings cannot necessarily be extrapolated to other types of institutions. In summary, a recommendation for osteoporosis treatment made by an orthopaedic surgeon to the patient's primary care physician resulted in an increase in the rate of bone-mineral density testing and in the rate of therapy compared with baseline. However, immediate initiation of osteoporosis care during hospitalization for the fragility fracture resulted in a higher rate of treatment—with two-thirds of the patients receiving therapy six months after the fracture—compared with delayed initiation (Fig 2).

▶ This is an extremely relevant study, with important implications for secondary prevention and treatment of osteoporosis in fracture care. Since 2007, the American Orthopaedic Association has made major strides to increase the awareness of orthopedic surgeons regarding the need for follow-up and investigation for low bone quality, in patients presenting with fragility fractures, and in a "Leadership in Orthopedics" position paper challenged them to "Own the Bone."[1] While this has resulted in improvement of the rate of counseling regarding osteoporosis to 90% and more frequent recommendations for bone mineral density (BMD) testing, the next step in evaluating the impact of this project is to look at actual implementation of osteoporosis treatment. In this particular study, the results of immediate in-hospital osteoporosis care (including evaluation by an osteoporosis consultant, initiation of appropriate pharmacologic therapy, and ordering of BMD testing) versus delayed osteoporosis care (consisting of recommendations to the primary care physician in the consultation letter by the orthopedic surgeon) were compared. The 2 interventions were stratified by hospital (both of which were academic institutions). After 6 months, according to telephone survey responses by 65% of the patients in each group, BMD density

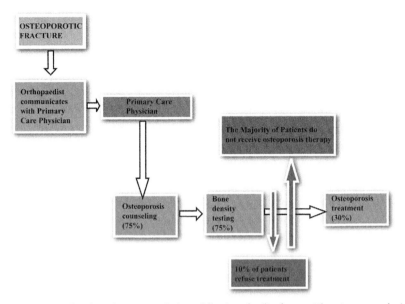

FIGURE 2.—Identifying the gap in medical care following a fragility fracture. The primary care physician did not counsel all participants. (Reprinted from Edwards BJ, Koval K, Bunta AD, et al. Addressing secondary prevention of osteoporosis in fracture care: follow-up to "own the bone". *J Bone Joint Surg Am.* 2011;93:e87.1-e87.7, with permission from The Journal of Bone and Joint Surgery, Incorporated.)

had been tested in 92% of the immediate care group and 76% of the delayed testing group, but significantly osteoporosis therapy had been instituted by the primary care physician in only 30% of the delayed care group compared with 67% of the immediate care group. There were several reasons for this, including failure of the primary care physician to initiate appropriate osteoporosis therapy after receiving BMD results and unwillingness of the patients to accept pharmacological treatment, either because of expense or because of perceived side effects. But the most important finding was a significant gap in medical care following a fragility fracture (Fig 2), identification of which will hopefully allow further targeted quality improvement interventions. Further research appears to be warranted to examine barriers to osteoporosis care by outpatient physicians. In addition, enhanced knowledge transfer and exchange strategies, for both physicians and patients, may help to increase compliance with, and adherence to, evidence-based guidelines for management of osteoporosis following a fragility fracture and prevention of secondary fractures.

C. Lebrun, MDCM, MPE, CCFP, Dip Sport Med, FACSM

Reference

1. Tosi LL, Gliklich R, Kannan K, Koval KJ. The American Orthopaedic Association's "own the bone" initiative to prevent secondary fractures. *J Bone Joint Surg Am.* 2008;90:163-173.

Article Index

Chapter 1: Epidemiology, Prevention of Injuries, Lesions of Head and Neck

Chapter 2: Other Musculoskeletal Injuries

Chapter 3: Biomechanics, Muscle Strength and Training

Chapter 4: Physical Activity, Cardiorespiratory Physiology and Immune Function

Chapter 5: Metabolism and Obesity, Nutrition and Doping

Chapter 6: Cardiorespiratory Disorders

Chapter 7: Other Medical Conditions

Chapter 8: Environmental Factors

Chapter 9: Special Considerations: Children, Women, the Elderly, and Special Populations

Author Index

Printed and bound by CPI Group (UK) Ltd, Croydon, CR0 4YY

08/05/2025

01864678-0018